Handbook of Clinical Social Work Supervision

Third Edition

Handbook of Clinical Social Work Supervision

Third Edition

Carlton E. Munson, PhD

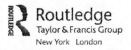

Routledge
Taylor & Francis Group
New York   London

For additional information about the contents of this book, video- and audiotape supplements, and supervision seminars contact:

Dr. Carlton Munson
Washington Area Supervision Institute
218 Mealey Parkway
Hagerstown, Maryland 21742
Telephone: (310) 733-3714

First published by
The Haworth Press, Inc
10 Alice Street
Binghamton, NY 13904-1580

Reprinted 2009 by Routledge

Routledge
Taylor & Francis Group
270 Madison Avenue
New York, NY 10016

Routledge
Taylor & Francis Group
2 Park Square
Milton Park, Abingdon
Oxon OX14 4RN

Case study identities and circumstances have been changed to protect confidentiality.

Cover design by Marylouise E. Doyle.

Library of Congress Cataloging-in-Publication Data

Munson, Carlton E.
  Handbook of clinical social work supervision / Carlton E. Munson. — 3rd ed.
     p. cm.
  Rev. ed. of: Clinical social work supervision. 2nd ed. c1993.
  Includes bibliographical references and index.
  ISBN 0-7890-1077-1 (alk. paper) — ISBN 0-7890-1078-X (alk. paper)
  1. Social workers—Supervision of. I. Munson, Carlton E. Clinical social work supervision.
II. Title.

HV40.54 .M86 2001
361.3'2'0683—dc21

2001039588

To my wife, Joan Smith Munson

ABOUT THE AUTHOR

Carlton Munson, PhD, is Professor of Social Work and former Doctoral Program Director at the School of Social Work, University of Maryland—Baltimore. He has served as a consultant to numerous educational programs, hospitals, long-term care facilities, and criminal justice programs and has conducted a number of workshops and seminars on clinical supervision throughout the United States and abroad.

Dr. Munson has published more than 70 articles in professional journals and is the author of seven books, including *Social Work Education and Practice, Family of Origin Applications in Clinical Supervision* (Haworth), *Social Work with Families,* and *Clinical Social Work Supervision* (Haworth). Dr. Munson's newest book, *Therapy for Traumatized Children: The Child's Perspective,* is forthcoming from The Haworth Press, Inc. He received the Maryland Society for Clinical Social Work's 1997 Educator of the Year Award for his work with children traumatized by domestic violence.

Dr. Munson maintains a clinical practice near Washington, DC, and directs the Washington Area Supervision Institute. An editorial board member for a variety of professional journals, he has been Editor of *The Clinical Supervisor* since its inception in 1983 and is Editor-in-Chief of The Haworth Social Work Practice Press.

CONTENTS

List of Visuals

Preface

Two events were paramount in my mind as I prepared this third edition of my supervision book, which was first published in 1983 by The Haworth Press. The first event was the new millennium we were about to enter. No other turn of a century created as much anticipation—positive and negative—concern, and speculation. The anxiety and concern over this event were a direct result of fifty years of rapid technological innovation and change that are unprecedented. Not everyone gets the opportunity to participate in the launching of a new century, and this event was reason to be reflective. In the past, people born in the first decade of a century had little chance of experiencing the turn of a century. With each passing century, the odds have improved. The characteristic rapid advances in technology of the twentieth century have improved the statistical likelihood that children born in the first decade of the twenty-first century will survive into the twenty-second century.

These technological advances have imprinted almost every area of existence. Social work practice has been deeply affected by technological changes, but the professional organizations and educational institutions have not made many effective adaptations to these changes; social work theories and research have not kept pace with the changes. The profession's resistance to change has taken the form of social work struggling to practice essentially the same way it did 100 years ago. The private practice of social work has changed somewhat under the mandates of managed cost organizations, but public-sector social work remains essentially unchanged. I believe that if social work practice and supervision do not make significant changes in the first two decades of this century, the profession, as we know it, will no longer exist and will be replaced by more adaptive disciplines. This view is based on my early grounding in sociological theory. The structural functionalists hold that societal institutions which no longer serve a function will cease to exist and be replaced by new institutions. I believe this will be social work's fate if it does not become more relevant to societal needs. Most of the changes made in the third edition of this book are designed to promote quality supervision, and the hope is that clinical supervision, in its small but significant place in the big professional picture, will contribute to the adaptations and advances that will ensure endurance of the profession.

The second event that is foremost in my mind is the advent of managed cost organizations. Most people refer to this phenomenon as managed care. This term is a misnomer. What has evolved in the United States under this concept is managed cost, not managed care. Genuine managed care would be a welcome event, but the transfer of mental health and health care services to private, business management firms has produced managed cost, not managed care. I have written articles about the distinction between the concepts of managed cost and managed care, and my chief concern is that the profession has allowed managed cost organizations to deflate our historic commitment to advocacy. The restoration of the advocacy role within the profession is key to our survival. I do not mean restoration of the old community organization model, which is alive, but not very active in promoting change.

Since the majority of social work graduates enter some form of clinical practice, one view is that they are abandoning social work's mission of advocacy. Harry Specht and Mark Courtney caused a brief professional debate in 1994 when they published *Unfaithful Angels*. They argued that social work's vast movement to private practice psychotherapy has been at the expense of social reform and advocacy. Many of the arguments made in the book are not supported by the facts. For example, private practice is not the predominant form of social work practice. Specht and Courtney were right to point out that the "undemanding" standards of the Council on Social Work Education and "the majority of social work scholars and educators have little interest in altering the direction of the profession" (p. 150). It is my view, that if the profession is to survive, a clinical advocacy model of social work intervention needs to be developed. While this new edition of my book does not articulate such a model, many of the concepts, procedures, and practices I recommend could help formulate a clinical advocacy model. I have argued for such a model (Munson, 1996e) but have seen no development of clinical advocacy models in academic programs. This is most likely because managed cost organizations cringe at the mention of the word advocacy.

This third edition of *Clinical Social Work Supervision* has many changes and additions. The entire text has been reviewed, with updated language provided where appropriate. Some of the older material remains because of its continuing relevance and enduring and reliable utility. New sections have been added to address the changes of the past ten years. The major additions are new material on diagnosis and assessment, treatment planning, practice protocols, practice guidelines, documentation, ethics, cultural diversity, disabilities, gender issues, domestic violence, substance and alcohol abuse, child and adolescent treatment, a model for managing organizational change, a partnership model of supervision, stress reactions, and an expanded review of the history of supervision. In addition, numerous case illustrations and case exercises supplement the text and can be used for classroom discussion or continuing education seminars. The appendixes have undergone major changes. All the scales have been revised and updated based on data gathered during the past decade. The assessment scale for becoming a clinical supervisor and the educational assessment scale have been revised. The ethics knowledge scale has been updated to conform to the revised NASW Code of Ethics, and the new edition of this code has been included, along with the Clinical Social Work Federation ethics code and the American Board of Examiners ethics code. The Short Form Stress Scale (SFSS) and the Supervision Analysis Questionnaire (SAQ) have undergone major revision and now includes guidelines for interpretation of scores. A supervision reporting form has been added. These are the highlights of the changes in the millennium edition of *Clinical Social Work Supervision*.

Ten-year intervals have passed between the editions of this book. When I think of all the changes that have occurred since the publication of the second edition in 1993, I wonder if the next ten years will see changes as rapid and as significant. In some ways, I hope they will be, but I hope also that we enter an era of relative calm so the profession can perhaps step back and be reflective about its future. However, I doubt the pace of change will slow. I only hope that I, and the profession, have the strength to keep up with the pace of change.

Carlton E. Munson

Acknowledgments

Doing the revisions for a new edition of a book is much more difficult than writing a book initially. For a book that is going into the third edition, the list of acknowledgments could be quite long. I want to thank my wife, Joan Smith Munson, for her many contributions to this project over the years. She did much work and spent much time alone while I was engaged in the solitary task of preparing this manuscript. Joan reviewed the text and offered gentle, but wise, suggestions on many aspects of the manuscript. Joan provided unwavering support for each of my writing projects over the past thirty-nine years and has never once complained about the struggles, frustrations, and separations that are associated with such projects. I can never completely and adequately express my indebtedness to Joan for her contribution to this and my other endeavors.

I want to thank the staff at The Haworth Press for their many contributions to this book. I have been working with The Haworth Press since 1983 and have always been impressed with their helpfulness and their pleasant, cooperative, and positive attitude. I want to acknowledge specifically Bill Cohen, President and Publisher of The Haworth Press, for his support, ideas, and guidance.

If psychotherapy supervision is really all that important, then why is training in how to supervise and become a supervisor so limited?

C. Edward Watkins
Handbook of Psychotherapy Supervision

Teaching is even more difficult than learning . . . because what teaching calls for is this: to let learn. The real teacher . . . lets nothing else be learned than learning.

Martin Heidegger
What Is Called Thinking?

Chapter 1

Introduction

This chapter is an overview of supervision. Background conceptions, a definition of clinical supervision, and the function of supervision are covered. The interactional framework that serves as background for subsequent chapters is summarized. Current issues and conditions that give rise to the need for supervision are delineated. Characteristics of supervisees and supervisors are summarized along with factors that need to be considered when becoming a clinical supervisor.

INTRODUCTION TO THE BOOK

If this book delineated all the things the supervisor must know and do in order to be effective, helpful, and appreciated, after reading it, most people would ask, Why would anyone want to become a supervisor? The answer to this question is complex, but to save time and space, it can be answered with, Because supervisors want to be effective, helpful, and appreciated. Otherwise, we would have chosen some other, less humane endeavor as a career. The actions of a supervisor have a ripple effect for the supervisee, the supervisee's client, the client's family, colleagues of the supervisee and supervisor, and others (Bradley and Ladany, 2001). These radiating effects can be positive or negative depending on the skill of the supervisor. This book is aimed at enhancing the skill of the supervisor and maximizing the positive effects of supervision.

Few supervisors have the luxury of devoting all their time to their supervisory roles, so they must be highly organized and efficient to be successful, helpful, and appreciated (Munson, 2000c). Some people find that supervision is more demanding than they expected, and they return to practice activities full-time. Others resign themselves to limited effectiveness, proceed through trial and error, become cynical and disillusioned, and pass this attitude on to their supervisees (Hess, 1992). Some struggle to do a good job and work harder and harder until they eventually succumb to distress. In all three of these situations, the knowledge and skills of good people are not passed on to the next generation of practitioners. The social work profession cannot afford such losses.

Some supervisors continue to be dedicated, calm, and steadfast in their commitment to helping others and remain a consistent source of support and inspiration for their supervisees. These are the supervisors who were identified and studied in depth, and what was learned from them became the basis for the content of this book.

This book is designed to help the profession avoid the loss of transmission of this knowledge and skill and to facilitate the passage of practice wisdom from one professional generation to the next. The desire is that the practices and guidelines presented here will make the supervisory job easier without sacrificing substance and quality. When supervisory responsibility has been abandoned or avoided, it has been because of inadequate coping mechanisms. It is simply less demanding or more rewarding for some professionals to devote themselves to other endeavors and not accept the responsibility of supervision.

Social work professionals are fortunate to live in an era and work in a professional generation that can trace its supervisory heritage directly to such people as Mary Richmond, Jane Addams, Bertha Reynolds, Porter Lee, Mary Conyngton, Lucille Austin, Ida Cannon, Frances Scherz, Yonata

Feldman, Fred Berl, Dorothy Hutchinson, Jessie Taft, Virginia Robinson, and Sigmund and Anna Freud. The author has interviewed, talked with, and read the published and unpublished works of many colleagues who studied under and were supervised by these great contributors to the profession's knowledge, skill, and practice. The author has been supervised and taught by people with such connections to the profession's heritage and feels a part of a legacy that sustains a commitment to the profession of social work.

Through the author's supervisory work, teaching, and through this book, the hope is to make a contribution to passing on this legacy and to promote the possibility of others doing the same. Many students and supervisees think social work began some time around 1960. If the social work profession is to endure, an understanding of and appreciation for social work practice and supervision history must be transmitted to the next generation of supervisors and practitioners. This book is focused on that transmission process, and Chapter 2 highlights the history of supervision.

The decision was made to write this book because there has never been one devoted exclusively to clinical social work supervision. That no such book has been written in the past is difficult to understand, given that casework has been the foundation of the profession since the beginning and that clinical treatment has, in the past decade, reemerged as the major practice area. Social work treatment has remained the major area of specialization among graduate students. Social workers are the largest professional group delivering psychotherapy services in the United States, and the National Association of Social Workers (NASW) has reported that social workers are the largest single professional group offering treatment services in mental health centers—and the numbers continue to increase.

From 1987 to 1997, the percentage of social workers practicing in mental health increased from 28 to 40 percent of NASW membership (NASW, 1991:5; Gibelman and Schervish, 1997), and by 1999, there were 192,814 clinically trained social workers in the United States, which is more than the combined totals for the other three core mental health professions: psychiatrists, psychologists, and psychiatric nurses (O'Neil, 1999). Approximately 48 percent of these clinically trained social workers have some form of employment in the mental health field. Approximately 44 percent of social workers who are NASW members report that they are supervising, and/or teaching and training (Gibelman and Schervish, 1997). These data indicate that a significant number of social workers are performing mental health practice and related supervisory functions. The few books that have been written on supervision have a much more general approach to the topic than is helpful to supervisors in such clinical settings and situations.

At a broader level, social work education has increasingly placed emphasis on generic skills, even though specialization in agencies has expanded greatly. This basic incongruity has led many agencies and organizations to place renewed emphasis on supervision as a means of overcoming this gap between educational focus and practice demands. Supervisors attempting to help new practitioners develop their skills have few guidelines to use. This book attempts to provide practical guidelines to assist the supervisor of clinical practitioners. The position taken in this book is that the era of generic practice has passed. Knowledge of human behavior and mental disorders is so vast, complex, and focused that generic interventions can be confusing and inadequate.

Most books on supervision have focused on what to learn and on how to learn clinical work through supervision. This book covers the essential aspect of supervision, but another component has been added by placing this material in the framework of the supervision process itself. What has to be learned about and done in practice is presented in the context of how the supervisor acts—what the supervisor says, hears, and writes. Organizationally, supervisors receive limited training, feedback, and support group help for what they do. This book is for and about supervisors.

BACKGROUND RESEARCH STUDIES

Throughout the book reference is made to research studies done by the author. Some of these studies have been reported in the literature, and they are cited and referenced in the text. Others have not yet appeared in the literature. Rather than repeat the details of these studies in the text each time they are referred to, the studies are listed here and are assigned an alphabetic reference code:

- A survey of thirty-four graduate students, representing a 10 percent random sample of students in one school of social work. The students completed questionnaires regarding their clinical activity and their supervisory activity (Study A).
- An intensive content analysis of the supervisory experience of three graduate social work students. Weekly one-hour research interviews were done over a nine-month period in which supervision activity was systematically analyzed based on the students' perceptions (Study B).
- A study of twenty-six field instructors selected at random from all the field instructors at one graduate school of social work. Each participant was administered an interview schedule that took an hour to complete. The supervisors were surveyed regarding their style of supervision, theoretical orientation, and philosophy of supervision and practice. In addition, demographic data were gathered (Study C).
- A survey of 183 workers and supervisors in a department of public welfare regarding their experiences in and attitudes toward super-

vision. The questionnaire also included a series of questions regarding the amount of stress the participants had experienced (Study D).

- A survey of eighty-two graduate students in a school of social work regarding the degree of stress they experienced in connection with classroom and field components of their educational program (Study E).
- A survey of forty clinical social work practitioners regarding their therapy work with respect to type of therapy performed, theoretical orientation, cotherapy activity, and conflict with colleagues (Study F).
- A survey study conducted through interviews with thirty practitioners regarding the styles of administration of supervisors and administrators. This study resulted in six administrative types that have been compared with over 300 practitioners to test the accuracy of the classifications (Study G).
- A content analysis study of videotape sessions of master therapists. The tapes of Ackerman, Bowen, Framo, Minuchin, Papp, Rubentstein, Satir, and Whitaker were analyzed for common techniques and themes. This resulted in the development of the SEES classification system (Style, Enabling, Encountering, and Shifting dysfunction) of intervention sequences (Study H).
- A survey of fifty social workers' knowledge of the National Association of Social Workers Code of Ethics through administration of a fifty-item instrument (Study I).
- A study of the structural, authority, and teaching models used in nineteen agencies in the Northeastern United States. The sample consisted of sixty supervisors and sixty-five supervisees. Numerous variables were studied in relation to the different models of supervision (Study J).

In addition to these formal studies, case examples are used as well as comments made by supervisors and supervisees in connection with teaching, consultation, and training done in various settings. Throughout the book, empirical research findings are blended with practical observations to form sound, logical, reasonable suggestions and recommendations for supervisors. Questionnaires used in some of this research can be found in the appendixes.

STYLE OF READING

Although many suggestions and guidelines are offered for use in supervision, the author has refrained from providing any suggestions on how to read this book to avoid hampering creative use of it. The only suggestion is to follow the advice of Virginia Woolf (1960/1932):

> The only advice, indeed, that one person can give another about reading is to take no advice, to follow your own instincts, to use your own reason, to come to your own conclusions. (p. 281)

Given Woolf's suggestion, only one recommendation is offered: the reader should avoid becoming defensive about his or her own practices in light of the new and different guidelines suggested in this book, because the moment a person become defensive, learning ceases. Again, Woolf advocates a point of view that is recommend to the reader:

> Do not dictate to your author; try to become him. If you hang back, and reserve and criticize at first, you are preventing yourself from getting the fullest possible value from what you read. But if you open your mind as widely as possible, then signs and hints of almost imperceptible fineness, from the twist and turn of the sentences, will bring you into the presence of a human being unlike any other. (p. 282)

Abstract discussion in this text has been minimized and used only to lay the foundation for the practical guidelines that are offered. The book is designed as a text for learning good supervisory practices through formal academic course work, but it can also serve as a resource for the practicing supervisor. The theoretical material and practice principles are interlaced with case material to illustrate major points.

Each chapter concludes with a list of suggested readings, including brief summary statements about the usefulness of each citation. These suggested readings were drawn on for much of the material in each chapter and can be used to supplement that particular chapter. These lists can be a quick reference tool for the busy educator and supervisor who does not have large blocks of time available to engage in many hours of extensive library research.

The concept of style is used a great deal in this book because it is a basic, but powerful, term that can be used to organize large amounts of helpful information. Style is defined and then used to identify the major styles of supervision. Little has been written elsewhere about style as a concept. In the research done for this book, the concept of style evolved as useful in formulating techniques for supervisory practice. The ideas about style used here have evolved over thirty years of clinical supervision practice and research activity.

In this book the terms *practitioner, worker, clinician,* and *therapist* are used interchangeably. These terms are used to refer to those actively engaged in short-term and long-term contact with clients for the purpose of intervention to resolve problems in functioning. The terms *client* and *patient* are used interchangeably.

Edgar Allan Poe believed that to make an impression, any literary work must be able to be read in one sitting. This rule of brevity has been kept in mind while writing this book. Each chapter is constructed as a reference source so that the supervisor and/or supervisee can come back to it many times until the suggestions and guidelines become a natural part of the supervisory process. Each unit within a chapter is designed to be read and mastered in one "sitting" in order to meet Poe's dictum.

ACTIVITY AND PRACTICE DIFFERENTIATION

The practice of clinical social work is difficult to achieve. Often, activity masquerades as practice. Immanuel Kant distinguished practice by noting that it is the "pursuit of a purpose which is thought of as application of certain general principles of procedure," and "there needs to be a connecting and mediating link between theory and practice"; but, at the same time, practice cannot be directly deduced from theory. Practice is disciplined conduct that rules out certain random activity. The Kantian conception of the relation between theory and practice that stresses rational, enlightened, practical conduct based on theory (Holzner and Marx, 1979:36) is of paramount importance to the supervisor. The supervisor's chief function is to minimize activity and maximize practice. Much of the interaction between supervisor and practitioner is related to transforming activity into practice. Inexperienced as well as experienced practitioners engage in activity that must be translated into practice if treatment is to be effective. In modern practice, the emphasis on task-centered, short-term, research-focused practice has made the distinction between activity and practice paramount in supervision. At times all practitioners need minor and major help in giving meaning, purpose, and discipline to what is done in relation to clients, and this is the function of supervision.

Supervisors, when working with adult learners, have taken Heidegger's concept of "to let learn," cited previously, to mean "let the learners alone." This is not what they need; in fact, it can be detrimental. Knowles (1970) has argued that when adults are given responsibility for their own learning, their initial reaction is shock and disorganization, and this reaction has been confirmed in a research study of andragogical methods (based on learning applied with self-directed, experienced, and problem-centered adults) used to train a group of social workers (Gelfand et al., 1975). When learners are asked to be more responsible for their learning, the supervisor becomes more important rather than less important. What is critical is the way in which the supervisor relates to the supervisee. The guidelines in the following chapters are focused on relating to supervisees as adult learners without abandoning them.

CLINICAL PRACTICE AND CLINICAL
SUPERVISION DEFINED

The term *clinical social work* is used because that is the most descriptive, in current phraseology, of what a certain group of social work practitioners performs. In the past, clinical social work was referred to as casework, social casework, psychiatric social work, social treatment, psychotherapy, and probably many other things. The desire here is to keep terminology from becoming a barrier to advancing knowledge and understanding of supervision. It has been argued that the term *clinical social work* became in the 1980s, "a euphemism for 'social casework,' treatment—oriented 'social group work,' 'social treatment,' 'psychiatric social work' and 'direct practice' "(Minahan, 1980:171). At the same time, efforts were being made to conceptualize a definition of clinical social work consistent with the social work heritage of evolving a coherent knowledge base and practice domains (see Goldstein, 1980; Simon, 1977).

The term *clinical social work* is relatively new (Ewalt, 1980:23). It still lacks specificity and has given rise to divergent definitions, as manifested in the proceedings of a national conference on clinical social work held in Denver, Colorado, in 1980 (Ewalt, 1980). In all of the definitions that have been offered, the common thread is work with individuals, families, and groups. The comprehensive term *clinical social work* appears to be designed to unite the diversity of practice that exists. One view is that clinical social work encompasses psychotherapy but goes beyond this form of practice. The tendency in the practice literature, and especially in the supervision literature, has been to use a broad definition of clinical practice based more on setting than on tasks. Some of the supervision literature mixes clinical psychotherapy and case management-oriented supervision (Kadushin, 1992). Practice literature indicates that agencies are making distinctions between case management practice and clinical practice. For example, practice in child welfare has been characterized as

> a conduit to private-for-profit or not-for-profit agencies that provide direct services rather than [a] provider of direct services. . . . Referred to as "case management," . . . child welfare practice . . . involves referring clients to appropriate external service providers, monitoring them, and maintaining liaison with external service providers. (Samantrai, 1991:359)

This observation is most likely associated with the reported increase in social workers in private practice, from 10.9 percent in 1982 to 16.1 percent in 1990 (NASW, 1991). By 1995, 19.7 reported private practice as their primary employment and 45.5 percent reported it as a secondary area of practice (Gibelman and Schervish, 1997). Such changes will require more precision in defining what constitutes clinical social work practice.

The definition of clinical social work has been evolving over the past three decades. This has resulted in refinement of the definition but also has led to some diversity, creating multiple definitions that are used by different organizations, which has resulted in some confusion (Kenemore, 1991: 83-93). For example, the National Registry of Health Care Providers in Clinical Social Work was guided by the following statement:

> Clinical social work practice includes provision of mental health services for the diagnosis, treatment and prevention of mental and emotional disorders in individuals, families and groups. Clinical Social Work Practice is based on knowledge and theory of psychosocial development, behavior, psychopathology, unconscious motivation, interpersonal relationships and environmental stress. Treatment interventions include, but are not limited to, individual, marital, family and group psychotherapy. (National Institute for Clinical Social Work Advancement, 1987:3)

The National Association of Social Workers uses a slightly different definition:

> Clinical Social Work shares with all other social work practice the goal of enhancement and maintenance of psychosocial functioning of individuals, families, and small groups. Clinical social work practice is the professional application of social work theory and methods to the treatment and prevention of psychosocial dysfunction, disability, or impairment, including emotional and mental disorders. It is based on knowledge of one or more theories of human development with a psychosocial context.
>
> The perspective of person-in-situation is central to clinical social work practice. Clinical social work includes interventions directed to interpersonal interactions, intrapsychic dynamics, and life-support and management issues. Clinical social work services consist of assessment, diagnosis and treatment, including psychotherapy and counseling, client-centered advocacy, consultation and evaluation. The process of clinical social work is undertaken within the objectives of social work and the principles and values contained in the NASW Code of Ethics. (NASW, 1987:1)

The American Board of Examiners in Clinical Social Work, a group formed to certify advanced practice, uses another definition:

Clinical social work practice is the professional application of social work theory and methods to the treatment and prevention of psychosocial dysfunction, disability or impairment, including emotional and mental disorders. It is based on knowledge and theory of psychosocial development, behavior, psychopathology, unconscious motivation, interpersonal relationships, environmental stress, social systems, and cultural diversity with particular attention to person-in-environment. It shares with all social work practice the goal of enhancement and maintenance of psychosocial functioning of individuals, families and small groups. (American Board of Examiners in Clinical Social Work, 1989:7)

For the purposes of this book, clinical social work practice is defined as follows:

Organized efforts by graduates of accredited schools of social work to assist people to overcome physical, financial, social, or psychological disruptions in functioning through individual, group, or family intervention methods.

The definition of clinical supervision in social work must naturally parallel the definition of clinical practice. With the previous definition in mind, the following definition of clinical supervision in social work is used by the author:

Clinical supervision is an interactional process in which a supervisor has been assigned or designated to assist in and direct the practice of supervisees in the areas of teaching, administration, and helping. The supervisees are graduates of accredited schools of social work who are engaged in practice that assists people to overcome physical, financial, social, or psychological disruptions in functioning through individual, group, or family intervention methods.

Supervisory assistance is not necessarily limited to these areas, but they are the main ones traditionally associated with supervision in social work. The key words in this definition that distinguish supervision from consultation are *assigned, designated,* and *direct.* A supervisor is assigned or designated by an agency, organization, or statute to supervise another's practice, and the supervisee is expected to be accountable to the supervisor. The supervisor is a person who has some official sanction to direct and guide the supervisees practice.

Consultation, on the other hand, has no such official sanction. The practitioner is free to decide whether to seek consultation, and whether to implement the advice and recommendations of a consultant. This is an important distinction because, in recent times, the tendency has been to use the two terms interchangeably. The trend toward referring to supervision as consultation to minimize the authority involved in supervision has been problematic for some supervisors and supervisees. (This difficulty is discussed in Chapter 7 in the section Authority and Supervision.) State statutes regulating the practice of social work are clear about the direct, assigned nature of supervision versus consultation.

FUNCTION OF SUPERVISION

Just as the scientific method can be applied to any problem or question, supervision can be applied to any clinical problem or question. Supervision can be superimposed on any theory or technique used in practice. Although supervisors do not have precise rules to guide them in supervision, as is the case with the scientific method, it is possible to identify some basic, general rules that can be useful in approaching practice situations and problems. A major purpose of this book is to identify those basic rules. The principles and guidelines presented in the following chapters can be applied by any supervisor, regardless of his or her theoretical orientation or the theoretical orientation of the supervisee.

Treatment often requires that the client and practitioner have faith in the process of treatment without much empirical evidence to justify this faith. Thus, because supervision becomes important it serves as the arena in which data are accumulated, documented, evaluated, and made known as measures of the success or failure of the treatment. Supervision is the only check and balance on the alliance of faith and action in treatment. The investment of faith is as important to the practitioner as it is to the client, and supervision is where faith is sustained and reinforced for the practitioner. The client must rely on himself or herself and the practitioner for perpetuation of therapeutic faith. For this reason, the supervisor is important to the practitioner as well as to the client, although the client rarely knows it. Thus, rules are crucial in supervision. In some respects, supervision is research on specific clinical practice that is abstract and defies concrete interpretation.

If supervision is viewed as the place where supervisors give answers, check up on the practitioner's work, and find solutions for the clinician, the supervisor will have embarked on a process that is of limited utility. Supervision should be a mutual sharing of questions, concerns, observations, and speculations to aid in selection of alternative techniques to apply in practice. This process of collaboration and facilitation on the part of the supervisor and supervisee is referred to as the *congruence of perceptions in supervision.* Practitioners should, and want to, participate in supervision rather than be recipients of it. Such mutual understanding requires mutual trust. If mutual trust is missing, then the supervisory relationship is bound to falter and eventually fail.

All of the material in this text is based on the assumption that the supervisor and supervisee trust each other. If such trust is uncertain, most of the guidelines provided in the following pages will be of little use. Supervision cannot proceed in a climate of mistrust. Where mistrust exists, the supervisory process becomes a stand-off, a struggle for survival. Supervision must be viewed as a safe place to share and struggle with concerns, weaknesses, failures, and gaps in skill. The supervisor must work to establish a trusting climate and be diligent to avoid using the information learned in the supervisory process against the supervisee. One must avoid the suspicious philosophy expressed by one supervisor in an initial session with a supervisee: "Different people bring different agendas to supervision." Fortunately, in this situation, the supervisee gave the right answer when she said, "My agenda is to learn."

There is nothing magical, mystical, or arcane about good supervision. Five basic propositions serve as the foundation of effective supervision, and these provide the basis of the material covered in this book. To be effective, supervision must have the following characteristics:

1. *Structured.* A formal structure for the supervision is made clear to the supervisee. Structure refers to the formats for conducting supervision, such as individual supervision, group supervision, or a combination of these formats.

2. *Regular.* Regardless of the structure used, the supervision should be conducted on a regular basis. It is easy for a busy supervisor to fail to formalize the regularity of supervision, and as a result, supervision is delayed or avoided completely.

3. *Consistent.* The supervisor should work to ensure that the style and approach used with the supervisee are consistent. A logical connection should exist between the style and pattern of decision making so the supervisee can anticipate the expectations related to a given situation. The supervisee left to wonder and guess how the supervisor will react to each situation will be limited in his or her ability to grow and learn through supervision.

4. *Case oriented.* Supervision, to be effective and efficient, should be case oriented at all times. All other matters are extraneous or secondary. Administrative issues, personal matters, and learning should all be connected to case material when discussed. This material does not have to involve only specific cases but can also be related to general case discussion. The objective is to keep the supervision focused. Any supervision discussion should be relevant to the practitioner's cases. If it cannot be related to cases, then, most likely, the supervision has lost sight of its primary focus.

5. *Evaluated.* The supervision itself should be evaluated. It is the responsibility of supervisors to periodically solicit formal and informal feedback about the supervision practice they are conducting.

SUPERVISION PERSPECTIVES

One can discuss supervision from several perspectives. The most prominent ones are listed here:

1. *Personality perspective.* This perspective involves the characteristics and traits that the participants bring to the supervisory situation and how these influence the practice activity and the supervisory relationship.
2. *Situational perspective.* This approach relates to the specific situations and problems that the participants encounter as part of the supervision process. The focus is on the situations and problems and how to deal with them.
3. *Organizational perspective.* In this model the emphasis is placed on the function of the organization and how the supervision serves to effectively implement the organizational goals and objectives.
4. *Interactional perspective.* This approach, which is the predominant model used in this book, focuses on the interaction between the supervisor and the supervisee. The emphasis is on how the participants interact and how interaction is varied to fit the specific content of the supervision.

Each of these perspectives is quite complicated. All can produce similar as well as different outcomes. It is common for participants to intermingle the various perspectives. This book is based on an interactional approach to supervision and the styles that emerge from interaction. Organizational, personality, and situational content are included in this perspective but are analyzed as interactional processes. The content is considered in the context of the interaction. The notion underpinning this book is that the process of supervisory interaction is as important as the content of supervision. Claude Levi-Strauss has succinctly described this view:

> [In] the social sciences . . . we are looking at things which are extremely complicated . . . to describe because of their complexity. Yet if instead of looking at the things themselves we look at the relations . . . between them, then we will discover that these relationships are altogether more simple and less numerous than the things themselves, and . . . can give us a firmer base for investigation. (1978:30)

Following Levi-Strauss's view, the focus in this book is more on the relationship between participants in supervision rather than on supervision as a concept.

Heidegger (1968) pointed out that becoming a teacher is much more difficult than becoming a famous professor. The supervisor's job is more difficult than that of the professor because, as Heidegger further argued, teaching is more difficult than learning since the teacher must know how to let learn. Supervisors have not always recognized the importance of the supervisor as a teacher. Rather than being viewed as a difficult task, letting a person learn has been perceived in much modern social work as a simple process of letting the supervisee alone.

When the supervisor is ill prepared for the role of teacher, the tendency is to shift the emphasis to interaction about administrative functions, which can create more social and professional distance in the process. This shift in focus illustrates the interactional nature of supervision.

This situation is illustrated by the case of Mary Newly* in supervising one of her supervisors who had not practiced for years and had slipped into administrative functioning at the expense of clinical supervision responsibilities.

Case Illustration:
The Case of Mary Newly

Mary is an MSW social worker who was recently employed to be clinical director of a large, regional mental health center that is part of a statewide mental health system. Mary has been working at the center for several months and a man, Lim A. Tations, who is the director of the substance abuse intervention unit, is having a functional difficulty.

The man has been employed by the agency for nine years. He was promoted to unit director at a time when the center was undergoing staffing problems and experienced many administrative readjustments. Mary asked Mr. Tations to do emergency intakes when none of his staff was available, and Lim stated that he feels uncomfortable doing intake assessments because it has been a number of years since he has done intake. He admitted to Mary that he has not kept up his credentials and supervises twelve workers. One supervisee is an MSW who is working toward advanced clinical licensure status under Lim's supervision.

Several of the workers Lim supervises have complained to Mary that Lim is not adequate in performing his supervisory duties. They complain that he has difficulty providing clinical direction, has difficulty setting priorities, and seems distracted during supervision. Mary talked to Lim about the importance of being able to perform the basic functions that he supervises, but Lim stated that he does not believe that he has a problem and that his "task is to be an administrator, not a clinician." Lim believes his workers like him, and he thinks they have no problems with his performance.

---

*A number of case examples are used in this book. All of the case examples are actual events, and the names have been changed to ensure confidentiality.

Mary has talked to the agency director several times about Lim's limitation, but the director has not been responsive to Mary's concerns. The agency director has known Lim for many years, has a degree in management and does not seem, to Mary, to appreciate clinical issues in depth. The director is a responsible man and generally supportive of Mary and other staff. Mary is having trouble sleeping because of her concern about Lim's limitations and the agency director's lack of response.

If you were Mary, what would you do?

WHAT GOOD SUPERVISORS DO

An important question is, What do supervisors do? A more difficult question is, What do good supervisors do? or, What should supervisors do? The answers to the first two questions are the following five basic actions of the supervisor:

1. *Reading.* It is essential that supervisors keep up with the literature and be prepared to guide supervisees to appropriate literature. There has been an explosion of practice research and a vast expansion of practice specializations. Supervisors must devise a systematical method to keep up with the literature if they are to be effective with and helpful to supervisees. Increasingly, practice guidelines and practice protocols are available for highly specialized modern practice areas. It is the supervisors' responsibility to be knowledgeable regarding these guidelines.

2. *Writing.* Supervisors are required to do various forms of writing in addition to charts and records that are a part of practice. This can vary from setting to setting, but preparing reports, drafting grant proposals, and writing articles for publication or presentation are common writing activities. Supervisors need to develop a system to manage all the writing tasks they must do. Supervisors can be effective role models by recommending works they have written to their supervisees. Engaging in joint writing efforts with supervisees can also be rewarding for both participants.

3. *Watching.* Supervisors need to be keen observers, using the same observational skills that are necessary for good clinical practice. Supervisors must continually be alert to the performance of supervisees. Not all observations need to become the focus of the supervision, but supervisors should be aware of more than what their supervisees present to them. Supervisors who rely completely on input from supervisees for judgments and decision making are at a disadvantage in the supervisory process.

4. *Listening.* This is a crucial skill for supervisors to possess. It is the same listening skill that is essential to good clinical work. The difference is that, at times, supervisors will need to be more active in supervision than in the clinical situation. Supervisees sometimes complain that, although su-

pervisors are good listeners, they do not provide enough direct information to assist the supervisee. Supervisors who "just listen" will be of limited help to the supervisees.

5. *Talking.* Most supervision activity is accomplished through discussion. Supervisors must possess skill at talking about material with supervisees. This same skill is also needed to be an effective clinician, but the discussion and the techniques used to promote participation must be altered from the manner in which they are used in the practice situation. Supervisees become uncomfortable and frustrated when supervisors treat them like clients.

Any action of the supervisor fits one of these five categories. This book deals with answering the question, What should supervisors do in these five areas to be effective? It is based on research about the actions of people who have been identified as good supervisors. Each chapter in some way deals with what to read, what and how to write, what and how to watch, what to say and how to say it, and how to listen.

SUPERVISORY THOUGHT PROCESS

Teaching in supervision involves an interactional process, but this must be based on a concomitant thought process. This thought process incorporates the following five components, which can provide a comprehensive approach to most supervisory practice situations:

1. *Perception.* This involves selection of stimuli in the environment, including both the obvious and the not so obvious. There will be areas in which the supervisor perceives that the practitioner needs improvement. This need may or may not be perceived by the worker. The need must be agreed upon before learning is pursued.

2. *Imagination.* This relates to creating ideas that were not known to the creator previously, regardless of whether the ideas are known to others in the surrounding environment. The supervisor must be able to translate for the practitioner accumulated knowledge and experience from the collective practice wisdom and practice literature and be able to apply it to unique practice situations. The supervisor can avoid problems by resisting the tendency to assume that accepted practice procedures will always be available to the practitioner in a common or uncommon practice situation. Knowledge of practice procedures must be confirmed or made known through the process of supervision.

3. *Analysis and redefinition.* This process requires separating elements of a complex whole and reorganizing them into a new whole, creating a differ-

ent form of understanding from what appears to be a known situation. This is the heart of supervisory interaction. Difficult cases can result in the practitioner's creating a complex orientation and comprehension of the case that is inaccurate diagnostically or results in ineffective treatment. For the practitioner to develop a new focus that will take him or her in a new direction with a case, the supervisor needs to guide the practitioner through an analysis to produce a new comprehension of the dynamics of the case.

4. *Pattern recognition.* The repeated elements of any situation form a pattern that permits consistent recognition and understanding and becomes the basis of focused intervention. As the supervisor engages in several case analyses with the practitioner, repeated patterns of client problems, client interaction, and worker interaction will become apparent and should be highlighted. This can occur over a series of cases or in a single case. If the worker is to learn to practice independently, recognition of these patterns of problems, interaction, and communication must become part of his or her observational and interventive skills.

5. *Prediction.* One can project outcomes or behaviors from known situations to unknown situations. This is the ultimate goal of independent practice based on learning in supervision. For learning in supervision to be successful, the practitioner must develop skill at achieving this transfer of learning. Once the supervisor has worked through the four previous elements with the practitioner, the supervisor must provide opportunities for the practitioner to apply what has been learned from previous cases to new cases.

These elements have been explained separately, but they become integrated in the supervision process to formulate a complex network of thinking and interaction that can be identified when the supervisory process is observed. One important factor that has become apparent from attempting to observe these elements in supervision interaction is that, for the learning to be successful, the elements should occur in the order that has been listed. None of the elements can be effectively applied unless the previous elements have been applied and understood. These five elements serve as the general principles of learning that are the basis for all of the other facets of learning covered in this book. The following supervisory case illustrates the components of the supervisory process.

Case Illustration:
The Case of Sally Smith

The following key elements of the supervisory thought process are illustrated in this case example:

- *Perception:* selection of stimuli by the supervisee and the supervisor that may or may not be obvious

- *Imagination:* creating new ideas from accumulated knowledge
- *Analysis and redefinition:* separating the elements of a complex whole and reconceptualizing them into a new whole
- *Pattern recognition:* becoming aware of repeated elements of a situation that permits consistent recognition, understanding, and basis of focused action
- *Prediction:* projecting outcomes or behaviors from known situations to unknown situations

Sally works in a mental health clinic, and she brought the following case to supervision for discussion:

> Charles Lawson, an eleven-year-old fifth-grade student, was referred to the clinic by the school counselor. Charles is a management problem at school but is not having any major academic problems, other than he becomes nervous and agitated when asked by the teacher to read aloud for the class, or when he is asked to perform academic functions in front of the teacher. When placed under such "pressure," he becomes oppositional and resistant.
>
> Charles's parents are receiving couples therapy and seem to be on the verge of separating. The parents have been married for seven years. Charles's mother was never married to his biological father. Her pregnancy with Charles was the result of "date rape." The father is still known to Mrs. Lawson and is reported to have a history of aggressive behavior, substance use/abuse, and alcohol use/abuse. When the Lawsons married, Mr. Lawson adopted Charles. Charles has never been told that he is adopted. Mr. Lawson is described as "a yeller" and disciplines Charles harshly. He is critical of Charles and has chastised him for making "stupid mistakes" during school football games. Mrs. Lawson becomes upset when her husband disciplines Charles and cries and argues with her husband about his actions. She feels caught in the middle of this family tension.
>
> Charles was recently released from a local psychiatric hospital after a seven-day stay for "anger and depression." The discharge recommendations included having Sally do individual psychotherapy with Charles that would include "helping Charles accept that his parents have many differences that may be so great that they may decide not to live together."
>
> Mrs. Lawson has a number of somatic complaints and suffers from severe migraine headaches. She was hospitalized the prevous weekend for three days for a severe migraine.
>
> The parents have had Charles in therapy previously with three different therapists, but the family changed therapists frequently because they felt no progress was being made. Charles reported he liked all of his prior therapists. The parents have also changed therapists several times for similar reasons. Mrs. Lawson has confided in Sally that she wants out of the marriage, because he "has been pressuring me to stay in the relationship." Mr. Lawson is not physically abusive, but he is at times verbally abusive of Mrs. Lawson. This pressure causes Mrs. Lawson to become "depressed," but she has not sought treatment for the depression.
>
> Charles is a management problem at school in that he cusses other children, spits on them, and "gives them the finger." This leads to alterca-

tions with other students and many trips to the principal's office. When Charles gets into such conflicts, he becomes sad and withdrawn after each incident. At the same time that he is aggressive toward other children, Charles shows signs of desperately wanting to be liked by other children.

Sally remarked to the supervisor, "I don't know where to begin with Charles, and I am looking for some direction" (PERCEPTION). The supervisor began with Sally by asking her to identify a theme or series of themes that appear to be central to all the many dynamics. With the aid of the supervisor, Sally was able to identify the recurring theme of tension and anxiety in the family relationships. This theme was arrived at by identifying the dynamics that Sally had reviewed in presenting the case. The review resulted in the following list of themes (PATTERN RECOGNITION):

1. Secrecy of the adoption. The therapist will need to deal with the parents' tension about the adoption. It is not clear whether the parents ever plan to tell Charles about his adoptive status. The parents may have tension about what to do regarding informing Charles. There may be tension about the possibility of the biological father showing up and declaring himself. There is the possibility that the adoptive father may reveal Charles's status during one of their frequent arguments. This seems to be a real possibility since the father is "a yeller" and prone to impulsivity.

2. The adoptive father's harsh discipline and chastising of Charles leads to tension and anxiety for each member of the family. The mother reports that she becomes upset when her husband disciplines Charles, and this leads to further tension and arguing.

3. The parental conflict leads to tension between the parents and causes anxiety for Charles. When the supervisor discussed this dynamic in supervision, Sally said it was "interesting" that Charles said to her that his parents "must stay together because I need them" (IMAGINATION). Sally discussed with the supervisor the discharge recommendations that included having Sally work with Charles to help him accept that his parents have many differences that may be so great that they may decide not to live together. The supervisory discussion led to the conclusion that Sally would not work to implement this recommendation. It was decided not to implement this recommendation since the parents were still living together and may not decide to separate. Also, it was concluded that the literature on divorce shows that children rarely accept that parents have separated forever and will often engage in numerous actions to get the parents back together.

4. There is little known about the biological father's background and mental health history. Anxiety may be a feature of his personality. His substance and alcohol use may be an attempt to self-medicate and self- soothe his anxiety and tension.

5. Charles's mother has much tension and anxiety. She has much marital tension. She has numerous somatic complaints. She feels conflicted and caught in the marital relationship.

6. The frequent therapist-changing activity of the parents appears to be an indication of tension, anxiety, and impassivity. It could be a manifestation of behavior that keeps the parents and Charles in an agitated, destabilized, but bonded state. The tension and anxiety could be serving as a function for the family's continued engagement.

With these themes of the supervisory presentation, Sally and the supervisor were ready to devise a treatment plan. What follows is the conceptualization of the treatment plan, and not the specific treatment plan items in the form of goals and objectives (examples of specific treatment plan items are presented in other sections of this book).

A. Sally will conduct several sessions with Charles's parents to clarify the following issues:

1. Sally will determine whether they have considered the possible consequences of Charles inadvertently discovering that Mr. Lawson is not his biological father. Sally will explore whether the parents have plans to discuss Charles's adoption with him.
2. Sally will explore the parents' view of the state of their marriage, and how they will plan to arrive at some consensus about living together or separating. She will determine whether they have discussed custody and visitation issues if they do separate. Sally will also explore with the parents how they will reassure Charles of their love for him if they stay together or separate.
3. Sally will discuss how Mr. Lawson could develop more sensitive parenting skills and use less harsh discipline, as well as how the parents can achieve consensus on how to and who will discipline Charles. There are indications that Charles is "triangulating" and "manipulating" the parents' disagreement about discipline. Sally will work to get the parents to form an alliance to produce more coordinated and effective discipline of Charles.
4. Sally will discuss directly with the parents the theme of tension and anxiety in the family and share this as an observation that will provide each parent the opportunity to "open up" about the tension.

B. In the therapy with Charles, Sally will work to decrease Charles's anxiety:

1. Sally will explore through play intervention techniques how Charles views his parents' relationship and how he perceives them as viewing him. This intervention strategy can be used to address any distortions that Charles may have regarding his parents. For example, Charles may believe that "if my parents separate they will not love me or care for me anymore." This is an alternative to addressing directly the psychiatric hospital recommendation that the possibility of parental separation be raised directly with Charles.
2. Cognitive interventions will be used to help Charles control his impulsive behavior toward other children. This will include the following:

    a. Sally will help to identify what triggers Charles's aggressive behavior.
    b. Sally will develop strategies for using behaviors other than spitting, cussing, and "giving the finger" to show displeasure with the acts of other children.
    c. Sally will use cognitive restructuring to help Charles see that his impulsive and aggressive behavior is resulting in the opposite of what he seeks from other children—being liked and accepted. (Sally struggled with this treatment plan item in supervision. She had told Charles that she "would be angry and upset" if he did the things to her that he does to other children. Sally believed this was a good strategy since Charles

told her he liked her a lot. She believed this would give him a different perspective on their relationship that would carry over to other relationships, but it did not work. With the help of cognitive restructuring in the supervision, Sally was able to conduct an ANALYSIS AND REDEFINITION in which Charles would have to imagine what it would be like for him and what he would do if someone behaved similarly to him. Sally was helped to develop an intervention in which Charles would have to identify specific acts he could do to get people to accept and like him, as well as behavior he would like people to exhibit toward him that would make him like them.

d. Sally will work with Charles in translating acts of aggression into language that these acts symbolized. Sally will then engage in a word search with Charles that will lead to development of language that could communicate to others acts he does not like. This will help him foster ways to express displeasure about the acts of others.

Sally and the supervisor worked on a set of measures that would serve as predictors of the success of the interventions. These included observations of changes in behavior and verbal measures of the reduction of tension in each family-member, and in the family as a whole. Sally would also rely on repeated use of standardized measures (PREDICTION).

COST OF SUPERVISION

Time and expense are rarely mentioned in connection with supervision, but they have become crucial to utilization of supervision. If more attention were devoted to them, more supervisors and practitioners would be conscious of the importance of making effective use of supervisory time. Depending upon the training, experience, and salary of the supervisor and supervisee, each hour of individual supervision can cost between $80 and $120. Over a typical professional year of weekly sessions, the cost can range from $4,000 to $6,000. If supervision involved more awareness of its cost, time would undoubtedly be used more effectively and efficiently. Tardiness, cancelled sessions, small talk, lack of content planning, and rambling clinical speculation on the part of either the supervisor or the supervisee are costly and unjustifiable. Every question, every interpretation, every comment should be clinically relevant and related to a treatment or learning goal. Another objective of this book is to offer some guidelines that aid in more effective use of supervision time.

In business and management, recent emphasis has focused on decreasing costs by eliminating supervision rather than increasing productivity through supervision. This has been the pattern in social work over the past three decades. Cost in administering treatment can be decreased by structuring supervision in a manner that decreases the need for it. Supervision should not be eliminated; it should be made more cost-effective.

The management field does have some conceptual ways of aiding supervisors in this area. In management, supervision focuses on what to do and how to do it, while in professional social work it is assumed that professionals know the basic functions of the work. In most cases, supervision has been obliquely focused on checking whether the work is being done, and, in some instances, supervision has been all but eliminated. More attention needs to be devoted to the "what" and "how" of doing treatment.

As financial demands for decreased administrative costs become more important in social work education and practice, supervision gets harder to justify. Ironically, more, rather than less, supervision is needed—more genuine supervision that is structured and specific to learning. This will not mean an overall increase in the amount of supervision since, in many settings, it is already being provided, but not on a sound basis. What is needed is greater effectiveness and efficiency within the existing time frame of supervisory practices and structures.

STYLE

Some attention has been devoted to style in clinical practice, but limited attention has been devoted to styles of supervision. The concept of style emerged as a natural and useful tool to organize the interactional perspective used in this book. There is a difference between structure of supervision and style. Style relates to the pattern of interaction that is fostered directly or indirectly by the supervisor. A thesis of this book, based on my research, is that the supervisor's style gives rise to the style that the practitioner adopts in supervision.

No theory of supervision exists, and no attempt will be made to create one in this book. Social work supervision knowledge and research are not sufficient to permit development of a substantial theory at this point. Instead, the attempt has been to create a paradigm of supervision based on interactional styles. (A paradigm is a set of concepts, descriptive categories, and a common language that allows researchers to work in a given area using consistent guiding principles [see Lachman et al., 1979:1-34]). Others are doing research within the paradigm; additional research and other paradigms will surely follow. Only with continued research efforts can supervision be utilized to contribute to quality treatment. (See Chapter 4 for a detailed discussion of style.)

Style as a concept allows analysis of the broadest and most detailed components of supervision. When asked to describe their style, supervisors cannot avoid describing the behaviors that constitute the relationships that exist with their supervisees.

NEED FOR SUPERVISION

A relevant question in the clinical practice of social work is, Why is supervision needed? This question is of importance because of the increased emphasis on the autonomy of the practitioner in a profession that historically has placed heavy emphasis on close supervision. The idea of consultation replaced the idea of supervision as the autonomous model of professionalism was developing. The focus on autonomy has emerged more as a supportive indicator that social workers are truly professionals than as a reflection of the self-directed practitioner. Certain characteristics of new BSW and MSW graduates support this view. The emergence of managed cost organizations (MCOs) has called into question the need for supervision. MCOs do not require supervision of the practitioner and rely on state licensure laws that mandate varying periods and types of supervision while working for licensed status.

Several general professional trends that support the need for clinical supervision can be identified: the resurgence of clinical practice, social work dominance in mental illness treatment, the theory explosion, changes in professional standards, limited supervision training, practitioner stress and burnout prevention, unethical practice, complex external controls on practice structure, complicated documentation, sophisticated outcome measures, and new highly specialized practice areas. These developments are beyond what social work education can effectively teach within the existing curriculum requirements and time constraints. New graduates need assistance to integrate the many practice demands that are marginally covered in educational programs. It is a mistake to assume that the recent graduate is totally prepared to be a practitioner. This book, in part, is designed to guide the supervisor in efforts to enhance and refine the functioning of the recent graduate.

Resurgence of Clinical Practice

Since the retreat of clinical practice during the 1960s under the pressure of social reform movements, resurgence of clinical practice has transformed what were called casework and group work into a more specialized classification of psychotherapy. Social workers functioning in this area do individual, group, and family therapy. By the 1970s statistics revealed that social workers were the largest single group providing psychotherapy; more than 29,000 social workers perform this service, compared with 26,000 psychiatrists; 18,000 psychologists; 12,000 nurses; and 10,000 other practitioners (Sobel, 1980). By 1990 this figure had grown to 60 percent, and by 1995 the number had grown to 65 percent (Gibelman, 1995). By 1999 this trend appeared to be slowing, but clinical social workers continued to outnumber all other mental health professionals. In 1997 there were 192,814 clinical social workers; 33,486 psychiatrists; and 73,018 psychologists in the United States (U.S. Substance Abuse and Mental Health Services Administration, 1998).

Surveys of social work practitioners reveal that mental health is the largest social work practice area, with 40 percent of the profession claiming clinical mental health as their primary practice area (Gibelman, 1995; Gibelman and Schervish, 1997). Although social workers deliver the majority of psychotherapy services, limited mention of this shift has appeared in the social work literature (Reisch and Gambrill, 1997). Even though the trend has been emerging for three decades, few schools have adapted to this change in practice function, and few schools prepare students exclusively for this form of practice. The profession and the schools will need to adapt to the significant changes in practice activity or risk being co-opted by other disciplines. There are indications that this co-opting process is emerging.

The growth of managed care has expanded the traditional core mental health professions from the three disciplines of psychiatry, psychology, and social work to include psychiatric nurses, addictions counselors, professional counselors, pastoral counselors, mental health counselors (Florida), and school-based guidance counselors. Federal government statistics indicate that in 1997 there were 96,263 counselors; 17,318 psychiatric nurses; and 44,225 family therapists in the United States (U.S. Substance Abuse and Mental Health Services Administration, 1998). Most of these practitioners have been added to the core of mental health practitioners since 1970.

Clinical Social Work in Mental Health

The trend of social workers as the predominant group offering mental health services and psychotherapy will most likely continue, since the definition of mental illness has expanded over the decades as mental illness has become better understood and as mental health treatment has become more accepted. As the number of psychiatrists declines, other professionals are starting to practice psychotherapy, and most of these are social workers. Social workers do most of the modern talking therapy for mild neurotic behavior, communication problems, and situational stress. With the decline in the number of new practitioners, psychiatric practice is focusing more on the severe mental illnesses (e.g., schizophrenia and mood disorders) and psychiatric research is targeting the biological aspects of mental disorders. Increasingly, social workers are treating situational and psychological dysfunctioning, and psychiatrists are treating biological disorders. This trend is a return to a service delivery pattern of earlier eras (Shorter, 1997). The only difference is the expansion of other disciplines competing with social work. This expansion is causing a redefinition and reconfiguration of psychotherapy practice.

At the same time that this is occurring, the schools and the professional literature have de-emphasized the teaching and practice of supervision. This, in part, has been the result of developing the concept of the social worker as a full-fledged professional and of the emergence of MCO control of mental health services. The view that a genuine professional must be independent and autonomous was believed to be necessary to professional status. Supervision and professionalism were seen as antithetical. The social work professional quest for autonomy converged with the managed cost organization view that clinical social work is an independent practice activity and the only necessary credential is a state license to practice. The need exists for a more balanced approach, and this book is an effort to help fill the gap in the supervision practice that has evolved over the past thirty years.

Theory Explosion

As these functional and structural changes have taken place, there has been a simultaneous increase in emphasis on practice theory to the point of confusion. Over 130 different theories of practice compete for utilization. Social work practice theory is in a period of diversified unrest. Some trends can be vaguely identified. Systems theory appears to have reached the apex of its contribution to practice knowledge, and along with it, Gestalt therapy and the ecosystems approach are reaching their theoretical limits. Resurgence of psychoanalytic theory has occurred in the broadest sense from an interactional perspective. Developments in communication theory and empirical research on linguistics-based theories have produced helpful results and insights. Cognitive and behavioral approaches are in ascendancy, while managed cost organizations are giving almost exclusive sanction to task-centered, short-term theories of intervention.

Social work in general seems to be fostering a plateau of theoretical dormancy and, in some respects, is returning to an earlier era of developing methodologies such as individual, group, and family treatment, rather than developing theories of intervention based on behavioral patterns. The era of "do your own thing" and philosophic "narcissistic"-focused intervention has ended, and the emphasis now is on symptom relief and optimal levels of functioning (Stone, 1997). Self-help and do-it-yourself approaches, which began with Karen Horney and bloomed in different arrangements during the 1960s and 1970s, gradually lost favor but are reemerging as public support for formal mental health services is declining. Supervisors need to keep abreast of these developments if they are to aid supervisees in their theoretical and conceptual learning. (See Chapter 8 for a more detailed discussion of theory in practice and supervision.)

Changes in Professional Standards

The responsibility for setting standards for entry into the profession has passed from the schools to the profession through licensing. The number of comprehensive examinations in schools has decreased as the number of states that have passed licensing laws has increased. Great variation exists in the supervision requirements for licensing. Although NASW has a recommended uniform licensure statute, a "states' rights" trend in licensing is creating diverse licensure requirements.

Learning and standards are being separated as licensing laws for social work increase. Over forty states now have laws regulating social work practice. Most of these laws require an examination for certification. Some do not have any requirements for supervision. The examinations are not associated with supervisory requirements, so there is no connection between learning, the examination, and supervision. Some examinations contain questions about supervision, but they have limited relationship to the supervision process and practice activity.

There is reason to believe that educational testing services have more experience than the social work schools in measuring competence today. The question remains whether examinations are sufficient to measure competence. In earlier times, social work relied more on supervision to monitor competence of practitioners. This was accomplished through discussion of cases, theories, techniques, evaluation, and administrative matters. Some states (for example, Virginia and California) used to require oral examinations but have eliminated them because of cost, time consumption, and inconsistent performance criteria. The profession now depends more on the licensing examinations to evaluate competence. With the decreased emphasis on verbal exchange to promote competence, the profession seems to have lost something, and must address these questions: What can be accomplished through such examinations? What are their limitations? Adler has pointed out that, "if the aim were to discover the student's familiarity with a specific branch of knowledge, one way to do that might be to test the individual's ability to use correctly a particular discipline's technical terms" (1981:16). This might be all that can be accomplished through licensing examinations. Written tests cannot deal with supervisees' fears, anxieties, and doubts; learning to recognize patterns of behavior; developing a philosophy of practice; identifying a basic effective style; and numerous other interactional factors. There is need for renewal of discussion of such areas in supervision if supervisees are to become truly well-rounded practitioners.

Continuing Education

Continuing education is taking on increased significance, as it is now required by many professional organizations and licensing boards to maintain professional standards and status. Some professionals consider these programs to be of limited value in promoting competence; to be of little importance or effectiveness; and, in some instances, actually to be detrimental, since there is minimal monitoring of what is learned, consistency of learning, and degree of application in practice. Supervisors have a responsibility to monitor continuing education courses attended by supervisees, and to evaluate how they contribute to learning about social work practice.

Continuing education programs are the chief source of learning for practitioners. They serve a valuable function in preparing for specialized practice areas. Continuing education is abstract learning since it usually is conducted outside the actual practice setting. Continuing education learning should be supplemented by structured application in the treatment setting, and supervision is the natural arena for this to occur. Continuing education should be viewed as a supplement to supervision, instead of a substitute for it.

Supervision Training

With increased pressure on schools to expand content in a number of areas, including minority concerns, women's issues, feminist practice, oppression, human biology, human behavior in the social environment, research, and policy, there has been a decrease in courses devoted to practice content and supervision. For clinical majors, 10 to 12 percent of the courses taken as part of a BSW or an MSW program are exclusively devoted to practice subjects. A two-year graduate curriculum is limited in its content. Committed students who recognize the limits of their practice knowledge are increasingly seeking third-year fellowship programs upon graduation, but few such programs exist. Given these conditions, supervision of the beginning practitioner will become increasingly important as a way of giving the social worker a unified view of practice and orienting him or her to the breadth of the profession.

That the schools are providing limited training to prepare workers for autonomous clinical practice is illustrated by the findings of a research project in which students undergoing a two-year graduate education averaged 15 to 20 cases and conducted 120 to 150 interviews, including an average of 120 individual sessions, 20 group sessions, and 13 family interviews (Munson, 1981b). This is hardly a basis upon which to base an autonomous practice.

The Council on Social Work Education's revised Curriculum Policy Statement, implemented in July 1994, does not cover clinical practice or technology (Commission on Accreditation, 1994). It does not mention supervision as a concept or require any curriculum offerings in the area of supervision. In a survey, it was found that only 13 percent of graduate schools of social work required a course in supervision (Munson, see Study C). At the same time, schools are placing emphasis on specialization (e.g., health, aging, mental health, rural practice). Cooper has argued that universities are not interested in developing clinical training programs and are incapable of adequate training for clinical practice because of disharmony between the schools and the field (in Mishne, 1980:29-30). This tension between the clinical practice community and educational programs has not changed significantly in the past forty years. As long as academicians and practitioners are so polarized, little hope exists for reaching any basic agreement about requirements for supervision of students and practitioners.

Supervision has made limited adjustment to changes in motivation of students entering graduate schools of social work. In one study, 53 percent of students indicated that they had undergone therapy themselves. A majority of these students indicated that they had entered graduate school because of a desire to emulate their own therapists (Munson, see Study A). This desire to accomplish a personal fantasy—rather than a strong, altruistic commitment to help others through social work—is consistent with Yankelovich's observation that "in our preoccupation with self-fulfillment we have also grown recklessly unrealistic in our demands on our institutions" (1981:5). The desire to enter the profession after a therapeutic encounter has been replaced by a diversity of reasons for seeking a professional social work degree.

As the emphasis on the role of supervision has decreased, there has been a failure to recognize both this change in motivation of practitioners and their tendency to draw on their experiences with their therapists as the model for their practice techniques.

Stress

This era of decreased emphasis on supervision, has witnessed an increase in concern about stress among practitioners (Munson, 1992). Although there is some question about the amount and degree of burnout (Streepy, 1981), it is ironic that the increased concern has occurred at a time when supervision is being de-emphasized, since good supervision has been held to be effective in preventing burnout. If burnout actually is accelerating, it possibly can be partly traced to the decline in emphasis on supervision. If this is the case, renewed requirements for supervision could be of value in combating stress. Burnout, in many instances, is associated with lack of coping mechanisms. When practitioners cannot cope with practice demands, they need to turn for help to a trustworthy source. The supervisor should be, and is, the most appropriate resource for dealing with such difficulties. Without supervision as a resource, practitioners will struggle on their own, turn to colleagues, or, as mentioned before, in some cases draw on experiences from their own therapy. Rarely do these measures aid the worker, and in some instances they can make the stress worse.

In supervision, as in any endeavor, anxiety, fear, frustration, and failure are the result of inadequate coping mechanisms. As was pointed out at the beginning of this chapter, graduates are being provided fewer coping strategies for practice and for supervision, even though practice demands are becoming more difficult. This could be the source of distress (Streepy, 1981) and disillusionment (Reiter, 1980) among practitioners and supervisors. Coping strategies are specific techniques to use in response to difficult situations and are discussed in detail in later chapters.

Research on stress in the workplace has repeatedly demonstrated that effective supervision is a powerful antidote to stress. For this reason, consideration should be given to reviving and expanding supervision in agencies. Administrators rarely associate stress prevention and supervision. More attention needs to be given to this function of supervision as excess stress, or "burnout," as it is commonly labeled, increasingly becomes a problem for practitioners and supervisors. (Chapter 10 provides a thorough discussion of stress and supervision as a way to minimize the negative effects of stress.)

Ethics in Practice

Unethical practices seem to be on the rise in society in general and among mental health practitioners specifically (Rubin, 1997). There is increasing evidence of sexual activity between practitioners and clients (NASW, 1982). Given the intensity of the therapeutic relationship and the lack of preparation in psychotherapy training programs to deal with sexual content (Edelwich and Brodsky, 1982), it is understandable that ethical problems are surfacing in this area. Supervision is an important arena for dealing with sexual content in practice and for helping the practitioner to develop appropriate and ethical ways of handling such material (Edelwich and Brodsky, 1982:135-138). With the increase in the number of private practitioners and the decreased emphasis on supervision, more practice is removed from monitoring by others. The unethical practices are an elusive problem, but exposure of practice through good supervision is the best safeguard against such problems. Some agencies have reinstituted supervision as a means of ensuring that abuse of the client-practitioner relationship is minimized.

SUPERVISOR PREPARATION

The indication is that the previous trends are giving rise to more complexity in supervision and practice. Formal learning about supervision and how to do it has been declining in the social work profession. In one survey, over 60 percent of the supervisors had no formal academic training in supervision. The majority of the supervisors reported that they learned to do supervision through an agency training program (20 percent) or through on-the-job training (28 percent) (Munson, see Study A). There is limited information about the quality or quantity of learning in such programs. The survey revealed that only 13 percent of the graduate schools required a course in supervision as part of the MSW curriculum; 28 percent did not have a course in supervision, and 58 percent offered a supervision course as an elective (Munson, see Study C).

These statistics reveal that, although most states that license and certify practitioners require a period of supervision, there is little assurance that the supervision will be of high quality or uniform from state to state or agency to agency, mainly due to a lack of consistent universal standards. Some states have made efforts to establish high-quality, uniform supervisory standards for licensure (see Munson, 1996a), but no national standards for supervisory practice exist. There is no national association of supervisors, and only since 1983 has there been a journal devoted to supervision practice *(The Clinical Supervisor)*.

Most supervisors tend to supervise in reaction to the way they were supervised. When asked how they developed their style of and attitude toward supervision, supervisors cite, about equally, the emulation of admired qualities and the avoidance of negative aspects of their past supervisors (Munson, see Study C).

CHARACTERISTICS OF SUPERVISEES

To understand the needs of supervisees, it is important that the supervisors have knowledge of the characteristics of supervisees. Each supervisee is unique, but it is helpful for supervisors to know general characteristics of supervisees as a group. This is especially important for new supervisors.

There is a 70 percent likelihood that the supervisee will be female (Kadushin, 1974:289; Munson, 1975:96). Supervisees on the average are thirty-four years old, making them ten years younger than their supervisors. There is a 60 percent chance that they are married, and on the average they have two children. The majority (43 percent) hold MSW degrees, while one-third (36 percent) hold BA degrees, and only 6 percent hold BSW degrees. The remaining 15 percent hold various degrees in related areas.

There is a slightly better than 50 percent chance that the supervisee is employed in a public agency; the remainder work in private agencies. The workers are employed in family and children's services (40 percent), health and mental health settings (30 percent), and social service (public welfare) agencies (29 percent). The supervisee will most likely have six years' social work experience, and half of that experience will have been in the agency where he or she is currently employed. The majority (54 percent) of supervisees report being supervised in the traditional, one-to-one, individual model of supervision, while 17 percent report undergoing group supervision, and 29 percent experience the independent model of supervision, in which they function autonomously and use supervision only occasionally. Over 60 percent of the supervisees report being satisfied with their supervisory experience. These are general characteristics of social work supervisees. They are summarized here to give the reader an idea of what the profession looks like and to give the supervisor something to compare with his or her individual situation. Each supervisee is unique and should be recognized as such.

BEGINNING PROFESSIONALS

With these general observations in mind, consideration is given to the nature and characteristics of beginning professionals who enter supervision. These neophytes will show wide variation in amount and type of clinical practice, techniques, theories, and supervision they have experienced. Some will have strong foundations in a theory or theories and will have experienced good, sound supervision in which specific clinical material has been explored and appropriate strategies and techniques of intervention have been applied.

Many more supervisees will have experienced poor, limited supervision in agencies that are under the practice gun and shoot from the hip, theoretically and practically. Such supervisees have been left with partially learned theory and techniques. Many of them have surveyed several theories and have mastered none, or they have developed a repertoire of fragmented and unrelated techniques that lack a coherent pattern. In many agencies, theories and concepts are used only as code words, which results in their misinterpretation and misapplication. Products of these settings make such statements as, "I am a Gestalt therapist" or "I am a systems person" or "I use paradoxing" or "I do TA [transactional analysis]." Such descriptions reveal little about what the practitioners know or can and cannot do.

For these reasons, the supervisor must do a thorough educational diagnosis as he or she begins supervision. In the past, educational diagnosis was equated with a personality assessment of the practitioner. This is too narrow for today's practice demands. An educational diagnosis measures what the person knows and has experienced. The more relevant questions that go into an educational diagnosis follow: What do supervisees know? What do they know about theory? What kind of practice settings have they worked in? What kind of and how many cases have they treated? How many in-depth cases have they had? What kind of outcomes have they produced in the cases they have treated? What do they know about diagnosis and assessment? What do they see as their practice strengths and weaknesses? What is their style of practice? What kind of and how much supervision have they experienced? What do they hope to accomplish from supervision? (Appendix II contains a form for doing an educational assessment of a supervisee.)

Many students enter graduate education today because of a personal problem they have experienced. Because of contact with a therapist they want to emulate, they have developed the desire to help others. This connection between being the helped and being the helper is perpetuated in schools through therapeutically oriented supervision. In cases in which this model is used, the student and beginning practitioner show a tendency to model themselves after the therapist rather than the supervisor. This can result in deficient practice style because the worker adopts as a general practice style the techniques that were utilized with him or her. These may not be appropriate to a variety of cases with diverse problems. Where the therapeutic model of supervision does not work for the supervisee, there is a tendency on the part of the supervisor to be leery of such practices in supervision.

Depending on their student supervisory experience, beginning practitioners either are eager for self-analysis in supervision or will resist it strongly. Research has demonstrated that the supervisor needs to encourage a healthy balance with respect to the amount of self-analysis, because some students seek self-analysis to avoid dealing with other important components of their practice, and others avoid self-analysis to the detriment of their growth and development as practitioners (Munson, see Study B). Self-analysis should always be encouraged by the supervisor in the context of how it will make the practitioner more effective in a specific case. Individual or group supervision focused only on the worker's personal dynamics to help him or her to learn abstractly about practice is inappropriate. Supervisors who focus primarily on supervisees' personal dynamics have been characterized as poor supervisors and poor therapists (Haley, 1976:187).

ORGANIZATIONS

Some have argued that under new demands of practice, clinical learning must be integrated with organizational theory (see Cottle and Whitten, 1980:3-19). This seems to be a generalization that confuses certain issues for practitioners. Organizations do have an impact on clinical practice, but this varies with the practice setting. The experiences of hospital patients differ from those of private outpatients in a group practice. Where there is an overemphasis on the organization in supervision, the organization can become the scapegoat for avoiding clinical issues or for justifying clinical failures. Organizational issues in supervision are relevant to the extent that they impede the progress of the treatment. Supervisees should be given full credit for any organizational obstacles they can identify. The supervision should be focused on the question, Given the organizational obstacles, what can be done to overcome them to the benefit of the client?

NEEDS OF SUPERVISEES

An extensive review by Hansen and Warner (1971) of research on counselor practicum supervision answers some questions about the impact of supervision and reinforces some old doubts. The survey revealed that supervisors rely predominantly on teaching through questioning as the interactional structure. Although supervisors do not like to rely on teaching of specific techniques, this is what supervisees perceive themselves as needing, especially in the early stages. Also, technique-oriented supervision produces more effective learning than supervision that has a therapeutic orientation. This finding has implications for supervisor styles that are discussed later.

Supportive supervision was found to produce more effective learning than nonsupportive or negative supervision. In the nonsupportive model, supervisees showed a significant tendency to shift the focus of the supervision interaction from the clients to themselves. This finding has implications for supervisees' reactions (discussed in Chapter 5). Also, supervisee learning is significantly greater when the supervisor's theoretical orientation is taken into account.

Social work supervisees show a tendency to prefer characteristics in supervisors different from those desired by supervisees in the disciplines of psychiatry and psychology. Respondents in a study of psychiatry and psychology supervisees ranked interest in supervision and experience as a therapist as the preferred characteristics, whereas social workers ranked genuineness and ability to provide feedback as the preferred characteristics (Nelson, 1978:548). Social workers tend to look for more specific characteristics in supervisors than do workers in other disciplines. The importance of feedback in supervision was highlighted and refined in a study by Thigpen (1979), who found that a group of supervisees in mental health settings preferred client-focused feedback and that they did not regard highly feedback focused on themselves.

Although these research studies indicate that supervisees can change on the basis of specific components of supervision, little is known about the specific reason for change, and it is not known what supervisors can do to make supervisees more effective with their clients. One of the problems has been lack of adequate research methodology in studies of supervision. Many variables remain uncontrolled. The need for more in-depth and extensive research on supervision cannot be overemphasized.

Research has begun to expose some of the inconsistencies that need to be addressed. In a controlled study of graduate social work students, Joel Fisher (1975) found that students who had received specific instruction in core practice conditions had higher levels of learning and performance and higher evaluative ratings by their field instructors than two control groups that had received less specific instruction. An unexpected finding in all three groups was that field instructors' evaluations of students' empathy, warmth, and genuineness were inversely correlated with academic grades.

A more disturbing finding came from two studies. In a study of sixty-five supervisees in various settings (Munson, 1975), supervisees perceived their level of accomplishment and various types of supervisory satisfaction to be highly correlated with the amount of interaction they had with the supervisor (see Visual 1.1). Another study, involving twenty-six field instructors of graduate social work students (Munson, see Study C), found no correlation between the amount of instructor interaction with supervisees and the instructors' own satisfaction with helping the supervisees grow professionally, sharing knowledge with them, and discussing administrative matters. The only variable that produced a significant correlation with interaction

VISUAL 1.1. Correlation of Supervisee Satisfaction and Level of Interaction with the Supervisor

Satisfaction Variable	Level of Interaction* (Correlation Coefficient)
Job satisfaction	.63
Helping satisfaction	.84
Teaching satisfaction	.81
Control satisfaction	.78
Administrative satisfaction	.84
General satisfaction	.83
Sense of accomplishment	.50

Source: Munson, 1975:288.

Note: Correlation coefficients are Kendall *tau.* All coefficients were significant at the .05 level or better.

*Level of interaction scale based on frequency of contact, approachability of supervisor, supervisor encouragement of discussion, ability of supervisor to put supervisee at ease, clarity of supervisor communication, and degree of congruence in supervisor and supervisee communication. All of these components are based on the supervisee's perception.

was their sense of obligation to direct the work of the supervisees (see Visual 1.2). These findings show that the factors that produce high levels of satisfaction and meet the needs of supervisees lead to little satisfaction for the supervisors. Although most studies reveal that supervisees are satisfied with their supervisory experiences, the findings of this study raise the question, At what price to the supervisor are these supervisee satisfactions being achieved? It is not known to what extent the supervisory role has negative impact on the supervisor. These findings could help to explain why some supervisors neglect and emotionally and physically withdraw from their supervisory responsibilities.

In many settings, workers express diminished perceptions or expectations regarding their supervisors when the supervisees experience supervisor withdrawal. When asked about the supervisor's performance, the worker will list numerous dissatisfactions, but when asked to rate the adequacy of the supervisor, the worker will indicate fairly high levels of satisfaction. When questioned about this inconsistency, supervisees will explain that they know they are not getting what they should from supervision but accept it because they understand that their supervisors are busy and overworked, and because they do not wish to burden them further. The supervisee adopts perceptions of supervision that lead to a diminished expectation of the supervisor. At this point, the supervisory process breaks down and fragmentation of learning sets in.

It is common to hear supervisees justify supervisor withdrawal and aloofness on the basis that more supervisory contact just creates anxiety in

VISUAL 1.2. Correlation of Supervisor Satisfaction with Supervisory Role and Level of Interaction with Supervisees

Satisfaction Variables	Level of Interaction* (Correlation Coefficient)
Helping supervisees grow professionally	.01
Sharing knowledge with supervisees	.14
Discussion of administrative matters	.07
Sense of obligation to direct and guide supervisees	.35

Source: Munson, Study C.

Note: Correlation coefficients are Kendall *tau*. The only variable that was significantly correlated with level of interaction was sense of obligation to direct and guide supervisees ($p = < .04$).

*Level of interaction scale based on frequency of contact, approachability of supervisor, supervisor encouragement of discussion, ability of supervisor to put supervisee at ease, clarity of supervisor communication, and degree of congruence in supervisor and supervisee communication. All of these components are based on the supervisee's perception.

the supervisee out of the fear of emotional dependence on the supervisor. It appears that, in reality, supervisee anxiety grows out of lack of mechanisms to cope with problems encountered in practice. The social worker who has difficulty tolerating clients who get upset, combative, and aggressive is like the medical student who cannot stand the sight of blood. Although medical students may be shocked at their first sight of blood, they learn and are taught to deal with it. Too often student clinicians are not taught to deal with highly emotional reactions of clients. As a result, these clinicians continue to be upset by these occurrences and conduct their treatment in a way that aims at preventing them, even if it is essential for the clients to have reactions of this nature. In both situations, these reactions negatively affect the treatment. Providing sound, helpful supervision through a trained, qualified, committed supervisor on a regular basis is the best antidote for practitioner anxiety about clinical activity.

In a series of surveys (Munson, see Study A), the following categories of learning needs were the ones most identified by graduating MSWs as they began their professional careers:

- Exposure to specialized cases
- Criticism of work
- Exposure to different practice approaches
- More exposure to theory
- Cotherapy experience
- Exposure to the work of others
- More direct supervision
- Developing more self-awareness
- Feedback on work
- Support and encouragement
- Training in group therapy
- Help improving diagnostic skills

It is clear from these responses that new supervisees recognize a need for help in developing their skills, applying theory, fostering self-awareness, being exposed to different practice modalities, and getting support as they struggle to develop self-confidence.

CLINICAL ASSESSMENT AND DIAGNOSIS

It is important for the beginning practitioner to learn to avoid attempting treatment before doing a basic diagnostic assessment. A diagnostic assessment is different from a diagnosis. A diagnostic assessment is a process of gathering various forms of information and permits planning sound treatment intervention; a diagnosis is a limited process of applying a label or diagnostic category to the client based on identifying symptoms and behaviors. Students and beginning practitioners can feel that they are under a great deal of pressure to apply treatment strategies and interventions. (The pressure may be imagined or real.) This results in interventions being made without an adequate information base to support them, which can lead the treatment astray. It is true that interventions are made without sufficient information upon which to base treatment. Beginning practitioners show a tendency to act without weighing the amount of information that serves as the basis for the intervention. The practitioner must be helped to understand that there is nothing wrong with asking questions until the client's problems are comprehended in the context of the therapy and the client's situation.

Educators, writers, managed cost organizations, and supervisors unwittingly contribute to this rapidity of treatment by minimizing the importance of the diagnostic phase and emphasizing that treatment begins as soon as the first interview starts. Although this is true, it is confusing to the practitioner because there is no clarity about the distinction between and the interrelatedness of the diagnostic and treatment phases. Beginning professionals feel a need to produce results for their clients and supervisors, which makes them vulnerable to questioning or engaging in weakly supported interventions. They are caught in a supervisory double bind of sorts: they are fearful of hesitating to intervene soon enough but are open to concerns about the basis for hastily planned interventions. The supervisor must be sensitive to this and help the learner balance the two realms. The supervisor has a responsibility to ensure that assessment and treatment are accomplished in a sound, thorough, and sequential manner.

This balancing act is important because prolonged diagnostic activity can be a barrier to intervening and learning about intervention. This is the basis for *persistent diagnosis*. Just as C. Northcote Parkinson (1957:2) observed that "work expands so as to fill the time available for its completion," so does diagnosis expand in direct relation to the time available for its completion. The supervisor has a responsibility to aid the beginning practitioner in adequately planning and preparing a diagnostic assessment, as well as giving it some form of closure, and in initiating treatment. When this process is clear, the client can also be reassured that the worker is proceeding in an orderly fashion.

In achieving an assessment/treatment balance, the supervisor must recognize that the beginning practitioner will tend to need to be in control and to be overactive in the treatment. The supervisor can guard against this by encouraging the neophyte practitioner to explore interactionally, rather than to explain, when the client asks questions about the quality, type, or purpose of the treatment, the program, or the agency. Chapter 6 provides a survey of how to teach assessment and diagnostic skills and apply them to treatment planning.

BEGINNING GUIDELINES

Research conducted with supervisees (Munson, see Study A, Study B, Study E) has revealed a number of factors the new supervisor must be aware of and prepared to handle. These factors are particularly appropriate to beginning supervisors and beginning practitioners, but they apply in most cases to any supervisory situation. These are the ten most critical factors:

1. Consider that the supervisee will likely have limited experience at applying theory, concepts, and techniques.
2. The supervisor should be prepared to demonstrate what he or she wants the practitioner to do.
3. The emphasis should be on evaluation of the supervisee's practice as well as on the evaluation of the supervision process itself.
4. The supervisor should observe the supervisee's practice periodically.
5. The supervisor should make the details of his or her expectations clear.
6. The supervisor should refrain from criticizing the supervisee's educational program, experience, or the profession.
7. The supervisor should refrain from using supervision as a forum to criticize other professions or other agency staff.
8. The supervisor should avoid comparing the supervisee's performance to that of other supervisees or other staff.
9. The supervisor should be willing to share his or her knowledge and skills with the supervisee.
10. The supervisor should remember that the supervisee is supposed to be working under the direction of a competent and informed master teacher and professional.

CHARACTERISTICS OF SUPERVISORS

Research has revealed that supervisors are, on the average, forty-two years of age and about ten years older than their supervisees (Munson, 1975). Supervisors have an average of fifteen years of social work experience, and an average of seven years of experience in the agency that currently employs them. Fifty percent of supervisors are female. A slightly greater percentage of supervisors are employed in public agencies (53 percent) than in private agencies (47 percent). The overwhelming majority (77 percent) hold MSW degrees. The majority (92 percent) of supervisors have some form of preparation for their supervisory roles, such as university-taught courses, agency training programs, and on-the-job training. One-third of supervisors carry a caseload in addition to their supervisory roles, 21 percent do not carry any cases, and 45 percent periodically carry cases. Of those supervisors who do see cases, one-third report that these cases are seen in private practice and are not connected with the agency in which they perform supervisory roles. (This probably accounts for the small degree to which supervisors share their practice with supervisees; this lack of sharing was reported by supervisees in the same study.) The supervisees reported that in the majority of situations (64 percent) they were satisfied with and valued their supervisory experience.

ON BECOMING A CLINICAL SUPERVISOR

Becoming a supervisor in clinical practice is somewhat different from becoming a supervisor in the more traditional management sense. Many subtle differences exist, but the major one occurs in the area of role and function in relation to authority. The traditional supervisor makes a complete shift from being a rank-and-file employee to assuming a new, full-time function as manager. This requires the mastery of a new perspective on work, new basic concepts, new emphasis on function, new sources of job satisfaction, new status, and new relationships with others in the organization (Reeves, 1980:1). The traditional supervisor must adjust to regulating the work rather than doing the work and must adapt to the authority that goes along with the new role. The most skilled worker can experience a high degree of difficulty in making the transition to supervisor and focusing on getting the job done through other people.

On becoming a clinical supervisor, the shift in responsibility is often vague and unclear. Most clinical supervisors are autonomous, professional practitioners rather than exclusively subordinate employees before they become supervisors, and upon assuming supervisory responsibilities, they often continue to practice. The assumption has long been that to be a good supervisor, one must be an active practitioner. This is undoubtedly a good premise, but it can create dilemmas for the supervisor carrying a dual role, such as the problems of time management and establishing priorities when the demands of practice and supervision conflict.

AUTHORITY

The role of authority is unique for the clinical supervisor. Since the supervisor is accustomed to working as an autonomous professional, and since the majority of the supervisees are trained professionals, the nature and extent of the supervisor's authority is vague, unstructured, and limited in sanction. Even with student practitioners, authority is vague because the supervisor is often a remote representative of the educational institution and because trainees are encouraged to prepare to be autonomous practitioners. The authority of the clinical supervisor is indirect. It resides in one's ability as a skilled practitioner, as in the sanction provided by the agency and the profession. The doing of the work remains in the hands of the supervisee, and the results are rarely seen by the supervisor. This is true in traditional supervision. In clinical supervision, learning to do a task or function is the focus, with a terminal point always in mind; whereas in traditional supervision, the regulation of the doing is ongoing even after learning the task has been accomplished. A problem for the clinical supervisor is determining when the learning is complete and regulation is no longer needed. The roles of authority and structure are addressed in Chapter 7.

AVOIDING SUPERVISION AS TREATMENT

The new supervisor is an experienced practitioner, but, unfortunately, this is all too often the only basis for assuming the supervisory role. The transition from practitioner to supervisor is an important change that often is lacking in adequate preparation. Usually, all the new supervisor has to draw on is his or her therapeutic orientation and experiences derived from supervision. This is unfortunate because the beginning supervisor is being asked to assume the most intensive teaching role imaginable.

Educational supervision is much different from teaching a course or presenting lectures to small or large groups. Instead, the clinical supervisor is in an intensive teacher-learner relationship (involving one or several students) that is vaguely defined, lacking in precise guidelines, and consisting of unstructured formats. Since most practitioners who become supervisors lack the knowledge or skills of general or specific teaching techniques, they fall back on their treatment skills to get by in supervision. This is especially the case when they encounter difficulty in supervising. This mismatch of needs and performance capability gives rise to many of the problems in supervision. The incongruence is heightened by the increasing belief that doing therapy with the supervisee leads to frustration, resentment, and anger for the supervisor and the supervisee.

Trust in the supervisor is essential to effective supervision, but evidence suggests that using therapeutic strategies as a focus in supervision results in distrust of the supervisor (Munson, see Study A, Study B). Supervisors who engage in this approach are simply attempting to develop skills to cope with the situation. The only problem is that such coping mechanisms rarely work. The function of this book is to provide alternate coping strategies based on sound educational principles.

SUPPORT FOR SUPERVISORS

In traditional management supervision, supervisors are supervised. They must account for their performance as well as that of their subordinates. Rarely do clinical supervisors have to account for their performance, either as practitioners or supervisors. Just as they do not have to account for their performance, there is little recognition of their accomplishments and little support when they encounter problems. Clinical supervisors need some form of support system as well as some accountability. When support is not provided from within the organization or from the outside profession, the supervisor will internalize problems, fail to acknowledge the difficulty, or perhaps seek support through supervisees. None of these alternatives is acceptable or appropriate; when utilized, each can lead to additional problems. When supervisors turn to their supervisees for support, they are open to manipulation. This does not mean that supervisors should avoid support by supervisees, only that they should not be put in or get in the position of having to depend upon supervisees for it.

UNANTICIPATED CONSEQUENCES

The clinical supervisor will encounter some unexpected consequences of the new role that are accepted in traditional management supervision. Practitioners will bring to supervision organizational problems, service gaps, and interpersonal staff problems that the supervisor, eager to provide clinical supervision, failed to anticipate and for which he or she has little tolerance. The differing expectations of the supervisor and the supervisee regarding the functions and purposes of supervision can be a source of frustration and disappointment for both sides.

In traditional management supervision, promotion to the supervisory position brings concomitant increases in pay benefits, status privileges, and access to higher-level members of the organization. For the clinical supervisor, assuming the supervisory role often does not result in any of these rewards; supervision is an added responsibility with few tangible benefits. Supervisory positions in psychotherapy are viewed more as a professional responsibility and an opportunity to make a contribution to the next generation of practitioners.

Although most traditional supervisors receive some form of training for or assistance with their new roles, clinical supervisors receive little, if any, training for their new responsibilities. Most have to rely on their judgment, experience, reading, and relationships with their own supervisors. The long-held assumption is that clinical experience can serve as a basis for and be converted easily to supervisory practice. This assumption can lead to problems. Some of the techniques and skills of direct treatment can be used in supervision, but they are insufficient for good comprehensive supervision practice. Weak practitioners rarely make good supervisors, and good practitioners do not necessarily make good supervisors. When clinical skills are relied on to conduct supervision, they can lead to problems because supervisees feel they are being placed unwillingly in therapy rather than being supervised. Thus, it is important that supervisors be trained in distinguishing therapy skills and supervisory skills. This book is devoted to identifying and applying the skills that are basic to good supervisory practice, so that some of the problems just mentioned can be avoided or overcome.

Many professionals enter the role of clinical supervisor without much anticipation of the adjustments required, but they should possess or be willing to develop certain characteristics. They should

- enjoy teaching others,
- have patience when others cannot understand,
- be able to make indirect suggestions,
- be able to plan effectively,
- have a positive attitude when expected to answer questions and explain actions,
- be able to discuss organizational problems in a constructive way,
- be able to tolerate others making mistakes,
- be able to give and take criticism,
- enjoy decision making,
- be able to work with others in a team approach, and
- be able to effectively manage paperwork.

Appendix I contains a scale that covers these areas, among others, in assessing suitability for clinical supervision. Anyone who is considering becoming a clinical supervisor should complete the scale and discuss it with others before accepting a supervisory position.

In addition, becoming a clinical supervisor involves some general shifts in attitude and functioning that one should be prepared in advance to accept (see Reeves, 1980:1-13). Some of these are

- assuming more responsibility for managing the work of others and doing less practice;
- assuming more responsibility in general;
- having more authority;
- carrying a broader decision-making role;
- having more status;
- having a changed relationship with co-workers;
- being privy to more "inside" information about the organization, its employees, and its functioning;
- having greater job pressures; and
- manifesting a greater commitment to the functions of the organization.

SUPERVISEE BILL OF RIGHTS

Many aspects of supervision considered collective wisdom have not been recorded or mandated by any ethical codes or social work licensure laws. The following Bill of Rights for supervisees was developed by the author in an effort to establish a basic foundation of expectations for supervision that could guide both the supervisee and supervisor. This Bill of Rights is the basis for all the material in this book. The supervisee Bill of Rights states that every clinical social work supervisee has the right to

1. a supervisor who supervises consistently and at regular intervals;
2. growth-oriented supervision that respects personal privacy;
3. supervision that is technically sound and theoretically grounded;
4. be evaluated on criteria that are made clear in advance, and evaluations that are based on actual observation of performance; and
5. a supervisor who is adequately skilled in clinical practice and trained in supervision practice.

Expectations of the Supervisor

The Bill of Rights based on the five criteria of consistency, growth orientation, stable requirements, clear evaluative criteria, and a knowledgeable, competent supervisor leads to the requirement for clear explication of expectations of the supervisor and the supervisee. The best way to explicate the basic ideas of a succinct Bill of Rights is by developing a list of expectations a supervisee should have of a supervisor. In addition to the basic rights, a supervisee can and should have certain expectations of the supervisor.

Supervisees have a right to know what to expect from a supervisor. This is especially true in the case of students. Although supervisees rarely inquire about this, supervisors should ask themselves this question as they strive to improve the quality of the supervision they provide. Given the nature and pattern of supervisee complaints about supervisors listed in evaluations and research studies, it would appear that supervisors should spend more time in reflection on how to best meet supervisee expectations.

Knowledge of what to expect of a supervisor is important for the supervisee as well as the supervisor. It is essential for the supervisee in order to be an educated consumer and to adequately evaluate the supervision. It is important for the supervisor because the primary method of training for supervision today is self-education.

Supervision is the most important educational experience any clinical practitioner undergoes. Classroom courses and workshops are abstractions that are remotely connected to the realities of practice. Student evaluations of educational programs overwhelmingly indicate that the practice supervision component of the program was the most helpful.

Even though the importance of supervision is acknowledged, in the past two decades its use as an educational experience has decreased (Hanna, 1992). Schools have minimal supervision time requirements; they increasingly give credit for work experience that has limited educational focus; they have downgraded qualifications to be a supervisor and have given marginal recognition and support to internship faculty and administrators. Agencies are de-emphasizing supervision because it is costly. Some professional organizations minimize emphasis on supervision because it is viewed as a threat to professional autonomy, and managed cost organizations do not require it.

Some argue that incompetent supervision is worse than no supervision at all. It is unfortunate that this point has been reached. Even though supervision is being used less, many practitioners in agencies must undergo supervision, and, of course, all students have one or two educational experiences on the path to a professional degree. The de-emphasis of supervision requirements at the agency and professional levels has decreased the pool of supervisors qualified to offer student supervision. In the past, schools could draw on the agency and professionally trained supervisors for internship supervision. Presently, schools are required to develop their own training and educational programs for supervisors. Most schools have limited resources to provide the level of training needed. This means that the educational supervisor is left to become self-educated about good supervision practices. It is the self-education process that the following expectations are designed to promote.

In an effort to assist supervisors in this important professional reflection, the following list of expectations is provided. The supervisee has the right to expect that a supervisor

1. is a master teacher;
2. is able to guide learning by virtue of superior knowledge and skill;
3. is able to transmit knowledge that integrates theory and practice activity;
4. has in-depth knowledge that can be applied to practice with precision;
5. is able to apply research knowledge and methodology to practice;
6. is confident in his or her knowledge, but open to questioning;
7. is able to accept criticism without becoming defensive;
8. is fair, honest, candid, but supportive and patient;
9. can provide cases that are appropriate, but challenging;
10. is appropriate in appearance, courteous, and clear in communication;
11. is thorough in providing orientation to the agency or setting;
12. is prepared for conferences and avoids wasting precious supervision time;
13. is involved in the agency, the community, and the profession;
14. is knowledgeable about the agency, the community, and the profession; and
15. is knowledgeable about the code of ethics and faithfully adheres to its tenets.

It is important for the supervisor to adopt these criteria as an internal code of self-directing principles because the supervisee normally has limited expectations of supervision. Schools, agencies, and the professional organizations offer little or no advance information about supervisee rights. Since supervision is increasingly conducted in private, there is no exposure of the activity. Supervisors do not experience supervision or consultation; thus their work as supervisors is not evaluated.

Expectations of the Supervisee

The supervision relationship is a reciprocal process, and the supervisor can have expectations of the supervisee. The supervisee should be on time for conferences, should be prepared with cases to discuss, should be open about difficulties and stress, and should be open about cases for which his or her abilities are limited.

In a study of supervisors (Munson, Study C), the expectations of supervisees that were repeatedly identified were that the supervisees would

- take that extra step in dealing with difficult cases,
- take responsibility for the job organizational matters,
- manifest a willingness to work hard,

- freely talk about problem cases and situations,
- be honest about how they are feeling,
- show respect for the supervisor,
- demonstrate basic interpersonal skills,
- have a genuine interest in learning,
- be willing to work with the supervisor,
- be motivated to learn,
- be able to set goals with assistance,
- be willing to discuss work and their thoughts about work,
- present themselves as professionals,
- be aware of themselves,
- have integrity,
- have a sense of respect for others,
- be able to effectively engage clients as well as agency staff members,
- ask questions on an ongoing basis,
- take notes on a timely basis,
- be willing to read up on topics in their area of practice,
- be open and curious about learning, and
- have an ability to assess their learning needs.

The rights and expectations listed here are general in nature, and supervisors and supervisees can draft their own list of rights and expectations based on the demands of individual or unique settings or situations.

SUGGESTED READINGS

Hoffman, L. W. (1990). *Old Scapes New Maps: A Training Program for Psychotherapy Supervisors.* Cambridge, MA: Milusik Press.
    Description of a system for training for psychotherapy supervision.

Holloway, S. and Brager, G. (1989). *Supervising in the Human Services: The Politics of Practice.* New York: The Free Press.
    An overview of primarily administrative supervision in public social services.

Jacobs, D., David, P., and Meyer, D.J. (1995). *The Supervisory Encounter: A Guide for Teachers of Psychodynamic Psychotherapy and Psychoanalysis.* New Haven, CT: Yale University Press.
    Overview of supervision practice from a psychoanalytic perspective.

Kadushin, A. (1992). *Supervision in Social Work,* Third Edition. New York: Columbia University Press.
    Overview of basic social work supervision.

Munson, C. E. (ed.) (1979). *Social Work Supervision: Classic Statements and Critical Issues.* New York: The Free Press, 1979.
Classic collection of thirty-one articles that serves as an introduction to the history and current practice of social work supervision.

Pettes, D. E. (1979). *Staff and Student Supervision: A Task-Centered Approach.* Boston: Allen & Unwin.
Classic overview for beginning supervisors, especially on the administrative aspects of supervision.

Reeves, E. T. (1980). *So You Want to Be a Supervisor!* New York: AMACOM.
Practical explanation of management-oriented supervision that can be applied to clinical supervision in some areas.

Rock, M. H. (ed.) (1997). *Psychodynamic Supervision: Perspectives of the Supervisor and Supervisee.* Northvale, NJ: Jason Aronson.
Survey of supervision topics from a psychoanalytic perspective.

Watkins, C. E. (1999). The Beginning Psychotherapy Supervisor: How Can We Help? *The Clinical Supervisor*, 8(2), pp. 63-72.
Overview of learning supervisory skills.

Whatever may be ahead, it is certain that the
new profession of social work is now being
given the greatest opportunity which has ever
come to it to aid in the directing of economic
and social change for the welfare of society.
And it does not seem likely that the social
worker will ever lose this advantage which he
has gained.

Esther Lucile Brown
Social Work As a Profession

Supervision . . . is entering a phase bright with
promise but also one in which supervisors will
have to stay alert to the political arena as never
before. It can be the best of times or the worst
of times—but it will be an exciting time for
making history.

Thomas Sergiovanni and Robert Starratt
Supervision

Chapter 2

History of Supervision

This chapter traces developments in the history of supervision in the
area of clinical practice, from the earliest conceptions of preparation for
casework practice to the latest views of clinical practice. There is as
much emphasis on the evolution of practice knowledge as on ideas
about supervision because the two areas cannot be separated. Several
themes have been central to every era of practice and supervision history: the art and/or science of practice, treatment versus social reform,
and the psychological versus sociological explanation of behavior.

What follows is not a comprehensive or rigorous analysis; social work
has a rich and diverse heritage that cannot be completely covered
briefly. This chapter is designed to give the practicing supervisor a summary understanding of over 150 years of history.

PRACTICE KNOWLEDGE

The history of supervision cannot be separated from discussion of the history of practice theory. Concern about supervision practices has increased and subsided over time in relation to development of, competition between, and conflict over intervention theories. Theories, and the people who develop and use them, change over time. What are judged to be problems and the best ways to approach them also change with time (Veroff et al., 1981:9).

The history of social work practice reveals a fairly consistent pattern of inductive reasoning to advance knowledge and deductive reasoning to measure effectiveness. Early efforts were focused on defining problems and identifying social ills. Later efforts were focused on searching for theories to explain the problems and to guide interventions, and on evaluating whether those interventions fit the theories. When a sweeping historical view of social work knowledge-building efforts is taken, this pattern becomes apparent. Supervision has played an important role in this process over the decades, and great social work theoreticians wrote about supervision as well as practice theory.

The history of social work practice is characterized by two recurring, related themes. The first theme has been the quest for a scientific approach to practice knowledge. In 1884 Josephine Shaw Lowell referred to social work as "our science" (Robinson, 1930:xii), and this characterization has continued to the present. In every era, social work leaders have striven to adhere to the scientific principles of the time. Until recently, supervision has been an important component in the application of the science and the evolution of social work knowledge. The second theme has been the shifts in practice orientation. These two themes are naturally related. The purpose of science is the evolution of knowledge. The continual application of scientific principles to a body of knowledge produces dynamic shifts in the way practice is defined and oriented.

This persistent quest to expand social work knowledge has brought about many of the changes in practice that are explored in this chapter. Clearly, not all changes are brought about by the pursuit of knowledge, but it is an important part in social work history that often goes unrecognized, and the evolution of social work practice has not been totally the reflection of economic or political forces, as some have held.

EARLY HISTORY

It is not known for certain where, when, or how the traditional model of social work supervision originated. It probably was based on the model of consultation and supervision developed in the field of medicine in England, which subsequently became the model for American medicine (Kaslow, 1979:1-24). It is reasonable to assume that the medical model of supervision was adopted by early social workers because they had many close connections with physicians. These connections were personal as well as professional. Some of the early social workers' parents and spouses were physicians. Physicians taught in the earliest social work training programs, a pattern that has continued in some schools to the present. Physicians served on the boards of various early charitable societies and had much influence on how these organizations were structured and operated.

Supervision, as conceptualized in clinical practice, began to emerge in the late 1800s within the Charity Organization Societies, in which paid agents became the model for casework practice. These paid agents were supervised within the agency as part of apprenticeship programs. There has been disagreement over the extent of administrative and educational focus of this supervision (Kaslow, 1979:28-34). When the apprenticeship programs became burdensome for the agencies to administer, perhaps because of increased focus on the educational component, leaders of the profession reluctantly agreed to having the training programs affiliated with universities. These programs did not become part of the university, but were appendages of them. This led to a modified version of the earlier apprentice programs, and field instruction, as it is known today, evolved from this arrangement.

The form and structure of supervision have remained fairly constant from the late nineteenth century to the present. The supervisor was responsible for a number of supervisees, who were provided supervision through periodic individual conferences. Much later the idea of group supervision was applied on a limited basis. Group supervision has not been widely adopted in clinical settings, although it has been conceptually confused with team approaches in some settings.

The structure of supervision has not changed significantly, but its content has evolved and shifted over the years. Social work practice has traditionally reflected the attitudes and values of society, and supervision has been the arena in which practice strategies and societal patterns are consolidated and integrated.

By 1840 more than thirty private organizations in New York City focused on moral uplift combined with the provision of relief. Society's response to this effort was mixed due to the fear that organized attempts to decrease poverty would actually contribute to its increase, an attitude that has persisted to the present in segments of society. In these early efforts, social work was associated more with the assessment of the deserving nature of the individual and with determining the extent of poverty than with offering moral uplift. The initial focus was on the individual and the characteristics that contributed to poverty. Later this focus shifted to the family and the effects of poverty on its members.

Institutional Supervision

During the era from the 1850s to the 1890s, the concept of supervision was more general than it is today. It dealt more with supervising institutions to ensure that clients or patients were being treated and that the institutions were being run effectively and efficiently. The role of the supervisor paralleled the societal concern with the need for and humane operation of asylums and poor houses. As the role of assessment emerged, the idea of individual case supervision developed. It was gradually recognized that to make a good assessment, to determine who was deserving, and to know what information was important in understanding problems, one needs training and practice under a skilled supervisor. This training function was carried by agencies for several decades before it was gradually taken over by universities and training facilities associated with universities. This process of transferring responsibility for training was slow, occurring over several decades, and raised many conflicts about whether agencies or universities were best prepared to train social workers (see Munson, 1979c:1-5).

Field instruction as part of educational programs has contributed a great deal to the evolution of supervision in social work. The earliest educational programs were agency-based apprenticeships. Classroom instruction emerged later and was "considered supplemental to rounding out of agency-based learning by doing" (Hollis and Taylor, 1951:230-231).

Assessment

At the turn of the century there was a quest for a theory of explanation of poverty and reaction to disease as medical social work emerged. This focus continued social work's emphasis on assessment. What had begun as work with poor persons served by relief agencies became the identification of the social and emotional elements of illness. It was in the move to develop medical social work that the psychological component was first introduced into the profession. At this stage, the emphasis was not on treatment but was still on assessment and identification of problems. Social work was founded on the basis of assessment, first in the area of relief and then in health. Soon after, the same pattern occurred in the area of psychiatric social work.

The social work profession emerged in direct relation to the quest for assessment in dealing with individualized social services. The assessment function of social work grew from the economic assessment of the Charity Organization Societies, to the physical assessment of hospital social work, to the diagnostic assessment of later work with psychiatrists. Ironically, but understandably, as the profession evolved through these forms of assessment it became narrower in focus. It can be argued that Mary Richmond recognized this trend and that her book *Social Diagnosis* was an attempt to reverse the trend. Within the profession, social assessment in individual cases was connected to the larger societal concern with social reform, and as society's concern with social reform waned after World War I (Weinberger, 1974:83), so did social work's interest in assessment.

Sociology and Social Work

During the decades that social work was struggling with assessment, it enjoyed a natural connection with sociology. In 1909, this connection was described:

> Charitable work has become so closely allied with all forms of social effort that general conditions must be taken into account before one can do good work, even among individuals. This involves some study of the whole situation, or in other words, some attention to sociology. (Conyngton, 1971/1909:326)

This connection is understandable. In the broadest sense, social work is a practice within society, while "sociology is not a practice, but an attempt to understand" society (Greenberg, 1971:4). When social work lost interest in assessment during the 1920s, its relationship with sociology deteriorated rapidly (Munson, 1979a; Siporin, 1980:14). Sociology and social work have since been toiling separately in their "little 'gardens of knowledge' " (Greenberg, 1971:10), but social work has been further divided in its devotion to individual treatment and social reform. This division has distracted it further from developing and refining systems of assessment.

Everett Dirksen, a sage senator from Illinois, said that "political parties do not defeat one another, but defeat themselves." The same is true of professions. The cause-and-function debate has distracted social work since its inception. Mary Richmond perceived this division and its destructive effect on the profession. She saw a place for both levels of functioning within the profession and advocated cooperative efforts in these areas. What Richmond proposed was only a beginning, but social work failed to recognize this dual functioning. Social work did not organize its social reform efforts around sociologists' succinct conception that "there are three requirements for a given social condition to be regarded as a social problem: (1) It must be social in origin. (2) It must be regarded by society as a problem. (3) It must require some form of social intervention" (Greenberg, 1971:13).

In the literature it has been held that a turning point for the profession was reached when Abraham Flexner addressed the National Conference of Charities and Corrections in 1915 and declared that social work was not a profession. Historians have accorded this speech more significance than it appears to have had at the time. In fact, Flexner's pronouncements were nothing new for social work and hardly came as a surprise.

The theory used during this era was practical and inductive. Psychological and sociological theories of poverty were not highly developed, and efforts to explain poverty on the basis of individual personality were not very successful (Robinson, 1930:10-11). Supervision, during this era of the development of assessment knowledge, was focused on developing skill at identifying and classifying individual problems and needs. Mary Richmond succinctly summarized the role of supervision at this stage of social work history:

> What should a supervisor look for in a case record in which the work has reached the stage of evidence gathered but not yet compared or interpreted? . . . Good supervision must include this consideration of wider aspects. . . . Every case worker has noticed how a certain juxtaposition of facts often reappears in record after record, and . . . this recurring juxtaposition indicates a hidden relation of cause and effect. . . . It is here that the "notation of recurrence" . . . becomes a duty of supervisor and case worker. . . . The getting at knowledge that will make the case work of another generation more effective may be only a byproduct of our own case work, but it is an important by-product. (1965/1917:351-352)

THE FREUDIAN INFLUENCE

At the time Richmond wrote of this view of supervision, a new era of theory building was emerging. Freud visited Clark University in the fall of 1909 and, along with others, gave a series of lectures on his theory. There is disagreement about the influence this visit had on the spread of Freud's ideas in the United States. Press coverage of the lectures was "spotty" and limited (Clark, 1980:259-276). It is apparent that the lectures had very little direct impact on social work. It took many years for Freud's influence on social work to become apparent, and it occurred in a way different from what is commonly believed.

Freud's ideas were promoted in the United States by people who traveled to Europe, were analyzed by Freud, and returned to the United States to work and lead the psychoanalytic movement (Strean, 1979). After World War I, Freud "had around him a flock of young Americans who came to Europe for training" (Roazen, 1974:378)—persons such as Horace Frink and Adolf Meyer. Horace Frink was a brilliant American who was analyzed twice by Freud and selected by him to lead the psychoanalytic movement in the United States. He was a tragic figure, however: he suffered from prolonged mental illness and died in a mental hospital. At one time he was treated by Adolf Meyer at Johns Hopkins. That Frink turned to Meyer is testimony to Meyer's reputation as a "famous psychiatrist" (Roazen, 1974: 380).

Born and trained in Europe, Meyer migrated to the United States at the age of twenty-six. Meyer, the son of a Swiss minister, rejected the biological view of psychopathology advocated by Emil Kraepelin, the German physician who is considered the founder of modern diagnostic systems. Meyer believed, in conjunction with the use of Freudian theory, that the biological and psychological aspects of functioning must be taken into consideration. Meyer introduced the case presentation method in the United States as a way to promote understanding of mental functioning and to develop staff sensitivity to needs of asylum residents (Shorter, 1997). Meyer was a believer in gathering the facts of the case in performing diagnostic and treatment decision making, and he was instrumental in the development of the first diagnostic and statistical manual of the American Psychiatric Association (DSM-I), although his influence has been gradually removed from the DSM system. Meyer had contact with famous Americans such as William James, John Dewey, Clifford Beers, and John Watson. Meyer helped Watson establish his famous behavioral laboratory, and he joined Beers, a former mental patient who became a reformer of hospitals, in establishing the mental hygiene movement in the United States (Stone, 1997).

Meyer was regarded highly by social workers and had much influence on their approach to psychiatric social work. He spoke before the National Conference of Charities and Corrections in 1911, and before the Smith College School of Psychiatric Social Work, the New York School of Social Work, and the Pennsylvania School of Social and Health Work in 1918 (Robinson, 1930:28-54). Meyer drew heavily on the ideas of Freud, but he had a much more comprehensive view of functioning. Meyer once remarked, "The main thing . . . is that your point of reference should always be life itself and not the imagined cesspool of the unconscious" (Lief, 1948:vii). Meyer's wife worked closely with him. She became the first volunteer psychiatric social worker and was the model for the first paid psychiatric social worker hired in New York in 1907. At about the same time, Richard C. Cabot in Boston was advocating utilizing social workers to work with psychiatrists (Lief, 1948). This brief example of Meyer's influence on social work illustrates the complex, but subtle, manner in which Freud's ideas found their way into social work. Also, Meyer was typical of psychiatrists who influenced the ideas of social workers in that the ideas shared by these psychiatric leaders were often sprinkled with Freudian conceptions but were much broader and not exclusively focused on Freudian conventions.

The Americans who traveled to Europe to study under Freud and then returned to the United States to practice introduced to social work the concept of exploring personal dynamics in supervision as well as the idea of group discussion, which became the forerunner of group supervision. An article in the April 1929 issue of *The Family,* titled "Supervision" and written anonymously by a Family Welfare Society worker, includes a description of a discussion group that paralleled Freud's Wednesday Society (which later became the Vienna Psychoanalytic Society) (Clark, 1980:213-219):

> Through the stimulus of lectures at the local school of social work, an evening reading group was organized, we discussed novels from the caseworker's point of view, and occasionally we studied books of a professional nature.

During this period, the "staff conference" was refined as "a method of supervision" in which a caseworker presented a problem case in the presence of the supervisor and staff from other disciplines, such as psychiatry and "home economics." The case was discussed at length, and treatment recommendations were made (Heston, 1929:46). This method of supervision became the model for the introduction of group supervision in social work and the team approach of several decades later.

The introduction of social work into the medical setting was promoted by Richard C. Cabot (Chaiklin, 1978:475). Cabot was advocating the social work role in medical settings in Boston at the same time that the psychiatrist Adolf Meyer and his wife were developing psychiatric social work as a specialty in New York (Lief, 1948:149-152). Cabot presented a broad view of the role of social work in medical settings:

> In our own case work in the social service department of the . . . hospital we are accustomed to sum up our cases in monthly reports from the case records by asking about each case four questions: What is the physical state of this patient? What is the mental state of this patient? What is his physical environment? What is his mental and spiritual environment? The doctor is apt to know a good deal about the first of those four things, the physical state, and a little about the second, the mental, but about the other two almost nothing. The expert social worker comes with those four points in mind to every case. It is of interest to notice that this fourfold knowledge is not the goal of the social worker merely; it is the goal of every intelligent human being who wants to understand another human being . . . Social work, as I see it, takes no special point of view; it takes the total human point of view, and that is just what it has to teach doctors who by reason of their training are disposed to take a much narrower point of view. They can safely and profitably continue that narrow outlook only in case they have a social worker at their elbow, as they should have, to help them. Each of us has his proper field, but we should not work separately, for

the human beings who are our charges cannot be cut in two. (Cabot, 1915a:220)

MARY RICHMOND

Mary Richmond was familiar with Adolf Meyer and his work. Until the appearance of Richmond's *Social Diagnosis* in 1917, social casework focused exclusively on social forces and the effects of large-scale economic need. The individual was seen in the context of larger social problems. Meeting individual economic need and character building were essential components of service, but there was no doubt in the literature about the societal causes. Historical analysis that attributes paramount importance to Richmond's *Social Diagnosis* as the initial and seminal work on casework practice is not completely accurate. Such analysis has caused more recent observers to neglect the evolutionary contribution of this work. Richmond's work is not the initial description of the comprehensive casework process. Seven years earlier, in 1909, Mary Conyngton published *How to Help: A Manual of Practical Charity* (1971), which was a comprehensive explanation of the nature of social casework from a sociological perspective. Richmond's book was more a synthesis of the psychological and the sociological in the context of the family. This view is epitomized in her observation that "a man really is the company he keeps plus the company that his ancestors kept" (Richmond, 1965:369).

Freud's visit to Clark University in 1909 went largely unnoticed, and he is not mentioned in Richmond's book, although American psychiatrists and psychologists are mentioned. Whether this lack of recognition was deliberate or due to lack of Freudian influence in casework circles will never be completely known. Much later Virginia Robinson argued that this was due to lack of Freudian influence (Robinson, 1930). There is reason to believe that Richmond did anticipate the gradual shift to exclusive focus on the individual and psychological determinism, and that her aim in *Social Diagnosis* was in part to offer some balance in this trend.

THE 1920s

Family Focus

In an analysis of trends in textbooks on the family, it was found that attention devoted to social work with families increased dramatically after World War I (Hart and Hart, 1935:vi). Many agency names were changed to reflect this trend (e.g., Associated Charities changed its name to Family Welfare Society in 1922). These two developments reflected two important trends—

training for supervisors and codifying supervisory technique (see Siporin, 1980).

It was during this era that it became apparent that supervisors needed more formal preparation. The failure to prepare supervisors adequately often led to "floundering" by workers, disillusionment of workers, and a frustrating "sink or swim" approach to treatment that caused deep frustration for workers. The situation was aggravated when workers suffering such self-doubt were promoted to supervisory positions. This situation was highlighted by a rare article, published in 1929 in *The Family,* giving one supervisor's account of these problems (Anonymous, 1929). It was at this time that "fieldwork teaching" as a requirement in schools of social work was begun in family welfare societies and spread rapidly to many other agencies (Brown, 1936:56). Also at this time, specific literature devoted to supervision techniques began to emerge. The idea of the staff conference as a method of supervision was devised as a way to be more effectively and efficiently oriented to the new knowledge, and it refocused service orientation (Heston, 1929:46-47).

Social Work As Art

The concept of art was introduced into social work practice and supervision after the concept of science. The idea of art was drawn on at points when science failed to further our understanding (see Chapter 15); it came to social work through our close ties with medicine, and was formalized with the publication of Richard Cabot's *Social Service and the Art of Healing* in 1915.

The concept was solidified in 1924 with the publication of DeSchweinitz's *The Art of Helping People Out of Trouble.* DeSchweinitz considered living an art, and he associated this with the art of helping. Several years later Porter Lee and Marion Kenworthy (a physician) further expanded the idea of social work practice as an art in their book *Mental Hygiene and Social Work* (1929). Subsequently, this concept has been applied loosely by those writing about practice.

The ideas of the art of living and the art of practice were used to unite personal growth and practice. DeSchweinitz explained:

> Growth is a product of the years. Man, being but part of the whole, may become impatient, content with what would be incomplete. Nature is comprehensive and eternal.
>   To have grasped this lesson is to have made a beginning of learning the art of helping. . . . Transcending the vicissitudes of experience is the challenge of the greatest of the arts. (1924:224-231)

Also, the emphasis on art as opposed to identifying the specifics of practice was observed by Dorothy Hutchinson in an article on supervision:

> The word "technique" as applied to supervision in social case work has a dull and rigid sound. The word "art" is more stimulating, if we can release ourselves from a certain shop-worn feeling in its presence. (1935:44)

During the same period, the participants at the Milford Conference, an annual meeting of social work executives and board members devoted to promoting social work as a profession (Trattner, 1999:268), concluded: "A social case worker whose own personality development is not furthered through his contact with his clients is probably not an effective social case worker" (NASW, 1974:31).

It was through this process of the connection among physicians, the concept of art, and social work that the analysis of personality found its way into supervision, rather than directly through the introduction of psychoanalysis into the United States.

The shift in focus to the client during this era led to the emergence of marriage counseling distinct from family treatment by social work and other disciplines. Also, prevention from a psychological perspective grew out of the new orientation. The literature of this period addressed premarital counseling in connection with marriage counseling as a preventive measure. Interestingly, the professional emphasis on prevention in mental health grew out of concern about what was termed *popular counseling,* which reached the public at large through newspapers, magazines, books, and radio. Karen Horney was typical of this movement, and her book *Self-Analysis* was most likely the first self-help book (1942) even though she cautioned against people engaging in self-help without the aid of a professional therapist. Such broad-based counseling was viewed as dangerous when offered by "professional lecturers" rather than professional practitioners (Groves, 1940), and this paralleled the modern concern over "pop psychology" available through the print and electronic media.

THE 1930s

A Shift in Focus

In the decade prior to the depression, a great irony occurred in social work. Relief efforts were pushed into the background when poverty was actually increasing. The depression resulted in the solidification of a dichotomy between public and private agencies that had been emerging for some time. Public agencies focused on relief, and private agencies were free to devote attention almost exclusively to treatment.

There was also a distinction in private agencies that resulted in some offering brief treatment, which has been rediscovered in recent times, with psychiatrically oriented agencies focusing on long-term treatment (Chapin and Queen, 1972/1937:18-22). Prior to the depression, professional education for social work declined, and with the onset of the depression, the professional schools could not supply enough practitioners to meet the need. This created problems for field instructors, who scurried to meet the demands for workers and raised the issue of generic training versus specialization for schools (Chapin and Queen, 1972/1937:91-95). These divergent forms of practice made it difficult to develop a uniform model of supervision and resulted in a supervision literature based on the broadest elements of supervision practice.

Rank-and-File Movement

An outcome of the depression was the rank-and-file movement, based on power through political and union groups. This led some to argue that this movement within the profession was at the expense of functional knowledge aimed at skillful analysis of service and social betterment (Chapin and Queen, 1972/1937:97). The rank-and-file movement gave new inspiration to trained caseworkers in private agencies, who had been dissatisfied "with the thinking of the social work establishment," and attracted employees of the public relief agencies, who were primarily untrained professionally (Fisher, 1980:93). The disgruntled professional caseworkers were reacting to the triumph in the 1920s of psychiatry and psychoanalysis in practice, with their emphasis on the role of the "individual psyche in human affairs." This division of practitioners was based on what was called "large-order problems" versus "small-order problems," and was epitomized by Mary Richmond's earlier view that "social work was in the retail not the wholesale business" (Fisher, 1980:17-18).

The division continued through World War II, as the split centered around large-scale political ideologies that became the essential struggle of the war. These ideologies were replicated in a somewhat different context in the 1960s in the United States during the Vietnam War and several social movements. In both eras these conflicts reached down to the basic levels of practice and often diverted attention from treatment issues in supervision.

Emerging Treatment Services

Social agencies made a shift to offering treatment services in the 1930s when the growth of public programs during the depression relieved them "of routine financial relief for clients" (Stevenson, 1940:131). A change of emphasis occurred in these agencies during the 1930s, causing an increase in demand for psychiatric social workers. The demand caught schools of social work off guard and "confused" about how to train such workers. This confusion has a modern-day equivalent in schools of social work (see Chapter 1). Psychoanalytic theory was used to fill many of the conceptual training gaps because it was readily available and was a "practical theory of interpersonal relationship" that fit the mental hygiene movement emphasis on "the personality needs of the client." There was concern that the renewed emphasis on psychological and personality factors was at the expense of "constitutional factors," but concessions were guardedly granted that such swings of the practice pendulum were necessary to advance knowledge. In this context the primary supervisory evaluative question became, "What is this experience with me (a worker) or this agency doing to the development (mental growth) of this client?" (Stevenson, 1940:131). This same question could be couched in the psychotherapeutic orientation specifically and was indicative of the shift away from diagnosis and environmental manipulation to a focus on treatment.

Field Instruction

By the 1930s, field instruction, which originated in the family welfare societies, was highly developed. The schools utilized several models. Some schools paid the salaries of supervisors of students in agencies, a few schools required faculty members to supervise students, and other schools had cooperative agreements with selected agencies that permitted their paid staff to supervise students (Brown, 1936:57). Field instruction was a significant portion of the educational program. In many programs students were required to undergo a general field placement before entering a more specialized placement. The emphasis in field instruction was upon developing practice skill through integration of "knowledge, philosophy and technique" (Brown, 1936:58).

THE 1940s

Therapeutic Eclecticism

It was in this era that the idea of therapeutic eclecticism emerged to fit the needs of the individual case rather than continuous commitment to one theory or approach that the case would be molded to fit. This trend was considered a change from the practices in the earlier child guidance clinics and was depicted as occurring rather rapidly. A survey of clinics reported by Stevenson showed a dramatic shift in practice orientation between 1936 and 1939. The sudden onset of this new focus was recognized by Jessie Taft in 1940, when she observed, "In the Philadelphia area, the past decade has witnessed a realization of psychological insight in terms of actual, day-to-day practice that was not dreamed of in 1930" (Taft, 1940:179). The new focus on the client—and not on the qualifications, emotional maturity, and mastery of psychoanalytic concepts of the worker—introduced a new balance of concern in supervision and required supervisors who had a broader perspective than had been the case in the past. The psychoanalytic model of supervision continued but was not as widespread, was concentrated in settings specializing in psychoanalysis, but did assume a broader focus of client functioning.

Child Guidance

The child guidance movement had begun in the early 1920s, spearheaded by psychiatrists who had traveled to Europe to study with Alfred Adler, who had invented the movement. Treatment of children was originated in Europe but developed in the United States (Barton, 1987:112). By the 1940s, the field of psychiatry, concerned over childhood responses to war, began a shift in focus from the children to the parents that laid the foundation for the family therapy movement. As Plant quipped in 1944, "Why talk of child guidance—it's the parents who need guidance!" This represented a shift in theoretical orientation from the intrapsychic psychoanalytic position to an interactional educational one. The concern about children was in part based on statistical trends revealing that delinquency had increased rapidly during the 1920s, had decreased in the 1930s, and had significantly risen at the beginning of the 1940s (Plant, 1944:1-2). It is interesting that when child-focused treatment was called into question, it was attributed to social work and not psychiatry. The following observation by a psychiatrist illustrates this:

> The "lost generation" of the depression is . . . doing our fighting now. One who remembers the dire prognostications of social-work group has to pinch himself as he reads today's news. Should we not temper all our theory with a healthy regard for the adaptability of the human being? (Plant, 1944:2)

Lawyers and judges viewed social workers in this theoretical debate from a different perspective. For them the idea of individual treatment was not fair. One judge went so far as to say, "Stripped of all its elaborate wrappings, the doctrine of individual treatment may be expressed by one word—injustice" (Perkins, 1944:47). The debate emerged around problems with adolescents because this group fit the transitions that were occurring in the theoretical perspectives. If the extremes of psychology and sociology did not satisfy all the requirements for a good approach to practice, a social psychology had to be shaped that would guide intervention.

The behavioral adaptations of adolescence fit the explanatory require-ments for the new theory that was needed. Hawkins described the behav-ioral adaptations necessary in an article that was a response to the attack on social work by the judiciary:

> Each adult ... must ... maintain ... balance between himself as an indi-vidual ... and himself as a member of society which makes ... demands upon him. . . . . [I]t is during the adolescent years that the psychological problem of achieving such a balance is at its peak, and ... difficulties of the adolescent can be traced to ... conflict over ... individuality and ... community as represented by his parents, other adults, such institutions as school, church, and law and society's customs in general. (Hawkins, 1944:129)

Through the professional conflicts, the new theoretical orientation was be-ing forged in the fires of the debate. The role of family in shaping the indi-vidual took on new meaning and the ideas developed during this era remain prominent in thinking about family intervention. The renewed theoretical emphasis on the role of family produced a tension between social workers and psychiatrists/psychoanalysts that had its beginnings in this era and, to some degree, continues to exist regarding who should be the unit of focus in assessment, diagnosis, and treatment. It is not clear whether social workers and psychoanalysts were ever as close theoretically as has been argued over the years.

THE 1950s

Psychiatry and Social Work

By the 1950s, social work had developed a conceptual basis for its con-nection to psychiatry generally and psychoanalysis specifically. In com-menting on the practice of field instruction during the 1950s, George Gardner, a physician, observed:

> It is comparatively of minor importance to cite that the present day indi-vidual supervisor-student method of instruction is but a reactivation of the old physician-medical student apprenticeship system or that it has borrowed heavily from the more modern psychoanalyst-analytic con-trol student approach. The fact remains that this educational device as it relates to students in the field of mental health has been brought to its order of excellence by educators in social work. (quoted in Garrett, 1954:iii)

Resurgence of Social Science Focus

Social work has not enjoyed as positive a relationship with medicine in general as it has with psychiatry. This is epitomized by the fact that in 1951 the president of the American Medical Association mounted a successful campaign to have unsold copies of Charlotte Towle's *Common Human Needs* (1965) destroyed and publication dropped by the Federal Security Administration because he interpreted the use of the word *socialized* to mean "socialistic" (Perlman, 1969a:12). The 1950s' reaction against psychoanalysis, expert helpers, and long-term treatment has been attributed to everything from mass transportation and mass media to the decline of religion and a reaction against science. In the eyes of many, the gains of half a century were in jeopardy, and many problems were thrust back on the community (Veroff et al., 1981:3-12). The shift back to the social sciences and away from psychiatry in practice and supervision in modern times was identified by Siporin in 1956. In 1959 Charlotte Towle gave a sweeping account of this and how social work had chosen psychiatry over social science as the source of its theoretical underpinnings at the turn of the century, but in the 1950s, she saw social work turning back to social science to conceptualize practice demands (cited in Perlman, 1969a:268-277). The "reunion" brought emphasis in practice to the nature of roles and functions. This carried over to supervision and led Towle to perceive the "process" of supervision as consisting of three functions: administration, teaching, and helping (Perlman, 1969a:166), a conceptualization that became the basic tenets of Kadushin's (1976b, 1992) model of supervision that has persisted to the present. A split in supervisory function based on orientations to practice that emerged over the decades resulted in a practical and theoretical distinction during this era that set the stage for the dominant theme of the 1960s. In some settings the social science/social reform model of intervention predominated, while in others the psychoanalytic model of supervision was used. These two models had coexisted for decades based on the orientation of the practice setting, but in the 1960s advocates of these models polarized the profession and produced significant conflict about the preferred model. This debate was especially intense in educational institutions. The result of the conflict has been that neither model has dominated, and the subsequent decades have witnessed the emergence of a new supervision model based on task and function.

Field Instruction

By the 1950s, the field instruction supervisor was viewed as a necessary and important link in the partnership of the classroom and the field. The way in which field instruction applied casework theory and developed technique was clear. Rather than focusing on differentiation, the emphasis was on integration. In her book *Learning Through Supervision,* which described the school-agency relationship in detail, Annette Garrett observed, "Theory without cases is empty; cases without theory are meaningless" (1954:5). There were "functional" and "diagnostic" theoretical orientations in different schools, but each school put much effort into ensuring that classroom and field learning were theoretically compatible. Close ties existed between the schools and agencies. By this time most schools of social work had become well-established within the university, and field instruction was considered an essential element of the educational program. Doctoral education for social work expanded during this era, giving educators a more theoretical and scientific orientation to practice, which resulted in further diminution of the agency-practitioner's approach to education. This shift in orientation had been taking place gradually since the turn of the century, when the first schools were being established, and this reorientation was fairly complete by the late 1950s (see Kahn, 1973:147-168).

Theory Integration

The Freudian influence continued in the 1950s and was highlighted by the publication of Gordon Hamilton's text on the psychosocial approach to casework in 1951. Based on Freud's psychology, this approach expanded the ideas to include the social context of behavior and became the foundation for the formulations of Florence Hollis (1966), which were published over a decade later. Hamilton's work called attention to the growing importance of environmental factors. The renewed attention devoted to social factors was also illustrated by the publication of Helen Harris Perlman's popular casework text in 1957 (Perlman, 1969a, b). Perlman drew on ego psychology, learning theory, and role theory from the perspective of the client's environmental or interactional problem. Internal dynamics were important for Perlman only in connection with the client's presenting problems (Strean, 1978:14-15). Perlman's work has had considerable influence on social work practice theory and serves as a forerunner of the problem-centered and interactionally based practice theories that emerged in the late 1970s. Perlman's (1957) work extended the practical approach to intervention that started in the era of Mary Richmond. Richmond and Perlman's work were precursors of the of managed cost organizations' (MCOs) "targeted" approach to intervention. Perlman's writings were the vector between Richmond's views and the task-centered practice approach (Reid and Epstein, 1972; Reid, 1978; Fortune, 1985; Reid, 1992) of social work developed in the 1970s that became the orientation of managed cost organizations.*

---

*The term managed care is a misnomer. These companies provide managed cost, not managed care, and in this chapter these companies will be referred to as managed cost organizations (MCOs). The abbreviations MCO and MCOs also refer to the philosophy and practice of managed cost organizations and do not refer to specific companies. This generic use of the term has been applied because public and private organizations have adopted managed cost methods.

Professional Status

It is ironic that, at the same time social work came into its own as a profession in the 1950s and 1960s, it diverted much of its concern from theory building and a scientific orientation to concern about the status of the profession. At a time when an organizationally unified profession was in great demand in many settings, the profession was questioning its validity and continued existence. During this era supervision concerns took a backseat, as professionalization was characterized as antithetical to supervision. The truly professional practitioner was viewed as independent, sufficiently if not completely educated, generically trained, and self-regulating with respect to evaluation, monitoring of practice, and being scientifically oriented. Towle, commenting on this trend in 1961, pointed out that the profession's orientation to causes, unhappily, had been lost. She observed that Mary Richmond and Jane Addams were "devoid of professionalism," that they went beyond it and "gave to their colleagues and subordinates a vital sense of something to work for, not just something to do in the way of performing a task" (quoted in Perlman, 1969a:280-281).

Interdependence

Systems theory emerged in the 1950s at the same time that sociologists and psychologists for the first time recognized that interdependence of individuals, governments, and societies was a basic fact. As this notion of interdependence gained ascendancy in American society, a reaction set in because the United States is a nation of individualists (Sharp et al., 2000). This reaction took the form of all sorts of self-development theories and do-it-yourself strategies and philosophies. It was in this societal context that the vision of the autonomous professional social work practitioner emerged.

Supervisors' Calm Existence

During the 1950s, supervisors had a relatively calm existence, compared with previous decades and with decades since. There was a general acceptance of the combined role of psychological and sociological factors as determinants of behavior. It was a relatively conservative period with a stable social structure. No massive social upheavals occurred. Social roles were well defined, and clinical practice was focused on clients' becoming adjusted to these fairly clear-cut role expectations. Practice theory was evolving systematically, concisely, and slowly, allowing time for integration of new knowledge.

The theories of the 1950s became the basis for much of the practice for the next two decades and remain as an influence on practice to this day (Strean, 1978:13), although the methods of casework, group work, and community organization forged during this era have been reconceptualized into generalist/specialist models.

THE 1960s

Change and Unrest

The 1960s saw massive political, social, cultural, and economic upheaval. Social roles were changing, and there was much experimentation with new lifestyles. The civil rights movement, the sexual revolution, the technological revolution, and the student movement all combined to bring new opportunities and new problems. Social agencies expanded to address unmet needs in a bold effort to combat poverty, and mental health centers focused attention on clients who were expressing feelings and reporting situational adjustment problems that also required new and bold interventive efforts.

A knowledge explosion in practice theory that had been gradually building since the 1950s erupted and crested in the 1980s. At the same time there was need for a unified profession of social work. Over the decades a number of organizations claimed to represent the profession. The central group that historically represented social workers was the Intercollegiate Bureau of Occupations, founded in 1911, which developed a social work department that became a separate organization in 1917, named the National Social Workers' Exchange. In 1921 this organization became the American Association of Social Workers. This organization merged with several other social work organizations and in 1955 became the National Association of Social Workers, which served as a stabilized professional force in the 1960s (Trattner, 1999). By the 1990s, the unification efforts had reversed and numerous organizations, such as the National Federation of Clinical Social Work, the American Board of Examiners in Clinical Social Work, the American Association of Social Work Boards, the Council on Social Work Education, and many other special interest social work organizations had emerged.

During this era, social casework came under attack from within the profession with more intensity than it had from outside during the early 1940s. During this decade supervisors had great difficulty integrating the vast new knowledge and fostering a commitment to practice at the same time, as the entire philosophical base of clinical practice was under attack. Some supervisors retreated; others persisted and struggled with consolidating the new knowledge and theory. Those who took the challenge seriously made commendable efforts not only to apply psychological and sociological theory to cases but to integrate this theory with social reform efforts in the tradition of Mary Richmond.

The integration of the new practice knowledge and resolution of the casework-versus-psychotherapy debate was greatly aided in 1966 with the publication of a casework text by Florence Hollis that cast casework in the context of "a psychosocial therapy." This book integrated the psychological and sociological in a usable manner and was evolutionary in relation to Perlman's (1957) earlier writings on social work intervention. At the same time the idea of casework as therapy or psychotherapy gave rise to renewed concern that such a conception of practice would tend to dissolve the knowledge base of social work practice that over the years had led to its being unique among the helping professions (Turner, 1978). Some would argue that although it has taken twenty years, today this dissolution of the social work practice base has, in fact, taken place.

Conflicting Views

For supervisors, the calm of the 1950s seemed far away. The new technology and increased emphasis on research produced conflicting views of what to do and how to do it in order to help clients. The old debate of residual treatment versus social reform intensified greatly, but even within the treatment field new theories and new methods escalated, along with conflicting and competing claims of how to intervene effectively. It is understandable that supervisors and practitioners alike began to question the efficiency of their practices. To some extent, the social work profession turned on itself during this decade.

The new lifestyles and freedom of expression of the 1960s in part contributed to the de-emphasis of supervision. This was the era of the popular slogan "Do your own thing" and its corollary of autonomous practice in social work. The feeling was that the schools needed only to arm students with enough of the new knowledge so they could go forth and forge it into effective independent practice. Faced with all the stresses that were emerging at the societal level, within the profession, and within agencies, supervisors were also willing to accept this view.

New Opportunities

The experimentation and research orientation of the 1960s produced a number of studies assessing the effects of different supervision structures. One, conducted at the University of Michigan (Sales and Navarre, 1970), found that individual supervision required more time of the supervisor than group supervision; student performance was equally good in group and individual supervision; the content of supervision was the same in both models; group supervisors were more likely to follow a prearranged agenda than individual supervisors; students were more likely to seek and accept advice in individual supervision; and supervisors were equally satisfied with both models.

Despite all the turmoil, the 1960s opened up exploration of and experimentation with new models and structures of supervision. Dual models of supervision and consultation, first discussed in the 1950s, were applied in many agencies. Mixed structures of individual and group supervision were used with much success. New models of field instruction were tried and the use of "faculty-based" field instructors became common practice in schools of social work based on the cooperative model developed in the 1930s. Employed primarily with federal grant money, field instructors were placed in agencies full-time to supervise students exclusively, individually and in groups. These field instructors worked side by side with "agency-based" field instructors, who were employees of the agency and supervised students as a part of their other agency duties. Even though the faculty-based model of field instruction was quite successful, it has been greatly curtailed because of decreased funding of social work training by the federal government.

Demand for Practitioners

The 1960s were similar to the 1920s in that the demand for trained practitioners was much greater than the supply that could be provided by schools of social work. This led to reemphasis in the 1960s on generic practice and reinstituting of training programs for BSW graduates to meet the manpower needs. Ultimately, and paradoxically, this led to more specialization among MSW practitioners in the decade of the 1970s, with BSW practitioners providing generic services. Supervision has become more specific in its functions when relating to the specialized nature of MSW practitioners. This orientation to practice has placed new demands on supervisors to be more job specific in their approach.

The renewed emergence of bachelor's level training for social work led to a conception in this era that bachelor's level practitioners would deliver services and master's level social workers would provide supervision exclusively. This model would have made master's level education highly specialized training for supervision. This structural change did not occur most likely because of the shortage of social workers during this expansionist era. The shortage forced master's level public agency social workers to stay in direct practice even though they were required to do supervision. The decreased demand for social workers in the 1970s forced many master's level practitioners into private practice and altered the demand for supervisors in public agencies.

THE 1970s

Disillusionment

In the 1970s the rapid changes of the 1960s slowly subsided. There was a growing sense of disillusionment when all the promises and hopes of the

1960s were not fulfilled (Yankelovich, 1981). This mentality characterized many of the problems clients presented. The economy began to decline, and for the first time in decades, social workers experienced cutbacks in the number of jobs available.

Technology and Specialization

Technology continued to advance. For example, new and dramatic medical treatments of the 1960s became commonplace in the 1970s. Organ transplants became routine. Drug therapies, renal dialysis, and radiation treatments became widespread. Such expansion created new, but highly specialized, jobs for social workers. Medical social work and geriatric social work were faced with new practice demands in the context of new technologies. The increase in specialization led the profession to reconsider the role of supervision in many settings. The historic broad-based version of supervision that began in the 1930s was no longer adequate and a more specialized form of supervision emerged. The 1960s' view of making large amounts of knowledge and theory available to students and then sending them off to practice independently gave way to the view that practitioners need help more than ever as they attempt to integrate so much knowledge as well as master a complex practice specialization, such as oncology social work or practice on a renal dialysis ward in a hospital.

Supervision for specialized practice became the dominant focus. The emphasis was on the role of practitioners as drawing on a common core of knowledge, at the same time recognizing the importance of individualizing treatment (Kahn, 1973:99). The specifics of this combined approach remained a challenge of integration for the profession and for supervisors. This dichotomy of orientation created a practical struggle for supervisors. There was doubt whether specialized knowledge and general knowledge were both being conveyed to practitioners. For example, in a study of a sample of social workers by Pratt (1969), it was found that knowledge of social factors affecting health was marginal. The decade of the 1970s was a struggle over how to integrate the general fundamentals of practice and specialized knowledge at the same time.

Field Instruction

This era, showed renewed interest in field instruction. With the renewal of undergraduate social work education and the elimination of faculty-based field instructors, there was increasing interest in the role of the agency-based field instructor (see Wilson, 1981). Increased interest in field instruction was related to concern about the limited specialized knowledge of beginning practitioners. The limitations of beginning practitioners and the growing concern about competence were epitomized by a position statement of the Family Service Association of America directors, formulated in

1972 (Anonymous, 1973:108-110). The directors took the stand that graduate schools of social work were providing "general" training that did not adequately prepare practitioners for work with individuals, families, and small groups. It was their view that theoretical learning was weak, that field instruction did not foster knowledge and skill that promoted a minimum level of practice competence, and that faculty were not adequately qualified to teach effective casework practice. The statement called for more cooperation between schools and agencies to overcome these problems.

No clear steps were taken to deal with this issue, and in many communities, the schools and agencies remain at odds about how best to prepare practitioners. This conflict had been building for over a decade and remained as a source of conflict throughout the 1970s. The debate over generic practice versus specialized practice continues, and the ultimate resolution of this issue will have significant effect on the social work profession in the second stage era of managed cost organizations that prefer and mandate specialty-trained practitioners.

Continued Professionalization

In the 1970s, the professionalization of social work continued mainly through passage of licensing and certification acts in a number of states. The National Association of Social Workers supported this legislation and strengthened its standards for membership in the Academy of Certified Social Workers. By the end of the decade, over two dozen states had laws regulating social work practice. State laws showed much diversity with respect to supervision and requirements for various levels of clinical practice, including private practice. The National Association of Social Workers worked to promote unified licensure laws and advocated their position through a model statute that was recommended to states. This effort was fairly successful in fostering standardization of licensure, but in the late 1990s, a "states rights" mentality in the political area resulted in renewed diversity in state licensure laws, as changes were made during "sunset" reviews required of statutes passed in the initial wave of social work licensure legislation.

Emergence of Private Practice

The essence of social work practice had remained essentially unchanged for fifty years. In the1970s two developments brought about fundamental changes in all that social workers do. The first was the development of private practice, and the second, renewed denial that social workers do psychotherapy. Briar and Miller pointed out that the debate over psychotherapy versus casework dealt not with practice method or orientation but with professional identity and legitimation (1971:22). Private practice increased on a full-time and part-time basis. Many private practitioners purchased supervision and consultation from practitioners in other disciplines, mainly psychiatrists. This was in part due to insurance company requirements that therapy performed by social workers be under the direction of a physician to qualify for reimbursement. The older consultative, collaborative relationship between psychiatrists and social workers evolved into a formal, official, supervisory relationship based on bureaucratic sanction.

These developments caused some social workers to raise concern about internal control of professional activity and the orientation of private practitioners to the social work profession. Others expressed the view that the profession needed to be more active in setting standards for private practitioners. For example, some MSWs began private practice immediately upon graduation, and the question was raised whether such practitioners possessed the knowledge, skills, and experience to offer competent private psychotherapy. Issues were raised about how to supervise private practitioners and what the content of such supervision should be. This debate diminished as the era of managed cost organizations emerged, along with their emphasis on the highest level of state licensure, which eliminated the need for supervision.

Social work has historically had high expectations for supervision without being rigid in its application. In some respects this era laid the groundwork for the current situation, in which the application is rigid but the expectations are not very high. Licensing, certification, vendorship, third-party payments, and various bureaucratic mandates have led to changes in structure and content, as well as creatng control of supervision that is external to the profession.

Focus on Relationship

Gradually, the focus in practice and supervision has turned to the relationship between the practitioner and the client. Research has supported the idea that, regardless of the theoretical orientation of the practitioner, the outcome of the treatment depends on the relationship the practitioner has with the client (Stein, 1961:94-127). In this era research revealed that supervisors placed paramount importance upon interpersonal skills of relating as opposed to theoretical knowledge, research knowledge, practice wisdom, and ability to relate to the community (see Brennan, 1976). The idea of relationship found its way into supervision through practice knowledge and was reified in practice by supervisors who drew on their practice knowledge in supervision. As Hutchinson put it in 1935:

> In the actual day-by-day process of supervision probably the greatest and most important factor for us is the kind of relationship we create between our workers and ourselves. We have heard a good deal about the worker-client relationship. . . . The relationship between super-

visor and worker has perhaps shown the same trend. (quoted in Munson, 1979c:36)

This is a succinct statement of the forces in practice and supervision during the 1970s.

Systems Theory

In the 1970s, the idea of systems theory became widespread in social work education and practice. This seems to have been a direct by-product of the obsession with science during the 1950s. It is interesting to note that in the social work interpretation of systems theory by Hearn (Turner, 1979, 1996), he traces systems theory to the 1940s and 1950s and does not mention the famous sociologist Talcott Parsons, although Parsons' work first appeared in 1937 and his second book, published fourteen years later, was titled *The Social System* (1951). The approach to systems that social work adopted came from biology, chemistry, and physics via psychology (Turner, 1979, 1996). It is interesting that social work adopted this limited approach to systems when Parsons' more comprehensive theory was available. This illustrates that the historical split between social work and sociology was greater than thought, or it could have been due to the cause-and-function split in the social work profession. Regardless, systems theory was adopted by social work from psychology and, in a more specific way, from the family therapy field in more recent years (Bowen, 1978).

Family Therapy Movement

The family therapy movement contributed significantly to social work practice and supervision in this era. Although there is no coherent theory of family therapy, the movement generated much information about the specifics of systems functioning, assessment, application of techniques, and interactional patterns in treatment and has developed new approaches to supervision. The diverse conceptual orientations developed by family therapy researchers during the 1960s through the 1980s provided rich conceptual material for social work practice and supervision. During the 1990s, the reduction of reimbursable practice modalities and rigid practice parameters set by managed cost organizations has limited the use and expansion of family therapy knowledge. Family therapy of intervention expanded greatly during the 1970s and social workers were prominent in the movement. The American Association of Marriage and Family Therapy (AAMFT), founded in 1942, has become a large organization, and social workers are its largest membership group. The old psychiatry/psychoanalyst tensions continued with the emergence of the AAMFT. The numerous professions within the AAMFT membership have not always agreed about what professions have the strongest theoretical orientations to practice family therapy. This is epitomized by Italian psychoanalyst Selvini-Palazzoli's statement, "Minuchin has a very shallow theory of family therapy. It's just a theory for social workers really." Selvini-Palazzoli later retracted her statement about Minuchin, but not about social workers (Simon, 1982:30). The AAMFT has developed supervisory and educational requirements, and tensions between social workers and this organization have increased as AAMFT has moved to achieve licensure status in some states, including efforts to restrict the practice of family therapy.

THE 1980S

Theory Stagnation

The 1980s showed more advances in specialized practice. The knowledge explosion of the previous decades produced many new specializations and subspecializations in the established areas of practice. This produced some confusion for the evolution of practice theory. Theory in social work has been historically generic, and education programs have followed the same model. The response in the 1980s was to emphasize functioning rather than knowing. This decade produced much information about how to perform in specific settings and no new comprehensive theories of intervention emerged. This trend had been occurring for several decades but appears to have reached its peak in the 1980s.

During the 1980s, social work expanded its use of systems theory, primarily because it fit nicely within the comprehensive orientation of social work. Some evidence from research suggests that, in clinical settings, clients had negative responses to the use of systems orientations to treat their problems (Howe, 1989). A range of theories has emerged over the years, and social work hopefully will engage in more outcome measurement research that analyzes the effectiveness of these differing approaches.

It remains to be seen whether there will be a return to more comprehensive orientations or increased emphasis placed on specialized, technical practice. Social work has always been recognized for its generic, comprehensive approach to the whole person in treatment. As the specialization trend continues, the challenge will be to maintain a balanced view of the two orientations.

The balanced, whole-person orientation of social work continued a dynamic tension between social work and psychiatry that was not always dynamic in the past, as was mentioned earlier. The negative tension had more to do with function than theoretical orientation, and has resulted from the increased number of social workers who are perceived to have "replaced" psychiatrists in many settings (Geller, 1996). This dynamic and negative tension often became the responsibility of the supervisor to mediate.

Credentialing

The 1980s saw continued expansion of credentialing of social work. By the end of the decade, forty-seven states had some form of regulation of social work at the state level (Kenemore, 1991:83). Credentialing has direct implications for supervision because the tendency has been to consider credentialing a substitute for supervision. This is understandable from an administrative perspective, since examinations and certification procedures are concise, clear, and time limited. From a clinical practice perspective, delivering effective practice is much more complex and time-consuming. The trend in some agencies is to reinstitute supervision practices to provide a balanced approach to ensuring effective and efficient clinical practice, but in many areas of practice, managed coat organizations have replaced supervision with credentialing.

The expanded utilization of social workers in mental health has led to demand for advanced credentials at the national level, and this has resulted in some confusion, as the profession has struggled to determine what would be the best way to provide a credential that would be a clear national standard for third-party payers to recognize. Clinical social work developments over the past three decades gave rise to the need for credentialing, as third-party payers demanded standards for payment. During the 1980s, certification of social workers was generic and concern emerged that the existing forms of certification were not specific enough. This trend resulted in more specialized credentials and multilevel licensure and certification in most states.

Licensure of social workers is approaching universality throughout the United States, but uniform standards promoted by the National Association of Social Workers eroded in the 1990s. Appendix III is a graphic presentation of the different forms and types of regulation of clinical social work.

THE 1990s

The 1990s were dominated by the emergence of MCOs. The growth of MCOs and their transformation of health and mental health services have had tremendous impact on the practice of social work. The rise of MCOs paralleled the general business trend of the domination of markets by large corporations. Continued consolidation of corporations reduced competition and increased the power and control of corporations over large segments of the population. By the 1990s the majority of mental health services in the United States were controlled by a few private businesses. This structural control did not exist previously. The transfer of mental health to private-sector control was the most significant development of the 1990s in relation to clinical social work, and the impacts on clinical social work in the 1990s are reviewed from this perspective. Each area discussed is viewed with an eye to the future and to the role of social work supervisors in shaping the profession in coming decades.

Trends

The 1990s continued and consolidated the explosion of theory and knowledge. Expanded research provided much insight about the origin and nature of mental illness. The diagnosis and treatment of mental disorders were refined. The medications to alleviate mental distress improved and their use increased significantly. At the same time, mental health services decreased in this decade due to MCO cost-cutting efforts. One of the ironies of this decade was that the significant increase in knowledge of mental illness was met with decreased programs to put that new knowledge to good use for clients.

Clinical Administration

Clinical practitioners and supervisors were increasingly required to become clinical administrators in many settings. This was typically viewed as integrating practice and administration but was mostly the result of funding cuts and managing workloads by combining functions. This practice resulted in clinical solutions being applied to administrative problems with detrimental effects on clients, practitioners, and supervisors. The problems associated with this dual role have received little attention. Little is known about the advantages and disadvantages of these role mergers and how clinicians reconcile the two roles. Supervisors perceive themselves as caught between the organization and the clinicians. This is not new, but the ways in which supervisors are being squeezed have a new and novel twist. A supervisor can begin to feel like a Ping-Pong ball if he or she becomes a mediator between the clinicians and the administration. Clinicians are rarely trained to fill clinical-administrative roles. If the trend continues, educational programs will need to include curriculum content and internship experiences that prepare for effective performance in this role.

Fiduciary Regulation

Medicaid, Medicare, and insurance reimbursement policies and procedures have effected clinical practice and supervision. Numerous requirements must be met before organizations will reimburse agencies and practitioners. Some have argued that unreasonable rules and regulations were utilized to cut costs by denying claims; others argue that such policies were merely designed to ensure quality of treatment. The larger issue is one of control. Many financial providers now dictate the timing of diagnosis, who does the diagnosis, who is qualified to provide treatment, and the length of treatment. The coding systems for diagnosis, interventions, and payment currently in use (DSM-IV-TR, ICD-9, and ICD-10) are highly variable from payer to payer and are complex to use.

In addition, the format and timing of social history data (initial database), treatment plans (initial treatment plans and review treatment plans), and progress notes (the author uses the term contact notes rather than progress notes for legal reasons; i.e., using the term progress notes with a client who gets worse is not accurate or appropriate) are mandated by these funding sources. The role of the clinical supervisor in assisting workers to develop initial data bases, initial treatment plans, review treatment plans, and progress (contact) notes has changed. Some funding agencies demanded the right to review treatment plans before paying. In some settings they required a periodic meeting with the therapist to evaluate patient progress. Some required the therapist to provide a copy of the treatment plan. Although MCOs declared that effective and efficient documentation had the goal to cut costs, little has been done to decrease the array of complicated and confusing documentation required by various MCOs.

Reimbursement by external sources increased record keeping. In addition to financial records, treatment records were mandated by funding sources. Although based on the premise that this would ensure accountability, little evidence exists to support that any effort is being made to use the clinical record to evaluate utilization of funds and treatment outcomes. The increased record keeping by clinicians in the 1990s has become a significant part of their workload. Studies indicate that 30 to 40 percent of practitioner time is devoted to record keeping and that much information is recorded as many as seven different times in each record. Clinical supervisors have a responsibility to work toward more effective and efficient record keeping. Caution is necessary in this area, however, because a plan to review record-keeping methods can result in the opposite of the initial objective and lead to more recording, rather than less.

Clinical supervisors in the 1990s were confined in planning programs, and creative, innovative programming was de-emphasized for fear of funding loss. Administrative mandates began dictating clinical judgments that were not always in the best interest of the client. If the understanding of mental health is to continue to evolve, ways must be found to mediate the financial providers' demand for accountability and the clinical need to plan treatment and to utilize innovative interventions.

Privatization

Public programs experienced increased privatization of services. This was viewed as a cost-effective way to provide treatment. The pressure for privatization of mental health services was increased as other social service areas demanded more funding. There were increasing calls for such programs in the mental health field for both institutional- and community-based care. Traditionally, mental health has not fared well, as various service programs engage in the political struggle to receive portions of federal and state appropriations. This has implications for clinicians and supervisors.

During the 1990s, clinical social worker's job security, benefits, and working conditions were compromised, and this produced ethical dilemmas for clinical supervisors, as programs shifted from the public to the private sector. As the gradual shift toward a privatized model continues, many factors will effect the functioning of the clinician and the supervisor. The trend toward a more equal mix of public and private services will most likely continue, and in some ways this is a return to a pattern of the past.

Task and Relationship

The intrusion of administrative and funding considerations in practice caused treatment to be increasingly dominated by behavioral and task orientations. Relationship lost recognition as a powerful curative factor. The supervisor's challenge now is to develop a model that integrates intervention task and relationship process. The traditional view has been that one has to be articulated at the expense of the other. This is not necessary, and to maximize treatment outcome, the two perspectives need to merge.

Supervisors must aid practitioners in developing skilled use of more techniques that enhance traditional relationship models. More emphasis should be placed on effective use of self-management models, cognitive approaches, psychoeducational methods, self-help groups, and prevention models.

Social workers have not been oriented to business models of service delivery (Austad, 1996). Unlike psychiatry and psychology, social work for the past seventy years has been practiced within the public sector. The return to a private-sector model or a mixed model requires individual practitioners and supervisors to change their attitudes and knowledge about business-based service delivery. Social work practitioners and supervisors are having to integrate the financial and practice aspects of decision making to survive in the new model. Methods need to be devised to develop a more rational connection between financial and intervention decisions.

The 1990s' MCO model shift from focus on relationship to task and outcome has ethical implications. Practice based on outcome-realted tasks negates ethics. MCOs are little concerned with how practitioners conduct tasks or how outcomes are achieved, because only tasks or outcomes have value. In the social work relationship model, ethics are central to the process because people always have expectations of how one should behave toward the other, regardless of the expected outcome (Munson, 1996a, 1996b, 1997a). This is a basic point that practitioners and supervisors who work for MCOs must remember. Supervisors need to mediate the task-versus-relationship tension in the practice relationship and continue to promote relationship-focused practice based on ethical standards. Supervisory ethical principles need to integrate technique-based ethical standards with a relationship-focused ethical model. Supervisors need to apply ethical standards to each technique that practitioners utilize in the practice situation. The increased emphasis on techniques and tasks requires supervisors to monitor the use of techniques to ensure that (1) techniques used are related to the diagnosis and assessment, (2) the practitioner is trained in the techniques being applied, and (3) the techniques are generally accepted and appropriate. These are the primary functions of the supervisor in the practice environment that emerged from the 1990s. Techniques that have not been subjected to clinical trials, or are not subject to regular and consistent monitoring, cannot be used in the new practice environment.

Supervisors need to assist supervisees in utilizing reliable techniques to counsel clients effectively under adverse conditions, such as trauma and loss. Supervisors should provide practitioners with skill in how to terminate with clients based on service cuts, not only because the intervention is completed. Practitioners are not trained in how to terminate for reasons other than completion of treatment, but MCOs frequently require practitioners to terminate before many client problems are resolved. Such shifts will require reorientation for social workers and can be accomplished only with the guidance and direction of a supervisor.

Diagnosis of Mental Conditions

In the 1990s, the issue of who is qualified to do a mental diagnosis was subject to multiple levels of review, but clarity still does not exist. In most states nonphysicians can do a diagnosis, but in some states the law requires the diagnosis to be done by a physician or psychologist. Because non-physician staff do intake in most settings, clients are required to make several visits to get an official diagnosis when only psychiatrists and psychologists can do a diagnosis. This is time-consuming, costly, and confusing. During the 1990s, mental health professionals were required by agency procedures to enter a DSM-IV diagnosis in their initial database (social history) reports. This was confusing for some practitioners and created much turmoil for staff not trained in the DSM system. The clinical supervisor faced a challenge in working to promote the use of sound professional practice principles when establishing and revising policies on diagnostic procedures.

The DSM-IV (American Psychiatric Association [APA], 1994) became the most widely used diagnostic system in the United States. The revisions the DSM system has undergone over the decades since its introduction in 1952 have made the system more medically focused and less socially oriented. The speculation before the release of the initial version of the DSM-IV in 1994 was that it would include recommended treatment plans and theoretical orientations to disorders, but these did not appear. Such changes could show up in future editions.

The DSM-IV-TR (APA, 2000a) was released in 2000, but no major changes were made in the manual classification system, with only the supplemental text for specific disorders being revised. Those interested in the possible future use of recommended treatments and theoretical orientations in the DSM system should refer to *Synopsis of Psychiatry* by Kaplan and Sadock (1998), which has a miniversion of the DSM-IV embedded in it and includes recommended treatments and theoretical orientations for all classes of DSM disorders. Some are concerned that such recommendations in a diagnostic system could limit who would be qualified to perform treatment, as well as the sphere of mental health professionals offering intervention. Clinical supervisors need to follow closely the evolution of the DSM system and take a role in training nonmedical staff in DSM-based diagnosis. As non-physicians gain acceptance in doing mental health diagnosis, educational programs will need to improve instruction that prepares students to perform diagnostic activities. Clinical supervisors will need to ensure that supervisees are adequately prepared to do thorough diagnosis that is accurate and appropriately documented. Clinical supervisors who work in settings in which mental health diagnosis is done routinely should refer to *The Mental Health Diagnostic Desk Reference* (Munson, 2000b), which provides detailed information on doing DSM-based diagnosis from a social work perspective.

Learning Assessment

The growth in the number of mental health practitioners has led to greater reliance on objective tests as the basis of credentials and to promote quality. Ironically, the use of testing is growing simultaneously with increased awareness that practitioners cannot be infused with competence through written multiple-choice question examinations, and that sound supervision cannot be replaced by a computerized test with the expectation of the same outcome. As testing emerged to measure competence, the belief developed that supervision could be replaced with examinations, just as it was perceived that relationship could be substituted with behavioral tasks.

During the 1990s, concern emerged about how to differentiate what can be expected from examinations and what to expect from supervision. There was a return to the idea that educational assessment was essential to good supervision planning with students, as well as with beginning and advanced practitioners. Research efforts focused on developing effective, thorough, accurate, and precise assessment scales. Such pursuits will need continuation and expansion if learning is to be enhanced at all professional levels and at all stages of practice experience.

Ethics

Ethics became the focus of general concern in American society during the 1990s primarily due to political scandals. Whether more or less unethical professional conduct existed in the 1990s than in the past is a moot question. There were sufficient reports of problems regarding ethical misconduct to warrant the attention of clinical supervisors. Some agencies considered videotaping all therapy sessions in case of allegations of misconduct by practitioners, but this practice did not become widespread.

Practitioners operating under increased stress can lead to poor judgment and ethical breaches. Most ethical violations are not committed by devious or malicious people, but by average practitioners who, because of stress, used poor judgment. Stress leads to frustration, decreased coping strategies, and, ultimately, poor judgment. The clinical supervisor can play an important role in combating stress-induced poor judgment.

Research indicates that a substantial number of mental heath professionals are not familiar with the mental health ethical codes under which they function. The supervisor has a responsibility to ensure that practitioners are aware of the ethical sanctions of their profession, their licensure body, and their agency or organization. Based on the ethics concerns that emerged in the 1990s, state licensing organizations are now mandating ethics continuing education for practitioners.

Stress

Stress is the disease of the modern age. As all forms of organizations search for ways to cut costs, workloads increase and clients as well as practitioners suffer more stress. A stressed practitioner cannot effectively counsel a client who is experiencing emotional turmoil.

Clinical social workers are stressed in many aspects of their work and personal lives. This trend, which began in the 1980s, increased in the 1990s. A study by Schor (1991) shows that, in the United States, people are working substantially more hours per year than in the 1960s. The average American worked 163 more hours per year in 1991 than in 1969. The increase in work time was significantly higher for women than for men. Women were working 305 additional hours per year, compared with an increase of ninety-eight hours for men. Other studies have confirmed this increased workload. During the same period, average wages declined 19 percent. One percent of families with incomes over $350,000 received 72 percent of total U.S. income, while the 60 percent of people in the lowest income category lost ground economically (Danaher, 1996). Professionals were identified as having been significantly affected by this trend. In the late 1970s and early 1980s, a series of studies focused on stress levels in social work practitioners, but studies of stress declined in the past ten years. There are continuing signs that stress levels are quite high in social work practitioners, but little empirical research is available to support the popular press and anecdotal reports of significant stress in practitioners.

A stressed, distracted, overwhelmed professional cannot be helpful to clients. Research has shown that supervision is effective in combating stress in professionals (Munson, 1993a). Supervisors have a responsibility to monitor workers and to assist them with work-related, stress-induced functioning. A study by Bissell and colleagues (1980) showed that social work supervisors are not sensitive to the behavioral manifestations of stress in practitioners, even when these behaviors are in the extreme form of arrests, hospital admissions, suicide attempts, alcohol abuse, and substance abuse.

Practice standards for supervision need to include visual and testing measures of stress in practitioners. Scales are available to assess stress in practitioners, as are specific guidelines for treating stress reaction through supervision (see Munson, 1993a), and such measures should be used in supervision practice. Supervisors should discuss with supervisees perceptions of stresses within and outside the work setting. Stresses associated with the work setting should be a focus in supervision, but reactions to stress in a supervisee's personal life should be referred outside the supervision for intervention. The basic rule to follow is, Supervise the *position*, not the *person* (Munson, 1993a).

Supervisors experienced increased stress during the 1990s due to administrative and practice demands documented in this book. Supervisors developed awareness of the increased stresses and were more attuned to the need to make efforts to reduce stress. Stress reduction efforts are difficult because professionals are not always sensitive to their distress. C. Northcote Parkinson (1957) said that the patient and the surgeon should never be the same person. This is true when it comes to addressing stress by practitioners or supervisors. Supervisors should form support groups to address the stresses they face and to share the reactions they have to stress. If a person is the only supervisor in the practice setting, then the supervisor should join a group outside the practice setting. There are a growing number of traumatic stress centers in the United States that supervisors can contact for referral to support groups.

Proximity

Practitioners increasingly became fearful of touching clients during this decade. They were afraid the touch would be misinterpreted and result in a grievance action or lawsuit. The author worked with a therapist who would not close his office door when interviewing a child or female client. He stated that the proximity issues, as well as the confidentiality issues, were of secondary concern to him. Clinicians reflected the general societal confusion about touch. The United States went from a low-touch society in the

1950s and before, to a high-touch society in the 1960s and 1970s, and back to a low-touch society in the 1990s primarily because of the fear about sexually transmitted diseases, especially AIDS. The United States remains a society conflicted about proximity. Mental health clients suffer from lack of closeness, and if practitioners keep them at a distance, how are people ever to recover? The challenge for the clinical supervisor is to assist clinicians in developing reasonable, balanced strategies regarding touch and closeness. Clinicians can touch people in nonsexual ways. Clients know when they are being touched and when they are being fondled.

AIDS

Concern about the AIDS "epidemic" reached its height in the 1990s but dropped from the public eye by the end of the decade. Practitioners and supervisors continue to deal with AIDS in their work daily. Many workers and supervisors are ill equipped to deal with the AIDS fear-threat potential in their caseloads. Although casual transmission has been ruled out, many remain skeptical and do not hold rational views about the disease. Clinical supervisors face tough educational as well as practice issues regarding AIDS. Some clients are putting those close to them at risk by engaging in high-risk activity without revealing it to others with whom they are intimate. The role of the clinician in honoring the client's confidentiality and at the same time assisting the unknowing who are put at risk remains an issue. Practitioners need to be trained to counsel people who lack knowledge and engage in high-risk behavior. This is especially the case when counseling adolescents and children because research indicates that sexual activity is occurring at an increasingly younger age. Some practitioners avoid any discussion of sexual activity since they admittedly lack knowledge about AIDS and experience discomfort with the topic.

There are reports that homophobia is fairly high among mental health professionals. This is a critical issue for the clinical supervisor who needs to assist practitioners in the development of nonjudgmental attitudes. Forming and practicing a nonjudgmental attitude takes more effort than reading or being lectured about it. Some clients bring to treatment very strong prejudices about homosexuality, and practitioners are vulnerable to subtle manipulation if they are not able to distinguish their personal and professional values. Clinical supervisors can help inexperienced and experienced practitioners to clarify and understand these issues. Supervisors will have to be honest with themselves as they work with these issues because they are subject to the same prejudices and weaknesses as the clients and practitioners.

Professional Language

The 1990's self-help books for adapting to MCOs advocated strategies that decrease professional control. For example, some clinicians (Corpt and Reison, 1994) advocate that practitioners should "behaviorize" the language they use in record keeping to please MCOs. The MCO "prescribed language" for practitioners goes to the essence of professional being because language is the fundamental connection between the individual and social functioning; it is the "ultimate social tool" (Allman, 1994:161). Supervisors must mediate the replacement of professional language with business-based language that occurred during the 1990s. Professional language is the common core that allows social workers to communicate and maintain a unique professional identity.

An old adage in supervision is that the role of the supervisor is to be symbolically present, looking over the shoulder of the practitioner as the intervention occurs (Munson, 1979c; Munson, 1993a). Unlike supervisors, MCOs do not share with practitioners the results of these evaluations, even though they are rating the practitioners' effectiveness. For the educative and evaluative functions of supervision to remain valid, the social work profession will need to maintain its language base in order to evaluate treatment outcomes and to transmit practice wisdom.

Scientific Orientation

Increased knowledge of disorders based on research enhanced intervention significantly during the 1990s. Differential diagnosis and diagnosis-specific treatment plans came into common use. Specific practice parameters, practice guidelines, practice protocols, practice standards, and standards of care emerged to guide practice in a number of professions, but the social work profession was slow to respond to these more precise measures. Outcome measures were increasingly used to justify the cost of intervention, and the social work profession lagged behind other mental health professions in developing outcome guides.

New understanding of the neurobiology of mental disorders and the development of effective and diverse medications were hallmarks of the 1990s, and these developments required clinical social work practitioners to have knowledge of research, neurobiology, and medications. The growing pressure for social work to develop practice guidelines will require supervisors to take into account diagnostic and intervention outcome studies. Such studies are currently done by psychiatrists and psychologists, and social work supervisors must develop practice guidelines unique to social work. Psychiatry has initiated practice guidelines (APA, 1996, 2000b) that can serve as models for the development of social work practice guidelines that take into account the unique psychosocial perspective of clinical social work. Social workers are being compelled to justify claims of effectiveness and appropriateness of interventions through practice guidelines based on outcome studies. Social work has been slow to produce studies that meet the projected requirements for scientific practice (Munson, 1996e). A more unified and effective initiative in response to demands by MCOs is for psychiatrists and social workers to collaborate on developing interdisciplinary practice guidelines. This would result in powerful comprehensive intervention genuinely based on biological, psychological, and social factors (Munson, 1997a).

Populations Served and Advocacy

Social workers have traditionally served the poor and middle classes. Practitioners have worked with all age ranges, and most clients have been female. The 1990s' trends indicate that the client population served by social workers is shifting and becoming more polarized at the extremes of the rich and the poor. Ozawa (1997) has conducted demographic research projects that indicate the subtle shifts of the 1990s will continue. The projections are that clients served by social workers will more likely be from the lower and the upper-middle classes. In the short term, children and adolescents and middle-class clients in general will be less served, and service to geriatric populations by social workers will increase in the long term. This will require a shift in the client orientation of social work practice and supervision. Social work education is focused on the poor and on younger clients. Less than 4 percent of social work students express interest in work with geriatric populations. The most significant need for mental health work in geriatrics is related to family support, resource development, referral, and advocacy for people who have difficulty receiving services through MCOs. This need has been created because the elderly account for the largest share of health care costs, and MCOs target this population for cost cutting.

Projections are that women will continue to be the largest portion of social work clients. The number of single-parent households will continue to increase. Women are vulnerable in relation to MCOs in the same manner as the elderly. Limits placed on hospitalization for childbirth and for mastectomy during the 1990s resulted in legislative regulation in some states and are indicators of the future need for advocacy for women.

Social work has historically been an urban profession. Although a slight redistribution occurred in the past decade, rural areas continue to be underserved by social workers. No scientific studies describe the urban-versus-rural differences based on MCO models of service delivery. As mental health care is privatized and such care becomes increasingly conected to the labor market, it is likely that service to the rural mentally ill will decrease. This area deserves further study because research has shown that the type and extent of mental disorders vary in rural and urban areas (Kessler, McGonagle, and Zhao, 1994).

Prevention

Prevention is viewed by many as the way to reduce social service delivery costs. Prevention became a popular fad during the 1990s, but in the mental health field, specific prevention models have not been devised or implemented, as in the general health care field (Public Health Service, 1994). The MCOs have no structures for promoting behavioral health prevention. Prevention can save money in the long term, but money must be provided in the short term for prevention efforts. The question remains: Who will pay for prevention? The MCOs are interested in only self-motivated prevention, not costly, large-scale, programmatic prevention. Prevention will most likely remain a slogan, rather than a service, unless supervisors compile data to support specific strategies for effective preventive services based on documented solutions. Social workers are not trained in prevention, but this may become an important practice area in the future if supervisors develop a supervision practice standard for collecting data to support prevention efforts.

THE FUTURE

In the social work profession, the recent increased restructuring of practice that is in excess of natural evolutionary change has been connected to the growth of MCOs. Social workers should always be looking for more effective and efficient ways to intervene, but the managed cost efficiency movement has produced a shift from process to procedure that is fragmented and significantly altering clinical social work practice. The process of rapid change will most likely continue. Schools of social work are continuing to teach a process, and, relationship model of intervention, whereas the MCO approach sanctions only mechanistic, task-oriented, linear models. Thus, social work graduates are entering a practice world for which they have not been trained, and this requires supervisors to aid practitioners in integrating the two conceptions. Because of this education-practice gap, the role of the social work supervisor will become more important to integration of practice.

Social work has made many contributions historically within the constellation of the primary helping professions, but four in particular stand out: (1) social reform; (2) focus on client advocacy; (3) a short-term, cost-effective model of intervention; and (4) an effective model of supervision.

Social work's strong emphasis on social reform was short-lived and peaked in the 1920s (Lundblad, 1995; Reeser and Epstein, 1990). Such efforts have been declining since the 1920s, with a few brief periods of increased activity. Social reform is no longer a part of individual practice or professional organizational emphasis (Specht and Courtney, 1994). The decline of social reform and advocacy has coincided with the development of the managed cost model in social work (Munson, 1998a). Targeting by MCOs of vulnerable groups for exclusion from participation to cut costs increases the need for client advocacy on a large scale. It remains to be determined whether the social work profession will play a significant role in the new advocacy movement.

Lerner (1986) argues that powerlessness corrupts people, and professionals are not exempt from such corruption. Professional powerlessness has been manifested through the belief that clients will become dissatisfied with the MCO system and demand changes. This has not occurred. When surveyed about health care priorities, people ranked mental health care eighth. People are more concerned about catastrophic health coverage, long-term care, disability, prescription drugs, routine medical treatment, eye care, and dental care (Psychotherapy Finances, 1996), and they show no inclination to organize against the MCO movement. The professional belief that clients will become the frontline advocates for reform is a significant indicator of the degree to which the social work profession has pulled back from its historic advocacy role.

Ironically, the social work profession evolved the short-term intervention model that is the hallmark of MCOs (Munson, 1998c). This can be traced from the works of Richmond (1917), to Perlman's (1957) problem-solving approach, to Reid and Epstein's (1972) task-centered model. The MCOs have added to this process the use of economic incentives to shorten intervention. This is illustrated by their use of "case rates" to decrease the length of intervention by paying standard rates for a predetermined course of intervention (Pollock, 1998). The MCOs have removed from the process the integration of individual intervention, advocacy, and social reform that was the hallmark of the social work profession. Supervision was the glue that held together these three functions. Before Mary Richmond, advocacy and social reform were the primary functions of social workers (Munson, 1993a). Richmond epitomized the shift to individual casework. She believed that reform, advocacy, and microintervention could be integrated by supervisors gathering data from supervisees and generating statistics that would be supplied to social reformers to influence philanthropists and legislators to meet social needs and promote prevention (Munson, 1993a). This is the integrative model that MCOs emphasize but make little effort to implement. If social work developed a model of supervision based on Richmond's earlier conception, it could play a key role in forging a new model of intervention. The dismantling of the historic social work model of practice and supervision has been accomplished by MCOs without significant resistance from the social work profession.

The role of supervision has changed as the restructuring of service delivery has evolved. Historically, supervision was an autonomy issue in the social work profession. The decreased emphasis on supervision of practice paralleled the social work profession's quest for professionalization through autonomous practice. Supervision has been replaced by multiple-choice examinations as the means of establishing competence. The monitoring function of supervision has been downgraded. Supervision is not required because the MCO model of accountability has no need for this function, which is not viewed as cost-effective. The face-to-face, individual, and group supervision provided by a seasoned social worker has been replaced by telephone and written contact with MCO case managers who often have no social work background. In this environment, practitioners lose control not only of the intervention process but also of access to the people who make the decisions regarding access to care, outcomes of intervention, and duration of intervention.

Americans live in a world that constantly threatens individual autonomy. A new business philosophy and strategy of increasing profits through downsizing, reorganizing, and merging dominates MCOs and further limits autonomy. People are increasingly at the mercy of the media and computers, even though people are presented with the illusion of "more options."

Lasch (1979) has historically argued, and Sullivan (1995) currently illustrates, that loss of control is the result of a complex mix of modern economic conditions, shifting family interaction and structures, and individual cognitive responses. The changes and resulting loss of autonomy have been in progress for the past three decades, and they are in part related to a long-term, slow decline in economic growth (Madrick, 1995). These changes are not due to the effects of short-term policies of political administrations, as individual professionals and professional organizations tend to believe. The professional focus on the short-term political, and not on the long-term economic, aspects of change, has caused professional groups to ignore and not challenge the changes that are significantly impacting professionals and their relationships with clients.

This economic restructuring has produced a revolution in information technology and communication methods that has affected the private, employment, and social spheres of all power relationships; it is redefining the rules for social life and the concepts of freedom and justice (Altheide, 1995). Advances in technology have accelerated change. Large-scale computers and small personal computers have made it possible to manage, control, manipulate, and predict in ways that present new challenges for the social work profession. Technology has produced an acceleration and streamlining of activity that increases stress for employees and consumers. For example, studies have shown that administrative monitoring units and payers for services have more sophisticated technology available to accomplish tasks than supervisors or practitioners, resulting in imbalances in information management systems that can be frustrating for and even harmful to supervisors, practitioners, and clients.

Evidence suggests that technology will give rise to future models of supervision and practice that will involve less human contact. Supervision will be conducted through video, telephone, and Internet connections. These changes will produce unique communication advantages and problems for supervision practice (Munson, 1997a).

Loss of individual control is taking place in professional life (Sullivan, 1995). As government and private industry restructure to cut costs, social work practitioners and their clients are faced with loss of autonomy. Health care and mental health care delivery systems have been the first segments of the social welfare delivery system to be affected by the large-scale societal loss of autonomy. The management, cost, and delivery of social welfare services have become chaotic, but people perceive themselves as being unable to promote more rational functioning of the system in spite of a general belief that the system is in crisis (Goodman, Brown, and Deitz, 1992).

Restructuring in the social service and social work sectors is taking the form of privatizing and/or contracting services to MCOs (Feldman and Fitzpatrick, 1992). A high degree of professional dissatisfaction with the restructuring exists (Psychotherapy Finances, 1995a, 1995b) due to a lack of reliable indications that privatization cuts costs, and because compelling evidence suggests that it does result in inadequate services for clients and hardship for professionals who work in the privatized environment (Motenko et al., 1995; Munson, 1993b, 1996e).

Restructuring and technology are producing larger, consolidated organizations, and corporate mergers and agency consolidations are creating larger bureaucracies (Schamess, 1998), as the globalization of economies continues and international alliances increase competition. All human service delivery systems are national systems and unconnected to global economic disasters, recoveries, or reforms that blur national boundaries and cause rapid fluctuations in national markets. Economic consolidation and globalization are relevant to human service delivery systems in the United States because the dominance of MCOs mandates labor market participation to be eligible for services. The mergers of hospitals, long-term care facilities, managed cost companies, and large group psychotherapy practices are a result of globalization and increased economic competition. These large entities can purportedly result in cost efficiency, but there is a question about any concomitant efficiency of social functioning in these quasi-monopoly environments. Although large organizations try to assure the public of their "entrepreneurial compassion" in dealing with consumers, clients, employees, and contractors (including human service professionals), when financial strains occur, profit becomes the ultimate criterion for action and change. In this climate, social work clients, practitioners, and supervisors will continue to experience frustration and disillusionment.

The role of government has changed from one of advocate, protector, and guardian of freedom, justice, and fairness to that of self-protective entity (Day, 1997). Since the 1930s, social workers in the United States increasingly have been employed by various levels of government as participants in the government mission to protect the general welfare. This trend is reversing, and government-based social work practice is being transferred to the private sector, with social work being practiced in large private-practice groups based on contractual relationships (Gibelman, 1995). The majority of government-employed social workers have practiced at the state and local levels (Donahue, 1989). Handy (1995, 1996) has predicted that future professionals will be a "portfolio class" of independent contractors who will work for multiple organizations. This is a return to the model of social work practice of 100 years ago (Munson, 1996e).

Governments are avoiding the citizenry through privatization of services. This highlights the need for a return to advocacy. Research has shown that privatization of government services does not increase effectiveness and efficiency; it can be detrimental to clients and staff, increases costs, and does not improve functioning (Schamess and Lightburn, 1998; Munson, 1993b; Nicholson et al., 1996; Warres et al., 1996).

At the same time, technologies have implications for "high-tech/high-touch" (Naisbitt, 1982) issues in which, increasingly, the client is unable to engage directly with the practitioner. Increased use of machines for communication will most likely lead to models of supervision and practice that do not include direct contact with the client or supervisor (Handy, 1995). Face-to-face contact with the client in a trusting relationship has been the hallmark of social work practice. As alternative models of intervention emerge, social work supervisors and practitioners will be required to utilize unfamiliar methods of intervention that limit contact or are based on no contact. The use of Internet counseling is an example of no-direct-contact intervention. Internet counseling raises licensing and supervision issues because Internet activity has no geographic boundaries. No studies have been done regarding the effects of these devices on the functioning of practitioners, no information is available about voluntariness in using such technologies, and no studies indicate whether these instruments actually increase response time or effectiveness of practitioners. Supervisors will increasingly have to work with such devices and guide practitioners to apply them effectively.

Advances in technology necessitate greater emphasis on ethics in supervisory practice. Increased reliance upon machines brings practitioners into closer contact with machine operators, designers, and analysts who have the "machine mentality," and practitioners can have their values compromised in such interactions. This is the case in large agencies and medical settings where machines are being used on a grand scale. Technology has increased electronic transmission of sensitive client information over telephone lines and the long-term archiving of information in computer storage devices. These developments offer new challenges to the supervisor and practitioner in relation to confidentiality and privileged information. Practitioners do not control much of the information generated about clients, and they do not always adequately inform clients about the use of confidential information by agencies and MCOs.

A number of books (Ackley, 1997; Alperin and Phillips, 1997; Aronson, 1996; Browning and Browning, 1996; Feldman and Fitzpatrick, 1992; Goodman, Brown, and Deitz, 1992) have been published in the past decade to assist professionals in how to "adjust" to the mandates of MCOs, but limited literature discusses the role of supervision in the transformed MCO practice environments. During this MCO era, supervisors must work to promote in practitioners the qualities of effective and ethical professionalism. Sullivan (1995) has reaffirmed the time-honored necessary components for professional status as specialized training, based on codified knowledge used to live out a commitment to public service that is carried out with a certain degree of autonomy, as perceived and accepted by the public. These principles should be the core of supervisory practice. The historical psycho-analytic models (Caligor, Bromberg, and Meltzer, 1984; Jacobs, David, and Meyer, 1995; Lane, 1990), psychodynamic models (Alonso, 1985; Rock, 1997), role theory models (Kadushin, 1992), task-centered models (Mead, 1990), developmental models (Stoltenberg, McNeil, and Delworth, 1998), and interactional theory models (Munson, 1993a; Shulman, 1993) of supervision are being replaced by specific intervention areas with specific standards for both practice and supervision. The challenge for the next generation of supervisors will be to create a balance between the general and the specific in practice to achieve the best possible outcome for clients. The profession has done it before and can do it again if it has the will.

SUPERVISION ISSUES

Supervision issues have diminished in the literature as supervision has been de-emphasized by managed cost and professional organizations. Supervision has become essentially a function of the licensure and regulation domain. This is one of the unexplained ironies of the social work profession. If social work science is real and social work theory an extension, reflection, and guide of practice, then supervision should be associated with ongoing debate and at the core of the social work profession. Supervision seems to get put aside during periods of intense theoretical adjustment and to re-emerge in times of theoretical dominance and security. It could be that supervision or control must be removed to advance theory through creative practice efforts, and that when a new theoretical perspective is accepted and applied widely, supervision and the control it provides are useful in indoctrinating new practitioners and in standardizing the theory. If this hypothesis is valid, supervision needs to be reconceptualized because it should foster creativity and not block it. What is clear is that cycles of concern with supervision and conflict over theoretical practice have been occurring for decades.

CONCLUSION

The author is neither a general historian nor a social welfare historian, but a social worker who has an interest in social welfare history generally and social work practice history specifically. When historians write about social work practice history, they bring an objectivity that is refreshing, but at the same time they lack a professional insider's perspective. When social work professionals write about their profession from a historical view, they lack the skills, tools, and techniques of a trained historian. As a result, a definitive history of the social work practice profession has not been written. This is a challenge that faces the social work profession. The history of the profession has much to teach that has not yet been explored.

This chapter is an attempt to establish some guidelines for uncovering the rich social work practice heritage. All present practice activities, including supervision, are connected to the profession's practice history. The technique employed here was to identify the threads of some of these connections, while keeping in mind an old dictum:

> The craving for an interpretation of history is so deep rooted that, unless we have a constructive outlook over the past, we are drawn either to mysticism or to cynicism. (Powicke, 1955:174)

An effort has been made to keep "a constructive outlook" and to avoid the extremes of "mysticism" and "cynicism." The author looks forward to additional efforts to explain and interpret social work history. This is not to promote a personal idiosyncrasy but is based on the belief that supervisors have a responsibility to know, understand, and convey to their supervisees a sense of the social work heritage. This heritage need not be conveyed in a technical sense; it can be transmitted in a philosophical and practical manner that provides the practitioner with a sense of mission that is part of an ongoing historical movement. Practitioners who experience supervision from this perspective can be inspired in a way that will make them more effective and more immune to the despair, disillusionment, and isolation that erode pride in social work professionalism.

A quote from over forty years ago about an incident that occurred at the turn of the century, which was reported in *The Survey,* a social work journal, serves as a metaphor for the modern supervisor:

> *The Survey* says that years ago in a midwestern orphanage was a ten-year-old girl, a hunchback, sickly, ill-tempered, ugly to look at, called Mercy Goodfaith. One day a woman came to the orphanage asking to adopt a girl whom no one else would take, and seeing Mercy Goodfaith, exclaimed, "That's the child I'm looking for." Thirty-five years afterward an official investigator of institutions in another state, after inspecting a county orphans' home prepared a report of which the following is a resume. The house was exquisitely clean and the children seemed unusually happy. After supper they all went into the living room where one of the girls played the organ while the rest sang. Two small girls sat on one arm of the matron's chair, and two on the other. She held the two smallest children in her lap, and two of the larger boys leaned on the back of her chair. One of the boys who sat on the floor took the hem of her dress in his hand and stroked it. It was evident that the children adored her. She was a hunchback, ugly in feature, but with eyes that almost made her beautiful. Her name was Mercy Goodfaith. (Fosdick, 1943:72)

To put it less dramatically, the modern supervisor has a responsibility, a heritage, a philosophy, a set of values, and knowledge to pass along to the next generation of practitioners, represented by their supervisees.

SUGGESTED READINGS

Alperin, R. M. and Phillips, D. G. (1997). *The Impact of Managed Care on the Practice of Psychotherapy: Innovation, Implementation, and Controversy.* New York: Brunner/Mazel.
    Two clinical social workers have edited this volume that addresses the impact of managed care on psychotherapy.

Austad, C. S. (1996). *Is Long-Term Psychotherapy Unethical? Toward a Social Ethic in an Era of Managed Care.* San Francisco: Jossey-Bass.
    Reviews debate of long-term and short-term psychotherapy in the managed cost era.

Ehrenreich, J. H. (1985). *The Altruistic Imagination: A History of Social Work and Social Policy in the United States.* Ithaca, NY: Cornell University Press.
    History of the complex connection between social work and social welfare policy.

Jacobs, D., David, P., and Meyer, D. J. (1995). *The Supervisory Encounter: A Guide for Teachers of Psychodynamic Psychotherapy and Psychoanalysis.* New Haven, CT: Yale University Press.
    A history chapter covers the European model of supervision. Some mention of social work supervision.

Kaslow, F. W. (ed.) (1979). *Supervision, Consultation, and Staff Training in the Helping Professions.* San Francisco: Jossey-Bass.
    The first two chapters of this book give a very good overview of the history of supervision in medicine and social work.

Kendall, K. A. (1982). "A Sixty Year Perspective of Social Work." *Social Casework* 63(September), pp. 424-428.
    A brief, but good, decade-by-decade summary of social work from 1920 to 1980 based on a review of articles that appeared in *Social Casework* during this period.

Munson, C. E. (ed.) (1979). *Social Work Supervision: Classic Statements and Critical Issues.* New York: The Free Press, 1979.
    Classic collection of thirty-one articles that serves as an introduction to the history and current practice of social work supervision.

Specht, H. and Courtney, M. (1994*). Unfaithful Angels: How Social Work Has Abandoned Its Mission.* New York: The Free Press.
    Controversial review of the debate over the mission of social work in the United States.

Stearns, P. N. and Lewis, J. (1998). *An Emotional History of the United States.* New York: New York University Press.
    Documents the history of emotions in various aspects of life in the United States.

Stone, M. H. (1997). *Healing the Mind: A History of Psychiatry from Antiquity to the Present.* New York: Norton.
    Interesting historical account of mental illness, diagnosis, and treatment.

Trattner, W. I. (1999). *From Poor Law to Welfare State: A History of Social Welfare in America,* Sixth Edition. New York: The Free Press.
    Comprehensive standard text on social welfare and the social work profession in the United States.

In the whole of philosophy, there is no
subject in greater disarray than ethics.

E. F. Schumacher
A Guide for the Perplexed

Chapter 3

Values and Ethics

Values and ethics are discussed in relation to the supervisory process.
Values and ethics are distinguished as concepts and the relationship between values and knowledge is explored. The discussion considers research on the knowledge level of supervisors regarding ethical tenets.
Specific sections of the 1996 NASW Code of Ethics are covered.

INTRODUCTION

Values and ethics are difficult to discuss under any circumstances. There are divergent views about the nature of ethical beliefs, both currently and historically. Interestingly, ethical behavior and beliefs have not been surveyed or researched. A national survey conducted by Patterson and Kim (1991) found a startling lack of research on people's beliefs. The survey revealed that either people are shifting beliefs, or they never really held the cherished traditional values. For example, the researchers found that people believe that America has no moral leadership; people are making up their own rules and laws; lying is viewed as permissible, and most lies are perpetrated on those closest to us; crime is 600 percent higher than government estimates; one in seven adults has been sexually abused as a child; people have generally lost belief in marriage as an institution; people believe that malingering and drug use in the workplace is substantial; the majority of people would lie, cheat, steal, and kill for money; people have lost respect for the property of others; and greed is accepted and advocated by consensus. At the same time that these responses were received, Patterson and Kim also found that people deeply love America and would make sacrifices to improve the country; people believe ethics and values should be taught in schools; and 90 percent of those surveyed believe in God. Ethics are no longer viewed as black and white, but as a large gray area where there is much latitude and doubt (Patterson and Kim, 1991).

It is not known what social workers believe as a group. Do social workers hold the values and beliefs revealed by Patterson and Kim, and therefore constitute a subgroup with different personal values, or do they hold these same beliefs but distinguish between personal and professional beliefs? This question remains to be answered by research. Merdinger (1982), in a study of 367 students, found significantly different global values for social work majors and non-social work majors. For the social work majors, no significant differences were found in global values for students at different points in the program. Measures of attitudes toward public dependency showed significant differences for social work and other majors, and students did develop more positive attitudes toward public assistance recipients as they progressed through the educational program. Much more research is needed before conclusions can be drawn about the values and beliefs of social workers and what implications they have for clinical practice.

Values in relation to supervision have received limited attention in the supervision and practice literature. Two areas should be of concern: first, the supervisor's role in orienting practitioners to values and ethics of the profession, and, second, the guidelines for ethical supervisory practices. Although the general field of ethics is in disarray, as Schumacher (1977) has observed, the problem of the field of specific professional ethics is somewhat different. Professional ethics are reasonably clear and concise. In an era of renewed concern with professional ethics, violations are on the increase. Although official reports of ethics violations are increasing, unofficial complaints about ethical breaches are heard in even larger numbers. These "minor" breaches undermine professionalism as much as sensational violations that result in criminal charges and negative publicity. Such minor breaches can be cumulative and can lead to the more dramatic cases. This chapter covers the theoretical aspects of values and ethics and draws on the results of empirical research to cover guidelines in the areas of practice and supervision regarding ethical and value sanctions and dilemmas.

VALUES

Values are viewed as such complex concepts and behaviors that, when one attempts to explore these areas, the tendency is to withdraw in despair or to forget the issue until it becomes problematic (Jones, 1970:35). The literature regarding values does demonstrate an evolutionary process, and a unified, clear conceptualization of values for use in practice can be documented. The articulation of values has evolved from the general to the specific. Early conceptions were based on global statements derived from such societal values as democratic participation, basic human rights of the individual (Hamilton, 1951:6-11), the importance of the family to individual growth and development, the role of religion in development of moral values and convictions (Towle, 1965:3-11), and the assumption that all individuals are concerned with biological and psychological survival as a basic necessity (Perlman, 1957:6-11). These conceptions were given more specificity by identifying concern for the well-being of the client, the uniqueness of the individual, the acceptance of the individual, the right to self-determination by the client (Hollis, 1966:12-13), noncoerciveness on the part of the worker, avoidance of social control of clients (Hamilton, 1951:6-8; Hollis, 1966:12-13), and client right to confidentiality (privileged communication). As society has become more complex and diverse, emphasis has been on value conflicts encountered by the helping professions (Briar and Miller, 1971:32-52). To deal with these value conflicts, more attention has been devoted to flexibility in professional activity and recognition that values constantly change and differ culturally and ethnically (Boyer, 1975:13-14).

Treatment of values in the literature has turned to operational referents and behavioral manifestations. This effort has led to identification of who possesses which values. In a sense, workers are surrounded by values: a worker's personal values, a worker's professional values, organizational values, client system values (the values of the client as well as the values of those in his or her environment, such as employers, friends, relatives, etc.), and prevailing societal values. Through interaction, people communicate these various value systems directly, indirectly, and symbolically (Goldstein, 1973:90-98). Conflicts frequently result. In interrelating values behaviorally, discussion has turned to ideas of social responsibility, how people are similar and different, means of achieving self-realization (Pincus and Minahan, 1973:38-39), group survival, recognition, security, identity, belonging, self-respect, competence, and privacy (Siporin, 1975:65-68). In explicating values more precisely, study has focused on how and why people develop values. Values are a result of complex socialization processes, and they serve as a means to introduce order into the world and provide a way of coping with it (Siporin, 1975:66; Jones, 1970:37).

Once the origins and functions of values have been defined, the question remains how they can be identified, changed, and reinforced in the worker-client relationship. Disagreement exists about how to categorize values in practice. Distinctions have been made between values and knowledge (Feibleman, 1973:14; Marsh, 1971:132-133) and values and beliefs (Scheibe, 1970:41-42) by writers who have studied functioning from cognitive and perceptual perspectives. The study of values in practice settings has tended to view values, knowledge, and beliefs without making clear distinctions. Pincus and Minahan (1973:38) hold that values are beliefs that cannot be verified as knowledge, and Bartlett argues that values are qualitative judgments that are not empirically demonstrable and are invested with emotions that represent a purpose toward which the worker's actions are directed (1970:63). Bloom (1975:109-110) believes that values can be studied empirically as persistent patterns of choice among alternatives. Practitioners are confronted daily in practice with these patterns of choice based on values.

Inexperienced workers frequently, and experienced workers occasionally, encounter value issues in practice that must be worked through in supervision. This is especially true in settings in which the practitioner is confronted with clients who deviate from the generally accepted norms and values of society. It is not always the younger worker who needs assistance with value conflicts. For example, older workers can experience significant value conflicts when confronted with the behaviors of adolescent clients.

VALUES AND KNOWLEDGE

Values and knowledge are interconnected through the choices people make. Although scientific knowledge alone is not sufficient to produce change in behavior, values in practice and supervision can be used to develop awareness of options, predict outcomes for each option, assess the importance of each outcome to the client, combine the outcomes, and measure the degree of goal attainment associated with the choice made (Bloom, 1975:102-113). It is important for the practitioner and supervisor to take into account this distinction between values and knowledge as well as their interrelatedness. For example, through lack of scientific knowledge of substance and alcohol abuse outcomes, a practitioner can subtly succumb to the client's belief that there is a distinction between drug use and drug abuse, and he or she may come to accept the client's self-generated value stance that casual drug use does not produce negative physical, psychological, and social outcomes. Much evidence suggests that even casual use can produce consequences, and the practitioner who does not find a way to communicate this to the client can contribute to the deepening of the client's problems.

Lack of such knowledge does not have to produce a value impasse between the worker and client or between the worker and the treatment organization, but knowledge is essential to the process of value clarification in any relationship. Through such value clarification, the worker can operationalize a belief in the client's right to self-determination (since the concept is based on the assumption that the client does have alternatives among which to choose), but the worker has to make the value judgment that the client does have viable alternatives (Briar and Miller, 1971:42). This process of values clarification is basic to supervision, and the supervisor has a responsibility to explore carefully client and practitioner options and alternatives in any given situation.

Knowledge and values merge in relation to confidentiality. For example, private interview rooms are not provided in many practice settings, resulting in constrained conversations when others are within hearing distance. Knowing this and at the same time wanting to ensure confidentiality, the worker can be placed in values conflict. The supervisor needs to assist the worker with reducing this conflict so that it does not disrupt the entire intervention process. In the past, little was done regarding clarification of privileged communication in the case of the practitioner. A client who shared content in confidence could be offered little assurance that the information he or she provided would be held in confidence in relation to law enforcement, criminal justice systems, and various other contexts. The supervisor's role in these situations is to clarify values and provide accurate, unambiguous information to the practitioner about safeguards and rights of the client so that these can be guaranteed. In June 1997, the supervisor and practitioner were provided assistance by the U.S. Supreme Court when, in the case of *Jaffee vs. Redmond*, the Court held that

> [T]he federal privilege, which clearly applies to psychiatrists and psychologists, also extends to confidential communications made to licensed social workers in the course of psychotherapy. The reasons for

recognizing the privilege for treatment by psychiatrists and psychologists apply with equal force to clinical social workers, and the vast majority of States explicitly extend a testimonial privilege to them. (U.S. Supreme Court, 1996:2)

This decision places confidentiality for social workers on the same level as other mental health professionals. All supervisors should be familiar with this court decision. A summary of the Supreme Court decision is provided in Chapter 11. Supervisors should read the entire opinion to get a sense of the positive response of the Court to the functions provided by clinical social workers that promote the good of society.

Values and Knowledge Congruence

Training programs for drug abuse counselors conceptualize the drug-abusing individual as having a medical-social problem (Trader, 1974:100). This is another illustration of how values and knowledge intersect. When counselors internalize this conception as a value, the result is quite often an impasse in the counseling situation. This situation was reported in a study of 224 addicts in which the staff viewed the clients as physically and mentally ill, while the clients did not perceive themselves as having either form of illness. Such disagreement was depicted as a block in staff-patient communication and was aggravated in cases in which cultural conflict existed. The researchers argued that successful drug counseling depends on complementary views between the two groups as well as similarity in background and experience of counselors and clients (Ball et al., 1974). This value stance is somewhat of a dilemma for practitioners in relation to acceptance of the client because other studies have demonstrated that dissimilarity of interactants leads to higher levels of verbal accessibility between the participants (Tessler and Polansky, 1975).

There are indications that dissimilarity between client and practitioner contributes to the change process. Halmos (1970:91) discusses this aspect of relationship by calling attention to research on Homans' hypothesis that interacting individuals tend to become more alike over time. If the therapeutic relationship is to promote change in the client, the worker must offer the client a different model of values, attitudes, beliefs, and behaviors at given points in the relationship. This view deviates in part from the traditional professional belief that the more similar the worker is to the client, the more likely the client will be to invest in the relationship. It also deviates from the tendency among paraprofessional counselors to mistrust their intuitive feelings, to minimize their street knowledge, and to resist imagined professional control of their activities (Dalali et al., 1976). What is needed in supervision is clarity about which differences and similarities between practitioners and clients need to be minimized and maximized to produce positive therapeutic outcomes.

A supervisor's failure to offer help to the practitioner with conflicts in identification with the client or the employing organization can lead to increased strains. This negative outcome is not inevitable, especially if the supervisor is innovative rather than traditional in orientation and is accepting of cultural differences in values and beliefs (Kaslow, 1972:58). Those who are responsible for supervision have an obligation to articulate clearly organizational and program values for practitioners as well as clients, so that the participants can understand expectations as well as make choices about the degree to which they want to participate.

Such openness and acceptance within the organizational context permit the practitioner to fulfill the advocate role that has been identified as appropriate to social work (Trader, 1974:101). The role of advocate must be clearly defined for the practitioner. Role clarity is important to the effective functioning of the practitioner (Kaslow, 1972:62-67), but advocacy is one of the poorly defined functions in the helping professions. The lack of definition of the clinician's advocacy responsibility is problematic in this era of managed cost organizations. When practitioners advocate for clients within the managed cost environment, they are put in conflict because these organizations view client advocacy as a threat and as a source of increasing cost of care. Advocacy can result in clinicians being removed (in essence "being fired") by the managed cost organization. When this conflict occurs, it creates a significant ethics problem for the clinician because the ethics codes that clinical social workers function under require advocacy for clients. This raises the question of whether a social worker can ethically practice within the confines of some MCOs' requirements (Munson, 1998c).

Values are important in providing role clarity for the advocate. The role of advocate has been argued from a value stance as being one of total commitment to serving client needs and interests in a social conflict (Grosser, 1965:18; Brager, 1968:6). If the practitioner perceives the advocate role as a one-sided struggle against an alien system and identifies with the frequently held client belief that the professional treatment system is not to be trusted, both the client and the practitioner are placed outside the system. The values of the advocate identified here differ from the conceptions of the role identified by Grosser and Brager. For example, drug-abusing clients often are in conflict with institutional systems or are totally out of contact with them. That substantial numbers of drug abusers are outside the system is illustrated by the wide discrepancy in demographic characteristics between clients surveyed in drug treatment programs (Ball et al., 1974) and patients treated for drug abuse in a hospital emergency room (Weppner et al., 1976). This difference is especially glaring in the case of women, who made up a much higher proportion of the drug patients in emergency room cases than in drug treatment programs (Weppner et al., 1976:172).

To bring about client involvement, the practitioner needs to be the client's advocate in other systems. At times the worker will have to confront the treatment system, the educational system, the law enforcement system, the client's family system, the drug culture system, and the economic system (e.g., employers) to bring about engagement, reengagement, or disengagement, depending upon the circumstances. At other times, the role of advocate will involve supporting and confronting a resistive client in relation to one or more of the aforementioned systems. In both cases the advocacy role requires providing information, and the practitioner must have substantial and accurate knowledge of his or her values to have genuine meaning for the client. In the first instance, the information will be used to interpret the needs of the client to the system. In the second instance, the client must be informed about what will or can happen or what will be done to him or her.

Through provision of information, the advocate can often promote equity in interaction between the client and the given system. This promotion of equity is one of the primary values of practitioners in general and advocates specifically. This kind of education is emerging as a significant variable in health and longevity (Comstock and Tonascia, 1977), and the application of these findings to social work settings needs exploration. To be successful in these tasks, the advocate must possess a great deal of knowledge about the functioning of treatment, education, family, law enforcement, drug culture, and economic systems. Practitioners who attempt advocacy roles without thorough knowledge will contribute to further resistance, hostility, and increased anxiety on the part of the client. The supervisor needs to be prepared to aid supervisees with these adjustments, especially in relation to work with managed cost organizations.

ETHICS

Values relate to what one believes, and ethics relate to how one behaves. Although values are hard to codify, social work ethics have become progressively more precise. A general one-page code of ethics adopted in 1960 by the National Association of Social Workers was superseded in 1980 by a longer document including a preamble and six major topical areas. In 1996 a more extensive code was approved. (For the complete NASW Code of Ethics, see Appendix IV.) The social work supervisor has a responsibility to be thoroughly familiar with the NASW Code of Ethics and other ethics codes relevant to clinical social work (see the full text of the Clinical Social Work Federation Code and the American Board of Examiners Code printed in Appendix IV) to ensure that supervisees understand and adhere to these codes. Such codes should be discussed and reviewed with new supervisees and referred to at points in the supervision process when value dilemmas or ethical issues emerge. The supervisor cannot assume that supervisees have become acquainted with the relevant ethics codes as part of their educational program, orientation to the profession, or prior work experience. Many problems can be resolved and much learned about practice from studying the codes that practitioners are mandated to adhere to in practice. The supervisor should approach such discussion in a sensitive, constructive manner but, at the same time, not accept practitioner resistance to, or defensiveness about, such discussion on the grounds that his or her ethics and professionalism are being questioned. Ethics exploration is mandated by the NASW Code in Section 4.01(b): "The social worker should strive to become and remain proficient in professional practice and the performance of professional functions" (1999:22).

There is no separate code of ethics for supervision or a section of the NASW Code of Ethics that specifically addresses supervision, but a number of passages in the NASW Code of Ethics do relate to supervision. Supervisors should be familiar with all elements of the code and the sections that deal with supervision, excerpted in the following pages, are presented here to aid supervisors in locating specific sections that deal primarily with supervision and consultation issues.*

Preamble

Social workers promote social justice and social change with and on behalf of clients. "Clients" is used inclusively to refer to individuals, families, groups, organizations, and communities. Social workers are sensitive to cultural and ethnic diversity and strive to end discrimination, oppression, poverty, and other forms of social injustice. These activities may be in the form of direct practice, community organizing, supervision, consultation, administration, advocacy, social and political action, policy development and implementation, education, and research and evaluation. Social workers seek to enhance the capacity of people to address their own needs. Social workers also seek to promote the responsiveness of organizations, communities, and other social institutions to individuals' needs and social problems. (p. 1)

Purpose of the NASW Code of Ethics

... For additional guidance social workers should consult the relevant literature on professional ethics and ethical decision making and seek

---

*The following material is reprinted with permission. Copyright 1999, National Association of Social Workers, Inc.

appropriate consultation when faced with ethical dilemmas. This may involve consultation with an agency-based or social work organization's ethics committee, a regulatory body, knowledgeable colleagues, supervisors, or legal counsel.

Instances may arise when social workers' ethical obligations conflict with agency policies or relevant laws or regulations. When such conflicts occur, social workers must make a responsible effort to resolve the conflict in a manner that is consistent with the values, principles, and standards expressed in this *Code*. If a reasonable resolution of the conflict does not appear possible, social workers should seek proper consultation before making a decision (pp. 3-4).

1.04 Competence

(a) Social workers should provide services and represent themselves as competent only within the boundaries of their education, training, license, certification, consultation received, supervised experience, or other relevant professional experience.

(b) Social workers should provide services in substantive areas or use intervention techniques or approaches that are new to them only after engaging in appropriate study, training, consultation, and supervision from people who are competent in those interventions or techniques.

(c) When generally recognized standards do not exist with respect to an emerging area of practice, social workers should exercise careful judgment and take responsible steps (including appropriate education, research, training, consultation, and supervision) to ensure the competence of their work and to protect clients from harm. (pp. 8-9)

2.05 Consultation

(a) Social workers should seek the advice and counsel of colleagues whenever such consultation is in the best interests of clients.

(b) Social workers should keep themselves informed about colleagues' areas of expertise and competencies. Social workers should seek consultation only from colleagues who have demonstrated knowledge, expertise, and competence related to the subject of the consultation.

(c) When consulting with colleagues about clients, social workers should disclose the least amount of information necessary to achieve the purposes of the consultation. (pp. 16-17)

3.01 Supervision and Consultation

(a) Social workers who provide supervision or consultation should have the necessary knowledge and skill to supervise or consult appropriately and should do so only within their areas of knowledge and competence.

(b) Social workers who provide supervision or consultation are responsible for setting clear, appropriate, and culturally sensitive boundaries.

(c) Social workers should not engage in any dual or multiple relationships with supervisees in which there is a risk of exploitation of or potential harm to the supervisee.

(d) Social workers who provide supervision should evaluate supervisees' performance in a manner that is fair and respectful. (p. 19)

3.02 Education and Training

(a) Social workers who function as educators, field instructors for students, or trainers should provide instruction only within their areas of knowledge and competence and should provide instruction based on the current information and knowledge available in the profession.

(b) Social workers who function as educators or field instructors for students should evaluate students' performance in a manner that is fair and respectful.

(c) Social workers who function as educators or field instructors for students should take reasonable steps to ensure that clients are routinely informed when services are being provided by students.

(d) Social workers who function as educators or field instructors for students should not engage in any dual or multiple relationships with students in which there is a risk of exploitation or potential harm to the student. Social work educators and field instructors are responsible for setting clear, appropriate, and culturally sensitive boundaries. (p. 19)

3.03 Performance Evaluation

Social workers who have responsibility for evaluating the performance of others should fulfill such responsibility in a fair and considerate manner and on the basis of clearly stated criteria. (p. 19)

3.07 Administration

(c) Social workers who are administrators should take reasonable steps to ensure that adequate agency or organizational resources are available to provide appropriate staff supervision.

(d) Social work administrators should take reasonable steps to ensure that the working environment for which they are responsible is consistent with and encourages compliance with the *NASW Code of Ethics.* Social work administrators should take reasonable steps to eliminate any conditions in their organizations that violate, interfere with, or discourage compliance with the *Code.* (p. 21)

3.08 Continuing Education and Staff Development

Social work administrators and supervisors should take reasonable steps to provide or arrange for continuing education and staff development for all staff for whom they are responsible. Continuing education and staff development should address current knowledge and emerging developments related to social work practice and ethics. (p. 21)

4.05 Impairment

(b) Social workers whose personal problems, psychosocial distress, legal problems, substance abuse, or mental health difficulties interfere with their professional judgment and performance should immediately seek consultation and take appropriate remedial action by seeking professional help, making adjustments in workload, terminating practice, or taking any other steps necessary to protect clients and others. (p. 23)

5.01 Integrity of the Profession

(c) Social workers should contribute time and professional expertise to activities that promote respect for the value, integrity, and competence of the social work profession. These activities may include teaching, research, consultation, service, legislative testimony, presentations in the community, and participation in their professional organizations. (p. 24)

Our modern, complex society generates many ethical issues for practitioners that should be addressed in supervision. Supervisors need to be well grounded in and knowledgeable about the NASW Code of Ethics (1996) and other ethics codes that may be relevant to supervisees' activity. It is now common for social workers to function under the mandates of several codes of ethics through licensing and membership in different professional organizations. The increasing legal and other mandated sanctions of social work practice present ethical problems for the practitioner that the supervisor should be prepared to address. Court-mandated duty-to-warn requirements, for example, present conflicts for workers and supervisors. A case example illustrates such a conflict:

Ms. Jones was receiving counseling in a public mental health clinic. She told her social worker that her teenage daughter had been raped by a man in the parking lot of a shopping mall. The man was found not guilty by a jury because of a technicality. Ms. Jones told the social worker that she would "give this man his punishment if she ever met him on the street." The social worker asked Ms. Jones the meaning of her statement, and she reached into her pocketbook, pulled out a hand-gun, and said, "This will be his conviction on appeal."

The supervisor should help the worker reconcile the worker's identification with Ms. Jones and the duty-to-warn requirements after a specific threat has been made against an individual. This is an example of the complex practice conflicts that supervisors and practitioners must resolve within current practice standards.

The actions of MCOs produce direct ethical conflicts for social work practitioners that can become a focus of attention in supervision. It is not surprising that the increase in professional concern about risk management and legal liability has paralleled the rise of MCOs. The NASW Code of Ethics (1990, 1996, 1999) contains contradictory statements that complicate its use, but it is the primary professional guide available, and the code does state that social workers who subscribe to it are required to abide by it. The NASW Code of Ethics includes the following guiding principles, which can create conflict issues for clinicians involved with MCOs as employees and contract providers:

1. Honor obligations to the social work profession, to clients, to employing organizations, and to the general public.
2. Foster self-determination of clients, respect privacy of clients, and honor confidentiality.
3. Retain responsibility for quality of service that is performed.
4. Act to prevent practices that are inhumane or discriminatory.
5. Provide clients with information regarding services.
6. Inform clients of risks and rights associated with service.
7. Withdraw services precipitously only under unusual circumstances.
8. Improve the agency employing them, and report unethical conduct by members of the profession.
9. Advocate for policies and legislation to improve social conditions and promote social justice.

These directives can be in conflict with common practices of MCOs. The profession has not provided practice standards or guidelines related to these conflicts. For example, is a social worker who contracts to provide services for an MCO an employee of that company? In the traditional sense of employment, this is not the case, but under current practices, it could be construed that the social worker is an employee of the MCO and therefore obliged to "work to improve employing agency's policies and procedures"

(NASW, 1999:21). Social workers do not have a relationship with MCOs that would allow them to advocate for policy changes, and if they did advocate for company changes, they would most likely be removed from the MCO provider list. Some state licensing boards are struggling with this issue as a supervisory and employee-employer issue, but the ethical requirements of the social worker and MCO relationship have not been clarified.

Some ethics conflicts related to confidentiality (Sabin, 1997), self-determination, and rights to informed consent remain unresolved. Supervision is an appropriate forum to resolve these differences because there are no structures for practitioners to communicate with MCOs regarding professional and practice issues. An adversarial relationship exists between MCOs and professionals that is filtering down to the relationships between practitioners and clients, and this can foster conflict and resentment in professional relationships. This flaw in the relationship between MCOs and providers will need to be resolved if the system is to work effectively. The difficult but traditional role of supervisors as midlevel managers who mediate the relationship between practitioners and administration may be needed to address the problems that confront the MCO-practitioner interface.

It has been argued that professional ethics codes are outdated and in conflict with managed cost policy and procedures to such a degree that the codes should be altered (Phillips, 1995; Wolf, 1994). The NASW Code of Ethics has been revised, and the new document (NASW, 1996) has modifications that reflect aspects of the managed cost view of ethics. Ethics codes, to be effective, must have clarity, show consistency, and be enduring (Munson, 1995b). Supervisors should work to identify the enduring aspects of ethics and strive to have them applied with clarity and consistency. These questions are complex and need to be resolved at the professional organization level. At the same time, supervisors must play a role in aiding supervisees in resolving ethical issues arising in daily practice. As the profession establishes supervisory standards of practice and guidelines to deal with such conflicts, the daily practice of supervision will become an easier task.

Psychiatry has taken initial steps to identify what is considered ethical practice in relation to MCOs (Macbeth et al., 1995), and many of the items they identify are relevant to social work. To practice ethically in connection with MCOs, the practitioner and supervisor should determine that the following conditions are met:

1. Clients make informed treatment decisions based on knowledge of
   a. their options,
   b. benefit limitations,
   c. authorization process,
   d. rights to appeal utilization decisions,
   e. limits on choice and co-payment requirements, and
   f. potential invasion of privacy by the review process.

2. No exaggerated claims of excellence or quality are made by the MCO.
3. Treatment is competent and meets client needs within benefit limits.
4. Utilization review process is not invasive of therapeutic relationship.
5. Reviewers are not financially rewarded for denying treatment or claims.

ETHICS KNOWLEDGE

The supervisor and worker must have a thorough knowledge of the code(s) of ethics under which they practice. This can be confusing because many social workers are licensed under several statutes and national bodies of professional sanction. It is common for practitioners and supervisors to be unaware of some of the codes. Most social workers are aware of and believe they should be guided by the NASW Code of Ethics. Fortunately, most of the lesser-known codes are quite similar in content to the NASW Code.

Before dealing with complex ethical and value issues, it is important to determine how much practitioners know about the ethical guidelines under which they operate. The assumption is that practitioners read, remember, and act on the tenets of the NASW Code of Ethics. The supervisor needs to evaluate this rather than assume the supervisees have such information and knowledge.

Research (see Munson, 1986) consisting of a fifty-item, true-false test to measure knowledge of the NASW Code of Ethics has provided some significant information about the knowledge and use of the code. The questions were simple, single-reference statements covering principles in the NASW Code. The instrument was given to a random sample of field instructors. The highest possible score was 100, and the mean score on the knowledge scale was 59.3. On the average, respondents were able to identify code items with just under 60 percent accuracy. Of the respondents, 32 percent answered less than 50 percent of the questions correctly.

Given the importance of the NASW ethics code in guiding clinicians' behavior, it is discouraging that 40 percent of the items were answered incorrectly by the respondents. There were no significant differences in the mean scores based on sex, religion, or perceived stress associated with work. Several groups have administered this survey to professional social workers, and the results have been similar. This same instrument was administered to several groups of graduate students, and the mean scores were consistently eleven points higher than the average scores of the field instructor groups (the mean score for the student groups was 71.1). It appears that practitioners and students have more knowledge of the NASW ethics code than supervisors (Munson, 1984).

A copy of the instrument used in this study is in Appendix V. The instrument has been updated to be consistent with the 1996 version of the NASW

Code of Ethics. Supervisors are encouraged to administer this instrument to all supervisees who practice under NASW sanction, and the results should be discussed. To do this will ensure a basic exposure to the elements of ethical practice. The NASW Code of Ethics can be a rich source of discussion of elements critical to effective clinical practice. Much of the content of the code refers to the specifics of practice and can serve as a guide for practice activity. By administering the ethics scale, the supervisor has a basis for discussing specific aspects of the code with the supervisee and avoids merely reviewing different sections of the code.

The results of this survey suggest that much needs to be done regarding the level of knowledge of the ethics codes. One question raised by the findings of this survey is, What would be considered an acceptable level of knowledge of ethics codes? Although it is not reasonable to expect that all respondents would score 100 percent on such a survey, it can be argued that practitioners should possess a higher level of knowledge of the ethics code than was demonstrated in the survey. And if supervisors are to contribute ethical models of practice for supervisees to emulate, they will need to possess a thorough knowledge of the ethics codes they utilize.

Much confusion surrounds ethics and ethical behavior. This is related to the failure of educational programs to systematically teach values, ethics, and statutory or mandated behavior. For example, in the survey just cited, 3.5 years had passed since respondents had read the NASW Code of Ethics, and the results showed they lacked accurate knowledge of the code's requirements. Even though most states now have statutes regulating social work practice, it is rare to encounter a practitioner who has read the statute under which he or she is licensed or certified. Many of these statutes mandate certain ethical behavior. This raises the question of what ethical guidelines practitioners and supervisors use when facing unusual or questionable situations. There are indications that they rely on what they consider common sense, logical, reasonable conceptions as well as vague remembrances and interpretations of ethics codes. Judgments based on such recollections are risky and at variance with ethics code requirements and statutory mandates.

Instead of relying exclusively on common sense, the practitioner can turn to codes of ethics to aid functioning in a complex practice world in which conflicting practice demands and legislative and court-ordered actions create ethical dualisms. Legal mandates are often contradictory to ethical codes. For example, duty-to-warn laws and child abuse reporting laws create ethical issues not covered by ethics codes. The use of video- and audiotapes of clients and the practice of leaving messages on phone answering machines when trying to reach clients raise privacy issues. Even modern practice theories raise ethical dilemmas, illustrated by the practice of paradoxing techniques, also referred to as "paradoxical therapy."

Paradoxing involves the practitioner encouraging the client to continue or increase dysfunctional behavior ("paradoxical injunction") in order to get the client to abandon the behavior (Kaplan and Sadock, 1998). It is similar to the concept of reverse psychology used in the 1950s with children. In paradoxing, the practitioner may be called on to advocate that the client take some action that would put the practitioner in violation of some codes of ethics. Paradoxing is viewed by some as "tricking" clients to do certain acts. Under the NASW ethics code, clients are to be told the "extent and nature" of services that are available to them and the "risks" associated with those services. If a practitioner tells a client about paradoxing, the intent of the technique is subverted. Some therapists use the paradox of suggesting suicide to a depressed patient in order to prevent the attempt. This is risky and counter to the NASW Code of Ethics. Although no formal research is available on the extent of paradoxing use, anecdotal reports from supervision and consultation would indicate that it is used by a fairly large number of clinicians.

The supervisor's role in these difficult situations is to present ethical codes as a guide, and the supervisor must be ready to assist supervisees in working through ethical conflicts. Practitioners need to become aware that laws regulating social work practice are not evolved in any logical manner, and that legal actions are not taken with professional ethics codes in mind. Such awareness of this fact can be extremely helpful to the bewildered practitioner confronting complex practice demands. It is a responsibility of the supervisor to address supervisee's confusion and the conflicts that can arise from ethical demands. This is one of the most critical functions that a supervisor performs, and it requires frequent review of ethics codes by the supervisor.

Case Exercise:
The Case of Arlene

Arlene graduated from the MidCity School of Social Work three years ago. Immediately after graduation, she began working in a public mental health clinic. While in school she did not think much about ethics, and when she joined the local chapter of NASW, she did not read the NASW Code of Ethics before signing the membership oath. She later recalled that none of her professors taught any content about practice ethics.

Two months ago Arlene, who is thirty-two, was assigned a male client about her age. The man was depressed and felt pressured in his job as a computer programmer for a large, health care technology supplier. He was intellectual and philosophical about his problems. Arlene was attracted to the man and told her supervisor about the attraction. Arlene asked the supervisor if she should transfer the case, and the supervisor said that she should. Arlene discussed the situation with the client, and he was transferred to another therapist. Two weeks after the transfer, the client telephoned Arlene, and they had a long conversation.

Arlene invited the man and his girlfriend to her home for dinner with her and her husband. The following weekend the couples went on a hiking trip through the local mountains.

Arlene denied any sexual contact with this man but admitted feeling strongly attracted to him. She decided to tell him this and explained that she would not agree to meet with him again socially. The man reluctantly agreed to this. Several weeks later, the former client told a psychologist, during a psychological testing session in the clinic where Arlene worked, about the social contact that had taken place between Arlene and him. The psychologist reported the remarks to the agency director, who consulted with the agency attorney.

You are Arlene's supervisor. (1) What would you recommend to the agency director regarding Arlene's actions in this matter? (2) What would you recommend Arlene do? (3) What do you see as the primary ethical issues in this case? (4) Do you believe anyone committed any ethical violations in this case?

EXTENT OF ETHICS VIOLATIONS

The extent of ethics violations is hard to determine for a number of reasons. An informal survey by the author revealed that people believe ethics violations have been committed against them at fairly high levels, but there is reluctance to pursue these breaches. These reactions could be highly distorted, since research reveals that awareness of provisions of the ethics codes is at a fairly low level. People could be the victims of ethics violations and not know it, or they could feel that they are victims of unethical acts when, in fact, those acts are not covered by the code.

Most professionals view ethical issues as internal to the profession, but, increasingly, ethical issues are externally driven, as private organizations determine much of the nature of social work practice. This trend is actually a return to the pattern of an earlier era, in that social workers are being employed in for-profit settings. Social workers are ill prepared for the ethical compromises they have to make as marketing and profits become the primary guiding principles. There are indications that this trend will continue. For example, one large hotel chain has used billions of dollars of "excess profits" to purchase long-term care facilities. This example illustrates the trend of long-term care facilities being owned by profit-making companies offering what they call "entrepreneurial compassion." Many times long-term care facilities and private, for-profit hospitals react to adverse publicity simply by countering negative accusations with massive marketing campaigns. As this form of care and helping expands, the old free enterprise concept of "caveat emptor"—let the buyer beware—is relevant. In addition to the individual ethical issues, supervisors and practitioners in for-profit settings have to develop coping strategies for dealing with organizationally induced ethical compromises.

ADVANCING ETHICS KNOWLEDGE

How can practitioners and supervisors further base their practice on ethical principles? Professionals should read, reread, and become familiar with the codes of ethics under which they are mandated to practice. They should become thoroughly familiar with the statutes under which they are licensed. Supervisors should require that supervisees become knowledgeable about ethics codes and statutes. One way to do this is to administer the ethics knowledge scale contained in Appendix V to new supervisees and discuss it with them. The supervisor cannot assume that the worker has read and understands ethics requirements.

Supervisors should insist that educational programs and accrediting bodies ensure that curriculum content includes orientation to ethics codes and state statutes. Professional organizations should be contacted and encouraged to require knowledge of ethics codes as a condition of membership. Redundancy and repetition of exposure to ethical mandates should be encouraged rather than avoided. It is unusual to encounter a practitioner who has been overexposed to ethical principles.

Case Exercise:
The Case of Donna

Donna has been working with Mike and his family as part of an intensive family service program. Mike, a bisexual man, is married and has a nine-year-old son. He has been married for seven years. Mike works sporadically as a drywall installer. Mike has been in treatment for six months for depression. He tearfully reported to Donna this week that he has tested positive for HIV. He does not know what to do, and he is obsessed with how he came in contact with HIV. He stated that he has not been sexually active outside the marriage for three years but did admit that recently he began to "cruise gays bars" occasionally, but he swears he has practiced safe sex with men and women.

His wife is not aware that he is bisexual. Donna encouraged Mike to tell his wife about his sexuality and his HIV-positive status. Mike said that he did not want his wife or son to "know about any of this mess." Donna then said she was going to check with her supervisor about what to do. She told Mike that she believed the supervisor "would most likely want me to contact your wife and schedule an appointment to interview her about the HIV-positive status." Mike became furious and said that Donna better not contact his wife. He then left the office in anger, slamming the door behind him.

(1) How would you supervise Donna in relation to this case and this specific session? (2) What would you recommend Donna do to reestablish communication with Mike? (3) How would you deal with Donna's use of the supervisor in the session with Mike?

SUGGESTED READINGS

Congress, E. P. (1999). *Social Work Values and Ethics: Identifying and Resolving Professional Dilemmas.* Chicago: Nelson-Hall.
    General survey of ethics in social work practice with cases examples.

Doverspike, W. F. (1999). *Ethical Risk Management: Guidelines for Practice.* Sarasota, FL: Professional Resource Exchange.
    Practical approach to integrating ethical principles in clinical practice. Includes forms and checklists for use in relation to ethics.

Jones, J. H. (1981). *Bad Blood.* New York: The Free Press.
    Excellent model for advocacy role of social work.

Linzer, N. (1999). *Resolving Ethical Dilemmas in Social Work Practice.* Boston: Allyn & Bacon.
    General survey of social work practice ethics with case examples.

Lowenburg F. et al. (2000). *Ethical Decisions for Social Work Practice,* Sixth Edition. Itasca, IL: Peacock.
    Good survey of ethical issues in social work practice.

National Association of Social Workers (1996). *Code of Ethics.* Washington, DC: NASW.
    Should be read and studied by all practicing social workers.

Stein, R. H. (1990). *Ethical Issues in Counseling.* New York: Prometheus Books.
    Overview of ethical issues in several helping disciplines.

Different supervisors have different supervisory styles.

Michael Blumenfield
Applied Supervision in Psychotherapy

The capacity to shuttle between levels of abstraction, with ease and with clarity, is a signal mark of the imaginative and systematic thinker.

C. Wright Mills
The Sociological Imagination

Chapter 4

Supervisor Styles

Style is a term that has been used indiscriminately in referring to aspects of supervisors' and practitioners' behavior. In this chapter the term is defined and described in a manner that permits the supervisor to use it to promote learning and guide interaction in supervision. General styles of supervisors are explained as *active* and *reactive*. The supervisors who use these styles can be further described as *philosophers, theoreticians,* and *technicians.* In addition to exploring these classifications and subclassifications of style, information is provided on how supervisors can use the concept to identify their style, which might be beyond the general categories described.

INTRODUCTION

Style is a concept that is taken for granted and is rarely defined or explained on a general or individual basis. More supervisory effort should be devoted to understanding style because much can be learned and effectiveness improved by studying style as supervisors and practitioners. As with the use of the word *art* in social work, the use of the word *style* conceals more than it reveals about a supervisor's practice. The following statement epitomizes this vague use of style as a descriptive concept:

> We view social work practice as an art that combines professionally mastered knowledge and chosen values with the individual attributes and style of the practitioner. (Kahn, 1973:98)

The author of this statement leaves to speculation the operational meaning of "art" and "style." To operationalize this conception, we would have to ask several questions: What knowledge? How do we know what has been mastered? What are the chosen values, and how were they chosen? What individual attributes? When we explore style with practitioners, these questions are answered as part of the process. This is why the concept of style is so important to practice supervision.

Style is simply *the patterns we use in attempting to communicate with others.* A refinement of this definition is that style consists of the recurring and consistent focus supervisors emphasize in supervision, the manner in which they articulate the theoretical orientation they hold, the philosophy of practice and supervision they hold, and how they convey this to their supervisees. In addition to using style as a generalized descriptor, it is also common to divide a supervisor's style into components. For example, the "evaluative style" (Eldridge, 1982:489) of the supervisor is one discrete component of style.

Some aspects of style are conscious and well-known, but other elements are unconscious (Munson, 1979e). Common elements of style are voice volume, voice tone, facial expressions, posture, use of arms and hands, examples used, questions asked, ways of responding to questions, interpretations given, organization and structure of sessions, physical setting of sessions, theories used, points chosen to intervene in discussion, how suggestions are made, and what suggestions are offered.

Research by Handley (1982) has demonstrated that cognitive styles of supervisors and supervisees affect the interpersonal relationship in supervision, but similarity of cognitive styles is not associated with supervisor rating of supervisee performance or competence. Handley concluded that it is important for supervisors and supervisees to develop awareness of their cognitive styles early in the supervision process in order to understand better the supervisory relationship and to enhance satisfaction with supervision. This study by Handley is one of the first empirical studies of style in supervision. It supports the author's research, reported in this chapter and in Chapter 5, regarding the importance of style in producing a positive outcome in the supervisory process.

OBSERVING STYLES

The best way to observe a supervisor's style of supervision is through viewing audiovisual recordings of supervisory sessions. Supervisors should observe themselves often to understand and improve their styles. During observation, the lesser-known aspects of style will be apparent to supervisors, and surprising. It is common to hear embarrassed supervisors say, "I didn't realize I do that, " or ask, "Do I always do that?" when observing themselves in action for the first time.

Supervisors should be exposed to the work of other supervisors in order to develop their styles, just as practitioners develop their styles from working with and viewing other practitioners. Supervisors need to emphasize the provision of supervision or consultation for supervisors for this purpose.

The supervisor needs to develop an orientation or frame of reference to supervision that incorporates his or her style. This relates to the focus of the supervisory interaction. The supervisor should consider his or her primary responsibility as being to the patient (Langs, 1979:18). If the supervisor keeps this focus, he or she will prevent the supervision from becoming vague or pointless and will avoid frustration for the supervisor and the supervisee. Use of this frame of reference helps to prevent the supervision from becoming focused on the practitioner rather than the treatment. Any interaction concentrated on the practitioner should be in the context of the work with clients. This is important because many practitioners who are having difficulty in their work with clients and are struggling in their therapeutic efforts attempt to deal with it by discussing themselves and their personal actions or motives with supervisors. (The implications of this are discussed in detail in the section Self-Analysis in Chapter 5.)

Practitioners who are having difficulty in their work may attempt to deal with it by attributing it to problems they are having with the supervisor. The supervisor should minimize such discussion and always relate it to work with the client or clients under consideration. It is the supervisor's responsibility to keep the focus on the client under discussion. When therapy and the resulting supervision become difficult, it is to the supervisee's conscious or unconscious advantage to shift the focus. It is the supervisor's responsibility to maintain the focus on the practitioner-client interaction.

STYLE AS A RESOURCE

Supervisees and supervisors use the term *style* indiscriminately and as a generalization. This is illustrated by a supervisor's comment in connection with a problem she was having with a supervisee: "Her style and mine are different; the problem of style is the way she talks about her cases." The supervisee responded to this comment by agreeing that the styles were different, and that she had difficulty visualizing how this could be reconciled. Before such a problem can be confronted, both the supervisor and the supervisee must specify the behavioral components of their styles.

An example of how style is differentiated by practitioners is illustrated by a comment made by a worker in an acute care hospital who was trying to explain how her style differed from that of her supervisor*:

> When I get a referral, I like to meet face to face with the spouse of the client as soon as possible. I arrange an interview. I want to see how the spouse is reacting. I want to get the spouse's impressions of how the client functioned before and after the initial onset of the disease. Usually, in our situation, the onset is an event, specifically a stroke. I see the spouse or family member's information as important to my assessment before seeing the client. Mary [the supervisor], on the other hand, likes to see the client first. She will visit with the client and then contact the family member by phone. She gathers information over the phone and sets up a meeting with the family member.

This illustration demonstrates a difference in structural or procedural style. Ultimately, the outcome is the same: both the client and the family member are sources of information for the assessment. This is often the case in instances involving differences in style. Supervisors and supervisees can become focused on stylistic differences and unable to see that the outcomes are often the same regardless of style. The supervisor should work to ensure that when supervisor and supervisee styles differ, no client dynamics or dysfunctions are overlooked in treatment and supervision.

Structural differences exist within the interview format. For example, the two workers just mentioned had different styles of note taking during the interviews. One took brief notes during the interview; the other wrote notes about the session immediately after the interview. The workers stated that they had tried the other's style of note taking without much success. The critical component is to compare the supervisor and practitioner notes to guard against missing important client dynamics.

Another difference in style can be in the interactional component. This relates to how the worker interacts with the client or family member during

---

*Similar examples given throughout this book are based on statements made by participants in research studies conducted by the author.

the interview. Again, different interactional styles can result in similar outcomes regarding assessment and intervention efforts. The supervisor needs to help the practitioner identify his or her style in practice and understand how it affects the outcome. In supervision, the supervisor should identify his or her style and explain how it affects achievement of the goals of the supervision.

The purposes for which the concept of style and categories of style are employed here are not necessarily the same as they would be in research, which focuses on precise definitions. To become overly detailed about style contexts in supervision would defeat the purpose, which is to explore interactions in a wide range of ways, rather than narrowly focusing people in precise categories, as research does, thus leaving no room for deviation, error, adjustment, alteration, or even complete reversal.

Supervisors who elicit feedback from supervisees about their supervisory style can gain much insight into their performance as supervisors without threatening the supervisees. Also, supervisors can gain insight into whether their supervisees perceive them in the same way as they view themselves.

STYLE AS A CONCEPT

Style as a means of understanding behavior is receiving more attention in the behavioral sciences. Steinberg and Davidson (1982) identified the "impulsive" and "reflective" cognitive styles in problem solving. Their view is that effective "problem-solvers are those who manage to combine both impulsive and reflective styles." Harrison and Bramson (1982) developed a comprehensive view of styles of thinking based on the five styles synthesist, idealist, pragmatist, analyst, and realist. They give an example of a casework supervisor that illustrates how the difference between her style and that of her supervisees can be problematic.

Jane, a social work supervisor with twenty years' experience in community agencies, tells of a problem she has with her younger caseworkers. The conversation goes like this:

JANE: I can't seem to convince them to do the job properly.

WE: They aren't performing?

JANE: Oh, they work hard. I can't say they're not performing.

WE: But they cause you problems anyway.

JANE: It's their attitude. They bring up all these ideas about casework that just aren't right.

WE: Such as?

JANE: Well, I was trained to practice non-directive counseling methods. Clients should be given the chance to work out their own problems. Caseworkers are there to help them do that.

WE: But your younger people do it differently.

JANE: Sometimes I can't believe what I hear. They act like Dutch uncles. They will tell a client what to do.

WE: Do they do it all the time?

JANE: Oh no. Just now and then.

WE: Do they get results?

JANE: Well, yes. For the short run, anyhow. But I wonder sometimes about the long-range effect on the client.

WE: *(persisting)* But the results they get are generally satisfactory? They meet agency standards?

JANE: Mm—yes. I can't really criticize them for that. But I just wish they would do it the right way.

> Jane was trained in idealistic, supportive casework. . . . Her younger employees . . . take a more pragmatic . . . approach. Jane's training and her preferred way of thinking about casework . . . make it difficult for her to acknowledge that anyone could succeed as a caseworker using [different] strategies.
>
> At the heart of Jane's problem is a commitment not only to a certain method and approach, but to a set of basic values. The method and the values go hand in hand. [T]hey define Jane as a professional. She is uncomfortable when others use methods different from her own, because that is a violation of her value system. To the extent that others succeed while using such methods, Jane's discomfort is increased.
>
> Notice that is true of all of us. The importance of the individual value system as one determinant of behavior and attitude is not peculiar to idealists, such as Jane. What is peculiar is the weight given by idealists to their values, to value judgments, to moral questions, and ethical principles. (Harrison and Bramson, 1982:39-40)

From this example we can see how style, the concept of intervention, and values all become integrated in a way that can dramatically influence what gets done in supervision and what people think about supervision see Chapter 1). It can lead to positive outcomes, negative outcomes, or, as in the case of Jane, an ongoing sense of adequacy but frustration.

Beels and Ferber were the first to identify therapist styles after studying videotapes of family therapists at work. They labeled two main styles: conductors and reactors. Conductors are more active in the treatment and direct the interaction. Nathan Ackerman, Virginia Satir, Salvador Minuchin, and Murray Bowen are classified as conductors. Reactors are viewed as "less public personalities who get into families playing different roles at different times." Carl Whitaker, James Framo, Jay Haley, and Don Jackson are examples of reactors (Guerin, 1976:17). In supervision, a parallel process of conductor and reactor supervisor styles occurs that replicates therapist styles. This is understandable because practitioners become supervisors, and their practitioner styles are transferred to their supervisory activities.

Main Styles

The transfer of styles from practitioner activity to supervisor activity led to asking the research question, Do clinical supervisors manifest styles that characterize their interaction in supervision? Based on content analysis of supervision, it was established that they do (Munson, Study B). Supervisors adopt one of two styles that have been identified as *active* and *reactive*. The active style consists of being direct with the supervisee and asking pointed questions, answering questions directly, and offering interpretations. Active supervision is problem focused, based on exploring alternative interventions, focused on client dynamics, and speculative about outcomes. The reactive style, on the other hand, is more subdued and indirect. The reactive style involves asking limited general questions and not giving answers. Reactive supervision focuses on the process of treatment, explores issues about interaction, and tends to focus on practitioner dynamics, providing a forum for practitioners to struggle with their own solutions.

Being active or reactive is not necessarily good or bad. It is merely a way of behaving. The style used can become negative if someone experiences it as negative. For example, as some of the respondents in the research reported, the quiet, passive supervisor who uses the "my door is always open" style is not always the best supervisor. The open-door policy often results in infrequent, inconsistent supervision that remains unstructured and operates on a crisis basis. This is a poor way to promote learning in supervision: it can lead to resentment on the part of the practitioner, or it can be graciously accepted by the insecure practitioner who is quite willing to let well enough alone. In this latter situation, the clients will be deprived of the quality services they are entitled to receive.

The first step in identifying supervisor style involves this general categorization of active and reactive styles. In a survey of graduate students, it was found that the majority of supervisors were viewed as being reactors (Munson, Study A). For the total group, 64 percent of the supervisors were identified as reactive and 36 percent as active. An interesting finding was that 74 percent of first-year students perceived their supervisors as reactive, while 66 percent of the second-year students perceived their supervisors as active. From a logical standpoint, the reverse should be true. Beginning students would appear to need more active direction of their work, while advanced students could benefit more from the reactive style as they emerge as independent practitioners. Since style is such a new concept in analyzing supervision, more research is needed to refine how these styles are differentiated and applied.

Substyles

After identifying the main styles, there was a need to refine these styles through the use of subclassifications. In the early stages of the research, the difficulty was in conceptualizing how to describe supervisors: How could you characterize what they do? How could you compare differences? At first an attempt was made to classify styles on the basis of personality, and it was found that such conceptions were inadequate. Some respondents would say, "My supervisor is anal retentive," because they had been trained predominantly in psychoanalytic settings, and terms such as *anal retentive* were readily available for expressions of negativism about supervisors. Such terms were not descriptive of what supervisors actually do. They might be poor supervisors, but calling them anal retentive did not describe their behavior toward the supervisees.

The second strategy was trying to determine styles on the basis of job description or on the basis of task: How could you organize what supervisors do? Do their tasks fit into any pattern? They did not, because the tasks are diverse. Only later was it realized that it is necessary to analyze the interaction that takes place in supervisory sessions: What does the supervisor talk to the supervisee about? How does the supervisor talk to the worker? The word *how* from this perspective means that some supervisors ask a lot of questions and never give any answers, whereas other supervisors give a lot of information and never ask any questions. In both cases, supervisors may never give any answers even though they give a lot of information, but the information they give does not necessarily answer the questions that the worker asked.

When the interactional process that took place in supervision was analyzed and categorized, patterns began to emerge. Some general categories of how supervisors tend to be described became apparent. Also, some ways in which the supervisees responded to the supervisors could be categorized. The three basic substyles of supervisors in addition to the main styles are *philosophers, theoreticians,* and *technicians.* Observation of supervisors at work revealed that each has an overall pattern of working that fits these styles. The combinations of the main style and substyles are shown in Visual 4.1. Some renowned practitioners, when in a teaching or supervisory

VISUAL 4.1. Conceptualization of Main and Substyles

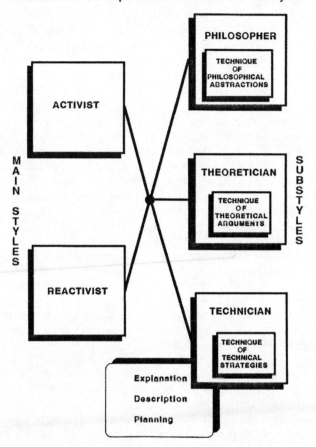

role, illustrate these styles. For example, Carl Whitaker can be characterized as a philosopher, Murray Bowen as a theoretician, and Jay Haley as a technician. Occasionally, one encounters a practitioner-supervisor who effectively combines components of all three styles. Descriptions of the early days of the Vienna Psychoanalytic Society (Clark, 1980:218-219; Roazen, 1974:176-179) leads the author to believe that Freud, in his role as leader of this group, assumed all of the styles, as theory, philosophy, and technique were explored. Although this was not a supervision group as we know it today, it was a precursor of approaches to group supervision and consultation currently in use. The same varied stylistic effectiveness can be documented in Freud's individual work with his pupils (Freeman, 1980).

APPLYING STYLE

Any attempt to categorize people will result in error to a certain degree. People do not fit into categories completely; there are always deviations. In terms of listening to the interaction and to the descriptions of the workers, it was discovered that supervisors fit into one of these three categories—philosophers, theoreticians, or technicians—based on what they do over time.

Before describing the three individual styles, the notion of style itself needs some elaboration. In social work we have placed much emphasis on the importance of self-awareness and use of self, but often we have no idea about what we really mean by these terms. The question is, How would one actually be self-aware in a session with a client? The same is true in supervision: How is the supervisor actually aware of what it is that he or she is doing? One way for the supervisor to be more aware is simply by asking himself or herself, What is my style? The answer to this question should not be found in the previous categories, but in self-description.

The author asked the question "What is your style?" of a supervisor who had been in social work for over forty years, had worked in the same agency for thirty-three years, and had been director of the agency for fourteen years. No one in her career had ever asked her that question. She was taken aback and said she would have to think about it because she did not know what her style was. She thought about it and came up with some words that she believes are descriptive of what she does and how she operates. In subsequent consultation visits, she injected the idea of style into the conversation repeatedly. She has thought about it and uses it to determine how she is relating to others and how they relate to her. The response of this supervisor reflects the utility of the concept of style. Application of the "style question" causes the person to reflect on all aspects of the supervisory interaction.

When asked to analyze their style, to consider how they perform in a given situation, and to put a label on it, supervisors assess what they have done in the past. Their answers have immediate impact on their present and future behavior. The author developed the idea of style originally in relation to treatment and teaching people about treatment. It was found that asking people, "What is your style?" (which practitioners do not think about while doing treatment) later affected what they did with clients. The practitioners were spending more time trying to determine what their style was than they were concentrating on what the client was doing. Eventually, the practitioners overcame this and became consciously aware of their style. In the long run, the benefits of practitioners going through this process far outweigh any harm to clients caused by the temporary distraction of concentrating on practitioner styles. Many practitioners and supervisors never stop to consider what it is that they are doing. By simply talking about style the supervisors can affect behavior directly.

The substyles of philosopher, theoretician, and technician are convenient models for describing techniques used in supervision practice. The philosopher substyle as a generalization can be transformed into the concept of philosophical abstraction to explain a specific segment of supervisory interaction, the theoretician style can be translated into theoretical speculation, and the technician style can be translated into technical strategy. The difference is that when talking about a supervisor's overall pattern of interaction, the tendency is to use the concept of style, but when talking about a specific unit of interaction in supervision, the terminology of a technique can be used. This dual focus gives the concepts more utility. The use of style as technique is illustrated in Visual 4.1 as "boxes" within the substyle "boxes" and is referred to as "technique of . . ." for each substyle.

SUPERVISOR STYLES

Supervisors tend to respond in three substyles that can also serve as specific techniques:

1. Philosopher/philosophical abstractions
2. Theoretician/theoretical arguments
3. Technician/technical strategies

These forms of response can be appropriate or inappropriate, depending on the practitioner's response to the supervisor (see Chapter 5). Each of these supervisor response forms is discussed separately in the following material.

Philosopher/Philosophical Abstraction

Rarely do supervisors use philosophy in its pure form—a profession of inquiry (Feibleman, 1973:14). Pure philosophy has been described as "a difficult subject that uses ordinary words" in strange ways and "has no practical application" (Feibleman, 1973:11). Philosophy can be used to intensify life and to support everyday activities. Sometimes, however, supervisors launch into philosophical abstractions that have little or no application from the practitioners' standpoint.

Practitioners will present everyday material from their practice that concerns them, and the supervisor can become philosophically abstract in response to such content. Although this type of discussion might be interesting and stimulating, it frequently has no immediate practical value for the clinician. In some instances, it can be helpful, even though it takes years for understanding to emerge. Supervisor responses can be lengthy explanations or brief, global statements. One example of a global statement of this type occurred when a practitioner "was bemoaning some ineffectiveness in [his] work as a therapist" and received the response, "It takes ten years before a therapist begins to know what he's doing." It took the practitioner involved "many years" to see the wisdom of this statement, and that "ten years" was a metaphor for "a lifetime" (Kopp, 1976:94). This example illustrates a philosophical abstraction of long-range impact that proved useful.

At times supervisors respond with lengthy statements of this type that the practitioners find of limited use, experience as frustrating, and view as a supervision strategy for avoiding the case material. An excerpt from a clinician's summary of her supervision illustrates this situation:

> We began today by discussing my patient, Arlene, who is undergoing resistance to family of origin work with her mother. My supervisor suggested I request the mother join the therapy for awhile. He mentioned that some people will do it on their own and some won't. I said, "Yes, like me," thinking to myself about parallel process in supervision and treatment. He asked me to repeat what I had said, and after I did, this led to a lengthy conversation which was philosophical in nature about family of origin material versus other ways of dealing with such material. We went on to talk about our own family of origin material. The discussion got heavy, and I think he sensed this and switched back to supervision. I started talking about another case. Afterwards, I felt frustrated and concerned that I did not get supervised on the original material.

Some supervisors make philosophical abstraction their major form of response. Such supervisors preface their remarks with, "I had a case like that once" or "That reminds me of a case where I . . .". If this becomes the major focus of the supervision, the practitioner will become frustrated and resentful after a while, especially when he or she actively seeks help with technical skill. If this cannot be worked out and congruence brought about between the supervisor's style and the practitioner's needs and expectations, consideration should be given to switching the practitioner to another supervisor.

The reactor-philosopher style of supervision is illustrated by the following description by a supervisee whose supervisor is much older than she:

> My supervisor, being the same age as my father, often treats me like a daughter instead of a social worker, which affects the structure and style of supervision he gives me.
>
> When I asked my supervisor about his style of supervision, he said, "I am eclectic." It is a cop-out; it is a way of avoiding a commitment. He is really a philosopher in supervision. He does not deal directly with my cases. He does not give me feedback. He does not take an active role. We have no specific times for supervision. He never gives straightforward answers.

My supervisor often engages in small talk by discussing his graduate school experiences and earlier times and work in the field of social work without directly relating any of this to my cases. I don't gain insight about my cases through this method of discussing his past experiences, and he never gives me a clue to the connection between the two. When I ask him to explain the relationship between his past experiences and my cases, he replies, "Well, what do you think the connection is?" I often try to make up a connection to avoid looking and feeling stupid. My supervisor usually agrees with my reply no matter how off-the-wall I feel it is. This style of supervision is frustrating and confusing, and it creates a feeling of incompetence about the supervisor.

In addition, my supervisor maintains a very relaxed and casual manner throughout supervision. He is rarely direct; he doesn't offer explanations or examples. Often I'm disappointed, angry, and frustrated with my supervisor as a person, [and] I don't perceive him as being a competent supervisor. I feel he has much knowledge and information to offer, but he has difficulty explaining what he does and why.

There are several characteristics that I truly like about my supervisor. For instance, my supervisor stands by me and offers me security and reassurance when I feel anxious due to the emotional impact of my work. In addition, I'm comfortable with my supervisor and feel free to ask questions, intervene in treatment, try new methods of therapy, express myself, and come and go as I please. Furthermore, I respect my supervisor because he tries his best to work independently from the larger system. Most importantly, I admire my supervisor because he enjoys his clients, and he's concerned about helping them. My supervisor finds hope in an elderly client when most people would give up. His clients often improve because he gives them hope and reassurance which motivates them to recover.

This is a typical response to this type of supervision. The supervisor is liked and disliked, is irritating in some respects and comforting in others. This excerpt illustrates how style is interrelated with the way supervision is structured and how authority is exercised. It also exemplifies how the philosopher style is problematic only when it is a consistent pattern of relating to the supervisee. This practitioner identifies how the philosopher style is helpful when she is feeling distress associated with her work. If this supervisor could shift into the other styles at different points in the supervision, he could avoid the supervisee's perception of his being incompetent.

Supervisors should think twice about using philosophical abstractions. When they are used, they should be brief, to the point, and clearly stated. To ensure that the practitioner has benefited from the philosophical abstraction, the supervisor should give the practitioner time to think about it and then ask him or her to attempt to make some connection between it and the case. To guard against the overuse or misuse of philosophical abstraction, the supervisor should reflect about the supervisory interaction and its content. Through such a conscious process, the supervisor can shift style to become more effective.

Theoretician/Theoretical Arguments

The use of theory in therapy is the primary focus of many supervisors. These supervisors believe mastery of theory leads to good practice. Some supervisors use case material as a means to the end of understanding theory. According to this style of supervision, once the theory has been mastered, the practitioner can deal with future case material on his or her own.

Theoreticians tend to be logical and orderly in their approach to case material. They are about evenly divided when it comes to being active or reactive. They are usually respected by their supervisees and are frequently viewed as "taskmasters" when it comes to dealing with clinical material. The only time the theoretician is viewed negatively is when he or she talks about theory in the abstract and does not relate it directly to case material and learning. Supervisees become upset if the theoretician tends to ramble from theory to theory or does not remain consistent to a theory after proclaiming it.

The following is a practitioner's description of an actor/theoretician supervisory style:

> My perception of my supervisor's style was that she was primarily a theoretician. She loved to discuss theory and at the time was taking a course on family theory. On numerous occasions she would point out to me various instances of maybe a client resistance or a triangulation. She was logical and organized in her approach. She would ask specific questions . . . Did I observe how the family was triangulating? or Did I pick up on the fusion in the family? I remember I was in awe of her style.

Not all theoreticians are active. Some stay focused on theory but remain reactive to the supervisee. The following account illustrates the reactor-theoretician style:

> My supervisor's style is that of a psychoanalytic theoretician. She fosters a growth environment as much as possible in our relationship. When I go in to discuss issues, she usually leaves it up to me to decide what I want to do. There are times when I know from her facial expression or body language that she does not agree with my conclusions or techniques. Unless she feels it's very important for the patient's well-being, she won't say anything.

Practitioners undergoing such supervision soon learn that the cases they present are secondary to the goals of the supervision, and any immediate help they get with presented cases is incidental. Practitioners adapt to this form of supervision and select cases for discussion that are amenable to theoretical speculation. The most difficult cases the practitioners have will be worked into the supervision, and the practitioners will present questions or theoretical comments that they hope will lead the supervisor to present some tangible ideas for dealing with these troublesome cases. In some instances, supervisees will deliberately misinterpret the theory or feign lack of knowledge of the theory when presenting difficult cases, with the hope of getting some tangible help from the supervisor who is attempting to "straighten the therapist out about the theory." This same pattern occurs in the philosopher style of supervision but is more common in the theoretician style, which lends itself to better getting the supervisor to be case specific.

Supervisors who rely heavily on this form of interaction use the Socratic method, asking questions that directly or indirectly cause the practitioners to see the connection between theory and practice. Such questions usually are not related to a theory as a complete set of propositions but deal with specific concepts from a theory. Questions take these forms: How can you help this client develop ego strengths? Are you sure you are showing unconditionally positive regard for this client? How are you going to use the here and now to lay the groundwork with this client? This type of questioning is viewed by such supervisors as shaking the concepts out of the theoretical rug. It is important to note that all three of these questions, derived from different theories, relate to the same dynamic of showing acceptance of the client and establishing a positive relationship, so that the conceptually based questions are related to the broader theoretical implications of the case. All of the questions are oriented to future actions of the practitioner rather than to strategies for dealing with problems already presented in the treatment.

In some instances, where conceptual questions based on theoretical orientations are necessary and helpful, but only when the practitioner is specifically asking for assistance with the broader implications of the case, or when the supervisor has determined that this is the needed focus in supervision. Such questions are limited of help in response to a specific question about problems in a case. This can be understood when supervisors realize that theories are not wrong, theories are not uncertain, and theories do not make mistakes. Only practitioners and supervisors commit these acts. Often supervisors help practitioners to circle the theoretical wagons to defend against practice mistakes. For example, it would be difficult to envision how supervisees could give incorrect answers to any of the three questions listed previously. Questions need to be worded in ways that require the practitioners to explore alternatives of actions and to select the best or potentially most productive alternative.

It is important to recognize that in supervision the practitioner will use inductive logic, while the supervisor tends to use deductive logic. In other words, the practitioner uses case points to derive a conclusion, and the supervisor uses a conclusion to identify case points. This produces learning gaps that must be overcome. Dealing with differences in orientation is not as difficult as it seems. The important factor is to identify which form of logic is being used and to have the supervisor and practitioner use the same form of logic. The supervisor and practitioner can openly discuss the direction they want the logic to take, and both can work at moving in the same direction.

Supervisors have been misguided by thinking that it is the theory that is important in practice. What is important is the way the theory is used, how well it is understood, how well it works, and that its limits are recognized. Theory in supervision should be viewed as a tool of knowledge. In turn, knowledge developed in supervision should be treated as both a dependent and an independent variable. This duality gives both the supervisor and the practitioner more flexibility.

After the discussion of theoretical implications and the resulting knowledge in a case, the supervisor and practitioner are still left with what to do about the case from a practical standpoint. This is similar to activity in the scientific method—the implications of a hypothesis must be explained after it has been found to be statistically significant. Rather than ending supervision with the theoretical significance of a case, this should be considered only the beginning, and the practical steps to be taken should be identified. (The purpose here has been to give an overview of the theoretician style and technique. For a detailed discussion of theoretical approaches, see Chapter 8, which focuses on the use of theory.)

Technician/Technical Strategy

The technician style of supervision is vastly different from the two styles just explained. Instead of being philosophical or theoretical in orientation, the supervisor deals almost exclusively with details of case problems and relates them to technical skills. In philosophical abstraction, the emphasis is on what ought to be known; in theoretical argument, emphasis is on the "why" of doing; and in technical strategy, the emphasis is on what was or should be done. This style is problem focused and interactionally oriented.

Good technicians are not cold, calculating bureaucrats. Good technicians are sensitive persons who can ask highly specific and focused questions in skilled, empathic ways. Without confrontation or threat, they can pressure supervisees to deal with difficult material. They have patience and respond in ways that encourage practitioners to find their own answers. These supervisors are respected by their supervisees but are also viewed as demanding and as having a no-nonsense approach to supervision.

Technical strategy takes three forms: planning, explanation, and description. These forms are described here.

Planning

This component of technical strategy is organized around working with the clinician to plan strategies and techniques of intervention that can be used in general as well as in individual cases. In many instances, this will be based on discussion of case material from past sessions and cases, but what distinguishes this from the descriptive form of technical strategy is that it is almost exclusively focused on future actions of the practitioner, rather than on reflection about past events. The chief focus of planning is teaching techniques that are to be utilized.

Technicians are active, although watching good technicians at work can give the impression that they are reactive, if only their verbalizations are counted. Good technicians listen, plan, and then strategically ask questions or make comments. When technicians do poorly it is because they have become too active and are controlling the practitioners. The technician must be alert to this problem and guard against it. Here is how one practitioner described her actor-technician supervisor:

> When we discuss a particular case my supervisor is very methodical, and she stays with the case material. We have a format. We talk about the client's appearance and feeling tone. We focus on the purpose of the session, topics introduced by the client, topics introduced by the practitioner, therapist interventions, and the client's response to the interventions. We talk about goals, about feelings. We explore possible questions, problems, and observations for the future. We talk about my resistances and how to unblock them. We always discuss where to go next in the treatment. We discuss themes, topics, and key issues in the treatment.

Explanation

This subcategory takes the form of the supervisor actually telling the practitioner what to say to the client. This would seem to be completely unsound educationally and to promote dependence. In certain situations, the practitioner presents specific concerns about what to say to the client, and the supervisor makes the judgment that explaining the appropriate and most efficient way to convey certain strategies to the practitioner can be the most helpful.

Occasionally supervisors will be so concerned that their supervisees make a good impression and be successful within the organization that they will coach them extensively in exactly what to say in treatment. This occurs in settings in which all practitioners have high visibility and do much cotherapy or collaboration. Such coaching, at best, is selectively ignored by practitioners (i.e., used only when they are in doubt and ignored when it is considered impractical) and, at worst, leads to practitioner frustration and eventual confrontation with the supervisor.

Description

Technical strategy based on description rests on after-the-fact exploration of case material. Most supervisors and practitioners explain their skills by describing processes rather than by focusing on behavior that occurred in the situation. Skill is more than description of practice, more than saying the client did better as a result of the interventions used. Skill involves timing in the situation and being able to articulate why a given intervention, action, or verbalization was used and how it promoted insight or moved the interaction into a helpful realm. It is only when the practitioner can differentiate the intent and the actual effect of any given intervention that learning and understanding occur. Most supervision is done in this context. It primarily involves learning from what has already taken place or is already known. The individual case conference or group conference is where most descriptive technical work takes place.

Some hold that although the case conference remains a primary method of teaching in psychotherapy supervision, there is no indication that this contributes anything to client improvement and evidence suggests that this method is relatively ineffective in producing learning (Bergin and Garfield, 1971:896). The case conference method should be used when appropriate and can contribute to effective intervention. Limited attention has been devoted to teaching in supervision, how the results of that teaching show up in practice, or how that teaching ultimately is acted upon by clients. This is a complex, multilevel process that requires sophisticated research strategies. In intervention and supervision, the goal is to improve techniques and to be more specific about what and how information is taught.

Integration of Styles

The primary style and the predominant substyle can be identified for analysis. Certain patterns of the main styles and substyles usually emerge. For example, reactive supervisors tend to be philosophers; active supervisors show a propensity to be technicians. These classifications are always just approximations and are designed only to help focus the supervisory interaction. As other research on style has indicated (Steinberg and Davidson, 1982:44), it appears that supervisors who are effective at combining and moving back and forth between the main styles and substyles at appropriate points in the supervision are the most successful.

It has been difficult to establish that supervisors adjust their style to accommodate the needs of individual supervisees. Since thinking about styles of supervisors as presented in this book is relatively new, it is possible that further research could lead to developing ways of adjusting to individual needs. For this reason, discussion of the supervisor's style is important, regardless of how the style is described or labeled. If supervisees are encouraged to discuss supervisory styles they prefer, supervisors can work at adopting variable styles based on individual need.

In exploring supervisor styles, the supervisor is not limited to the styles that have been identified in this chapter (e.g., see Shulman, 1982, 1993). Exploring the concept of style enhances supervisory interaction regardless of the label that is used. It is important to understand that assigning a label is necessary, but not sufficient. The supervisor must give a description of the behavior that is associated with the label applied to the style. When a supervisor describes his or her style as "a teacher," for example, the supervisor, in order to become more aware of this style and what it means to him or her and the supervisees, must answer these questions: How do I teach? What do I teach? How do I determine what should be avoided in teaching? What do I do when teaching fails to achieve the desired result? These are just a few of the key elements that make up a supervisor's style, and making this style known to oneself or to others is more than using a label to describe it.

STYLE AND THEORETICAL ORIENTATION

Guerin (1976) speculated about the relationship between the idea of style and theoretical orientation. He asked whether theory sets limits on the clinician's style. He observed:

> Beginning family therapists inevitably go through stages in which they mimic the styles of the masters. Only if this remains a fixed phenomenon does it become an obstruction to the development of the therapist as a clinician. A well-defined, open-ended theory does allow a family therapist to evolve his or her personal style of operating with a family. (Guerin, 1976:17)

More needs to be known about the style-theory connection to make any definitive statements. The following questions should be explored: Do supervisors develop supervisory styles similar to the styles they use in treatment? Do supervisees copy the styles of their supervisors? What role does theory play in contributing to and determining styles of treatment and supervision? These are questions that must be addressed as efforts are made to improve the effectiveness of supervision.

· *SUGGESTED READINGS*

Cohen, B. Z. and Laufer, H. (1999). "The Influence of Supervision on Social Workers' Perception of Their Professional Competence." *The Clinical Supervisor,* 18(2), pp. 39-50.
Analysis of supervisee's reactions to supervision.

Haley, J. (1996). *Learning and Teaching Therapy.* New York: Guilford.
A good discussion of techniques used in practice as well as an informative chapter on supervision.

Harrison, A. F. and Bramson, R. M. (1982). *Styles of Thinking: Strategies for Asking Questions, Making Decisions, and Solving Problems.* Garden City, NY: Anchor Press/Doubleday.
This book describes five styles of thinking. It is a good introduction to the concept of style from a cognitive perspective, with some ideas for the supervisor on how to approach styles and thinking processes.

Webster, E. and Haler, P. (1989). "Effects of Two Types of Direct Supervisory Feedback on Student Clinicians' Use of Consequation." *The Clinical Supervisor,* 7(Spring), pp. 7-26.
Report of student reactions to different supervisor styles.

It has required 20 years of supervisory work to generate these current discoveries. Interacting with direct observations of patients and the unfolding of an interpersonal-intrapsychic theory of both the treatment experience and emotional disturbance, the detachment of a supervisor studying the therapeutic experience offered by student therapists to unknown patients proved to be indispensable. (It is impossible to learn how to do psychotherapy without such supervisory help.) However, insight emerged only because these student therapists would present the details of their therapeutic exchanges in strict sequence. This permitted not only observation and formulation, but also prediction and validation. It embedded the supervisory work in interactional considerations.

Robert Langs
The Psychotherapeutic Conspiracy

Chapter 5

Practitioners' Reactions to Supervisor Styles

Supervisees develop interactional reactions to supervisory styles. Supervisee reactions can be positive, or they can become problematic, if they form patterns that thwart learning. Eight reactions the supervisor should be conceptually aware of and prepared to handle are (1) reasoned neutrality, (2) perceived organization constraints, (3) overwhelming clinical evidence, (4) persistent diagnosis, (5) oversimplification response, (6) pseudo criticism desire, (7) theoretical speculation, and (8) self-analysis. Each of these reactions is explained, and suggestions are offered for dealing with all of them. A set of three basic supervisory questions is presented for use in organizing ways of focusing supervisory interaction that can offset the negative effects of supervisee reactions.

INTRODUCTION

Although supervisors develop styles, practitioners generally do not develop styles in their role as supervisees that are unique or unrelated to the supervisors' styles. In fact, most practitioners' styles in supervision are reflections of the supervisors' styles. Evidence suggests that practitioners change styles when they change supervisors. Some practitioners who have had two different supervisors simultaneously use different styles with each supervisor. It was while working with practitioners in this unique position that the discovery was made that practitioners adopt styles in supervision that are reflective of the supervisors' styles. These workers were able to adapt quite well to the differing styles encountered in dual supervision.

Further study of practitioners' styles in supervision revealed that their personal styles or professional styles as practitioners had little correlation with their supervisee styles. The key to the worker's style in the supervisory setting was the style of the supervisor. Supervisors must remember that they have power by virtue of their position; therefore, they do not have to work as hard as the supervisees to establish the supervisory relationship. The author's research has shown that regardless of practitioners' personal or therapeutic styles, in supervision they followed the lead of the supervisor. This accounts for the high levels of satisfaction with supervision that have been reported in a number of research studies.

SUPERVISEE EXPECTATIONS

In a study by Webster and Haler (1989), the style of the supervisor produced different interactional responses from supervisees. Supervisees expect that the supervisor will set the style for the supervisory interaction, and they follow that pattern with a high level of acceptance. This interactional congruity is not always consciously planned or directly recognized as the supervision process unfolds. In other situations supervisees are aware of their reactions, as the following remarks by a supervisee reveal:

> My supervisor tends to use me as a sounding board. Maybe that is because he sees a lot of patients and doesn't have anyone else to talk to. I have some difficulty because I never know what role I'll be playing when I go in for supervision. So what I do is just adjust my mood to his. If he is laid-back, I'm laid-back. If he is hyper, I'm hyper. If he is reflective, I become reflective. I take responsibility for this behavior, but it's not comfortable sometimes not really being myself.

When the practitioner is unable or unwilling to conform to reflecting the supervisor's style, difficulty develops in the supervisory relationship. If, for example, a supervisor is a philosopher and the practitioner assumes the style of technician, difficulty will soon follow if both persist in their preferred styles. Failure to work through varying perceptions of supervisor and practitioner can lead to conflict and frustration. The following summary of a supervisee's perception of his supervision illustrates this problem:

> I never knew where I stood with her. Everything was a power issue with her. She told me to take more initiative, and when I did, she accused me of "usurping authority" and "resisting direction." She also saw my time as having no value. What I mean by this is that when I was late for supervision sessions, it was a crime and I was told I was avoiding supervision, but when she was late, and that happened often, "it was just one of those things." I think she is really too busy as a therapist to have supervisees, but I never dared say that to her. When the situation got unbearable, she decided I should be evaluated by the staff. I agreed to this, but the problem with this was that I wasn't involved with the other staff. They really didn't know me. When the evaluation took place, I felt "ganged up on" and got defensive, so I didn't come out looking too good.

When this difference in style occurs, it rarely is recognized or discussed as an interactional stylistic problem. The problem is attributed to many other factors—most commonly, personality clashes, theoretical differences, or authority struggles. If the participants could recognize and explore the differences in styles covered in this book, much frustration, conflict, and lost learning opportunities could be avoided. Many supervisors and practitioners have been assisted in overcoming their relationship problems by identifying clashes of style. In this process, personality variables, theoretical conflict, and authority struggles should be avoided, since these types of differences are harder to reconcile. These factors can be addressed after the style issues are resolved. With genuine effort, styles can be altered and made more compatible. Understanding and recognizing styles in supervision are also important because practitioners who eventually become supervisors usually adopt the style that was predominantly used in their most significant supervision. This leads to particular styles being perpetuated in supervision, which is the chief reason for weak and ineffective practices being repeated and passed along.

Although the practitioner mirrors the style of the supervisor, he or she does develop different interactional strategies at times to deal with the supervisor. Within these styles, practitioners utilize what are defined as *interactional reactions* that occur periodically and episodically and often become patterns that can be identified and addressed.

INTERACTIONAL REACTIONS

The supervisor, as well as the practitioner, must be aware of and alert to the fact that supervisee interactional reactions can create obstacles to learning in supervision. This does not mean that clinicians deliberately avoid learning. Most of the resistances are unrecognized as clinicians are required to develop new techniques and new strategies in treatment. It is safer and easier to rely on familiar methods even when they are therapeutically naive or neutral.

The adjustments in style made by supervisees, either for encounters with different supervisors or as distinct from the supervisees' practice styles, are quite subtle, but they can influence the supervisory interaction and outcome. When supervisees must alter interactional styles to accommodate to supervisor styles, the adjustment can be problematic because the ability to alter core patterns of relating is difficult. The limited ability to adapt has been described by Harrison and Bramson:

> When we approach problems or decisions, we employ . . . specific strategies. . . . Each of us has a preference for a limited set of thinking strategies. Each set of strategies has its strengths and liabilities. Each is useful . . . but each can be catastrophic if overused or used inappropriately. Yet almost all of us learn only one or two sets of strategies. . . . (1982:1)

Although the predominant cognitive styles and resulting interactional styles used as coping strategies are limited in range, the techniques or specific interactional reactions employed in adjusting to supervision are somewhat broader.

In considering the following supervisee reactions, it is not intended that these responses be viewed as negative. Each one can be positive when employed rationally, logically, and specifically in a case situation. The categories of reactions can be considered resistances, but this is the case only when they become an inhibiting pattern or a block to learning.

The forms these interactional reactions take are varied, but the following are the most common ones that practitioners manifest:

1. Reasoned neutrality
2. Perceived organizational constraints
3. Overwhelming clinical evidence
4. Persistent diagnosis
5. Oversimplification response
6. Pseudo criticism desire
7. Theoretical speculation
8. Self-analysis

Some practitioners repeatedly use one or two of these reactions, although in cases of severe blocks to learning, the practitioner will use all eight forms—and usually in the order that they have been listed. Each of the obstacles is discussed separately here.

Reasoned Neutrality

In this form of resistance, the practitioner will balk at a supervisor-suggested intervention on the basis that it will make the practitioner appear to the client as if he is "taking sides." This is a quite reasonable response, since there is general agreement in treatment training on the importance of practitioner impartiality. However, when it is used in response to a supervisor's attempt to deal with a specific segment of clinical intervention, it is a distortion of the practice dictum. Patterns of activity and consistency—not single episodes of intervention—are important to the neutrality rule (see Haley, 1973:36). When reasoned neutrality is invoked by the practitioner, the supervisor needs to make the distinction between patterns and portions of interaction in practice. The supervisee must learn that intervention that is to make a positive difference in clients' lives requires taking a stand on issues or dysfunctional client behavior. "Taking sides" is not negative unless it is unbalanced through the course of the therapy and is indicative of a clear pattern of preference for one client.

Perceived Organizational Constraints

Often practitioners resist implementing certain interventions on the basis that the agency would thwart or not permit a recommended intervention. Consider this case example:

> A twenty-four-year-old woman sought help in a mental health center at the insistence of the man with whom she was living. It was the worker's assessment after the initial diagnostic interview and supervisory exploration that the woman was functioning quite well and that the boyfriend was really the one in need of help, but he refused to enter treatment. The supervisor suggested that the worker share this with the woman in a subsequent interview and not offer further treatment unless the boyfriend agreed to participate. It was the supervisor's view that to offer the woman treatment individually would confirm the boyfriend's motives. The practitioner agreed with this reasoning but was reluctant to implement such a strategy because this would be against agency policy of offering treatment to those who desired it. This view was reinforced and voiced by the agency director frequently in staff conferences. The supervisor pointed out to the practitioner that the client was not being denied treatment, that conditions were being set on the treatment contract, and that such a strategy could be defended. The practitioner could make a case for the view that he was acting in

the best interest of the client, and he reluctantly implemented the strategy. Two weeks after the follow-up interview, the woman phoned the worker to make an appointment for herself and her boyfriend. This resulted in a successful course of joint therapy.

If the supervisor had not supported the practitioner in overcoming this perceived organizational obstacle, this woman could have been destined for a course of therapy that would have perpetuated her perception of a nonexistent individual dysfunction.

The supervisor should be prepared to deal with perceived organizational obstacles. The practitioner should be allowed to identify any organizational constraints he or she can, but the practitioner should also be required to search for ways to overcome them. Since there are no supervisory injunctions in educational supervision, the practitioner has a wide-open clinical field to explore freely. Although the field may be surrounded by an organizational fence, it is the responsibility of the supervisor to help the practitioner to find legitimate ways to climb the fence. This does not mean that organizational constraints should be discounted. They need to be separated from clinical material so that the emphasis can be placed on the clinical issues. Although more information is often needed and organizational rules are can real obstacles, it is interesting how often practitioners find solutions when they focus solely on understanding the client's needs.

When viewing supervision as a learning enterprise and dealing with organizational issues, it is often easier to explore organizational dynamics through what can be called *office pathology* and *office rationality,* rather than talking in abstract and theoretical terms associated with organizational theory. Freud is reported to have applied clinical concepts to organizations (Freeman, 1980:91). Practitioners think best in clinical terms, and at times it is easier to provide understanding through using familiar concepts and theories to aid learning about unfamiliar material. Clearly, such a strategy has limits, and organizations do not in reality take on characteristics of humans or operate on a rational basis. There are many glaring and tragic examples of this. It is in this area that the supervisor can help the practitioner to see the distinction between organizations as entities and the individuals that make up the organization. Practitioners are trained to do treatment and to work with clients, and many times they are naive in their understanding and expectations of organizations. Perhaps more emphasis should be placed on understanding therapeutic organizations in training programs, but supervisors still need to work with practitioners as they encounter organizations in their therapeutic efforts.

Overwhelming Clinical Evidence

In this reaction, the practitioner presents to the supervisor a series of symptoms, problems, and behaviors that make the case seem hopeless. This reaction can be signaled by a supervisee statement such as, "I tried everything with this case and I don't know what else to do." When the supervisor offers help with a portion of such complex situations, the practitioner responds with more dynamics that seem to put the case out of therapeutic reach. The supervisor can become overwhelmed by such cases, and such feelings of hopelessness should be an indicator to the supervisor that this reaction is occurring. The supervisor should work to get the practitioner to organize and categorize the problem areas, then to assign priorities, and finally to explore a strategy for dealing with the specific problems selected for intervention. The supervisor should aid in the selection of problems to be treated by thinking in terms of which ones cause the most pain or impairment of functioning but, at the same time, have the best chance of amelioration.

Also, in some cases, it helps simply to confront the practitioner with the hopeless nature of the case. Asking if the case is hopeless usually draws forth "No" in reply. When this occurs, the supervisor can move to having the practitioner identify what leads him or her to believe that the case is not hopeless. This strategy breaks up the interactional sequence of clinical hopelessness and transforms the negative to a positive approach to the case. If the supervisee responds with "Yes," the supervisor needs to explore with the supervisee the basis of such an attitude. Such exploration can lead to a philosophical abstraction (see Chapter 4) form of discussion that can open other insights into the case for the supervisee.

Persistent Diagnosis

Persistent diagnosis occurs when the practitioner continues to gather in treatment and provide in supervision information about the case, as if a point will be reached at which enough information will be accumulated to make interventions and solutions apparent. This is especially a problem in group supervision, and it is also a reaction to which the supervisor is highly susceptible. It is interesting to discover facts about cases and to speculate about the meaning of events. The supervisor needs to make a judgment about how much information is enough in order to move to planning intervention strategies. There are no easy answers to knowing when this point is reached. This is why it is so easy to get caught up in a persistent diagnostics interaction.

The supervisor should remember that it is sometimes necessary to act on the basis of insufficient information. There will never be as much information available as one would like to justify an intervention. Once the judgment is made to press the practitioner to move from diagnostic effort to intervention planning, this can and should be done simply and directly. The supervisor should keep in mind that practitioners cling to persistent diagnosis tenaciously. Often, even though they have been asked by the supervisor to move beyond diagnostic activity, they respond briefly but return to it. It is common for a supervisor to have to confront persistent diagnosis several times in one supervisory session.

Persistent diagnosis can result in speculation about patient behavior that remains undocumented and in unfair judgments of the client. For example, in group supervision a case was presented and the group persisted in asking questions about the client and speculating about a diagnosis. One group member commented, "It sounds as if she is a potential drug abuser." Now the practitioner not only had a problem that was not clear but also an unsupported speculation about a potential problem. This is unfair to the client and causes the practitioner to pursue a course that can be damaging to the treatment and the therapeutic relationship, as the practitioner becomes concerned with potential problems rather than existing problems in the case. The supervisor has a responsibility to guard against such speculation and to focus the supervision on identified problems that constitute the basis of treatment.

If persistent diagnosis is allowed to continue for a protracted time, it can lead the participants to conclude that there is *overwhelming clinical evidence* that moves the case into the realm of hopelessness. When these two categories of interaction are combined in this manner, cases can be subtly dropped from supervision attention without ever being considered from the perspective of attempted interventions to help the client.

Oversimplification Response

Oversimplification response occurs when the practitioner presents a complex case. The worker is bewildered by all the dynamics, and the supervisor has difficulty in gaining a comprehensive view of the case or in locating specific and appropriate points of intervention. In such a situation, supervisors often focus on a specific piece of clinical material that is the most troubling to the client and that can be used for the treatment focus, or they integrate less significant aspects of the case. The practitioner is offered simple strategies to guide initial intervention.

The oversimplification response occurs when the practitioner responds to the supervisor's comments and suggestions with, "I think your response is an oversimplification of what is taking place in this case." Inexperienced supervisors can be intimidated by such a response, withdraw their initial observations, and launch back into the quagmire of clinical complexity. This often leads the supervisor and practitioner to revert to the earlier categories of *overwhelming clinical evidence* or *persistent diagnosis* and a stalemate. Practitioners use this strategy and supervisors succumb to it easily; as Scheflen (1972) has pointed out, middle-class Americans seem to have a tendency to engage in oversimplification when explaining behavior. Supervisors should be prepared, when faced with such responses, to articulate that they are not oversimplifying but are offering points for initial intervention in a complex situation. The practitioner should be asked to suspend judgment of oversimplification until the proposed intervention is attempted.

Not all suggestions made by the supervisor will be valid, but this can be known only after intervention is attempted with the client by the supervisee. The supervisor can concede that the practitioner might be right, but neither the supervisor's attempt at simplification nor the practitioner's perception of oversimplification can be determined until the strategy offered is tested out in the practice situation. However, if the worker persists in the belief that what is being offered is oversimplification, he or she might influence the patient to view the use of the strategy in practice as an oversimplification. The supervisor should point this out, stand firm if committed to the need for use of the strategy, and remind the practitioner to avoid being defensive about the supervisory response.

Pseudo Criticism Desire

Practitioners at times take the stance that they want critical analysis of their work by the supervisor, with the implied assumption that the supervisor is failing to give them sufficient feedback. Often this is the case, and the supervisor simply needs to spend more time doing case analyses with the practitioners. When more case analysis is done, the practitioners can become defensive of therapeutic action. The supervisor becomes confused and frustrated because he or she thought this is what the practitioners wanted. Even when practitioners ask for criticism or evaluation, they are often seeking confirmation of their existing level of performance, and when, instead of complete support, genuine criticism and evaluation are offered, the practitioners resist.

This practitioner reaction occurs as a pattern over time rather than being episodic. Supervisors often withdraw from such conflicted communication and respond only when necessary and in a positive way. This lessens the conflict and gives practitioners what they were seeking—no real evaluation of their practice and predominantly positive feedback, even when it is inappropriate. When this state of affairs is reached, the supervision is stalemated and learning ceases.

To reinstate a learning process in the supervision, the supervisor must reorient the focus of the interaction. The supervisor needs to place responsibility on the practitioners for bringing to the supervision case material that is troublesome. (The Practitioner Self-Assessment Form explained in Appendix VI is a good way to initiate this.) However, if the supervisor assumes responsibility for identifying the problem areas, the practitioner is more likely to become defensive and to shift the focus on the basis that these are not the real problems.

Theoretical Speculation

Intellectual and academically oriented practitioners are likely to derive satisfaction from theoretical speculation about cases. They will be interested in the exploration of the theoretical implications of case dynamics or in demonstrating how patient behavior is illustrative of theoretical concepts. These practitioners are delightful to work with in supervision and are especially welcomed by the supervisor who uses the theoretician style or theoretical speculation technique. The use of theory in supervision is important, but the supervisor must avoid having it become the major focus of supervision, causing both participants to lose sight of the client's efforts to change. The practitioner and supervisor can easily move away from the clinical material at hand and shift to a debate over the meaning and significance of theoretical concepts.

Sometimes young practitioners want to use supervision to learn more theory, but limits should be placed on this activity by the supervisor. The use of theory in practice is important, but it can become a dangerous obstacle. As one supervisor stated, "many practitioners have difficulty boiling theoretical water and struggle long and hard to do it." Theoretical discussions often lead to speculation about concepts the practitioner marginally understands, has difficulty precisely defining, and has difficulty relating to theoretical origins. The supervision in such circumstances can lead to intriguing, but lengthy, continuing, unresolved debates. The supervisor should limit the discussion of theoretical material that is directly and inconsistently applied to the case material. (For detailed information on how to deal with discussion of theory, see Chapter 8.)

Self-Analysis

Self-analysis is a common response among practitioners. Practitioners are taught throughout their education and supervision the importance of self-awareness to being a good practitioner. Little attention has been devoted to how much self-awareness is enough and what kind of self-awareness is appropriate. The pattern has been to believe the more self-awareness, the better. Practitioners should be taught limits to self-awareness so as to avoid becoming therapeutically immobilized. Just because practitioners indicate a desire to develop more self-awareness does not necessarily mean that this is what they need. The supervisor should ask, What kind of self-awareness, and for what purpose? Development of self-awareness in the practitioner promoted by the supervisor should be case specific. Encouraging self-awareness outside the context of practice material increases the risk of placing the practitioner into therapy, a situation that should be avoided.

Given the emphasis placed on the importance of practitioner self-awareness to treatment, it is understandable that many practitioners fall back on self-analysis when faced with a difficult case in supervision. Supervisors trained in the same way find it easy to deal with practitioner dynamics rather than relating to client dynamics. The practitioner is present in the supervision, and his or her behavior is directly available for observation and interpretation; the client is once removed and only presented through the eyes of the practitioner, giving the supervisee more knowledge and control than the supervisor.

Supervisees tend to block out positive feedback from the supervisor about their work. In some cases this is due to inconsistency between the worker's self-image and the supervisor's feedback. This causes the worker to retreat psychologically from the positive feedback. The supervisor can overcome this by making sure that the supervisee has heard the feedback and requiring the worker to give a response to it. In supervisory interaction, exploration of client dynamics should precede discussion of practitioner dynamics. That is, practitioner dynamics should be discussed only in the context of case material. Orienting discussion in this manner prevents practitioner behavior from becoming the primary focus of the supervision. When worker dynamics become the predominant area of exploration, the practitioner can develop the belief that supervision is a form of "being put on the hot seat" and can become defensive.

Self-analysis can take several forms, but the result is always the same—an avoidance of treatment issues. One form of self-analysis is focusing on worker "burnout" or distress (see Chapter 10). The supervisor should separate such discussion from discussion of case material.

In supervision, therapy should be avoided even if the practitioner asks for it directly or indirectly. Supervision is supervision, and therapy is therapy. There is limited value to a practitioner's learning to do treatment from being in therapy. Haley has taken a strong stand on this issue by stating, "There does not appear to be a single research study showing that a therapist who has had therapy himself, or understands his involvement with his personal family, has a better outcome in his therapy" (Haley, 1976:178). Therapy is education, but it does not necessarily follow that education is therapy. This is a mistake in logic that supervisors sometimes make when attempting educational efforts in supervision.

There should be some personal reference in supervision, but the supervisor must be careful how this is done and how it is stated. The supervisor must ensure that personal references are related to the practitioner's work. It has been known for quite some time that when practitioners are placed in therapy in their supervision, they begin to act like clients, especially in group supervision (Beukenkamp, 1956:82).

Ambush Interaction

Practitioners who are having difficulty in supervision or who are resistant to it engage in *ambush interaction,* using any or all of the reactions just covered. The practitioner will set the supervisor up with case material that he or she knows cannot be effectively dealt with, and each attempt to assist the practitioner will be met with an excuse or an explanation that the strategy being suggested has been tried to no avail. Practitioners who have a craving to know and master theory in supervision are at times avoiding committing themselves to an intense set of practice relationships. The interactional reactions of supervisees do not have to be identified or discussed as such, but the supervisors must be aware of them conceptually and, when they become problematic, find ways within their own styles to deal with them.

THREE FUNDAMENTAL QUESTIONS

In general, all of the reaction categories just discussed can in part be guarded against, dealt with, and overcome by focusing on the following three questions in supervision:

1. What are the major areas in which the client needs help?
2. What are the genuine problems the client has encountered?
3. What are the positive and negative patterns of relating that the patient demonstrates?

These three questions alone can be helpful in focusing large segments of supervision.

INTEGRATING SUPERVISOR STYLES
AND SUPERVISEE REACTIONS

The suggestions for developing effective supervisory styles discussed in Chapter 4 can be helpful in dealing with all the practitioner reactions covered in this chapter. A matrix of supervisory styles and supervisee reactions is provided in Visual 5.1. This visual indicates the outcome when a particular supervisor style and supervisee reaction coexist in the supervisory process. Both supervisors and supervisees can use this visual to assist in overcoming or enhancing style-and-reaction combinations. Each style has a corresponding supervisee reactions. The supervisor can identify a given style and connect it with a particular reaction that the supervisee is prone to use in order to determine a likely outcome. If the outcome is limiting the learning, the supervisor may want to shift style slightly or organize the supervision so that the supervisee will be required to shift reactions. For example, if a supervisor uses the philosopher style and the supervisee responds

VISUAL 5.1 Matrix of Supervision Styles and Supervisee Reactions

SUPERVISOR STYLE

Supervisee Reactions	Philosopher	Theoretician	Technician
Reasoned Neutrality	Moderately helpful if justification is avoided	Helpful	Helpful
Perceived Organizational Obstacles	Can be helpful when rationalization and justification of inaction are avoided	Moderately helpful	Helpful
Overwhelming Clinical Evidence	Can be helpful if duplicity that leads to mutual frustration is avoided	Can be helpful if duplicity that leads to mutual frustration is avoided	Helpful
Persistent Diagnosis	Avoidance of genuine clinical issues can result	Can result in avoidance of genuine clinical issues and narrow focus	Helpful
Over-simplification Response	Can be helpful if unclear, frustrating, and defensive interaction is avoided	Moderately helpful when used to move beyond supervisee reaction	Very helpful
Psuedo Criticism Desire	Use to avoid genuine clinical issues should be guarded against	Can result in distraction from clinical issues, conflict, and distortion of treatment	Can result in avoidance of genuine clinical issues
Theoretical Speculation	Use to avoid genuine clinical issues should be guarded against	Can result in avoidance of genuine clinical issues and distraction	Helpful
Self-Analysis	Can result in duplicity and mutual frustration	Can result in distraction from clinical issues, conflict, and distortion of treatment	Helpful

with clinical hopelessness this can result in duplicity. In this context, duplicity means that the style and the reaction are compatible but the combination results in mutual floundering and lack of focus, leading to frustration for the supervisor and the supervisee. When this occurs the supervisor should shift to another style. If the supervisor shifts to a technician style, this could be more helpful to the practitioner when he or she remains in the clinical hopelessness mode.

Case Exercise:
The Case of Doris

Doris is a recent graduate and her first job is in a public program that serves adults. She is bright and articulate. She performs tasks with promptness and has much clinical insight. She presents a case to you in supervision in which she is doing family intervention. The father is alcoholic and the mother appears to be mentally impaired and in need of inpatient treatment. There is one son in the home who is eighteen and has a drinking problem. Doris says she "dreads" sessions with this family. She has no focus during the sessions and does not know what to talk about with the family. During supervisory discussion she states that the father reminds her of her ex-husband, who was an alcoholic. She feels this is interfering with the intervention and suggests transferring the case to another worker.

(1) What approach would you take with this supervisee? (2) Would you recommend transfer of the case? (3) How would you characterize Doris's reaction to the client?

SUGGESTED READINGS

Cohen, B. Z. and Laufer, H. (1999). "The Influence of Supervision on Social Workers' Perception of Their Professional Competence." *The Clinical Supervisor,* 18(2), pp. 39-50.

Analysis of supervisee's reactions to supervision.

Harrison, A. F. and Bramson, R. M. (1982). *Styles of Thinking: Strategies for Asking Questions, Making Decisions, and Solving Problems.* Garden City, NY: Anchor Press/Doubleday, 1982.

To date, no books are devoted exclusively to the role and function of style as an interactional process. The only related book the author is aware of is this book on cognitive styles of thinking, and it is highly recommended to the supervisor interested in the concept of style.

The processes and the changes in processes that make up the data which can be subjected to scientific study occur not in the subject person nor in the observer, but in the situation which is created between the observer and his subject.

Harry Stack Sullivan
The Psychiatric Interview

Just being in a supervisory job means that one is assumed to be knowledgeable.

Jay Haley
Learning and Teaching Therapy

Chapter 6

Technique in Supervision

This chapter focuses on the concept of technique in supervision. It is not a listing of techniques supervisors can use but an orientation to the idea of supervisory technique, along with general examples that can act as guides for individual supervisors to use in developing their own techniques. Assessment of learning needs is presented as a supervisory technique through exploration of areas relevant to initiating supervision. Case material and technique are explored through ten basic questions that can serve as a starting point for any supervisor. Guidelines for case presentations as well as sources of distraction in case presentations are identified. The importance of focus is illustrated through discussion of four sets of patterns that can be utilized to guide supervisory discussion. Questioning is one of the chief techniques that the supervisor can use, and guidelines are given for developing good questioning technique. Contracts are being used more in supervision and are discussed as a form of technique. Even good supervisors resist performing certain functions at times, and a way in which this resistance can be turned into a positive technique is explained. As a conclusion to this chapter, nine elements of good supervision and eleven techniques to encourage learning in supervision are listed. Much of the discussion in this chapter is oriented to the development of supervisory techniques that promote good practice techniques.

INTRODUCTION

Certain supervisory techniques can be used with each of the supervisory styles mentioned in Chapter 4. It should be kept in mind that each of the supervisory styles can also be used as a technique when applied to a specific unit of interaction in supervision. Many techniques are included throughout this book. This chapter is devoted to general techniques that can be helpful in a broad range of situations.

EDUCATIONAL ASSESSMENT

There is renewed interest in supervision within many disciplines that make up the helping professions. An aspect of this trend is new interest in the role of educational assessment: What does the student or new supervisee know as he or she enters the new situation? What does he or she need to learn? Years ago this was referred to as "educational diagnosis," but this terminology was abandoned because it seemed to suggest doing therapy with the learner.

In the past, the tendency was to focus the educational diagnosis on the personal aspects of the learner's functioning. When this approach was eliminated, the tendency was to do very little assessment of the new supervisee. The belief was that the learner was a blank slate, and it was assumed that the program staff or the supervisor knew what the supervisee needed to learn without much review of the supervisee's level of functioning or knowledge. When assessment began to reemerge, it took the form of relying almost exclusively on strengths and weaknesses identified by the learner. The general belief was that the learner was the person best qualified to establish what was needed to enhance learning. In other words, the focus shifted from the view that the learner knows little about his or her own needs to the position that the learner knows precisely what is needed to promote learning.

When educational assessment as a concept began to be formulated, a more balanced view of what constituted a good assessment evolved. The focus now is aimed at a mutual evaluation of the goals of the learning experience. There has been an effort to identify the major areas that are basic to a good educational assessment.

Educational Assessment Concepts

An instrument that can be used to organize educational assessment is printed in Appendix II. The instrument focuses on the following assessment areas. After the practitioner completes the instrument, it should be discussed in supervision and become a part of the supervision record. It is reviewed at key evaluation points during the educational experience.

1. *Previous experience.* It is important for the supervisor to know exactly what work and volunteer experiences the supervisee brings to the situation. This has become more important, as supervisees increasingly come to the practice situation with substantial experience. It is common to encounter supervisees who have held several practice positions prior to entering an advanced educational experience. In most educational programs, almost three-fourths of the students are part-time and have employment associated with the helping professions. Some supervisees have significant experience in positions related to the learning situation. At the same time, however, the supervisor cannot assume that the learner has mastered all of the elements of a position that he or she has held. In this age of specialization, the exposure of a practitioner in a given position can be quite narrow. For these reasons the supervisor needs to explore thoroughly all past positions the learner has held. This should include paid as well as volunteer positions and positions held within and outside the helping professions. Supervisees who have had substantial work experience in business and other non-human service positions sometimes have difficulty knowing what to expect from clinical supervision and how to react to clinical supervisors, and expectations should be clarified with such supervisees.

2. *Ethical awareness.* Ethical practice is of paramount concern in most aspects of our society today. Much confusion exists regarding what is ethically appropriate behavior in many settings. All disciplines have ethical codes that guide practice. It is the supervisor's responsibility to determine the learner's knowledge of the ethical code or codes he or she is required to conform to in the current practice position. It is a good idea for the supervisor and learner to engage in a detailed review of the relevant codes that apply to the situation.

3. *Theoretical knowledge.* There has been a large expansion of theories of behavior and intervention in recent decades. The practitioner may have varying exposure to theories from past educational and work experience. Educational programs and agencies place varying emphasis on theories and theoretical knowledge. The supervisor needs to know what theories the practitioner has knowledge of and the depth of his or her knowledge of each theory identified. The supervisor needs information regarding what theoretical orientations the clinician is currently exploring and how the clinician is integrating theory in practice.

4. *Assessment and diagnosis.* The key question in this area is, What experience and skill has the clinician accumulated regarding assessment in general, and specifically in a given treatment area or specialty? In-depth assessment involves more than being able to compile a social history or initial database. Assessment involves the ability to integrate knowledge of behavior, personality, social functioning, educational development, health, economic status, and spiritual activity. The specialized aspects of assessment

can be troublesome for practitioners. For example, in mental health agencies, the supervisor needs to know the practitioner's level of knowledge and skill in using the American Psychiatric Association diagnostic and statistical system (DSM) and manuals used to reference medications. Some clinicians resist developing knowledge in these areas even though demands for skills in these areas of assessment are increasing. To do competent and risk-limited practice, the supervisee and supervisor must have thorough and complete knowledge of assessment, diagnosis, and uses and actions of mental health medications.

5. *Intervention skills*. The supervisor cannot assume the supervisee has extensive knowledge of intervention strategies even if the supervisee has prior clinical experience. The supervisor should inquire about the supervisee's specific abilities related to forming alliances, engaging clients, and dealing with client confusion, hostility, and resistance. Information should be gathered about ability to perform specific techniques, such as making interpretations, seeking clarification, being supportive, and asking sensitive questions. The review of intervention skill should include an assessment of ability to identify transference and countertransference issues and skill at planning termination.

6. *Organizational understanding*. Supervisees usually have some degree of experience in organizations. The supervisor needs to learn how the practitioner has come to view organizations and their formal and informal structures. Clinicians can have unique perspectives on their own experience in an organization. One of the author's supervisors wisely stated that a person can have ten years of experience in one agency or one year of experience repeated ten times. In this example, the practitioner with ten years of genuine experience can build on the cumulative insights he or she has gained, and the clinician with one year repeated ten times will need to be assisted in developing a broader perspective on the significance of experience in an organizational context. It is critical for the supervisor to determine what type supervisee he or she has in order for an effective organizational educational experience to evolve. Some supervisees have limited knowledge of organizations and have no experience with the formal and informal organizational structures that can enhance or impede practice activity.

7. *Agency functioning*. Organizational understanding is more comprehensive and global than agency functioning. The supervisor needs to assess the supervisee's knowledge regarding the nature of the agency he or she is about to enter. Each agency has a unique structure and atmosphere. A practitioner can have general knowledge, but the clinician has to be able to apply this general knowledge to an individual setting.

8. *Attitudes and values*. Supervisees with work experience have undoubtedly developed values and attitudes toward working with clients. It is not just social agency experience that gives rise to attitudes and values about cli-

ents. The supervisor needs to be aware of negative attitudes and conflicting values as the supervisee enters the agency, so that accommodation can begin to avoid problems for clients and the practitioner. Such practitioner attitudes are often subtle and unconscious. Once identified, clinicians are able to change these attitudes and remove them as barriers to effective relationships with clients.

9. *Goals and objectives.* It is important that the supervisor know about the practitioner's general goals. Frequently clinicians have difficulty identifying specific skills and knowledge they want to acquire but are able to state their career goals. Through identifying career goals, the supervisor can learn much about what the practitioner hopes to achieve as part of the current position and supervisory process. The types of interventions, modalities, methods, and specialty areas that are of interest to the clinician are factors the supervisor can explore to help the practitioner refine precise learning goals. The supervisor should foster integration of supervisee learning and career goals with the supervisory process.

10. *Previous supervision.* Practitioners have usually undergone some form of supervision in their positions in the helping professions and general employment areas. The supervisor should explore with clinicians their perception of the quality of past supervision and as well as its duration and structure. Past experience shapes people's expectations. Supervisees who were given much independence in a past position may resist meeting regularly with the supervisor. Supervisees who have been oversupervised may make excessive demands on the supervisor's time. By knowing past supervisory experiences, the supervisor is in a much better position to establish current expectations.

11. *Learning impediments.* Practitioners have very active lives. Balancing all of life's demands can be a juggling act for anyone. When demands become too great, the job is usually the first area to be compromised, and family the second. The supervisor needs to have accurate information about the overall functioning of the practitioner. The supervisor should avoid intruding or imposing on the practitioner's life outside the agency but does need to be aware of events that could influence professional functioning.

The supervisor should cover these general areas with any practitioner before he or she begins practice. After completing an assessment, the supervisor is much better prepared to develop a supervisory plan for the supervisee. Developing educational plans that are not based on information in these areas puts the supervisor in the position of blindly assuming what the practitioner does and does not know.

Different supervisors have varying ways of doing educational assessment. The most common method is to interview the person and evaluate the practitioner's responses to a set of loosely organized questions. Some supervisors have practitioners make a list of strengths and weaknesses. These are effective ways of doing an assessment, but there needs to be a record of the practitioner's participation in the process, as well as a way to review with the clinician periodically the degree to which the educational program and supervision are meeting his or her learning needs. The criteria provided previously and the assessment instrument in Appendix II can be effective tools in assessing and meeting supervisee learning and developmental needs.

CASE MATERIAL

Case material is the foundation of supervisory clinical techniques. Case material should be the focus of supervision and techniques should derive from this focus. In considering case material, the supervisor should use general areas for practitioner reflection that can help the supervisee gain a comprehensive perspective of the case, regardless of the supervisee's specific concerns. The supervisor can help the practitioner plan assessment and treatment sessions by asking the following questions:

1. What do you like about this client?
2. What do you think the client likes about you?
3. How much of yourself do you see in this client?
4. What do you feel inside yourself when you are with this client?
5. What thoughts do you have when you are with the client?
6. Theoretically, what is the basis of what you have presented about this client?
7. On what basis did you decide to use the techniques you did in this session with the client?
8. What was the major focus of this session?
9. What worries you the most about this case?
10. What are you going to do next with this case?

The supervisor should cover these areas in some format. The supervisee needs to grapple with these questions, but the supervisor should assist the practitioner when the response is, "I don't know."

The question "What do you like about this client?" might be dismissed as insignificant, but this question can elicit a great deal of helpful information about the client to which the practitioner has not given much thought. This is similar to Harry Stack Sullivan's observation that mental health professionals know a great deal about their patients that they don't know they know. For example, caught off guard by the offhand question of a friendly colleague—"Yes, but damn his difficulties in living! What sort of PERSON is this patient of yours?"—the psychiatrist may rattle off a description that would do him honor if he only knew it. (1954:14)

This example relates to the idea of the "level of knowing" in practice, and the previous ten questions relate to "knowing" that goes beyond professional knowledge. The questions are designed to be clear, simple inquiries that reveal the essence of the treatment relationship.

CASE PRESENTATIONS

Case presentations are one of the most effective ways to promote learning in supervision. Case presentations have been de-emphasized because they are considered time-consuming and not cost-efficient. This attitude is unfortunate because case presentations are one of the most effective supervisory techniques when applied appropriately. Practitioners who are asked to present cases or share their practice are being expected to take risks and can feel threatened. This anxiety can be lessened when the supervisee is given time to prepare, organize questions, and consult with the supervisor in advance. The practitioner may have two fears regarding case presentations: fear of not meeting expectations and fear of losing existing autonomy. The supervisor should support and reassure the practitioner to lessen both fears. When a supervisor can accept that he or she cannot be responsible for the practitioner's performance, but is responsible only for clarifying the expected standards of performance, the door is opened to interaction that allows the supervisor and practitioner to engage in a process of genuine growth and development.

To help the practitioner who is struggling with a case, the supervisor should identify with the client and assist the practitioner in understanding what the client may be experiencing and how the client may be responding. If the supervisor has difficulty identifying with the client, he or she should ask the practitioner to describe and imitate or role-play the client. Through this process the practitioner will be forced to identify client patterns of relating, and the supervisor will gain access to client characteristics that he or she can then feed back to the practitioner. Langs strictly adheres to this view of supervision, seeing the central focus of supervision as the therapist-patient interaction, and considering all else to be peripheral: "I spend much of my supervisory time attempting to identify with the patient and what he is experiencing both within himself and from the therapist . . . because I . . . wish to experience the therapeutic interaction as it unfolded for the supervisee" (Langs, 1979:15).

Any presentation of a case for supervision should result in the supervisor's asking the practitioner to explain all efforts to deal with the problem before giving assistance. This helps avoid the practitioner response, "I tried that, and it didn't work."

Not every act of the practitioner can be scrutinized in supervision, and not every case can be explored. Priorities should be set for which cases and which case material will be reviewed. Priority should be given to areas of practitioner concern, but provision should also be made for reinforcement of the practitioner's strong points to avoid an exclusive focus on areas of weakness and vulnerability.

The following guidelines for case presentations are offered to assist supervisors and supervisees in keeping presentations focused. Remember, case presentations can be threatening. Anxiety about case presentation can be lessened by the following:

1. The supervisor should present a case first.
2. The supervisee should be granted time to prepare the case for presentation.
3. The presentation should be based on written or audiovisual material.
4. The presentation should be built around questions to be answered.
5. The presentation should be organized and focused.
6. The presentation should progress from client dynamics to practitioner dynamics.

In addition, several common distractions occur in case presentations of which the supervisor should be aware:

1. Presentation of several cases in a short session
2. Presentation of a specific problem rather than the case in context
3. Presentation of additional problems in a single case
4. Therapist dynamics preceding case dynamics during discussion
5. Intervention expectations beyond the capabilities of the therapist

---

Case Exercise:
The Case of Paul

Paul is an MSW graduate who graduated one year ago. He worked in an adult treatment center for one year before coming to work in child and adolescent foster care, where you have been assigned to supervise him. Paul has been working for nine months and several workers have expressed concern to you about Paul's performance. He does not do well at presenting his cases at staff conferences. He rambles and often goes into great detail, but many times does not get basic information from clients (e.g., medications, previous treatment information, details of family history). Other workers see this as a waste of valuable time. You have discussed this with him, but it has not helped, and he seems to be getting more disorganized. In meetings he seems distracted and tired. You do know that recently he took a job at nights selling insurance to earn extra money to make a downpayment for purchase of a house.

(1) What, if anything, could you do to deal with this situation? (2) How could you assist Paul in doing better in gathering background information? (3) What could you do about Paul's unfocused presentations?

LEVEL OF KNOWING AND TECHNIQUE

Level of knowing can be generally divided into two types—technical skill and perspective (Lachman et al., 1979:4). Technical skill in this context relates to specific units of activity; perspective deals with understanding the relationship among sets of units of activity that allows comprehension of the whole. A bus driver can be a good driver without understanding the total functioning of a mass transit system. By the same token, the director of a mass transit system can understand the complex operation and large-scale issues without being a good bus driver. Technical competence is possible without perspective, and perspective is possible without technical skill. It is helpful if one has both, but it is not always a necessary condition. Practitioners can develop technical skill without a great deal of perspective about treatment, and supervisors can supervise with perspective while having limited technical skill, although this is much harder to accomplish. It is important to promote both levels of knowledge in both supervisors and practitioners.

In treatment-oriented supervision, problems can arise when the practitioner and supervisor are aiming at different levels of knowledge. Practitioners are more often interested in technical competence—in improving their practice skills—while supervisors frequently focus their attention on perspective—on philosophical and theoretical issues. When the practitioner's level of knowledge or inquiry is different from the level at which the supervisor wishes to work, supervision becomes, at best, benign and ineffective and, at worst, frustrating, tense, and conflictual.

To avoid this mismatch of knowledge development, the supervisor should be sensitive to the fact that the two levels exist and be aware of how each is presented in supervision. At times it is appropriate to focus on one level in supervision so that learning can be maximized. For example, younger, inexperienced practitioners are more likely to be interested in learning technical competence; older, experienced practitioners are more interested in perspective from a philosophical and theoretical stance and will be annoyed when supervisors force them to focus exclusively on technical skills. At the same time, practitioners at times raise perspective issues to avoid discussing technical competence. This is not always a deliberate shift of focus. Sometimes it is a subtle erosion of the appropriate learning process to which the supervisor must be alert, and against which he or she must guard.

It is a good general policy to begin with technical skill learning and then move to perspective learning. One helpful way to picture this in supervision interaction is to view technical learning as the *horizontal* aspect of supervision, and perspective or philosophical and theoretical learning as the *vertical* component of supervision. Technical competence, then, relates to activity on a horizontal level with individual cases, and perspective or insight comes as one moves up the scale of complexity and integrative understanding in a series of cases.

It is best to begin with development of technical skill because traditional learning theory has taught us that technical obstacles should be removed (in therapy this translates into mastery) before the higher level of perspective learning can occur.

CONTINUITY

Supervision should have continuity, just as treatment does. A case should be presented sequentially, beginning with identification of patient dynamics and problems, a tentative diagnosis, alternative intervention strategies, selection of a general intervention approach, and follow-up of the case. Supervision that focuses on only specific problems will not maximize learning for the practitioner. Observation of supervision sessions often reveals that the supervisor failed to follow a comprehensive process, which results in confusion and frustration for both supervisor and practitioner. The supervisor cannot perform the supervisory function effectively if one of the previous elements is missing or slighted.

Most often, follow-up is the missing component. Failure to do follow-up deprives the supervisor of an opportunity to evaluate the effect of the supervision on the practitioner and the treatment. When follow-up is not done, the supervisor has no way of knowing if the efforts of a considerable amount of supervisory time were ever applied. A case illustration highlights how harmful failure to follow-up can be:

> A child welfare supervisor in reviewing a case with a family service worker arrived at the conclusion that a child should be removed from a mother's care and placed in foster care because of indications of neglect by the mother. The worker reluctantly agreed to the removal but did not implement the plan. Several weeks later the mother's male companion physically abused the child and emergency shelter care was arranged for the child.

The supervisor was upset when she learned the removal plan had not been implemented, but the burden was on the supervisor because she did not follow up with the supervisee regarding the original removal plan.

Thorough follow-up can serve as ongoing evaluation of the practitioner, the therapy, and the supervision. Some strategies worked out in supervision are wrong and inappropriate, and this needs to be made known. Many errors of supervision are repeated because of failure to do follow-up.

UNIFYING ASSESSMENT, DIAGNOSIS, TREATMENT PLANNING, AND OUTCOME MEASUREMENT AS SUPERVISORY TECHNIQUE

Clinical supervision technique is moving toward a more unified process rather than exclusive concern with individual techniques. Helping supervisees master the requirements to do assessment and diagnosis of clients is an important function of the supervisor. Supervisees should be aided in understanding how to integrate unifying principles of assessment, diagnosis, treatment planning, and outcome measurement.

Assessment and Diagnosis

Diagnosis and assessment are critical to the new standards of practice. Clinical social workers need to develop standardized assessment for the client groups that are served, and the intervention plans used must be directly connected to an extension of the assessment and the diagnosis.

Supervisors need to be highly qualified in assessment and diagnosis and prepared to assist practitioners in developing good diagnostic assessment skills (see Munson, 2000b). Supervisors need to be skilled in the use of the *Diagnostic and Statistical Manual of Mental Disorders* (DSM-IV-TR) classification system of the American Psychiatric Association (2000a) and the person-in-environment system developed by the National Association of Social Workers (Karls and Wandrei, 1994). Standardized assessment screening instruments are necessary in assessments, and standardized measures of mood, anxiety, and various other mental disorders are essential for diagnosis and justification of interventions.

Strategies for rapid assessment and diagnosis are becoming the hallmark of effective and efficient evaluation. Models for rapid assessment are emerging (Olin and Keatinge, 1998), and standardized formats are being adopted. Social workers historically have not developed specific intake measures and client screening procedures beyond global categories of assessment. Supervisors need to develop "initial database" standardized measures to replace the traditional "social history" categories. Many models for evaluation and assessment exist and can be easily adapted for social work settings. The intake and screening measures developed by MCOs are generic and unreliable for many settings that employ social workers. Supervisors need to develop screening instruments unique to specific practice settings. Screening instruments are easy to develop and do not have to be standardized on large populations when they are designed for specific settings. For example, the screening instrument for potential for domestic violence in Visual 6.1 was devised by the author based on the literature and the needs of the specific shelter program that needed a screening instrument for staff.

VISUAL 6.1. Domestic Violence Rapid Assessment Scale

Name of Client: _____

Name of Interventionist: _____

Date/Period of Report: _____

Instructions

Assign a score for each item that represents an overall rating of the item for the report period. Brief comments can be entered to the right of each item. After assigning a score for each item, sum the items and enter the number in the blank for the total score. Do this for each group of measures.

1. Degree of domestic violence
   (Including verbal and physical assaults)
   1....2....3....4....5....6....7....8....9....10
   LOW   HIGH

2. Arrests for domestic violence
   (Including police intervention)
   1....2....3....4....5....6....7....8....9....10
   LOW   HIGH

3. Treatment for physical harm
   (Including ER Tx., Physician Tx., Self Tx.)
   1....2....3....4....5....6....7....8....9....10
   LOW   HIGH

4. Flight to avoid harm to self, others
   (Including shelter care, family care, leave
   and return)
   1....2....3....4....5....6....7....8....9....10
   LOW   HIGH

5. Protective order issued
   1....2....3....4....5....6....7....8....9....10
   LOW   HIGH

DOMESTIC VIOLENCE LEVEL SCORE (sum of 1 through 5)
(5-10 = low, 11-20 = mild, 21-30 = moderate, 31=40 = high,
41-50 = severe)   SCORE_____

6. No assaults, but disputes
   1....2....3....4....5....6....7....8....9....10
   LOW   HIGH

7. Adult partner assaulted
   1....2....3....4....5....6....7....8....9....10
   NUMBER OF INCIDENTS

8. Adult partner assaulted and child witness
   1....2....3....4....5....6....7....8....9....10
   NUMBER OF INCIDENTS

9. Adult partner assaulted and child assaulted
   1....2....3....4....5....6....7....8....9....10
   NUMBER OF INCIDENTS

10. Child assaulted and adult partner witnessed
   1....2....3....4....5....6....7....8....9....10
   NUMBER OF INCIDENTS

NATURE OF DOMESTIC VIOLENCE LEVEL SCORE (sum of 6 through 10)
(5-10 = limited, 11-20 = concern, 21-30 = moderate, 31-40 = intense,
41-50 = extreme)   SCORE _____

11. Violent person can access victim(s)   1....2....3....4....5....6....7....8....9....10
                                                 LOW   HIGH

12. Violent person's whereabouts unknown   1....2....3....4....5....6....7....8....9....10
                                                 LOW   HIGH

13. Violent person not remorseful   1....2....3....4....5....6....7....8....9....10
                                                 LOW   HIGH

14. Adult victim's continuation of relationship 1....2....3....4....5....6....7....8....9....10
                                                 LOW   HIGH

15. No treatment sought by violent person and victim 1....2....3....4....5....6....7....8....9....10
                                                 LOW   HIGH

POTENTIAL FOR VIOLENCE LEVEL SCORE (sum of 11 through 15)
(5-10 = low, 11-20 = mild, 21-30 = moderate, 31=40 = high,
41-50 = severe)   SCORE_____

Teaching Diagnosis

Supervisors should survey new supervisees regarding their knowledge of diagnosis before orienting the supervisees to the system. An important aspect of helping supervisees to understand the DSM system is that it cannot be approached in the same way as traditional learning of a theory, an orientation, or a set of principles. The DSM-IV-TR is a classification that has been inductively derived from data collected from various sites under varied conditions. As a result, the system has evolved over many years and has been modified in a fragmented way that has resulted in limited conceptual foundation, no theoretical underpinning, and a numbering system that has inconsistencies, lapses in organizational coherence, a unique and inconsistent structural presentation of disorders and symptoms, and unique grammatical construction. This is not mentioned as criticism of the DSM system. It is mentioned because if a clinician is to master the system he or she must understand how such a complex document is constructed and that a search for the logic of the system will lead to only frustration. The person should approach the DSM as a collection of disorders and an array of symptoms that characterize each disorder. It is a system of matching symptoms, behaviors, and characteristics with a defined set of criteria for inclusion within a disorder of any given person's presentation to the clinician. When the learner understands this basic nature of using the classification system, the learning process becomes easier. Various sets of conventions are associated with each disorder, and these are explained in the first sections of the manual. These sections include Introduction, Use of the Manual, DSM-IV-TR

Classification, and Multiaxial Assessment. It is essential that the learner read, reread, and master these sections of the manual before moving to applying the system clinically. The details of teaching specific diagnostic skills are not covered here. A number of good books exist for learning the DSM system. It is suggested that the supervisor and supervisee refer to *The Mental Health Diagnostic Desk Reference: Visual Guides and More for Learning to Use the Diagnostic and Statistical Manual* (DSM-IV-TR) (Munson, 2001b) for a detailed step-by-step method for mastering diagnostic criteria. This book also lists other major diagnostic learning aids.

Relationship of Treatment and Diagnosis

The supervisee should be oriented to connecting diagnosis and treatment planning. Changes in the monitoring of practice over the past ten years have led to increased emphasis on demonstrating, as part of the client chart, a direct connection between diagnosis and treatment planning. In many cases payers will not authorize or pay for treatment without documented evidence of a connection between diagnosis and treatment. Some agencies have established formats for recording this connection, but most have no such guidelines. The supervisor should remember that for psychiatrists, the treatment plan is related to Axis I, Axis II, and Axis III; for psychologists, Axis I, and Axis II; and for social workers, Axis I, Axis II, and Axis IV. Even though social workers are the specialists in relation to Axis IV, clinicians frequently fail to relate the treatment plan to data reported on this axis. Each item mentioned on Axis IV should have a corresponding treatment plan segment. This is a general rule when correlating diagnosis and treatment: each diagnostic symptom or behavior and each psychosocial and environmental problem noted should have at least one corresponding treatment plan entry. Treatment plans should have at least three categories of corresponding entries: (1) problem statements, (2) goals, and (3) progress in goal attainment. These treatment plan items should be measurable and observable.

Treatment plans must be connected to a diagnosis, and treatment plan items should be directly related to the diagnostic criteria for the specific diagnosis. This is difficult for practitioners to do initially. The supervision should help the clinician to start treatment planning by referring to the DSM-IV-TR criteria for the disorder or disorders the client has received as part of the multiaxial diagnosis. New clinicians need assistance in making this connection. Visual 6.2 gives a graphic illustration of the process of connecting specific diagnostic criteria to formulating problem statements and generating long- and short-term goals and interventions.

After seeing the connection between diagnostic criteria, problem identification, and interventions, the clinician is faced with how to craft problem statements and treatment goals. Practitioners frequently do not know how to begin the process and become frustrated. One way the supervisor can be

VISUAL 6.2. Integration of DSM-IV-TR Diagnosis and Treatment Planning

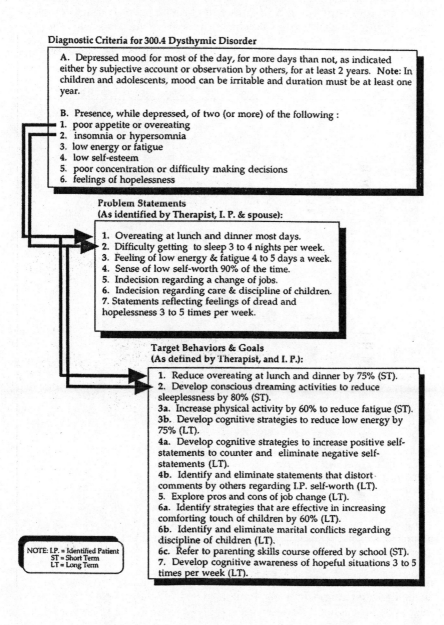

Diagnostic Criteria for 300.4 Dysthymic Disorder

A. Depressed mood for most of the day, for more days than not, as indicated either by subjective account or observation by others, for at least 2 years. Note: In children and adolescents, mood can be irritable and duration must be at least one year.

B. Presence, while depressed, of two (or more) of the following :
1. poor appetite or overeating
2. insomnia or hypersomnia
3. low energy or fatigue
4. low self-esteem
5. poor concentration or difficulty making decisions
6. feelings of hopelessness

Problem Statements
(As identified by Therapist, I. P. & spouse):

1. Overeating at lunch and dinner most days.
2. Difficulty getting to sleep 3 to 4 nights per week.
3. Feeling of low energy & fatigue 4 to 5 days a week.
4. Sense of low self-worth 90% of the time.
5. Indecision regarding a change of jobs.
6. Indecision regarding care & discipline of children.
7. Statements reflecting feelings of dread and hopelessness 3 to 5 times per week.

Target Behaviors & Goals
(As defined by Therapist, and I. P.):

1. Reduce overeating at lunch and dinner by 75% (ST).
2. Develop conscious dreaming activities to reduce sleeplessness by 80% (ST).
3a. Increase physical activity by 60% to reduce fatigue (ST).
3b. Develop cognitive strategies to reduce low energy by 75% (LT).
4a. Develop cognitive strategies to increase positive self-statements to counter and eliminate negative self-statements (LT).
4b. Identify and eliminate statements that distort comments by others regarding I.P. self-worth (LT).
5. Explore pros and cons of job change (LT).
6a. Identify strategies that are effective in increasing comforting touch of children by 60% (LT).
6b. Identify and eliminate marital conflicts regarding discipline of children (LT).
6c. Refer to parenting skills course offered by school (ST).
7. Develop cognitive awareness of hopeful situations 3 to 5 times per week (LT).

NOTE: I.P. = Identified Patient
ST = Short Term
LT = Long Term

helpful is to provide a list of key words that can be used to stimulate thought about target interventions. Visual 6.3 provides a list of helpful words. These words are commonly used by clients and clinicians in conversation but are not always recalled when attempting to prepare a written treatment plan.

VISUAL 6.3. Descriptive Words Used in Documentation and Treatment Planning

Word/phrase	Used by: Client	Used by: Practitioner
Admitted	✓	
Advised	✓	✓
Alluded	✓	
Announced	✓	
Answered that ...	✓	✓
Ascribed	✓	
Asserted	✓	
Affirmed	✓	✓
Characterized	✓	✓
Cited	✓	✓
Clarified	✓	✓
Commented	✓	✓
Communicated	✓	✓
Conveyed	✓	
Declared	✓	
Delineated	✓	
Depicted	✓	✓
Described	✓	✓
Detailed	✓	
Disclosed	✓	✓
Divulged	✓	✓
Emphasized	✓	✓
Explained	✓	✓
Expressed	✓	✓
Gave details of ...	✓	
Gave an account of ...	✓	
Illustrated	✓	✓
Implied	✓	
Indicated	✓	✓
Informed	✓	✓
Listed	✓	✓
Mentioned	✓	✓
Narrated		
Noted	✓	✓
Painted a picture of ...	✓	
pointed out	✓	✓
Portrayed	✓	✓
Proclaimed	✓	
Rectified	✓	
Recounted	✓	
Related	✓	✓

Remarked	✓	✓
Reported	✓	✓
Represented	✓	
Retold	✓	
Revealed	✓	✓
Reviewed	✓	✓
Said	✓	✓
Specified	✓	✓
Sketched	✓	
Suggested	✓	✓
Summarized	✓	✓
Told	✓	✓

Use of this list can assist the practitioner in preparing treatment item statements. The strategy of preparing written statements from words used by the client and the practitioner can heighten the clinician's attention to language used during the interview process. The words can also be used as qualifiers in clinical notes and evaluation reports. Visual 6.4 carries this word use method a step further by providing key words that can be used to begin the actual statement of a treatment plan item. The words are loosely organized by the DSM-IV-TR axis to which they are most closely related.

Intervention and Measurement

The evolution and expansion of diagnostic knowledge, as well as the expectation that practitioners should connect diagnosis and treatment planning, require social work supervisees to develop more sophisticated research literature, behavior-based practice skill, and documented practice wisdom. These are roles that the supervisor should carry. The repertoire of intervention techniques needs to be expanded for every practice situation and repeatedly tested. Development of practice guidelines and diagnosis-based recommended treatment plans makes it difficult for MCOs to exclude social work interventions from care plans and reimbursable services and procedures. Diagnosis is difficult for practitioners and requires much training, practice experience, and supervisory support for mastery and confident skill to emerge.

Intervention needs to be measurable and outcome focused. The profession has not devoted much attention to outcome measures or what constitutes successful intervention. More attention to objective measures and quantifiable outcomes is being demanded by service payers and monitoring organizations. The supervisor carries a primary role in promoting successful intervention. When external payers or regulators do not mandate standardized outcome measures of intervention, the supervisor has an obligation to work within the agency or practice group to devise outcome instruments specific to the practice setting. Visual 6.5 contains a psychotherapy outcome scale designed by the author for a psychotherapy setting.

VISUAL 6.4. DSM-IV-TR-Based Assessment Outcome Terminology

	Axis I	Axis II	Axis III	Axis IV	Axis V
Problems	Clarify Determine Document Establish Identify Observe	Disclose Elicit Explore Probe Test	Document Gather Request	Report	Evaluate Establish Document Review
Goals	Counsel Develop Enhance Encourage Help Improve Plan	Assess Build Compliance Facilitate Foster Oversee Process	Observe Consult	Assist Focus on Overcome	Elevate Improve Increase
Intervention	Answer Arrange Attend Challenge Change Conduct Confront Decrease Demonstrate Design Discuss Eliminate Enact Express Implement Increase Interpret Overcome Postpone Praise Read Reduce Refocus Replace Reinforce Require Restore Specify Terminate Utilize Verbalize	Accept Acknowledge Assign Conduct Cooperate Coordinate Describe Educate Facilitate Inform Instruct Maintain Manage Monitor Recommend Regulate Set limits Self-manage Self-soothe Stabilize Stop Teach Train Transport Urge	Compliance Inform Observe Refer Report	Adjust to Improve Provide	Document

VISUAL 6.5. Psychotherapy Outcome Scale

Name of Client: _____

Name of Interventionist: _____

Period of Report: _____

Instructions

Assign a score for each item that represents an overall rating of the item for the report period. Brief comments can be entered to the right of each item. After assigning a score for each item, sum the items and enter the number in the blank for the total score. Do this for each group of measures.

1. Degree of depression during treatment this report period
   (Including crying spells and anger outbursts)

   1....2....3....4....5....6....7....8....9....10
   LOW   HIGH

2. Anxiety evident during treatment this report period
   (Including eating and sleep disturbance)

   1....2....3....4....5....6....7....8....9....10
   LOW   HIGH

3. Dissociation evident during treatment this report period
   (Including daydreaming and inattention)

   1....2....3....4....5....6....7....8....9....10
   LOW   HIGH

4. Stress evident during intervention process this report period

   1....2....3....4....5....6....7....8....9....10
   LOW   HIGH

5. Psychosis evident during treatment this report period

   1....2....3....4....5....6....7....8....9....10
   LOW   HIGH

SYMPTOM LEVEL SCORE (sum of 1 through 5)
(5-10 = low, 11-20 = mild, 21-30 = moderate, 31=40 = high, 41-50 = severe)

SCORE_____

6. Resolution of precipitating problems with this report this period

   1....2....3....4....5....6....7....8....9....10
   LOW   HIGH

7. Reported school/work performance during this report period

   1....2....3....4....5....6....7....8....9....10
   LOW   HIGH

8. Level of adequate ADLs during this report period

   1....2....3....4....5....6....7....8....9....10
   LOW   HIGH

9. Appropriateness of relationships with staff this report period

   1....2....3....4....5....6....7....8....9....10
   LOW   HIGH

10. Appropriate relationships with residents this report period

   1....2....3....4....5....6....7....8....9....10
   LOW   HIGH

LEVEL OF FUNCTIONING SCORE (sum of 6 through 10)
(5-10 = inadequate, 11-20 = poor, 21-30 = average, 31-40 = good, 41-50 = excellent)

SCORE_____

11. Compliance with treatment focus established by therapist

   1....2....3....4....5....6....7....8....9....10
   LOW   HIGH

12. Responsiveness to therapist's reframes of problems

   1....2....3....4....5....6....7....8....9....10
   LOW   HIGH

VISUAL 6.5 *(continued)*

13. Acceptance of intervention efforts by therapist	1....2....3....4....5....6....7....8....9....10 LOW HIGH
14. Insight and understanding of issues leading to placement	1....2....3....4....5....6....7....8....9....10 LOW HIGH
USE OF THERAPY SCORE (sum of 11 through 15) (5-10 = inadequate, 11-20 = poor, 21-30 = average, 31-40 = high, 41-50 = excellent)	SCORE_____

Court Appearance and Diagnosis

Increasingly, social workers are being required to give court testimony related to the diagnoses they perform and the treatment plans they devise. In many instances social workers are ill prepared to testify in court. This is especially true in relation to the act of diagnosis. Lawyers are becoming more familiar with the DSM system and can ask more technical questions about diagnosis than has been the case in the past. The supervisor can be helpful to the supervisee who is faced with giving court testimony related to diagnosis by actually preparing the practitioner through role-play of testimony. In some cases it may be possible to have the attorney who is involved in the case prepare the clinician for testifying.

There are several pointers to give the practitioner. Testimony related to diagnosis goes through a process in the courtroom. If the practitioner is aware of this general process, then he or she can be prepared for and anticipate each step.

The first step is qualifying as an expert witness through review of the practitioner's credentials. It is helpful for the practitioner to have a written summary of his or her credentials to provide to the attorneys and the court prior to testimony. The summary should contain the practitioner's name, current position, education and degrees, credentials (licenses, certifications, etc.), consultantships, number of times qualified as an expert witness, past experience, publications, research experience, and specialized training. The statement should be limited to one typed page. If too much detail is included, the practitioner runs the risk of having items questioned. The practitioner should have a copy of this summary in front of him or her when stating the credentials for the court, if the attorneys will allow it. . . . A written summary can help defend against memory lapses by the clinician, but a good attorney can work from his or her copy to assist with memory lapses if the clinician cannot keep one with him or her. Some attorneys will ask that the clinician not use such a list to testify from. It is surprising how many times clinicians forget their experience and credentials when not accustomed to giving testimony. A written summary can help defend against memory lapses by the clinician, but a good attorney can work from his or her copy to assist with memory lapses if the clinician cannot keep one with him or her.

Step two often involves questions about the practitioner's knowledge of the DSM system and manual. The clinician should always have a copy of the manual with him or her while giving testimony. Attorneys may ask specific questions about different disorders or about organization, structure, or meaning of different aspects of the manual. For example, a common question is, "What is the difference between Axis I and Axis II?" It is best to give answers that are technically accurate, but in layman's terms. A good response to this question is, "Axis I deals with disorders that have acute onset, are made up of symptoms that can occur in reaction to external factors, and are amiable to treatment, while Axis II covers disorders that are the result of the developmental process, are a part of the person's total character and functioning, are enduring, and are less responsive to treatment generally." This is sufficient to clarify the distinction without being too technical. If an attorney asks a specific question about the manual, the clinician should ask the court for permission to refer to the manual and ask the attorney to be specific about what is being asked.

Step three will be the practitioner's statement of the diagnosis. Any challenge about the practitioner's qualifications to make a diagnosis should be left to the attorneys to argue. However, the clinician should alert the attorney with whom he or she is working about differences in the use of terminology, for example, using *diagnostic impression* rather than *diagnosis*. This sometimes can get beyond the challenge to the practitioner's qualifications to do "a diagnosis," and the court interpretation of this can vary from jurisdiction to jurisdiction. The diagnosis given should come from a written report, and the clinician should be prepared to state how he or she arrived at the diagnosis. This will include identification of specific symptoms and behaviors.

Step four, depending on the nature of the case, can be the connection between the clinician's treatment approach and the diagnosis. This can vary depending on whether the clinician has been required to testify as an expert who performed an evaluation of the person at the request of someone else or is testifying as the person who has been providing ongoing treatment. Again, the practitioner should work from notes to explain how the intervention was focused on the diagnosis, including the treatment process, how progress was measured, and presentation of precise documentation of actions and behaviors of the therapist. It is helpful to distinguish statements of the client, observations of the therapist, and interpretations made by the therapist.

In general, the practitioner should answer questions directly; not volunteer information; not attempt to be humorous; speak clearly, distinctly, and loudly; look at the attorney when he or she asks questions; look at the judge or the jury when answering; and pause before answering to give the attorneys time to object. It is easy to become confused about whether to answer when the judge sustains or overrules an objection. The practitioner should try to remember that "sustained" means to be silent and "overruled" means to give an oral response. These are general rules, and the clinician should follow the advice of attorneys in specific cases. In the absence of any guidance from the attorneys involved, the clinician should try to apply these rules.

Planning Successful Intervention

Models of planning for and assessment of successful intervention strategies through supervision have not been developed. The following guidelines can be helpful in creating treatment plans and articulating successful intervention:

1. An intervention is identified by the practitioner that can be understood by the client.
2. An identifiable connection exists between the problem and the intervention.
3. The practitioner and client can implement the intervention with reasonable effort.
4. The practitioner, supervisor, and client can identify possible outcomes of the intervention in advance of its implementation.
5. The client has an identifiable reason or motivation to comply with the intervention.
6. An alternate intervention can be identified by the practitioner.
7. The possible outcomes (intended and unintended, positive and negative) of the intervention can be observed and measured.

TREATMENT PATTERNS

In supervision it is important to focus on patterns that occur in the treatment. It is only through identifying patterns that the supervisor and practitioner can be confident that they have a comprehensive grasp of the client and his or her life situation and problem. Focusing on isolated behaviors of the client can lead the treatment astray and cause it to become fragmented and frustrating. Four forms of patterns in the patient can be identified and interrelated:

1. Patterns of personality or behavior
2. Patterns of life events and interaction

3. Patterns of interaction during a single treatment session
4. Patterns of the treatment process

MECHANICS OF THERAPY TECHNIQUE

The supervisor who wants to learn the mechanics of how to teach therapy technique to practitioners must consider several factors. First, techniques cannot be taught in isolation or without regard to the total therapeutic process. Techniques are never entities in and of themselves. A technique taught as a self-contained activity will leave the practitioner holding the bag interactionally once it is introduced or used in the treatment.

Second, techniques must be identified and taught as a series of actions so that the process of beginning with a client includes developing techniques for setting up the initial session, greeting the client, putting the client at ease, discussing fees, explaining how treatment works, gathering information, helping the client verbalize difficult material, formulating a diagnosis, setting priorities for problems, and mutually establishing treatment goals. Techniques for accomplishing these tasks can be taught and practiced individually, but this should be done within the context of initiating the treatment process.

Third, a series of techniques should be arranged from the simple to the complex. It is difficult to identify the ordering of techniques because certain techniques will be difficult for some practitioners and quite easy for others, depending on their level of experience, training, self-awareness, and emotional orientation.

In discussing practice skill, most practitioners and supervisors give descriptions of process rather than talk about skills developed and used in connection with behavior that occurred in the situation. This is what Haley refers to when stating that "the therapeutic process is such that one cannot go directly from the problem at the beginning to the cure at the end" (Haley, 1976:121). Skill is more than description of practice; it is more than saying that the patient did better as the result of the techniques used or the skills applied. The supervisor can be the instrument through which the practitioner develops awareness of skills he or she possesses or needs to develop.

Finally, teaching therapeutic technique can be like the job of a swimming instructor teaching small children. The supervisor who wants to learn how to teach technique should observe this process of teaching swimming. The instructor demonstrates basic arm strokes, leg action, and head movement individually out of the water, and then each activity is demonstrated and practiced individually in the water. Head movement and arm strokes are practiced while the learner walks in shallow water. Leg kick is practiced using a kickboard for buoyancy. In many respects, the kickboard is to swimming instruction what audiovisual teaching aids are to supervision. The students then put all these strokes together while the instructor observes them from in the pool and outside and offers comments about incorrect use of movements. Sometimes the instructor will swim alongside the students and point out misapplications. Then the students practice, practice, practice.

OVERCOMING DIFFICULTY

There are many parallels between what the swimming instructor does and what the supervisor needs to do to teach a series of techniques for mastery of an intervention strategy. The supervisor can learn much about style and technique from observing how technique is taught in other disciplines. Musical instruction, dancing classes, drama rehearsals, painting classes, and baseball and football clinics are common learning situations that can be helpful to the social work supervisor in treatment-oriented settings.

Any technique worthy of the term can be described and explained. More effort needs to be devoted to describing and labeling techniques that are in use. Focus needs to be placed on why a particular technique is used, how it is used, what the response is, and the outcome of its application.

If practitioners use any technique in treatment long enough, it will eventually backfire on them. Because of this, supervision should emphasize developing alternative strategies in advance.

Practitioners can go sailing along in a treatment session with their style and technique serving them effectively, but then they enter a difficult interactional sequence that is sufficient to get them completely out of style and cause them to lose sight and command of their most reliable techniques. When this occurs, practitioners withdraw verbally, ask questions that are not relevant, or become supportive of the client regardless of the appropriateness of such support. If such sequences can be identified and explored openly in supervision, the practitioner can be helped to develop strategies for overcoming such situations rapidly and can readjust more quickly.

Therapy sessions that have been moving toward a productive outcome can be totally altered and flounder when practitioners do not work their way out of such setbacks. This pattern has potential for occurring as the number of clients in the treatment increases. Cotherapy activity is one good safeguard against this pattern.

Clients can resist change and consciously and unconsciously attempt to thwart the worker. The practitioner is at a knowledge disadvantage when treatment begins because the client has more knowledge of his or her problems, feelings, concerns, and conflicts than the practitioner who learns only what the client chooses to reveal. This remains the case throughout treatment. Thus, the supervisor should evaluate with the practitioner the availability of corroborative sources of information to verify the accuracy of client views. At the point when powerful interventions are taking place, the client will resist with strategies equal to the practitioner's best interventive efforts. The practitioner frequently will underestimate the power of the client to resist. The practitioner's reluctance to recognize the client's pattern of efforts to maintain dysfunctional behavior can slow the progress of treatment.

When practitioners are distracted by difficult material, discussion of what happened, why it happened, and how it can be prevented in the future can take many forms, and creative suggestions are limited by only the practitioner's and supervisor's ability to dissect the material. Several general guidelines can be offered to practitioners when they sense that their style is shifting or being disrupted due to discomfort or overwhelming content:

1. Stop the interaction and focus on analyzing the meaning of the most recent interaction.
2. Withdraw temporarily and think of an alternate way to return to the difficult content. This should be accomplished fairly quickly. The therapist must develop skill at thinking fast.
3. Avoid admitting to feeling uncomfortable or overwhelmed. This can diminish trust in the therapist or reinforce the patient's dysfunctional pattern in the treatment. It is better to attempt to relate to the possibility that the patient is uncomfortable or that the focus of the interaction is upsetting.

Case Exercise:
The Case of Heartha Viands

You are the clinical supervisor for a twenty-six-year-old pregnant therapist, who was called to the local hospital to arrange shelter care for a seventy-nine-year-old woman, who was brought there after her eighty-three-year-old husband attacked her with a knife while she was preparing dinner. The therapist works for a family crisis resource center, and you are her supervisor. The worker arranged the shelter placement, transported the woman to the shelter, and conducted an intake interview with her at the shelter. The woman stated that her husband had never attacked her during forty years of marriage, but six months ago he fell down the cellar steps. She stated that since that time he has become violent and has hit her and threatened her many times. The husband was charged by the police and then allowed to return home. The woman was very anxious and wanted to return home herself. She feels she needs to care for her husband who, she reported, "gets confused at times." She stated that she has one daughter who is married and has children. The daughter lives in a town seventy miles away from the client's home. The client stated she does not want to bother her daughter with "this thing because she is very busy." The worker is "nervous" about this case because she has never handled a spouse abuse case for a woman this old. She states to you that the woman "reminds me of my grandmother." The worker does not know how to proceed in this case. She feels that she does not want to keep the woman in the shelter against her will; at the same time, she is concerned about the woman returning home.

(1) As the supervisor, what areas would you address with this therapist? (2) How would you deal with the worker's identification with the client as being like her grandmother? (3) What factors would you expect the worker to consider in assessing the possibility of the client returning home?

TECHNICAL DIFFICULTY

Supervisors who use technical strategies as part of their supervisory style can experience *technical difficulty,* and this is to be expected. At times the strategies they use fail to work or are completely ineffective. This should not immobilize the supervisor. When good supervisors encounter such difficulty, they shift to another strategy and continue to shift techniques until they reach their objective.

Practitioners are prevented from accomplishing goals or applying techniques through interventions if they are unable to carry them out practically or to control the treatment. For example, a practitioner cannot do intensive intervention with the family of a terminal cancer patient if the practitioner works on an open cancer ward and has no private office to interview the family. The good technician will be sensitive to this kind of issue.

The "if-then" proposition is a good linguistic and interactional technique to use in approaching much case material explored in supervision, especially when technical difficulty is encountered. Statements should take this form: "If the client is this way, then this technique should result in . . ."

Every statement of the practitioner should be well thought out and incisive. Each comment should elicit more than one possible response. The practitioner, like the good writer, should be precise, to stimulate a variety of responses. As Thomas Wolfe said of Hemingway, he "says one thing and suggests ten more."

Supervision of cases on a weekly basis provides continuity and follow-up of specific techniques and is well suited to individual supervision; cases reviewed only periodically or during one session are better suited to theoretical and conceptual learning, and this can be better achieved in group supervision.

QUESTIONING TECHNIQUE

Questioning is one of the chief techniques supervisors use to help practitioners reflect about their own work. Limited attention has been devoted to the use of questioning in supervision. When and how a question is asked can be one of the most valuable forms of interaction used in supervision. Supervisors attempting to evaluate their questioning technique should review tapes of supervisory sessions and evaluate their style of questioning on the basis of the following guidelines:

1. Questioning is one of the best techniques the supervisor has available to help practitioners articulate knowledge (both manifest and latent) of cases.

2. Questions should be simply stated, clear, and concise. The supervisor should avoid prefacing a question with a lengthy introductory statement. Good questions stand on their own.

3. Questions should be general in nature, but the practitioner's answer should be specific. This should be a basic rule of the questioning that is made clear to the supervisee. A general question avoids locking the practitioner into a predetermined perspective held by the supervisor. A general question allows the practitioner to answer in one of several ways, usually in relation to a specific aspect of the case.

4. A general question that is answered in a general way should be repeated. The supervisor can repeat and rephrase the question again and again until a mutually agreed upon response is achieved.

5. Questions related to diagnostic understanding should be more specific than those related to treatment strategies and techniques. Diagnostic questioning will require a series of specific queries that will result in a generalization or conclusion about the case. A treatment-oriented question should be general and singular, resulting in a series of answers that will reveal various techniques or strategies.

6. When the supervisor is not certain that the practitioner has adequate knowledge of the case (diagnosis) to make treatment decisions, the supervisor needs to move from general to specific questions. If the practitioner demonstrates lack of knowledge, it is appropriate to delay discussion of the case until the practitioner becomes familiar with the case. Too often supervisors pursue cases for which adequate information is not available, and this can lead to idle speculation, misguided treatment, and poor learning. Adequate information is important because the more the practitioner knows about the case, the less likely it is that errors in treatment will occur.

7. When general supervisory questions result in answers that reveal thorough knowledge of the case, the supervisor can move to questions related to treatment and intervention strategies. If diagnostic questions repeatedly reveal lack of knowledge of cases, the supervisor needs to shift the focus of the supervision temporarily to deal with problems the practitioner is having in grasping the dynamics of cases. Excuses or substitution of speculation for lack of knowledge of cases is unproductive in supervision.

Case Exercise:
The Case of Martha Shepherd

Martha Shepherd is one of your supervisees at a local women's shelter. In a regular supervision session, Martha asks you about a case in which she is counseling a twenty-four-year-old woman. The woman has been abused by her boyfriend in the past. The boyfriend is not currently physically abusing her, but he regularly abuses her dog. Martha is an animal lover, and she is very upset. She inquires whether you would support her desire to report the man to the local SPCA. She believes reports to the SPCA are accepted anonymously. Martha has not discussed this with her client.

What questions would you ask Martha in the process of making a supervisory decision in this situation?

CONTRACTING AS A TECHNIQUE

Contracting in clinical settings was in vogue during the 1980s, and this carried over into supervision to the point that most schools of social work require student-field instructor contracts, and some agencies require contracts for professional-level supervision. There has been emphasis on the procedures in negotiating supervisory contracts (Wijnberg and Schwartz, 1977; Munson, 1993a). The contracting literature has not taken into account the power difference in the supervisory relationship that places limits on the ability of the supervisee to negotiate a contract. Any structure, technique, or issue the supervisee wishes to negotiate must always be judged in advance by the supervisor as to whether it is essential to learning and, therefore, nonnegotiable. Under these circumstances, anything that is deemed nonessential to learning is negotiable, but any item that falls into this category can be easily perceived by the supervisee as unimportant. It is difficult for a supervisee to take such a contract negotiation seriously.

The advocates of contracting in supervision have not provided guidelines regarding what to do when conditions of the contract are not followed. If contracts are to have any value, they must be honored. Supervisors must confront supervisees who do not meet conditions of contracts, or they risk loss of authority and respect. The situation is more complex when supervisors do not live up to the contracts. Most supervisees feel uncomfortable confronting supervisors about such lapses. For this reason, supervisees regard contracts as rather one-sided documents. Given these problems, it is good to include in the contract what procedures can be used if either party does not meet the conditions of the contract. Contracts should be general and limited to short periods. Six months or one year is an appropriate time period.

Contracts in clinical settings should include, at minimum, reference to the following:

1. *Timing element.* This section should include items such as frequency of supervision, length of sessions, and duration of supervision process.
2. *Learning structure.* This would include any learning structures the supervisor may use, such as joint interviews, audiovisual techniques, consultants, continuing education, etc.
3. *Supervision structure.* This section would include the type of supervision to be used, such as individual, group, or a combination. If mentoring is used or rotation through different agency units or services is required, then this should be documented and lines of authority made clear to the supervisee.
4. *Agency conformity.* Items such as dress codes, listing of phone numbers, licensing requirements, work hours, and holidays should be covered in this section.
5. *Special conditions.* These are requirements that are unique to the setting, such as doing DSM diagnosis, being familiar with medications, providing legal testimony, or any activity for which the practitioner lacks training or familiarity. In such cases the contract should state how the agency expects the practitioner to acquire the knowledge and skill required.

READING AS A TECHNIQUE

Reading books is rarely associated with supervision. Supervision has always been perceived as highly personalized teaching with a "hands-on" and "learning by doing" approach. Reading about practice has been reserved for the abstract classroom aspects of learning. Even continuing education programs have focused mostly on practical, rather than "bookish," learning. Supervisors rarely use books in supervision and express reservations about trying it. With supportive discussion, and suggested techniques for how to begin, the resistance subsides. This reluctance is mainly due to lack of assistance and encouragement in using this as a teaching method.

Some supervisors, when discussing their own development as practitioners, comment on cherished and truly integrative learning resulting from books that their supervisors had suggested they read. Passages, concepts, and ideas from some of these books still guide their clinical and supervision practice at different times. One supervisor commented:

> I draw on my reading that my supervisor suggested. It is not extensive, a few very essential books and articles. I cannot say I remember or use any of the textbooks from my classroom days. I cannot recall any of the reading my supervisor suggested turning out to be a negative. I realize now the supervisor reading assignments were embedded in and

grew out of the supervisor's own practice. For example, Sidney Jouard's *The Transparent Self* and *Disclosing Man to Himself* are two books my supervisor introduced me to that deepened and expanded my learning and continue to influence my understanding. Another book I go back to often is Wilhelm Reich's *Listen, Little Man.* This is a book about freedom, oppression, and authority that can promote understanding of practice, clients, and the inherent conflicts supervision produces. Brief, clearly written books can be the most helpful and memorable. The books do not have to be serious to make a somber point. This is the case with Greenburg and Jacobs' *How to Make Yourself Miserable,* which can be recommend to supervisees and to clients. Book suggestions can be customized to the individual.

Supervisors should suggest that supervisees read books to supplement their learning. If supervisors promote reading as a learning method, supervisees will come to associate reading with their own self-development long after teachers, supervisors, and educational programs have become a fond memory. Practice, even in an agency, can be a very lonesome endeavor. Although colleagues and continuing education programs can be a rich source of stimulation and learning, the act of reading, discovering commonalities with others' experience, and applying the techniques and thoughts of others to your own practice can be the most rewarding and comforting form of growth.

A good feature of reading as a supervisory technique is that it does not require a lot of formal mastery of educational methods or techniques. It emerges out of the supervisor's past or present reading experience. There does have to be a logical connection between the circumstances surrounding the supervision and the books the supervisor suggests, as well as follow-up of connections made between the reading and the supervision or practice dynamics. This is essentially all a supervisor has to do. Of course, there are many variations on the theme. Supervisor-assigned reading can stimulate interaction and reciprocal exchanges in supervision. The supervisor can use readings as a basis for follow-up discussion in supervision. In response to supervisor-suggested reading, a supervisee can mention other texts with which the supervisor may be unfamiliar. This allows the supervisee input in the supervisory process and contributes to the supervision being a genuine reciprocal process.

This form of learning is available to us at all times. It is only as far away as the nearest bookshelf. Learning through reading does not have to wait until the next supervisory or consultation appointment, the weekly staff meeting, or the continuing education workshop next month. This form of learning is truly convenient and completely under the control of the practitioner. By promoting reading in supervision, the supervisor can genuinely contribute to giving rise to the "self-directed" practitioner who has a research orientation to practice.

This form of learning is not the passive learning of the traditional model utilized in training programs and continuing education programs. We have so ritualized the teacher-student model that self-induced learning is foreign to and difficult for many practitioners. This is not the fault of the practitioner. It is a systemic problem. For example, licensing and certification bodies lack provisions for granting continuing education credits for reading, but they are beginning to allow such credits. The difficult lies in monitoring such learning. The irony is that the most significant learning can stem from experiences that cannot be monitored by organizations and supervisors. Supervisors should work to keep the supervisees from becoming too dependent on externally monitored learning. Supervisors can assist in limiting overdependence through encouraging supervisees to use reading to enhance learning.

LATENT SUPERVISION

Supervisors must be aware of and take into account in their supervisory interactions forms of what the author refers to as "latent supervision." Latent supervision refers to any aspect of the supervision in which the supervisor makes decisions or judgments about the practitioner's work in which the practitioner has no say, or of which he or she is unaware. This occurs, for example, when the supervisor reviews the case summaries or tapes of the practitioner's work. Another example is when the supervisor discusses one of the practitioner's cases with another clinician or another supervisor. Although such activity can be beneficial to the practitioner under supervision, in the long run, it can also lead the supervisor to unsubstantiated and unjustified evaluations of the practitioner and his or her work. In any judgment or evaluation of a supervisee's practice, the supervisor should ensure that the supervisee has had a fair opportunity to defend the action taken in the case or to document its basis.

A subtle form of latent supervision occurs when the supervisor holds a particular philosophical or theoretical perspective that the practitioner finds alien. In this situation, the supervisor can indirectly and unknowingly foster discussion in a way that will force the practitioner to present cases from the supervisor's preferred orientation. In some instances, simply the choice of cases the supervisor asks the practitioner to present in supervision can shape the nature of the supervision.

To promote supervisee creativity, flexibility, and adaptability, supervisors need to monitor their own actions to ensure that practitioners are not being "pushed" or "pulled" into viewing their work in a manner not of their own choosing. Practitioners at times will be aware of such latent supervision without the supervisors recognizing that this form of suggestion is taking place.

Supervisees who experience discomfort about raising such issues with their supervisors will develop a sense of frustration and adjust their activity in supervisory sessions by presenting material in a framework that the supervisors find pleasing. When this occurs, the supervision becomes a game for the practitioner and the focus shifts from genuine learning to the secondary purpose of developing congruence with the supervisor's style. By encouraging open discussion of the supervisor's and the practitioner's respective orientations, and by identifying points at which these orientations converge and diverge, this form of latent supervision can be decreased. This is an important point because, as was discussed in Chapter 5, supervisors develop their own styles (reaction) in supervision as a response to their supervisors' styles.

SUPERVISOR RESISTANCE

In the author's research, supervisors have reported times when they have tended to resist teaching what the young, struggling practitioners need to know. This is a withholding of knowledge, an unwillingness to share one's style, techniques, and strategies. Clinical supervisors shared similar feelings about this phenomenon, but they were unable to offer much help in identifying the reasons for this vague reluctance in teaching. This withholding occurs more in group than in individual supervision and is experienced mostly just after a supervisory session when the supervisor is reflecting on a difficult case or a clinical process with which the supervisee and supervisor were struggling. At these times, supervisors reported awareness of much information that could have been helpful but that was not shared with their supervisees. Sometimes this reluctance occurs during the supervisory session. Even though supervisors indicate awareness of this pattern, it can happen repeatedly. Grotjahn hinted at this reluctance: "I have had a terrible time revealing group interaction and the private life of the group and its members. It feels like being disloyal to one's own family" (1977:6).

It appears this process occurs because the supervisor recognizes the complexity of the situation, and the time and energy required to make it understandable and useful to the supervisee would be greater than the supervisor is willing to invest at the time. Rather than attempting to explain, understand, or overcome this supervisory weakness, the supervisor can compensate for it by making detailed notes about the material and bringing the information to the supervisee at the beginning of the next session. The supervisor can then admit the lapse to the supervisee, explain what happened, and present the new information. This strategy can lead the supervisee to share a parallel process that occurs in his or her therapeutic work. The strategy can serve as a model for developing a similar technique for the supervisee to use in his or her practice when lapses occur with clients. By admitting the lapses to the supervisee and sharing reflections about the case material that occurred outside the supervision, the supervisor communicates to the supervisee that the supervision is taken seriously, and that thought is given to the process outside the supervisory hour.

GUIDELINES

As a summary set of guidelines for the supervisor to keep in mind in relation to techniques used in supervision, the following elements of good supervision and methods to encourage learning in supervision are provided.

Elements of Good Supervision

1. Supervision should be based on the needs of the practitioner.
2. Supervision should be based on the premise of education for what to do.
3. Stand for and manifest commitment to good practice. Practitioners have difficulty committing themselves to something to which the supervisor is not committed.
4. Give answers when the situation demands it.
5. Authority should be de-emphasized rather than explicated.
6. Avoid relying on nonverbal communication. *Spell it out!*
7. Limit teaching through analogies or stories.
8. Use case material as a teaching tool, not as a threat.
9. Adequate interaction with the supervisor is a key to practitioner unity and understanding.

Techniques to Encourage Learning in Supervision

1. Allow the practitioner to select a portion of the case material that is presented.
2. Encourage practitioner self-development of learning material.
3. Focus on skills in which the practitioner is strong, and then move to weaknesses.
4. Give recognition to the practitioner for overcoming weaknesses.
5. Remove technical obstacles to practice and supervision.
6. Develop strategies to simplify complex material.
7. Use varied learning techniques.
8. Encourage lively discussion.
9. Set goals.
10. Use positive control.
11. Stress the enjoyment of doing treatment.

Technique and Best Practices

The following recommendations are made for implementation by supervisors to ensure that the quality standards and guidelines for supervision identified in this chapter are applied. Supervisors using a standards-of-practice model should implement these guidelines in applying techniques in supervision:

1. Supervise practitioners only for tasks and functions the supervisors have performed.
2. Have documented professional training in the areas supervision is provided.
3. Have documented formal training in supervision before assuming a supervisory position. On-the-job training should not be counted as sufficient supervisory training.
4. Be thoroughly knowledgeable regarding the code or codes of ethics the supervisor and supervisees are functioning under and ensure that supervisees have read and understand the code(s).
5. Ensure that the supervisees understand the role of advocacy and are able to identify when the need for client advocacy exists.
6. Be knowledgeable about and monitor stress reactions in supervisees.
7. Identify agency/organization policy and professional organizational ethical conflicts and call them to the attention of supervisees, employing organizations, and professional organizations.
8. Have written risk management policies for supervisees.
9. Have written requirements for intake procedures, diagnostic formats, assessment and evaluations criteria, and informed consent policies for clients.
10. Be knowledgeable about screening measures and familiar with basic standardized tests and measures relevant to populations served.
11. Have clear criteria for written treatment plans and foster supervisee understanding that treatment plans are related to diagnosis and initial assessment.
12. Have clear policies regarding the use of techniques during intervention. Supervisees should be able to explain, justify, and document existing research for techniques that are used.
13. Have clear criteria for evaluation of intervention that is applied equally to all supervisees.
14. Have clear protocols for termination with clients under differing circumstances (e.g., successful completion of intervention, loss of funding, client failure to pay, client failure to keep appointments, departure of the social worker).

15. Require supervisees to be aware of practice standards of other disciplines that may be relevant to the supervisees' practice (e.g., those of the American Psychiatric Association, American Psychological Association, and American Association of Marriage and Family Therapy).
16. Be aware of the role of culture, race, ethnicity, lifestyle, preferences, and vulnerability in relation to clients and practitioners and monitor intervention to ensure that all practitioners and clients are treated with fairness and equality.

Case Exercise:
The Case of Helen

Helen received her MSW twenty years ago, and after graduation she spent the next fifteen years raising three children. During this time the family moved several times because of the husband's occupation as a military officer. When all of Helen's children were grown and gone from home, she reentered practice in 1998 in a public child and adolescent foster care program that serves primarily abused children and adolescents. Helen is overwhelmed. She is shocked by the beliefs, experiences, and language of the children and their families. She is having difficulty mastering the DSM-IV-TR and resists giving cases a diagnosis as a part of the intake evaluation required by the agency. She has difficulty doing systematic intervention and struggles with developing intervention plans. Helen is likable and asks many questions. Many times she seems to forget the suggestions various staff offer her and has trouble applying the concepts learned in one case to other cases. You are assigned to be her supervisor. Staff, and Helen herself, have become frustrated with these limitations but are tolerant because she is so likable. Though more experienced, you are younger than she is and you feel intimidated.

(1) How would you assist Helen to become reoriented to practice? (2) How would you assist Helen in mastering doing DSM-IV-TR diagnosis? (3) How would you approach Helen regarding her forgetfulness?

Case Exercise:
The Case of Calgare

You are Jack's supervisor in a mental health clinic, and a fifteen-year-old female named Calgare has been referred to Jack by a school counselor because of failing grades and anxiety about boys who "stalk" her. Calgare has experienced a sudden onset of symptoms. She recently moved from Florida to Maryland with her twenty-year-old brother, her mother, and the mother's live-in male companion. Calgare is failing all of her subjects. She went to the school counselor and told him during a series of interviews that a boy her age was "after her" and had made "a crazy statement about giving me some jelly beans to come to his house with him." She claimed that two older men were "stalking" her and a friend when they went to a store after school to get soda. She observed these two men following her in a pickup truck over several days. The counselor notified the police, and they interviewed Calgare at the school, but no action was taken.

Calgare is afraid to go home from school and stays at school as late as she can. She has trouble going to sleep at night during the week but sleeps all day on weekends. Calgare said she would jump out of her second-story bedroom window if anyone came into the house after her. She knows she can do this because she has jumped out the window before. Calgare does not like one of her teachers, who is very tall, is loud, and "stands over my shoulder watching me work, and this gives me the creeps." Calgare also said that her brother is about to enter prison for car theft.

Jack is a beginning social worker who graduated from an MSW program six months ago. He is very interested in this case and wants to help Calgare but does not know "where to begin."

(1) How would you initiate supervision with Jack on this case? (2) What recommendations would you have for Jack regarding needed information about Calgare and her family as part of the initial assessment? (3) What would you view as essential elements of a treatment plan for Calgare?

SUGGESTED READINGS

Haley, J. (1996). *Learning and Teaching Therapy.* New York: Guilford.
  Covers technique in therapy and supervision. Haley uses examples from his own supervision by Milton Erickson.

Kadushin, A. (1992). *Supervision in Social Work.* New York: Columbia University Press.
  Overview of basic social work supervision with specific techniques.

Watkins, C. E. (ed.) (1997). *Handbook of Psychotherapy Supervision.* New York: Wiley.
  A collection of articles on a broad range of supervision topics. Can serve as a reference book for the supervisor.

The difficulty in elaborating this intuitive sense of authority is the idea of strength on which it is based. I have never known a bad or inept musician who managed to preserve . . . authority over an orchestra for very long.

Richard Sennett
Authority

The powerful lobbyists who represent professional organizations have persuaded legislators that a therapist must be licensed by them to earn an income . . . . So now the law requires therapists to listen to supervisors if they are ever going to make a living.

Jay Haley
Learning and Teaching Therapy

Chapter 7

The Role of Authority and Structure

This chapter covers the basic concept of authority and how it relates to the supervisory process, as well as its role as an inherent part of organizations. The interactional manifestations of authority are explored along with the ways in which authority orientations vary with respect to different supervision structures. Guidelines are provided for appropriate use of individual and group supervisory structures.

INTRODUCTION

The quote from Sennett's excellent study of authority epitomizes the essence of what supervisors must keep in mind as they embark on the supervision process: *never attempt to direct the work of others when you are not good at doing that work yourself.* This rule is the basis of this chapter.

Authority has always been troublesome. Perhaps, as has been observed, Don Quixote expressed a universal desire with the words, "I would have nobody to control me, I would be absolute" (Marcus and Marcus, 1972:234). But at the same time, Don Quixote was depicted as a man who had "lost the Use of his Reason" (Cervantes, 1950/1605:3). Freud expressed the other side of this desire when he wrote, "The great majority of people have a strong need for authority which they can admire, to which they can submit, and which dominates and sometimes even ill-treats them" (Freud, 1967/1939:139-140).

Balancing these two opposing desires is a dilemma that is a part of the human condition. Clinicians, in their lives and in their supervision, have not been spared this dilemma. Practitioners and their supervisors overtly and covertly grapple with independence and accountability issues daily in practice and supervision. The personal and professional struggle with authority has been described in the literature by Endress (1981).

Endress points out that "exhorting a beginner to model himself after the experts can prove to be more discouraging than motivating" (1981:305). Instead, workers must be helped to discover a style and method of their own. Because the authority issues were handled in a sensitive manner and Endress had an effective role model, she evolved a different perspective:

> Because I am not out to prove I am the best, I can be more relaxed with my clients, listen to them more effectively, and give of myself in a way that encourages them also to give of themselves. (1981:308)

That a student has to point this out is indicative that supervisors have forgotten something over the years. In 1929, the same statement about the idea to "let learn" was apparent:

> Students who are given responsibility as an opportunity for them to learn will themselves provide teachers with plenty of opportunity to teach. We believe it to be true that students learn more from teaching which they have sought because of a consciousness of need than from any offered by a teacher because he knows something which he thinks the students ought to know. (Lee and Kenworthy, 1929:187)

ORGANIZATIONS AND AUTHORITY

The growth of organizations and the formalization of the profession of social work have led to the dilemma of the modern-day practitioner as a creature of organizations. The nature of authority and autonomy have evolved through Durkheim's belief that the division of labor would not destroy the notion that "to be a person is to be an autonomous source of action" (Durkheim, 1933:403), and through Weber's early description, as organizations emerged:

> [T]he principles of office hierarchy and of levels of graded authority mean a firmly ordered system of super- and subordination in which there is a supervision of the lower office by the higher ones . . . [but] hierarchical subordination . . . does not mean that the "higher" authority is simply authorized to take over the business of the "lower." (Schuler et al., 1971:348-349)

William Whyte describes the "social ethic" that defines the struggle of the individual for autonomy in organizations through a summary that fits professionals in organizations:

> If individualism involves following one's destiny as one's own conscience directs, it must for most of us be a realized destiny, and a sensible awareness of the rules of the game can be a condition of individualism as well as a constraint upon it. . . . I speak of individualism WITHIN organization life. . . . Every decision he faces on the problem of the individual versus authority is something of a dilemma. . . . We do need to know how to cooperate with The Organization but, more than ever, so do we need to know how to resist it. . . . Organization has been made by man; it can be changed by man. (1956:3-14)

Professionals have come a long way since Don Quixote, and this chapter deals in part with ways of changing the organization with respect to supervision of professional practice so that authority and autonomy become less of a dilemma. Supervisors tend to overlook authority issues until they become seriously problematic, but authority is increasing in organizations rather than decreasing. In addition to all the traditional areas in which authority is exercised most, such as record keeping, statistical reporting, work hours, caseload size and type, and case management, there is increasing authority associated with peer review, utilization review, accreditation, and third-party payers (Rock, 1990:29; Munson, 1980a, 1996b). This increased control is occurring at a time when the profession is again raising concern about its degree of professionalism because autonomy is limited and shrinking (Veeder, 1990:33; Munson, 1998). This requires supervisors to be skilled at dealing with authority issues and comfortable with their own degree of authority and autonomy.

AUTHORITY AND SUPERVISION

Supervision is the arena in which a great deal of the knowledge regarding the limits of and creative capabilities in practice are worked out. The definitions of professionalism associated with practice come from externals, such as status, esoteric training and knowledge, sanction through licensing, remuneration, and professional organizations. Little attention has been focused on the interactions that constitute professional behavior among participants within the professional group. Elements of this aspect of professionalism can be identified and articulated through the exercising of authority in supervision.

Authority issues repeatedly have been overlooked and pushed into the background in the social work literature and in actual practice of supervision. In some instances, group supervision (Munson, 1976) and peer group supervision (Hamlin and Timberlake, 1982) have been used to sidestep authority issues, but these issues remain and can erupt in these forms of supervision (Hamlin and Timberlake, 1982:87). Supervisors must remember that they have power by virtue of their position; therefore, they do not have to work as hard to establish the supervisory relationship as do supervisees. Some hold that anxiety in the supervisee grows out of fear of emotional dependence on the supervisor. Supervisee anxiety can just as easily grow out of lack of mechanisms to cope with problems encountered in practice. In general, the use of authority in supervision of clinical social work practice should recognize the role of authority and its limits while placing emphasis on the function of creativity in practice.

Hughes epitomized the issue of authority in supervision when he asked, "What orders does one accept from an employer, especially one . . . whose interests may not always be those of the professional and his client?" (1963:658). The problem of control in conjunction with the teaching and evaluation functions in supervision of professional practice leads to a number of important questions: What are the limits of control in teaching and evaluation through supervision? What are the best means of carrying out the teaching and evaluation function in relation to professional autonomous practice? What is appropriate to teach and evaluate, and how is supervision to be designed to help experienced and inexperienced practitioners differentially? These are the questions covered in this chapter.

Social workers have always functioned predominantly within the confines of organizational necessities (Barber, 1963:678-682). Supervision is the arena in which much of the conflict regarding professional autonomy versus organizational authority is confronted. Mandell (1973) has pointed out that this conflict has increased within the profession in conjunction with the "equality revolution" that has taken place at the societal level and sees only limited opportunities for autonomous social work practice. Epstein (1973) holds the same view but argues that limited qualified autonomous practice is possible if authority can be decentralized and teaching de-emphasized in supervision. Levy (1973) has suggested that the question of authority can be partially resolved through application of a code of ethics to supervision. Kadushin (1968) has related authority problems to interactional games played by supervisees to avoid risk and loss of control; Hawthorne (1975) has applied the same framework to supervisors who play games categorized as power and abdication. Most of these writers describe the process that takes place, but not much progress has been made to reduce authority conflicts substantially, and only limited theoretical and practical models have been developed to resolve the issues. A dual model of supervision and consultation (Munson, 1979c:336-346) has been devised to decentralize authority and to maximize professional autonomy in organizational settings to deal with these issues.

The question of authority and autonomy in practice through supervision is an issue that is on the minds and in the discussions of workers who are in active practice. Briar summarized the issue that faces the social work profession:

> Ninety percent . . . of all caseworkers practice in bureaucratic organizations, and the demands of such organizations have a tendency to encroach upon professional autonomy. Every attempt by the agency to routinize the conditions of professional practice amounts to a restriction of professional discretion, and for that reason probably should be resisted, in most instances, by practitioners. . . . There are, of course, realistic limits to the amount of autonomy and discretion an organization can grant to the practitioner, but no one knows just where that limit is, and we cannot know until we have tried to reach it. (1970:96)

The problem of control in modern professions and organizations leads to a number of questions especially appropriate to social work. Supervision has traditionally been summarized functionally as administration, teaching, and helping (Pettes, 1967:15). If this is the case, what are the limits of control in these functions? What are the best means of carrying out these functions structurally? In clinical settings, there is a growing sense that autonomy is decreasing and much clinical activity is being dictated by third-party payers. Cost, length of treatment, type of treatment, who is qualified to do the diagnosis and treatment, and who is included in the treatment are essentially determined by the payers in many settings. Supervisors play a difficult role in helping practitioners reconcile these autonomy issues. Such issues can cause a great deal of confusion and frustration if practitioners fail to accommodate to the amount of internal and external control of practice that exists in a profession which, in recent years, has been extolling its autonomy.

INTERACTION AND AUTHORITY

Much can be accomplished by applying individual and group supervision differentially according to experience, education, and preference of workers. This alone does not seem to be sufficient to bring about optimal congruence between the worker, the supervisor, and the organization. Analysis of the extent and nature of interaction in supervision, regardless of the structure used, is helpful in sorting out authority issues and conflicts. How the supervisor interacts with the supervisees has been demonstrated to be the crucial variable in psychiatric studies of supervision, which are substantially more controlled and empirical than those which have been conducted in social work (see Munson, 1979c: 337-338).

The interactional framework can be applied to the structure of supervision in terms of how the supervisor will exercise authority in individual and group supervision. A supervisor can exert a great deal of control in both types of supervision, although it does appear that control is more difficult to exercise in the group situation. Regardless of the model, authority can be dealt with directly by establishing at the outset what the roles of the supervisor and worker will be. The following are nteractional issues that deal directly with authority: Who sets the agenda? Who establishes the frequency, time, and length of the session? Will emphasis be placed on case discussion, worker growth, or both? Will the supervisor present case material? Who will make which decisions? Who establishes the structure of presentations? Who establishes the content of presentations? These examples can be applied to either individual or group supervision and have less to do with how the supervisory process is structured in general and more to do with authority and interaction.

Supervisees can use interactional strategies to subvert the authority of the supervisor. This is illustrated by a group supervision situation. A supervisee presented in the supervision group a case of a Mexican-American family, with an acting-out child, who was to come for an initial interview the following week. The supervisee expressed concern because she had never interviewed a Mexican-American family. In setting up the appointment, the father was resistant and noncommittal about coming for the interview. The supervisor and several members of the group offered the practitioner suggestions for working with Mexican-American families, as well as how to deal with her concerns about the father's resistance.

During the next supervision group session, the supervisor asked the practitioner how the interview with the family turned out. The worker said that it had gone very well and indicated that one of the members of the supervision group had offered her additional advice after the group session. The worker made it a point to state that the advice she had received from the other worker outside the group was the opposite of the advice she had received in the group. That worker did not offer her comments in the group but chose to share the information outside the group. The supervisor in this case was good, highly trained, and well liked by the supervisees. The supervisor felt circumvented in this situation, and the group had difficulty moving ahead after the worker gave this feedback.

The supervisor chose not to comment on this attempt to subvert the purpose of the supervision group and did not share her feeling of being undercut and made to look foolish in the eyes of the other supervisees. The supervisor did the best thing by not commenting on this and not making it a direct issue of authority in the supervision. The supervisor moved on to the next case and was able to recover without much loss of power or respect. However, if this type of worker behavior became a pattern, the supervisor would need to deal with it directly by requesting this individual to share her observations in the group.

It would be best to discuss this privately with the worker and not make it a group issue. The worker might not be consciously aware of the effect her behavior is having on the supervisor and the group. The supervisor can directly ask this particular worker to comment on specific material during group supervision to minimize the possibility of such material being discussed outside the group.

Studies of interactional issues regarding presentation of case material and sharing of clinical material deserve more attention than they have been granted in the past, for such issues can be important to practice outcome. In a study of eighty-nine patients treated by psychiatric residents, Burgoyne and associates (1976) found an inequity in the cases presented in supervision. Those presented differed significantly from others in that the patients were younger, were better educated, had higher incomes, were better liked by the residents, and were given longer-term treatment. Dressler and associates (1975) found that residents showed more warmth toward patients with low suicide risk and limited overall psychopathology, and that they felt anxious about patients with high suicidel risk and significant pathology. The authors used supervision interaction to modify these attitudes, thus improving the equity of service delivery (1975). These studies involved psychiatric residents. No comparable studies of social work students or practitioners exist, but if such studies did exist, the results most likely would not differ, since social workers often work with the same patients and families as psychiatrists. These studies demonstrate the importance that supervision can have for adequate service delivery purely on clinical grounds and involve interactions that should be shared free of administrative constraints and evaluation.

AUTHORITY AND STRUCTURE

Many of the issues surrounding supervision and development of the profession have focused on the structure of supervision and the use of authority. The arguments regarding structure of supervision have centered on whether group supervision is more effective than individual supervision or mixed models, without much empirical research to support the theoretical arguments. The same pattern has occurred with respect to authority in supervision. With increased emphasis on independent professional practice, debate has centered on how much autonomous practice is possible (Epstein, 1973:6). At the same time that the case for control in supervision has been getting more difficult to make (since emphasis on autonomy has increased in education and practice), there has been a trend to license social workers, and the licensing laws mandate varying degrees of active supervision. A connection between structure and authority does exist, since much of the supervision literature indicates that the structure of supervision has been varied to dilute and redirect authority in supervision. Little progress has been made in resolving these issues, and not much is known about worker attitudes toward authority in and structuring of supervision.

It is difficult to discuss the use of structure and authority in supervision separately, and, historically, supervision literature has made few, if any, distinctions between the two concepts. A certain degree of authority is inherent in the supervisory relationship. Pruger has pointed out that the worker must be attentive to and understand legitimate authority, but that "there still exists significant autonomy for the individual, if he consciously recognizes and uses it" (1973:28). For social workers to grow and at the same time recognize the limits of autonomy, a distinction needs to be made between the structure of supervision and authority. Pruger unites the two concepts by stating that "if . . . autonomy is lost, it must be because it was . . . given up, rather than because it was structurally precluded" (1973:28). The idea that authority and structure in supervision are two different but related concepts is supported by research, which found that structural models are independent of authority models, that structural arrangements do not produce significantly different outcomes, but that the perceptions of authority models do result in major differences (Munson, 1975:131-186).

Although there have been increasing demands for worker autonomy, the research indicates that the struggle for less control has had little impact on the structure of supervision (Mandell, 1973:43). Group supervision has been viewed as an alternative structure to promote autonomy. In spite of the claims for group supervision, evidence suggests that group supervision has not been implemented on a broad basis, and where it is employed, use of authority is a better predictor of outcome than use of group or individual structures in supervision. Kaslow (1972:117) attributes this to supervisors lacking the skills or confidence to engage in supervision that requires group methods. If this is the case, the issue becomes one of how competent the supervisor is perceived to be by the worker. The failure to use group methods widely in supervision could be related to the supervisor's fear of loss of control and authority in the group setting. Supervisors can manifest specific behaviors that will promote worker regard for their competence to decrease the resistance to group supervision and increase the degree of autonomy the worker can have through the group approach. This view is consistent with the finding of Cherniss and Egnatios that the ideal supervisor is one who "knows when to ask questions and when to give advice without always doing just one or the other" (1978:222-223).

Widen defined supervision as a creature of agencies rather than as a professional enterprise. His view was that supervision literature had explored the supervisory process, but little attention had been paid to supervisory structure, which "is particularly sensitive to the life-style of the agency as a social institution," with the result that "each agency that has a formal supervisory structure has a philosophy of supervision" (1962:79). Often the problem of autonomy and supervision gets expressed as a conflict between the individual professional worker and the agency. The supervisor, who is usually a member of the same professional group, is put in conflict when expected to mediate this relationship. As long as the issue is viewed as a worker-agency conflict with the supervisor as mediator, little substantial change will occur. Kadushin found that the greatest discrepancy between supervisors and supervisees regarding the role of the supervisor existed around the mediation function. Workers wanted the supervisor to mediate more than the supervisors were willing to (Kadushin, 1974:294). Supervisors' failure to use the mediator model could be the result of a conscious attempt to avoid role conflict and strain, since most supervisors in the social work profession know the consequences of such role performance. The supervisee is left with the problem of how to confront the organization. Only when the social work profession as a group addresses this issue through its professional organizations will systematic, standardized principles be established to guide agencies in their practices. Organizational issues can be resolved only at the organizational level.

In addressing the issue of supervision at the professional level, the unit of analysis should not necessarily be the structure of supervision itself; it should be the content and means of implementation, regardless of the model used. Autonomy will be achieved best when the worker is free to select the model to be used rather than having one imposed by theoreticians, agencies, and supervisors. Given the diversity in agency resources, agency size, worker education, worker experience, personalities, and worker supervisory preferences, it seems unrealistic to seek one best model of supervision. It is realistic to select a model that is best suited to a given situation. When the supervisor and supervisee are willing to work at it, such a flexible system is attainable.

STYLE AND AUTHORITY

The supervisor needs to strive for a model of exercising authority that will be accepted by supervisees. Supervisee perceptions of how supervisors exercise their authority produce different outcomes for supervisory interaction and satisfaction (Munson, 1975). The styles of authority identified in one study fell into two main types: sanction and natural competence. The sanction style is the traditional style in which supervisors are perceived as relying on the official sanction and power granted to them by virtue of their hierarchical position in the organization or profession. The competence style was perceived as originating from supervisors' knowledge, skill, and ability as competent practitioners who derived power from their self-confidence. In other words, the sanction style is used by supervisors who view their power as originating externally, and the competence style is used by supervisors who view their power as originating internally from their own performance and skill. Research (Munson, Study B) shows that the sanctioned approach of authority is more often associated with the overall philosopher style of supervision, and the natural approach of authority is more likely to be found in relation to the theoretician and technician styles (see Chapter 4). This research suggests that supervisors should strive to achieve a perception of their authority based on natural competence rather than through organizational sanction. Supervisory interaction and supervisory satisfaction are higher in the competence than the sanction model, and the competence model of authority as perceived by workers is the more productive model in all respects.

The research cited previously on the relationship between authority and structural supervision models is similar to that of a sociological study of supervisory styles of authority in which an association was found between authority styles, verbal aggression toward the supervisor, productivity, and job satisfaction (Day and Hamblin, 1967). If this distinction is valid, agencies, the profession, and supervisors must strive to attain the perception by workers of competent supervision to achieve the most effective functioning of the organization and to promote worker satisfaction. Given these findings, the most difficult task remains for the profession and agency managers. If the natural competence model produces the better outcome, supervisors must define what produces workers' perceptions of their supervisors as competent. Worker responses in the structural/authority research cited earlier indicate that such perceptions involve personal characteristics that the supervisor brings to the situation. These characteristics include genuine interest and support of what the worker is doing; organizationally manipulable behaviors, such as availability and appropriate levels and timing of control; and superior skill and knowledge with respect to the task and position to be supervised. Agencies need to make well-grounded decisions about who becomes and remains a supervisor, and supervisors need to make firm choices about what and when to control and not to control. Authority involves the ability to influence, but the subjective responses of workers indicate that workers should also be able to influence their supervisors. When this is taking place, supervisors are viewed as true mediators with respect to authority. This conception of authority has been succinctly described in relation to organizational functioning:

> A greater amount of total control, whereby subordinates can actually influence their supervisors, will heighten, not lower, the organization's performance. However, when subordinates obtain a measure of expertise but are given no control, morale and willingness to contribute to the organization decreases. (Marcus and Marcus, 1972:234)

Workers say that they continue to look for supervisors "who are smarter than we are," and want to feel that "We work for our supervisor, not the agency." At the same time, they contend that supervision is no good if the clinician has to tell a client, "I will have to talk this over with my supervisor and let you know," and they say that good supervision exists "when you know you are supervised, but you are not aware of it every moment" (see Howe, 1989, for examples of client views of authority of practitioners and supervisors).

Case Exercise:
The Case of Ellen Maze

A supervisor in a community-based mental health intervention program for abused children supervised Ellen Maze, a clinical social worker supervisee who became upset during the Christmas holidays when a child she treated was removed from foster care because the foster parents were taking a vacation and did not want the child to go with them because the child "was not really a member of the family." The department of social services worker could not find another foster home, so the child was placed in a psychiatric hospital on the grounds that she was "oppositional" about the foster family decision not to take her on the vacation. The child remained in the psychiatric hospital for fourteen days. Ellen visited the child in the hospital and was concerned about her condition. She was angry, refusing treatment, and said she wanted to go home to her "real mother."

This was not possible because the natural mother was intellectually limited, neglectful, and her parental rights had been terminated by the department of social services.

Ellen was concerned about the child's status and wrote a letter to the local legal aid society to seek legal assistance in getting the child released from the hospital. When Ellen told her supervisor about her action, the supervisor reviewed the child's file and found an information release that was dated but did not specify a termination date authorization of the release. The supervisor supported Ellen's writing the letter to the legal aid society regarding the child's status.

Two weeks later Ellen received a letter from a department of social services supervisor. The letter stated that Ellen had broken state law by contacting the legal aid society because the social services department had legal guardianship of the child. The social worker had breached confidentiality because the department of social services had not authorized release of the information to the legal aid society. The letter indicated that any further "breaches of this nature" would result in legal action. Ellen was extremely upset and brought the letter to her supervisor. The supervisor took the letter to the agency director.

Ellen indicated that the department of social services worker frequently did not keep appointments with the child, and when she did see the child, she would try to undermine the progress Ellen was making with the child in weekly sessions. The child was released from the hospital and sent to live with a new foster family.

If you were the supervisor in this situation how would you respond to the following questions:

1. What are the major administrative, policy, and interagency issues in this situation?
2. What intra-agency policy would you emphasize as a result of this incident?
3. What actions would you take to resolve this issue?
4. What would you say to your agency director, if anything?
5. What would you say to Ellen, if anything?
6. What are the major clinical issues in this case?
7. What would you request the agency director do about this situation?
8. What action, if any, would you take in relation to the social services agency?
9. What would you see as the next step in this case?

AGE AND AUTHORITY

Authority can become a problem when the supervisor and supervisee differ in age. Authority problems can emerge when the supervisor is much older or much younger than the supervisee. The problem can originate in the supervisor or the supervisee, but the supervisor has the responsibility to be alert to such issues regardless of the origin. The problem of the older supervisor and younger worker was identified many decades ago by Bertha Reynolds (1965/1942:193); she assigned responsibility to the supervisor for recognizing and overcoming it.

Less attention has been devoted to the difficulty that arises when the supervisor is much younger than the supervisee. This is illustrated by the situation in which a twenty-eight-year-old MSW was assigned to supervise a forty-nine-year-old, untrained, but experienced woman. Although the supervisor was highly competent and had much to offer the supervisee, she felt inadequate to contribute to this older woman's growth and learning. The supervisor became sensitive and immobilized when the supervisee made such comments as, "If I were in charge, I would not do it that way." It was suggested that the supervisor handle such a paralyzing comment by asking, "If you were in charge, how would you do it?" This question released the authority blockage in the relationship, providing the supervisee the opportunity to have input into the decision-making process. It also allowed the supervisor to learn that her ideas and the ideas of the supervisee were not as different as she had thought. This approach opened up exploration that led to a more positive relationship. Not all situations can be resolved as easily, but this illustrates the point that such differences must be brought out into the open in order to be resolved.

Paralleling the authority approaches and structures of supervision is the model of intervention that supervisors use. Some supervisors see themselves as antecedent to the practitioner's interventions. Other supervisors view themselves as intervening between the practitioner and the client as the practitioner tries to change. Others see their role as parallel to the ongoing change efforts of the practitioner. Each of these models can be effective if applied in a sensitive and consistent manner. The models are illustrated in Visual 7.1.

AUTONOMY

A significant historical contribution that social work has made to the helping professions is the supervision model it developed. In the early years of social work, the model the profession adopted was based on medical education. Social work soon deviated from that model, but for a long time, it followed a strong model with formal supervision. Initially, social work deviated from the medical model in one significant respect: after people graduated from educational programs, close supervision continued in practice for a year or two. Some people were known to be supervised longer, for example, there were reports of practitioners being supervised for an hour a week for as long as fifteen years. Social work deviated from the medical model in that the profession did not recognize practitioners as having the ability to practice autonomously.

In 1955, when NASW was founded (Dinerman and Geismar, 1984), the notion was developed that to become a full-fledged professional one had to

VISUAL 7.1. Models of Supervisory Intervention

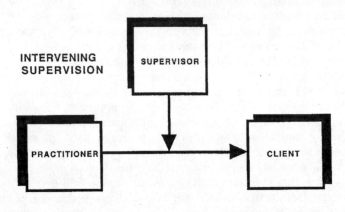

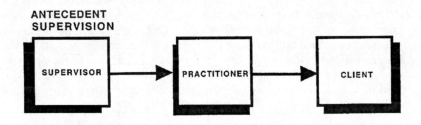

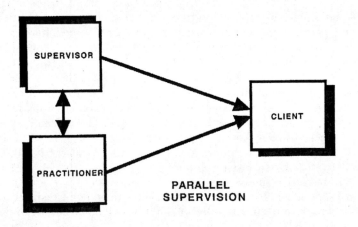

function autonomously. The term *autonomy* was exploited to promote professionalism. Autonomous practice evolved over the next forty years. Schools and agencies promoted the idea of autonomy without much regard for its consequences for the practitioner, supervisor, or client. Supervisors and practitioners experienced confusion about the role of supervision in relation to the idea of the fully trained, autonomous, professional practitioner. The situation became confused over the past decade as managed cost organizations altered the status of autonomy that the social work profession devoted 100 years to developing (Munson, 1998a). Other mental health professions have had their autonomy diminished as well.

The word *autonomy* is inappropriately used in relation to the nature of most social work practice settings under managed cost auspices. There is no such thing as a completely autonomous practitioner. The word *autonomy* means that one functions without regard for anyone or anything else. Practitioners tend to view the autonomous practitioner as totally out of the control of others, and social work practitioners do not function that way. The majority of social workers are employed in agencies that put severe constraints on their activity. Even private practitioners are required in most states to have their work reviewed by psychiatrists for insurance reimbursement, and managed cost companies micromanage most aspects of clinical social work practice.

Social work students are told that upon graduation they will be autonomous practitioners, but indications are that beginning practitioners do not believe in this autonomous, professional image (Munson, Study A and Study B). The confusion that results from academic portrayal of the autonomous practitioner is illustrated by the reflection of one beginning practitioner several years after graduation:

> What happens is after you have graduated you go to the door of the agency, and you are assigned a supervisor, if you are lucky, and the supervisor will then say, "Well, now you are an autonomous practitioner; you are competent. You've had two years of graduate education, and really, the only thing I'm here to do is to help you if you have any personal problems," or "If there is anything I can help you with, just let me know." Nobody is going to admit or own up to the fact that they are not ready to do this all by themselves and that they need help. I had a limited number of cases in school; now here I was faced with this. I had five cases my second year of school, and now the supervisor says I'm going to do twelve intakes this week. But I never admitted that I needed help with that. Also, I was led to suspect that I should resent supervision. I should resent that somebody should want to try to tell me how to practice. But they are really not telling us how to practice. What they are supposed to do is help us learn those additional things that we didn't learn in school, but my supervisor didn't say that.

This practitioner's statement illustrates the confusion on the part of the supervisor and the practitioner about the role of supervision and what to expect from it. Graduates want to develop their skills. They want to test what they have learned theoretically and abstractly. Some have never had a group or family therapy treatment experience. The many areas of specialized practice a beginning social worker can enter means that no practitioner will know all that is necessary to be an effective clinician.

Autonomy is something supervisors need to be clear about. The practitioner has to ask, "How much autonomy does one really have when functioning in an agency?" It is unrealistic to think that you can function autonomously and do only what you want to do. For example, in many public agencies, such as probation, officers are required to have their phone numbers listed in the phone directory. Some agencies have rules against making home visits, even if the practitioner thinks one is appropriate. In other agencies, supervisors open supervisees' mail. Many agencies have detailed and restrictive dress codes. The increase in practice standards, practice guidelines, agency practice protocols, and organizational policy and procedure manuals limits autonomy in significant ways. These factors illustrate the illusion of autonomy. It must be recognized that work in an agency places constraints on practitioners and supervisors. If these constraints and limitations are kept in mind in clinical work, difficulty, confusion, and frustration can result. The trend in public and private agencies, and in private practice, is less autonomous functioning based on increased accountability, documentation, competency testing, utilization reviews, and peer reviews. Insurance companies and other referral services often place constraints on what mental health professionals do.

Because autonomy has been defined in reaction to authority in the social work profession, authority is often viewed as the opposite of autonomy. This is the basic issue that faces anyone who enters supervision today—students and practitioners. Supervisors and supervisees can get locked into authority struggles and not understand what is happening. Some social workers and agencies do not like authority. It does not go along with democratic principles. However, democratic principles have limits in practice, and failing to face the reality of their limits in supervision can lead to difficulty, especially in the student-field instructor relationship. Field instructors have authority. They have a degree of control over students' destinies, and this should be recognized by both parties in each relationship. Some supervisors try to avoid authority issues by referring to themselves as consultants. This is not a good practice. There is a difference between a supervisor and a consultant. A consultant gives recommendations or suggestions. When a supervisor makes a suggestion, the worker does not necessarily have the freedom to reject it, since it may be a directive.

In certain situations, in which the supervisor may have to order the worker to perform tasks, saying, "You will do this." From the beginning, supervisors should accept their authority and acknowledge it as a fundamental aspect of supervising. The supervisor must not first say, "I'm your consultant, and I'll help you with this, but you are not under any real obligation," and then, when something goes wrong, say, "You have to do this—I'm your supervisor." It is too late to change the rules then. The rules should be stated clearly at the outset.

The limits to autonomy and the resulting confusion is discussed by Wells (1999) in a lengthy case example. A brief excerpt is presented here to illustrate the point about degrees of autonomy:

> ... I had a dizzying number of supervisors. . . . Above and beyond that, [the] director . . . had announced . . . that she would be meeting with the social workers as a group, on occasion, to provide direct training in social work. This would be interesting because Dr. Knight had no training in social work. . . . None of my supervisors had . . . training in social work. Perhaps that is why . . . not one of them gave me the foggiest idea what I was supposed to be doing with my job. . . .

Now I not only wanted some direction; I also wanted some support. . . . I wanted to develop social histories for children . . . but my local supervisor, Lou Bachus, had directly told me not to do them. . . . I had asked Martin Murdock whether he would talk to Lou about it, as Martin was . . . officially Lou's boss. . . . But he didn't get back to Lou Bachus to support my request. I had asked Lou about that . . . and Lou just looked blank. . . . Then he had gone into his "guns in the closet" routine again. . . . A bit disgruntled with the supervisors I had contact with, I decided to try consultation—peer consultation. . . . So I took my questions and frustrations to Gertrude Baker, the full-time social worker in Kingston. . . . I asked Gertrude . . . whether I could talk to her for a while after work. I explained that I had noticed some strange contrasts in evaluation procedures . . . that I wanted to talk over with her, and I expected I would be needing a good hour or so of her time. Gertrude grinned and suggested a rendezvous in a local tavern. (pp. 44-45)

GROUP SUPERVISION

There is not much evidence that structure or content of supervision is significantly changing, but frequency and duration of supervision is decreasing. The individual and group models, or a mix of the two models, predominate. Group supervision is used less than in the past and some state licensing boards have eliminated it (for example, in Missouri) or placed limits on its use (for example, in Kentucky) through specifying a majority of supervision time for licensure must be accomplished through individual supervision (see American Association of State Social Work Boards, 1998, for the requirements of individual states). The content of supervision has evolved from a psychological to a sociological orientation in the sense that the emphasis has shifted from supervising the *person* to supervising the *position*. Most of the material covered in this book can be applied to individual or group supervision, but factors unique to group supervision are covered in this section.

Group supervision can be a valuable and rewarding experience, but a positive outcome is highly dependent upon how the supervision is presented, set up, and carried out. It requires more preparation and organization than is recognized by supervisors. Group supervision often occurs through default, rather than design, in that it is entered into because it seems to be the most practical and time-saving way to accomplish supervision, rather than being utilized because it can produce the most positive outcomes for specific clinical material and practitioner tasks. Any structuring of supervision should be based on the needs of the practitioners. Group supervision should not be entered into simply to relieve time pressures of the supervisor. When a supervision group is used by the supervisor to learn to do this form of supervision, the supervisor needs to be supervised or provided with consultation.

Supervisors need to be aware that many practitioners undergoing group supervision for the first time have never been in a group, even though they may have read about group process. Some have experienced group therapy as clients or practitioners and may respond to group supervision in the same manner as group therapy. Others will treat group supervision as a class in which they are to be lectured or taught didactically. In other words, most practitioners do not know what to expect from group supervision, and the supervisor must make the expectations clear. Many practitioners and supervisors who have not experienced group supervision view it as a sound idea theoretically but question its utility from a practical standpoint. Once they have experienced good group supervision, this resistance dissipates. In moving from individual to group supervision, something is gained and something is lost. In group supervision, less time is available for each practitioner's individual cases, but more information is generated for discussion. The supervisor should evaluate which approach is best suited to the practitioner's needs.

It is easier for the individual practitioner to escape evaluation in group supervision. Some practitioners who resist group supervision initially may later use the group setting to avoid exposure. The supervisor will need to work with such practitioners to aid them in appropriately using group supervision.

Basic Questions

The supervisor contemplating group supervision needs to think through basic questions before embarking on such an effort:

1. Will it be defined as supervision or peer consultation?
2. What methods will be used to get practitioners to risk exposure in group supervision, and how will anxiety about such risk be handled?
3. How will competitiveness be handled?
4. How will overly verbal and reticent members be handled?
5. How do you deal with the different backgrounds and skill levels of practitioners in the group?
6. How will case monitoring be handled?
7. What are the advantages of group supervision in comparison to individual supervision?
8. How will transference and countertransference material be handled?
9. What techniques will be used to initiate the supervision successfully?
10. Who will be supervised in the group or groups?
11. How large will the group be?
12. What day and time will the group meet?
13. What limits will be set on the group, and how will they be presented?
14. How will resisters be handled?
15. What impact will the group have on other elements of the agency or organization?
16. Who will be responsible for setting the agenda?
17. How many supervisors will be in the group?
18. How many groups will be used?
19. What are the main purposes for establishing a group?
20. How will the goals of group supervision differ from the goals of individual supervision?
21. In what different ways will the supervisor interact in group supervision and in individual supervision?
22. How will the supervisor structure the group?
23. How will feedback be channeled?
24. How will group commitment and identity be fostered?
25. What kind and amount of record keeping will be done?
26. How will therapy be avoided, if it is to be avoided?
27. How will the group be used to improve working relationships?
28. Should the supervisor present cases?
29. How will poor presentations be handled?
30. Will the group be time limited or open ended?

Practitioner Experience Level

Even skilled practitioners need advice and support at times. Inexperienced practitioners need and prefer individual supervision more than experienced practitioners. This varies with years and types of experience, but often the needs of both groups are not adequately addressed in supervision. The less-experienced practitioner usually needs help with the specifics of practice and aid in developing a repertory of techniques; this is often better suited to individual supervision. The experienced practitioner desires broad, general evaluation of practice and opportunities to apply different and complex treatment modalities, which is more appropriate to group supervision. When supervisors focus on the problems of the young, inexperienced, and inept practitioner at the expense of the experienced practitioner in a mixed supervisory group, the potential for innovation in supervision and treatment is decreased.

Experienced and prestigious practitioners should not be denied supervision. If experienced practitioners are to be genuinely autonomous, they do not have to be anonymous and left with no way to make a contribution to the learning of their colleagues and their profession. This should be kept in mind when planning group supervision, especially when the supervisor is responsible for experienced and inexperienced practitioners. Including both types of practitioners in a supervisory group can be beneficial if the supervisor is sensitive to their needs and provides a healthy balance in the content of the group.

Supervisor's Role

The supervisor's chief responsibility in group supervision is to keep the group on task. The aim of group supervision is to present clinical material in an organized fashion so that new and alternative practice strategies can be developed. The whole process assumes that problematic and difficult material will always be before the group. Practitioners resist dealing with difficult material. After the basics of a difficult case are presented, the group will often attempt to gather more information from the presenter or begin telling the presenter what to do. Without assistance from the supervisor, the group can struggle for a diagnosis to no avail. The leader must intervene and encourage the group to move beyond this point, asking members to relate the case to their own practices. This is why the supervisor has to be more skilled than the group members. In this situation, the supervisor does not give answers; he or she simply reminds the group of its task and asks questions that move the group beyond information gathering.

Once the group experiences the freedom to struggle at being clinically competent, a sense of trust will develop. A good indicator of this is the feeling of freedom to externalize concerns about case material. Members will begin to express fears and problems they would not share before. For some, this is the first time in their professional training and career that they will have shared real questions about their practice.

The leader must be careful of what he or she says and how it is stated. Even skilled workers, when discussing difficult clinical material, will take clues from the supervisor. One simple statement by the supervisor, which is designed only to elicit further information about the case, can result in the group's moving in a specific direction that becomes the focus for the intervention. Such questions as, "Do you think they have a symbiotic relationship?" or "Has the marriage always been this combative?" can influence the focus of the group so that broader aspects of a case are missed. The supervisor has a responsibility not only to comment on specific material but also to organize and guide the discussion.

Once trust is established, the supervisor usually has a new problem. Group members tend to become quasi-supervisors. The supervisor must guard against this. The emphasis should be on continued sharing, with the presenter articulating the significant material that is applicable to his or her own case. What is being sought is a judgment-free learning environment. The group members should be made aware that they are not at risk with the supervisor or other group members, but only with themselves and their clients. The client is at risk secondarily in group supervision, but the outcome can benefit both the client and the practitioner. To achieve beneficial learning, the group must go beyond what the case presenter *should do* to what each group member can gain from the discussion and apply in practice. This self-directed, self-selected learning results in independent clinical competence.

When one supervisor works with several practitioners separately in individual sessions, a certain amount of practitioner competitiveness and curiosity frequently develops. This is healthy as long as it does not develop into intense rivalry or game playing. When supervision is conducted exclusively in a group setting, competition within the group also develops, and the supervisor has a responsibility to prevent this from becoming a negative experience for one or more members of the group. When two supervisory groups exist simultaneously in the same setting with one supervisor, intergroup competition and curiosity can develop, and the supervisor must be alert to this.

The issue of liability is not clear when group supervision is utilized. The NASW Code of Ethics (1996) states that "social workers should seek the advice and counsel of colleagues whenever such consultation is in the best interest of client" (p. 16). Group supervision is an appropriate area for seeking such advice. Court decisions have held that any professional who offers advice or guidance to a practitioner can have liability for the case outcome. This could be problematic for group supervision since numerous participants make input during group supervision. There are no professional guidelines for how to conduct group supervision and how to determine lia-bility regarding decision making that results from group supervision. Can an individual practitioner be held liable for a case action decided in group supervision even if the practitioner contributed nothing to the discussion, was absent the day the case was discussed, or opposed the decision that was made? Under these circumstances, it is recommended that the group partici-pants have individual supervision, with the group supervision considered supplemental to the individual supervision. The group should be referred to as group consultation, not as group supervision. An agency should not rely exclusively on a group process as a supervision vehicle. The designated leader of the consultation group should have documented expertise in the ar-eas of practice that are under discussion in the group (see NASW, 1996, p. 16). Supervisors should ensure that the same criteria for effective and ap-propriate supervision used in individual supervision are applied in group consultation. This includes the criteria for case review procedures, identify-ing problems, prioritizing problems, selecting interventions, and documen-tation of the decision-making process.

CONCLUSION

The supervisor must give thought to the role of authority in supervision, how that authority will be used, and how it will be perceived by the supervisee. Authority is inherent in the supervisory relationship and must be recognized as such. It should be discussed openly when supervision is initiated and at relevant points in the supervisory process, especially when it threatens the learning component of supervision. Supervisors should not be reluctant to use their authority but should apply it with caution and sensitiv-ity in the context of the needs of the supervisee. Supervisees welcome con-structive use of authority and accept direction from the supervisor when it originates from the supervisor's skill, knowledge, and confidence. The practitioner is under ethical mandate to seek supervisory assistance and the NASW Code of Ethics (1996) states, "social workers should provide ser-vices . . . only within boundaries of their education, training, license, certifi-cation, consultation received, supervised experience, or other relevant expe-rience" (p. 8).

Case Exercise:
The Case of Marcie

Kathy came to supervision with the following case, stating, "I don't know what to do with this case. The mother and grandmother are problematic."

The identified patient is Marcie, the seven-year-old, only child of Connie Mathews. Marcie was sexually assaulted six months ago when being cared for by Connie's boyfriend in his home. The assault was perpetrated by a fourteen-year-old nephew of the boyfriend. No charges have been filed by the department of social services.

Four weeks ago Marcie told Kathy that her mother hit her for "not listening." The child reported that there were marks on the back of her legs, but these could not be seen by Kathy. Kathy reported the abuse to the department of social services and informed the mother of the report. Connie is now angry at Kathy and will not respond to her questions but continues to bring Marcie to therapy. Kathy stated in supervision that the mother is "passive-aggressive when I try to talk to her." Kathy suggested referral to another therapist, but Connie has refused a referral.

Marcie's paternal grandmother, Marsha, brings Marcie to therapy about 50 percent of the time. Marsha has tried to get Kathy to "straighten my daughter out." Connie resents the intrusion of her mother into her life, even though she depends on her mother to care for Marcie while she is at work as a postal carrier. Marcie's mother and grandmother's main conflict revolves around how to care for and manage Marcie. Connie reported that she is a survivor of childhood sexual abuse but has refused to talk with Kathy about the abuse.

Kathy believes that Marcie is angry with her mother for allowing the abuse to happen and for hitting her. She added that Marcie manipulates the conflict between Connie and Marsha. The supervisor agreed with this observation and commented that children can observe and make associations that adults often overlook.

Last week Connie reported to Kathy that she is breaking up with her boyfriend. She also stated that she is about to begin parenting classes that she was ordered to attend after the physical abuse charges were investigated by the department of social services. Connie stated that the classes may interfere with her bringing Marcie to therapy since "the classes are held on the other side of town and I do not know if there is enough time to get here from there."

Kathy is seeking help with what steps to take next in the therapy and you are the supervisor. (1) What areas would you explore with Kathy to assist in planning the next steps in this case? (2) Would you make any recommendations regarding the role of the grandmother? (3) What would you suggest with respect to the parenting classes interfering with the therapy sessions?

SUGGESTED READINGS

Rock, B. (1990). "Social Worker Autonomy in an Age of Accountability." *The Clinical Supervisor,* 8(Summer), pp. 19-3 1.

    Discussion of the tension regarding professional autonomy and organizational accountability.

Sennett, R. (1980). *Authority.* New York: Knopf.

    A general study of authority and its origins. The historical analysis of authority can be related to the authority issues that face the social work profession.

Veeder, N. W. (1990). "Autonomy, Accountability, and Professionalism: The Case Against Close Supervision in Social Work." *The Clinical Supervisor,* 8 (Summer), pp. 33-65.

    Summary of the authority and autonomy issues facing the social work profession.

Theory cannot, in reality, create the world:
it can only help in explaining what we
have chosen to be interested in.

Joe Bailey
Ideas and Intervention

Chapter 8

Use of Theory

The use of theory in practice has long been advocated in the social work profession. This chapter deals with how to use theory in supervision to enhance practice activity. There has been confusion about theory and the terms that are associated with it. To clarify these issues, this chapter begins with explanations of the terms *technique, methods, modalities, philosophy of practice, theory, ideology, practice theory,* and *theory of practice.* The elements of theory are explained and include a discussion of facts, concepts, and hypotheses. The functions of theory are covered through explanations of the functions of organizing, explaining, and prediction. The components of theory are explained as utility, verification, comprehensiveness, and simplicity. The use of theoretical speculation in supervision is discussed, as well as the use of occasional theory abandonment to aid learning. Theory application and supervisory interaction are explored along with a list of guidelines for using theory in relation to clinical material in supervision.

INTRODUCTION

In clinical practice there has always been a polarity between the philosophical and the scientific, which in one form or another can be traced to the earliest philosophers and theoreticians. Chessick (1977) described this polarity as the empirical view versus the invisible view, which is reminiscent of Spengler's thesis that the pendulum swings back and forth between these orientations.

This historical polarity is re-created in supervision, and rather than occurring over decades or centuries, it can take place in a matter of minutes. This is to be expected during an endeavor that grapples constantly with ways of resolving problems in human functioning, while drawing on numerous theories and strategies. To avoid confusion and frustration, supervisors must control such rapid swinging of the pendulum in a smooth, orderly fashion that promotes understanding and learning.

This chapter addresses how to bridge the philosophic-scientific polarity in supervision through the use of theory.

THEORY IN SUPERVISION

Theory in supervision is a tool used in making knowledge apparent and understandable. In a sense, supervisors need literally to shake the concepts and examples out of the theoretical rug. Supervisors can commit the classic error of confusing terms by inadvertently referring to a theory as treatment modality.

Clinically the practitioner is faced with more data than can be dealt with effectively or efficiently. Consciously and unconsciously, clinicians and supervisors are selective about the data chosen to act upon. The data chosen are related to the theory in which the professional has been trained or to which he or she subscribes. Theory has an impact on the diagnostic phase, and, in turn, the diagnosis determines the direction taken in the treatment phase.

Practitioners who have been exposed to and know a smattering of theory develop a practice orientation that takes the form of a mixed application of a variety of concepts that can result in therapeutic confusion for the supervisor, the practitioner, and the client. When there is an inadequacy of theory in use in a given practice area, obscure and gimmicky techniques expand and are elevated to the level of quasi-theory. This results in a narrow and limited approach to practice. The elevation of paradoxing techniques in family therapy to the level of quasi-theory is an example of this phenomenon.

In supervision, theoretical constructs are often used rather than empirical concepts. This is accepted practice in science when it is known that something exists but cannot be explained completely. If astronomers and physicists can do this in the name of science, so can mental health professionals. Science should free practitioners and supervisors to learn more, rather than lock them into a system that places solutions out of reach.

CONFUSION ABOUT THEORY

It is common for supervisors to confuse theory with practice methods, modalities, philosophies, and techniques. To avoid such confusion here, these various concepts are clarified in this section, as are the definitions of theory used in this chapter.

Techniques

A *technique* is the basic tool of practice. It is a specific action taken by the practitioner to promote change, give insight, or gather information in treatment. A technique is a highly specific, singular action. It is meaningless to ask a supervisee, "What is your technique?" Practitioners don't use one technique all the time, and if they did, they would be ineffective. A better question would be, "What are several techniques that could be used in this situation?" or, if the supervisor is more interested in the practitioner's general pattern of relating, "What is your style?" Questioning, interpretation, comment, and paradoxing are all techniques. A simple way to separate theory from technique for exploration in supervision is that *what* is said during treatment relates to theory, and *how* it is said is related to technique. This is not a hard-and-fast rule, but a quick way to sort out issues in the midst of supervisory discussion.

Techniques can be analyzed on the basis of those which deal with the *structure* of the treatment, those which deal with *content* of the treatment, and those which deal with the *process* of intervention. The general categories of techniques related to structure are

1. composition of therapy (pertaining to clients and practitioners),
2. length and number of sessions,
3. setting in which the therapy occurs,
4. rules related to degree and level of interaction, and
5. type of therapy itself (i.e., individual, group, or family).

Techniques related to content can be categorized as

1. support,
2. confrontation,
3. encounter,

   4. interpretation,
   5. comment,
   6. questioning,
   7. focus,
   8. reflection,
   9. recapitulation,
   10. restructuring,
   11. sculpting or choreography,
   12. conflict, and
   13. paradoxing.

Techniques related to process can be categorized as

   1. projecting outcomes,
   2. predicting the future, and
   3. expressions of trust.

Methods

Methods deal with the broad structure of practice and describe practice orientations. Casework and group work are methods. When a person says, "I am a caseworker at the mental health clinic," he or she is describing an overview of the role and the structure of the work.

Modalities

Modalities are limited forms of practice. Family therapy and group therapy are modalities. Caseworkers and group workers might engage in family therapy or group therapy from time to time, or they may even specialize in these modalities.

Techniques are used in all of these forms of practice. Some techniques are common to all, and some are unique to one form.

Philosophy of Practice

A *philosophy of practice* is a belief system that guides a person's activity. It is a generalization that determines why a person performs in a given way in the practice situation. A family practitioner might say, "It is my philosophy that people can be treated only in the context of the family." A philosophy determines the modality to which a practitioner limits his or her practice. A philosophy is connected to both personal and professional belief systems.

Most practitioners believe it is important to have a philosophy of life that is applicable to their practice. Supervisors need to be aware of these beliefs. To be helpful to supervisees, supervisors must ask supervisees to articulate their philosophy. In asking practitioners to state their philosophy, supervisors can get access to a great deal of information that can be helpful in gaining insight about workers and their level of practice functioning. When practitioners state their philosophy, it should contain a cluster of five elements:

1. Workers have a *motivation* to make a contribution to the welfare of people.
2. Workers have a degree of *idealism* about people and the belief that clients have a desire to do good in life and to grow and change. As one supervisor stated, "The practitioner must accept that the clients we see lead the best lives that they can."
3. It is important to have a desire to *help* others and to recognize the many ways of helping different clients.
4. Workers have a sense of *caring* about others and genuine concern for them and their problems.
5. Practice must have an element of *suspense* to keep it lively and focused. In this context, suspense is a belief that in the practice situation clinicians are always striving to make the unknown known, and that this process of discovery will make the treatment effective and successful.

These five values, which are the elements of a philosophy of practice, can be used to promote learning and growth on the part of the supervisor and supervisee in the process of supervision. These elements can be applied to the supervision process as well as to the treatment process.

Discussion of philosophy can be related to specific issues in supervision and may be helpful to the supervisor in addressing a particular problem the worker is experiencing. This is illustrated by the case of a child welfare supervisor who strongly disagreed with a young, inexperienced worker about removing a child from the home:

> The supervisor felt that the child was in danger if allowed to remain in the situation. The supervisor realized that all the specific points about the situation had been resisted or rebutted by the worker. The supervisor then asked the worker, "What is your philosophy about removing children?" The worker gave a lengthy, but articulate explanation revealing that she did not believe in removing children under any circumstances. This had not occurred to the supervisor or the worker before, and further discussion revealed that this was due in part to her lack of confidence as a worker. It also helped to explain problems she was having in other cases and led to insights about negative attitudes the worker had toward the agency, her clients, and her job. The supervisor was then able to focus with the worker on the details of handling a removal and placement, and how to handle feelings about such a drastic step.

The worker was then able to accomplish the removal and change many of her attitudes that had emerged about herself and her job.

If this philosophical discussion had not taken place, the worker might have left the agency eventually or, even worse, gone on for years as a disgruntled practitioner who put many children at risk.

Social workers in supervision usually operate from a philosophical stance rather than a theoretical stance. This hierarchical stance emerged from Freudian theory as a philosophy being applied to the worker as well as to the client, rather than empirically matching philosophical and theoretical stances with the client problems.

Ideology and Theory

Stevenson makes a distinction between theory and ideology, stating that "a system of belief about the nature of man which is thus held by some group of people as giving rise to their way of life is standardly called an 'ideology' " (Stevenson, 1974:7). Since Gestalt therapy has been called a form of treatment as well as a way of life by many of its proponents, it could be argued that it is an *ideology* rather than a theory of treatment. Various implications of this holistic or unified approach of Gestalt therapy that remain unaddressed by many of its advocates. When a theory becomes an ideology and gives rise to a way of life for a particular social group, it is difficult for the members of the group to consider it objectively (Stevenson, 1974:12). This lack of objectivity can become problematic in applying theory in supervision. Learning through theory is most effective when the supervisor and supervisee embrace a theory objectively rather than as an ideology (Amada, 1995).

A *theory* is a set of propositions that are designed to describe, explain, and predict. Two forms of theory are theories of personality and theories of human behavior. Many of these theories grew out of theorists' experiences working with individuals in therapeutic relationships, and examples are the theories of Freud, Jung, Adler, Sullivan, Hôrney, and Rogers (Hall and Lindzey, 1970:526). All of these theories are well codified in extensive literature. In the discussion of using theory in supervision in this chapter, this form of theory is used as well as the unsystematized form of theory referred to as practice theory.

Practice Theory

Practice theory, also referred to as theory of practice, is a highly generalized term used in connection with the individual theory utilized by various practitioners. "A *practice* is a sequence of actions undertaken by a person to serve others, who are considered clients" (Argyris and Schon, 1980:6). Practice theory is what distinguishes helping professionals from other professionals. Horney observed, "A saleswoman will heed other qualities in a customer than a social worker will in a client applying for help" (1942:115). A clinical theory of practice is a highly individualized set of propositions aimed at communicating how change is produced in relation to clients, while a salesperson operates from a set of goals and behaviors that will maximize sales and profits.

There is a distinction between formal theory and practice theory. Formal theory is the highly organized conceptions that constitute textbook explanations and that practitioners can describe. Practitioners can give articulate accounts of Freudian, cognitive, behavioral, existential, and other theories. These descriptions bear little resemblance to what practitioners do in their practice. Although formal theory is used to initiate clinical discussions, practitioners quickly launch into what they do and how the client acts in treatment. Supervisors must listen closely to these descriptions because supervisees' practice theories emerge from them.

Practitioners have an "espoused theory" that they use when asked how they would behave in a given practice situation and a "theory in use" (Argyris and Schon, 1980) that actually governs their behavior. This distinction is important for a discussion of supervision and how to manage theory exploration in supervisory sessions. For example, a clinician's espoused theory might be made up totally or in part of descriptions of the various theories of personality and human behavior that exist in the literature, but his or her theory in use, which is made known to the supervisor through direct observation of practice behavior, might be quite different. For the theory in practice to be effective, it must be congruent with the espoused theory. Promoting this congruence is the main task of the supervisor in the theory exploration component of supervision.

TEACHING THEORY

In teaching theory, supervisors tend to use conceptual perspectives at the same time as supervisees are attempting to apply experiential material. A natural incongruence is built into this situation. The supervisor must find a way to promote congruence. This gap can be lessened, but rarely eliminated, by

1. *connecting* the conceptual material with experiential material;
2. *translating* the conceptual material into experiential material before and while presenting it to the supervisee; or
3. *abandoning* the conceptual material, presenting exclusively experiential material, and checking that the supervisee has made the association.

Completely eliminating the gap between the two areas means telling the supervisee what to do and why to do it. This is ineffective because it fosters dependence and should be differentiated from the third procedure of abandoning.

Learning a theory and learning to apply a theory are two different matters. These two forms of theory learning involve different skills, and it is primarily the application form with which the supervisor will need to deal. In this process, the supervisor must constantly keep in mind three salient factors in relation to the supervisee. The supervisee

1. knows only what can be stated,
2. knows only what is manifested by behavior, and
3. knows more than can be told and more than behavior consistently shows. (Argyris and Schon, 1980)

Initially there seems to be a contradiction in these factors, but they could be adopted as a functional creed for the supervisor. The supervisor must focus on having supervisees state what they know as well as stating something so that they can know it; exploring supervisees' knowledge about their behavior as well as discussing their behavior will improve their knowledge of it. This is the essence of the supervisory process, and repeated circular discussion of factors one and two leads to that unknowable component of practice contained in factor three.

THEORY AND PRACTICE CONNECTION

The connection between theory and practice has worried social work educators and supervisors since the beginning of education for practice. This concern grows out of the supervisor's desire to have students and practitioners proficient in theory as well as practice. In efforts to achieve this, there has not been ample recognition that attempts to mix theory and practice randomly are more likely to result in confusion than in solutions. Research has demonstrated that educational techniques for the integration of theory and practice are different. To achieve this integration, which has been called "dynamic intellectualism," requires use of educational models that promote systematic comprehension of both theory and practice (Williams, 1982:168-169).

In part, the confusion of the past has been fostered by the direct and indirect use of the term and process of *eclecticism*. It is common to hear students and practitioners say, "I don't use any one theoretical orientation; I am eclectic." The word *eclectic* is loosely borrowed from the arts. It means "selecting what appears to be best in various doctrines, methods, or styles";

eclecticism is "the theory or practice of an eclectic method" (*Merriam-Webster's Collegiate Dictionary,* 1994:365). Eclecticism relates more to techniques or components that make up a theory rather than being a theory itself. Once the best components have been organized into a new constellation, they constitute a theory of eclecticism that can be explained and described. This new description is the espoused theory, and the applications of eclectic components are the theory in use described earlier. In supervision it is insufficient for supervisees to say, "I am eclectic." Supervisors must require supervisees to state the set of propositions that make up their espoused theory of eclecticism.

In the past conceptual thinking was limited by the belief that it is the theory itself that is important in supervision and practice. The real task is using the theory, understanding and applying it, being able to observe when theory is relevant, and recognizing the limits of theory in practice.

Theory alone without connection to behavior or without connection to case examples is of little value. Not making this connection has been responsible for repeated shortcomings in applying theory to practice.

In social work education programs, much time is devoted to talking about theory. Some discussions present theories accurately, but at times there is confusion because what is presented as theory does not genuinely meet the criteria of theory. This confuses students about theory and its relevance to practice. This confusion carries over when graduates begin practicing. Many practitioners say that they use theory, but if their work is observed, there is no connection between the theory that they say they use and what they actually do.

This chapter is an orientation to theory utilization that can be helpful in the supervisory process. In this approach, theory is not just an abstraction, not just a set of concepts that somehow gets presented in supervision but never used in the agency or with cases. Supervisors actually connect few theories with the behavior seen in clients and practitioners. When such a connection is made—a concept from a theory is used to understand or explain actual dynamics in a case—it is one of the most exciting and fascinating events a supervisor and supervisee can share; it is one of those rare instances in which the abstract world comes together with the real world. This is the essence of learning through supervision.

For theory to be helpful, it must be useful. Practice theory must be at the level of relating all aspects in the theory to what takes place in practice. In order for the theory to be helpful, the concepts must be constantly related to behavior. If abstract theory is all the supervisor has to offer, it would be better just to teach people techniques. As supervisors begin to use theory as a learning tool in supervision, they need to know the basic, traditional approaches to theory. Supervisors must learn about theory before learning a theory, and they must teach about theory before teaching a theory.

ELEMENTS OF THEORY

What is a theory? Theory is the explanation of the interrelatedness of concepts. Theory has been defined in various other ways, but essentially this is what theory is for the practicing supervisor. A theory is made up of a set of conventions, and almost all theories—or, at least, the theories used in the be-havioral sciences—have three basic elements: facts, concepts, and hypotheses.

Facts

Every theory has facts. There are various levels and types of facts. The only level of fact that is of concern in practice theories is that of verifiable observations. General facts can exist on several levels in clinical practice. A practitioner could say that the person is a twenty-eight-year-old white man. That is a set of three facts—twenty-eight years old, white, and male—and this could easily be verified. Another level of fact is that this man is having difficulty in his social relationships, especially with his wife and his em-ployer. Most of the time this would be accepted as a fact, and it is a form of fact, but it cannot be verified in the same way as his age, race, and gender.

At another level, one could say that this man seems to have suicidal ten-dencies. Some would declare this statement as a fact, but facts can get fuzzy in supervision. Does this mean that the person has to commit suicide before these tendencies can be verified as a fact? No, that would be absurd. A cer-tain general level of fact is accepted in practice as theory is used in supervision. The critical point is that any "statement of fact" accepted in supervision should be able to be verified from the practice activity. To accept suicidal tenden-cies as a fact in supervision and theory, observations and statements from the treatment session must verify such tendencies.

If something cannot be verified, it is an assumption or interpretation. If a supervisor and supervisee do not agree on the verification the supervisee of-fers regarding a case dynamic, it remains an assumption until they can agree on an alternate verification. This is an important basic process that the su-pervisor and supervisee engage in as they go about amassing factual infor-mation that becomes the foundation for theory application.

Concepts

The next level moves from the realm of facts into that of concepts. Con-cepts are symbols used to describe objects, events, characteristics, traits, etc. The symbol is expressed as the equivalent of the phenomenon it repre-sents (Lastrucci, 1967:77). For example, professionals talk about concepts such as anxiety, and anxiety cannot be seen or verified. However, it can be verified that clients sway back and forth in their chairs constantly, or that they keep tapping their feet on the floor, or that they sit on the edge of their chairs and rock. This constitutes the manifestation of a concept. There is a statement of the concept that a person suffers from anxiety, and that symbolic meaning has been connected with a fact, or a series of facts, that is then used to describe that concept.

Hypotheses

The third important element of a theory is a hypothesis or hypotheses. A hypothesis is the statement of relationship between concepts. One can now see how facts, concepts, and hypotheses are interrelated. It can be said that a man's mother died when he was three years old, that he was shifted from foster home to foster home, that this left him with a great deal of instability and insecurity, and that this seems to be generating much of his current anxiety about raising his children. In this hypothesis, an attempt is made to connect the idea of anxiety and early childhood experiences. A hypothesis is formulated that these three factors are related. The possibility exists that these factors are not related. In the practice situation, the task is to test this hypothesis by helping the man to see this connection and to overcome it. His anxiety should decrease if the hypothesis is valid.

The concepts themselves do not become facts; they are still concepts. Concepts and facts taken alone are of little value. It is only when the connection is made between concept A and concept B that they have any use. This is the practical explanation of theory in supervisory practice.

Supervisors often teach theory by essentially saying, for example, "This is psychoanalysis, which was founded by Sigmund Freud. He developed concepts such as the unconscious, the preconscious, the conscious, the ego, the id, the superego, transference, countertransference, and insight. If people gain insight, they get better." Rarely do supervisors or teachers connect those concepts with real events in the lives of clients. For example, when the concepts in the case of the man mentioned earlier are applied, part of the equation exists: anxiety is present and has been observed. The supervisor can say that what needs to be done is to help the man develop insight. Many times, however, one of the problems with teaching from a purely theoretical approach is that knowledge of how to give rise to insight is lacking. How do you do it? How can one relate what is going on unconsciously with this person to his anxiety? In terms of how supervisors teach theory and its utilization for practice, concepts often are not connected to the behavior, and the distinction between what are the facts in the case, what are the concepts, and what are the hypotheses is overlooked.

The problem is that, at times, a supervisory hypothesis is generated, an intervention is made, and no support is found for the hypothesis. When this happens, the tendency is to continue to apply the same hypothesis and intervention. To keep testing the same hypothesis over, with a slightly different result but nothing that confirms the hypothesis, is not effective. Evidence suggests that clinicians can stray from the theory in use at this point, causing the intervention to flounder. All hypotheses are predictions, and the outcomes of the hypotheses should be held up to the theory in the supervision to keep the practice focused. The supervisor should strive to adhere to the idea of what the facts, concepts, and hypotheses are and how they work in relation to theory. Use of this strategy is necessary to meet the outcome and effectiveness expectations that are hallmarks of what managed cost organizations advocate but do not know how to implement.

Another way to think of a hypothesis, rather than as the interrelationship between concepts, is that a hypothesis is always, "If A, then B." The connection could be causation or association. Most of the time the behavioral sciences do not operate on the basis of causation. There is limited knowledge of what causes the behavior that clients present—although it is interesting that much is known about what causes problems to subside, that given certain conditions, B will cease. For example, if a client is psychotic and is given human contact, concern, and care, psychosis can remit. In many instances, when psychotic persons are severely withdrawn and flooded with contact—touching, holding—they will improve. It is not known what causes the psychosis to subside, or whether it will return, but this hypothesis has been tested time after time, and it works. This hypothesis cannot be reversed to say that if concern and touching and human contact cause psychosis to subside, lack of human care, concern, and touching must cause psychosis. Information is not available to make the causative statement, but based on the testing of the connection between A and B, it is possible to act on the association between the two concepts.

Another way of approaching hypothesis testing in practice and supervision is for the supervisor to use the idea of *paired concepts* or *dual concepts*. This means that the supervisor should limit the supervisee's discussing one concept. For example, the supervisee who spends much time discussing the symptoms and behaviors that describe a male client's depression is dealing with a single concept. (This occurs in the supervisee reaction of persistent diagnosis described in Chapter 5.) Two concepts should normally be the basis of discussion, so that when a man's depression is under exploration, so should be at least one other concept. The second concept could be self-esteem at a given time in relation to his children, to his wife, to his employer, or to his parents. Depression might occur in cycles and be associated with any of the concepts described. Depression might be associated with the loss of a significant relationship. It could be due to life stage changes and a loss of meaning and goals. The point is that in the diagnostic phase or the treatment phase, discussion of a single concept is of limited value; it is only when one concept is explored in relation to another that supervision can give meaning, direction, and focus to the supervisee's treatment effort. Karen Horney commented on this process in treatment: "The chain of associations that reveals a connection need not be a long one. Sometimes a sequence of only two remarks opens up a path for understanding" (1942:121). This is a simple way to approach concepts, but it is a down-to-earth description of hypothesis testing. Also, observation and content analysis of supervisory sessions reveal that much time is wasted engaging in single-concept approaches rather than dual-concept approaches. Dual-concept case exploration produces more positive supervisory interaction and higher levels of accomplishment and satisfaction than single-concept discussion.

FUNCTIONS OF THEORY

How is theory used in supervisory practice? Theory is used primarily in three ways: to organize, to explain, and to predict.

Organization Function

First, theory can be used to organize what practitioners do. In terms of the theories used, the daily practice activity that practitioners go through begins with gathering the social history. When the practitioner gathers social history information, unless there is a way to organize the array of information, and a theoretical basis for understanding the information, the process can be confusing. Theory helps to decrease the confusion and will determine the approach to that particular case. The practitioner's orientation will affect the kind of information he or she gets from the client, and the theory used in part determines how the information is presented to the practitioner.

For instance, in many psychoanalytic agencies, emphasis is placed on determining the relationship that a client had or has with his or her father or mother, and what relationship the client's parents had with *their* parents, as this is considered to be important to the client's current difficulty. If the practitioner uses Gestalt theory, more emphasis is placed on what is going on in the client's present environment. If cognitive-behavioral theory is used, the focus is on identifying dysfunctional behaviors.

Even when a client makes a simple statement about not getting along well with his or her mother, the theory will determine how the practitioner responds. According to differing theories, the practitioner could say, for example, "And how does that make you feel?" or "Do you know why you are angry at your mother?" or "Is there anybody else in your environment who reminds you of your mother?" or "How would you know the relationship with your mother was getting better?" or "What prevents you from having a good relationship with your mother?" The list could go on. Theories do determine the focus of the interaction. Nothing is wrong with that. Focusing on a unit of analysis is the function of theory. Theory helps organize intervention, provides a perspective for understanding clinical content, and gives treatment focus. If practitioners hold that they use a theory, then the questions asked should establish a direction for gathering the facts that fit the theory, formulating concepts, and testing hypotheses. If this is not the goal, then there is no reason for using theory.

Situational theoretical orientations in supervision promote more analysis of the interactional process in treatment. The use of intrapsychic theory increases discussion of affect in the treatment. The same is true of systems-oriented supervision, which promotes focus on interaction and psychodynamic orientations that encourage expression of affect. The supervisor must recognize this difference and use different theoretical orientations depending on the practice needs of the supervisee.

In the diagnostic phase, the tendency is to assume that problems are manifested as feelings and that feelings and problems are the same. For example, a practitioner begins an initial interview by stating to the client, "What feelings brought you here in relation to your marriage?" The assumption the practitioner has made, and the perception the client might well develop, is that the feelings about the marriage problems are more significant than the marital events that are conflictual and give rise to certain feelings. Separating problems from feelings about problems helps to sort out the complexity of the diagnostic phase. In the treatment phase, the practitioner can relate the two areas.

Explanation Function

The second function of theory is that it explains behavior. This is a simple, but valuable, point. The more behavior the theory explains, the better it is. Some theories do this better than others.

Theory is something that has always been used by interventionist professions to organize explanations of how they intervene. In many respects, theory has been independent of practice. For sociologists, a much different framework exists in that practice for them is dependent upon the theory because theory has been so basic to the discipline. Sociological knowledge has always been organized through theories and their subsequent concepts, whereas social work knowledge has been, and continues to be, organized around behavior and action (Gordon, 1981; Reid, 1981). The unit of analysis has presented problems for both professions. The failure of both groups to recognize the origins of their orientations and the impact of orientations on outcomes has prevented creative problem-solving efforts from emerging. In social work, the mixing of theoretical orientations with action orientations has resulted in confusion. The intermingling of psychological and sociological theories and action (character structure, role, and social structure) has been described by Chescheir. She concludes:

> As social workers, we need a number of different theories of personality and social systems to understand all the different events, behaviors, and conditions that we encounter in practice. Sorting through this wealth of theories, methods, and techniques can be a confusing process for the practitioter and this difficulty remains a principal concern of the profession. (1979:94)

Prediction Function

The third function of theory is to predict what the outcome will be. Clarity about the level of predictability is different, but the theory itself should predict an outcome. For example, systems theory predicts that if one part of the system is changed, all the other parts will also be affected and will change. That is one level of prediction. Proponents of this theory say that an action is going to have an effect on the system without explaining what the effect will be. Prediction at this level of abstraction is of limited value. The supervisor should assist the practitioner in reducing the theory to the level of specific behavior in order to be of value in supervising a practitioner. For instance, a practitioner is working with the family of a retarded child and they are trying to decide if they should institutionalize the child, and the supervisee will mention the impacts on the family. What impacts? There could be negative impacts; there could be positive impacts; there will probably be both. Do the positive impacts outweigh the negative impacts? This is where predictability comes into consideration. Other parts of the system must be known before the level of predictability can be defined. The basic tenet from systems theory is true: If one part of the system is changed, the other parts will also change. What becomes important in supervision, however, is what will change and how it will change.

COMPONENTS OF THEORY

Organize, explain, predict—these are the three main functions of theory. The supervisor and practitioner have to be able to use theory to organize what is done, to explain what happens, and to predict what could happen or might happen. In addition, good theory has four other components.

First, it has to have *utility.* This concept means the theory must be useful in treatment and in supervision.

Second, it has to be *verifiable.* That is, there must be a way to verify that the things the theory postulates do in fact exist or happen. This is one area in which psychoanalytic theory has been accused of being weak. Many times practitioners who are not closely associated with psychoanalytic theory will use the unconscious as a way to avoid verifying conclusions they have drawn. Current psychoanalytic writers are moving from the exclusively unconscious model to an interactional model. They are attempting to make elements of the theory more verifiable (Langs, 1979; Schafer, 1976). There is no necessary connection between utility and verifiability. For example, many of the concepts of existential theory are highly abstract. They do not have a lot of verifiability, but they do have a lot of utility. Any theory that has both utility and verifiability is more useful.

Third, theory has to be *comprehensive*. How much of the behavior shown in the treatment situation is the theory able to explain? Psychoanalytic theory is strong in this component. It is a comprehensive theory, which in turn gives it much utility, although its limited verifiability weakens it. Perhaps this weakness will be overcome as current and future writers and researchers report their findings. Empirical verification of psychoanalytic theory is increasing.

Part of the problem historically has been that Freud used the inductive method, and most people who do academic research use the deductive method. Most practice theories, which come from the inductive method involves going out into the world and gathering evidence, and from that evidence drawing conclusions upon which to formulate concepts and theories. The deductive method remains abstract: one states certain hunches, or formulates certain hypotheses, and then goes out into the world to see if reality conforms to one's conception of it.

Some theoreticians do not think that the inductive method is as acceptable as a scientific method. They believe one has to use the deductive method to be scientific. Theories in practice have been formulated mainly through the inductive method. However, future verification of these theories will come from the use of the deductive method. In the supervision process, both inductive and deductive methods are used in case analysis.

The fourth component of theory is *simplicity*—not that the theory is simple, but that it explains complex information in a concise, accurate, and understandable manner. Great artists in any field have as the essence of their creativity and greatness the ability to create simplicity out of complex material. No less is true of the good supervisor who is able to discover simplicity in complexity, allowing information to be communicated and understood by the supervisee.

The basic discussion of theory has been stated in simple form, and much detail has been left out because the objective has been to describe theory in terms that the supervisor can readily use in the supervisory process. The aim has been that, using this material, the supervisor can quickly and easily promote learning through the ideas of fact, concept, hypothesis, organization, explanation, prediction, utility, verifiability, comprehensiveness, and simplicity. The first six components can be used to guide the supervisory inter-action, and the last four can be helpful in selecting established theories to apply in supervision.

THEORETICAL SPECULATION

Practitioners show varying ability to apply theory to their practice. As noted in Chapter 5, some practitioners have difficulty "boiling theoretical water," while others can apply theory to practice with much effort. Rarely will a supervisor encounter a practitioner who can apply theory with ease. In assessing the practitioner's level of theoretical knowledge and ability to ap-ply it, the supervisor must keep in mind that using theory in supervision pre-dominantly relates to the teaching and learning roles and has minimal rele-vance to the solving of immediate practice problems. Educational programs indoctrinate the importance of espoused academic theory that can hamper insight regarding immediate and difficult problems that occur in practice. This manifests itself as theoretical speculation (discussed in Chapter 5).

Practitioners will introduce theoretical speculation into supervision when they lack coping strategies to deal with practical problems. Supervisors must be aware of this and repeatedly bring the practitioner back to technical therapeutic issues. The supervisor must keep in mind the economy of super-vision and its focus on aiding the supervisee in being more effective with the client. Clients do not care about theory and its relationship to the problem. This is illustrated in a study of family therapy outcome done in England in which the families made it clear they did not care about systems theory—they just wanted to be viewed as individuals in a family with problems that needed help (Howe, 1989). From this perspective, the supervision should focus on what to say or what to do next in the treatment. Any use of theory should be based on the practical aspects of the case. If theory can be used to predict an outcome or can guide the sorting out of problem areas, its use is warranted. The supervisor needs to monitor the supervision interaction con-stantly to ensure that theoretical speculation is being used to enhance the treatment rather than to resist confronting sensitive problems or concerns.

TIMING

The use of theory for long-range learning purposes must be reserved for less immediate points in the supervision. Cases used to teach theory need to be selected carefully. When the supervisor feels that the supervisee needs to develop more theoretical knowledge, timing is important. Cases cannot al-ways be dealt with on a crisis basis. This is important because practitioners who resist learning theory show a tendency to present cases on a crisis basis and will jump from case to case in supervision. This must be guarded against, and the supervisor will need to control the rapidity and fragmentation of case presentation. In such situations, the supervisor must keep in mind his or her guidance role. The teaching of theory can leave the practitioner with the impression that theory is the important factor in supervision, and this will logically lead him or her into using theoretical speculation at times when a crisis or difficulty occurs.

THEORY AND TECHNIQUE

A basic question is, Can one learn techniques of intervention that have been found effective without presuming such techniques can be directly related to a body of theory? The answer to this question is yes, but at the same time, this does not imply that theory is unimportant to practice and supervision. Theory is important, especially in helping practitioners develop self-confidence in their orientation to treatment and in articulating and communicating that orientation to colleagues, supervisors, and clients.

Use of theory is only indirectly apparent within the treatment process but is directly applicable to consideration of the treatment process outside the actual treatment situation. One underutilized vehicle for improving treatment skills is increased articulation outside of treatment of what is done in treatment. One reason this does not occur is that students of therapy have not been provided adequate, consistent models and theories to use in organizing explanation of their therapy. For example, some teachers and supervisors place heavy emphasis on the concept of equifinality from systems theory to argue that regardless of the theory used, the outcome is often the same. This brings the use of theory into serious question, but at the same time, people who hold this view have students survey many theories and master none. This approach is confusing to learners and gives them little incentive to organize their orientations and descriptions of practice.

Supervisors should avoid expecting supervisees to apply specific theoretical material when supervisees lack adequate knowledge of the theory or lack sufficient practice experience. A good rule to follow is exploration with supervisees of their practice theory before progressing to exploration of an espoused academic theory.

Supervisors should avoid attempting to apply theories with which they lack thorough familiarity. It is inappropriate for supervisors to pass on to supervisees a heritage of defective theoretical knowledge. Supervisors who do this take the risk of losing supervisees' trust and respect. This problem is epitomized by one supervisee's comment: "My supervisor has not read anything in ten years, but she is constantly telling me to become more familiar with the literature."

Learning theory necessitates a delicate balance that avoids confronting the supervisee with too large or too small increments of information. If the increments of learning are too large, confusion results, and if the increments are too small, frustration arises. There is no specific formula for the correct size increments because they must be based on an assessment of the knowledge, skill, and ability of each supervisee.

Solid grounding in one theory is preferred by most supervisors, as well as applying it to practice before moving to comparing and contrasting it with competing theories. Pressure can be made less for the learning practitioner by articulating what has taken place or will take place in the treatment situation in a theoretical context, rather than insisting that the theory be used directly in the actual treatment session to determine the course of the therapeutic interaction. This is not a rigid rule, but a guiding principle. It is based on the repeated discovery in research that it is the wisdom and experience of the practitioner and the nature of the relationship he or she has with the client that are the crucial variables related to outcome, rather than the theories or techniques used. A major point in this context that the supervisor must remember is that *supervisors must help practitioners set up a theoretical hook on which to hang their practice hat.*

THEORY ABANDONMENT

One strategy for being more specific, and therefore more helpful in supervision, is to ask the practitioner to abandon conceptual thinking temporarily and to focus exclusively on treatment interaction. Conceptual and theoretical thinking require a Gestalt thought process in the generic sense of the term. Gestalt thinking requires understanding the whole to understand the parts. This process can be complex for practitioners at certain stages. Nonconceptual thinking moves from the parts to understanding the whole. Theory and concepts can be applied later.

An case example illustrates this:

> A practitioner was having difficulty understanding a client's pattern of behavior. The supervisor asked him to move to simply describing what events were apparent. He described the client as going to college, then dropping out. Soon after, she met and married an older man. Two years later the marriage was dissolved. Shortly after the end of the marriage she returned to school, and soon after completing her education, she became anxious and doubtful. Soon after graduation, she remarried. The woman sought treatment as this second marriage was

collapsing, and she was contemplating returning to school to pursue a master's degree. This pattern of events was brought to light through a set of careful questions by the supervisor. Only after this pattern was identified could the supervisor help the practitioner see the relationship between marriage and education in providing structure to this woman's life.

Even though this person was a good practitioner, he failed to see the conceptual connection until he was required to identify the empirical events in sequence without reference to any pattern. He felt much better about the case after the supervisory session and returned to the therapy situation with renewed confidence of understanding a major dynamic that occurs in many cases. Follow-up revealed that this material resulted in a breakthrough in the treatment and facilitated identification of related patterns of functioning.

An example of abandoning theory can illustrate the relationship between theoretical argument and technical strategy:

A supervisor and beginning practitioner sought consultation on a case that involved the involuntary court order that a child-abusing family receive treatment at a mental health center. During an initial interview the family members appeared quite nervous, especially the father. The worker sought supervisory assistance with this specific manifestation because he had encountered similar problems of nervousness in cases of this nature in the past, and he had had difficulty dealing with the material.

In other words, the practitioner had identified a specific problem area in his practice and was requesting help in developing a technical strategy. When such material is presented for consultation, a component of the supervision has become problematic in addition to the case material that is presented, and the consultant should approach the situation in a way that will promote direct or indirect identification of possible supervision obstacles.

The consultant began by asking if this problem had come up in supervision before, and the reply was that it had. The supervisor indicated that he had focused on how the worker felt about the client's nervousness. The worker, with difficulty, admitted that seeing agitation in clients, especially a family, made him nervous. The supervisor then pursued what made the worker nervous. The supervisor's approach was based on his stated orientation as a Gestalt theorist that the practitioner needed to deal with his "here and now" feelings and what was making him nervous. This approach simply made the worker more nervous. The consultant asked the supervisor and worker to abandon this theoretical orientation, which had resulted in a dead end and, in fact, was making the situation worse. Instead, the focus was placed on the treatment interaction and establishing goals for the treatment, as well as on how the worker could keep the interaction focused on the family and its problems. It came out that the worker was not clear about how to proceed with certain content, especially sexual content. Once the worker learned specific strategies for focusing on the family and handling its nervousness, his tension subsided, and his confidence as a practitioner grew.

In this example, theory-based exploration was a block to learning and needed to be abandoned to promote growth. Supervisors need to be alert to such situations to avoid allowing theory to block growth. Supervision should be guided by theory, but the discussion does not always have to be in theoretical or conceptual terms. One purpose of theory is to provide a frame of reference or a focus. It is necessary to return to the theory only periodically to ensure that the discussion is within the theoretical framework. Some theories focus on internal dynamics, others focus on environment influences, and others focus on a combination of the two. If the theory is used as a checkpoint for the discussion, it can be a valuable aid in keeping the supervision focused and consistent.

How theory can inadvertently lead to a block in the discussion of case material is illustrated by a supervisee's observations of a component of her group supervision:

> Larry, one of the other interns, is caught up in this struggle with the supervisor over theory and who knows the most about it. They'll get into a debate over some little point from the theory. The supervisor will give Larry some readings, and Larry doesn't read them but he will still argue about the points. It's an ongoing thing. The rest of us get tired of this and feel we aren't getting what we should out of the group. Sometimes the supervisor is accommodating toward Larry and concedes points rather than address the real issue.

This supervisor is caught in the trap of theoretical speculation and does not know how to cope with it. If the supervisor in this example does not get help, he will eventually lose the respect of the entire group, and perpetual frustration will be the result. In this situation, neither the interns nor the clients are getting what they deserve from supervision. The technique of theory abandonment would help this supervisor. The real issue of authority, power, and knowledge could be better dealt with by putting theory aside and focusing on the case dynamics.

CREATIVITY AND THEORY

Creativity and use of theory in practice are antithetical. Theories place boundaries on what supervisors and practitioners do. Theorists consistently hold users of theory to established concepts, especially in deductive theory, while inductive theory forces a constant search for patterns. Creative artists, on the other hand, cherish the freedom to go wherever their art takes them. Boundaries are not the companion of the artist. This does not mean that the artist works unfettered. Artists must master their craft. For the artist, method and technique are the means to creating and producing original outcomes. For the clinician, theory predicts the outcome. To the extent that creativity is possible in practice, it is limited to the confines of the theory, whereas for the artist theory and technique are prerequisites to creating new forms.

This basic inconsistency of theory and art in psychotherapy has never been resolved. Some practitioners have called for abandonment of theory; others consider it folly to do so and believe such a strategy invites chaos, inconsistency, and incompetence. This issue should be explored and could help advance knowledge of the use of theory in practice. If theory were abandoned, how would this contribute to the art of social work practice? What are the foundation techniques to be mastered that would guide creativity? If these questions were confronted, perhaps mental health intervention could become genuinely artistic without fear of producing merely unrestrained performances.

THEORY APPLICATION

Haley believes that supervisors tend to supervise from the same theoretical orientation that they use in therapy (1976:170). Although this may be the case, a slightly different perspective is required when defining good clinical supervisory practices. Supervision involves common use of techniques and strategies regardless of the supervisor's theoretical orientation. Supervision can be superimposed on any theory of practice, just as the scientific method can be applied to any research topic. Some content and the focus of supervision may vary according to the theory, but how the supervisor asks questions, makes comments, and offers interpretations should remain consistent. This provides the supervisee with a systematic, consistent way of approaching supervision over time and can reinforce and solidify learning.

There has been debate about the role of theory in treatment. Rogers held that attitudes and feelings of the practitioner are more important to treatment outcome than theory or technique (Stein, 1961:98). Bowen views theory as important; Whitaker believed the use of theory isolates the practitioner, dichotomizes the treatment, makes the practitioner an observer, and stifles practitioner creativity (Guerin, 1976:154-164). Little systematic study focuses on how theory is actually used in therapy and how it affects what is said and what gets done. There is little conscious use of theory in the actual practice of therapy. Beginning practitioners, who are struggling with the intensity of the treatment situation, have little energy to invest in the skilled use of theory, and the experienced practitioner focuses on the therapeutic interaction and issues to be explored without conscious consideration of the theoretical implications of this activity. This does not mean that theory is unimportant in clinical practice. What practitioners have been taught about theory does show up in their work, but this is seldom consciously recognized. It is the role of the supervisor to make this conscious awareness, so the supervisee can have it under his or her control to use for the benefit of clients.

Videotapes of good practitioners at work show consistent patterns of interaction that can be traced to their theoretical training and to the "theory in use" that they claim to hold when outside of a practice situation. For purposes of supervision, this becomes an important observation. To give practitioners the technical skill to know how to deal with therapy content, the supervisor must have a way to organize the analysis of therapy content. Although the practitioner may not always be aware of the use of theory in the practice situation, effective supervision for practice must be theoretically based. Carl Whitaker has pointed out that research suggests that nontheoretical practitioners can be effective when given good supervision (Guerin, 1976:163). A good rule to follow is that the more nontheoretical the therapy becomes, the more important theory is in supervision.

THEORY AND SUPERVISION INTERACTION

The supervisor must be careful of using theory in the abstract. Abstract use of theory occurs for a number of reasons. Supervisors in some instances lack the skill to apply theory effectively because they have never been trained in this way. Some supervisors feel it is their responsibility to identify and explain theory, and it is up to the practitioners to make the connections to practice. Some supervisors use theory abstraction to avoid dealing directly with difficult or unfamiliar case material. Weak supervisors use this pattern consistently, but even good supervisors will occasionally handle difficult supervisory material this way.

Supervisors find it easier and more stimulating to talk about theory rather than cases, and supervisees respond in the same way. Supervisors focus on theory sometimes out of resistance, but more often they use it to combat boredom with clinical material. Supervisees often use theory to resist clinical material. Where both sides have so much to gain from abstract theoretical discussion, the supervisor must constantly be alert to theory in the abstract.

If the supervisor and the supervisee work consciously to apply theory to practice, much of the boredom and resistance can be overcome. These problems emerge because the participants do not work at applying theory to clinical material. Research observation of supervision sessions demonstrates that the supervisor explains theoretical concepts and the practitioner presents a case summary, but seldom do they interrelate the two. The functions of theory are to describe, explain, and predict. These concepts should be the basis of applying theory to clinical material. The theory should be used to describe what exists, to explain what is taking place in the case, and to predict or project what interventions the practitioner must make.

Theory and practice material must be defined independently before they can be integrated. The supervisor and practitioner must develop a *joint style* of how they will segment the supervision to contain the three components of theory, clinical material, and integration. Some like to lay out the theory, then summarize the case material, and finally apply the concepts to the case. Others reverse this process, and some alternate between the two styles. There is no best way to accomplish this, but it is a good idea for the supervisor to identify the three methods and allow the practitioner to select the style with which he or she feels comfortable.

It is important that the supervisor and practitioner work together to select a procedural method and stay with that method until they discuss and select an alternate style. This prevents the supervision from becoming unfocused or imbalanced in favor of theory or case material. The supervisor has ultimate responsibility to ensure that the procedural method is being followed. This does not mean that all supervisory sessions will be stylistically segmented. At times this format will not be appropriate to the content.

GUIDELINES FOR APPLYING THEORY
TO CLINICAL MATERIAL

1. Theory as such cannot be applied to clinical material; only concepts from theories can be applied. The supervisor needs to point this out to the practitioner and structure the discussion around specific concepts in relation to specific clinical examples. The supervisor should avoid the approach, for example, "How does Bowen's theory apply to this case?" and instead use, "How do Bowen's concepts of individualization and separation apply to how this couple present themselves and the verbal conflict in their marriage about child care?"

2. Theoretical material must be related to clinical material. A good rule for the supervisor to follow is that no theoretical concept should be presented without one or more clinical examples.

3. It is easier for practitioners to handle criticism of their work when it is presented in relation to practice theory.

4. It is easier for practitioners to understand the implications of an action in theoretical terms rather than simply in terms of practitioner or supervisor behavior or feelings.

5. Supervisors frequently complain that it is difficult to apply theory to practice, and that there are no good guidelines for doing this. It can be complex and difficult to relate theory and technique, but to get started the supervisor need only ask the supervisee two questions: (a) What would you do in this situation? and (b) What are your reasons for doing it? The first question relates to technique, and the second relates to theory.

6. Beginning practitioners can believe that if concepts from a theory are summarized and a case history presented, the theory has been applied to practice. This is only a beginning step. Theoretical concepts must be clearly and consistently integrated with practice material. When theory and practice are being learned simultaneously, it is the supervisor's responsibility to foster integration.

7. Supervisors tend to talk about terminology, facts, and problems much less than they discuss theories, theorists, ideas, and concepts. For example, it is common for a supervisor to say, "We mainly use Minuchin's structural model here and some of Erikson's strategic methods," without any specific explanation for the young practitioner of precisely what is meant by this. This leaves practitioners to make whatever they want of such statements, which becomes the information they pass on when they become supervisors. When discussing a theory or a theorist, both the supervisor and practitioner must know exactly what theoretical concepts are under discussion.

8. After discussing the theoretical implications of a case, the supervisor and supervisee must decide what to do about the case. This is similar to the process in research of explaining a hypothesis after having provided statistically significant support for it. Rather than theoretical discussion being the ending point in supervision, it should be the beginning.

9. Knowledge developed in supervision must be explored as both an independent and a dependent variable until a logical understanding is derived. This relates to the idea of dual-concept exploration explained earlier in this chapter. Sometimes the ordering of the concepts must be reversed to understand the correct sequence of occurrence and association.

CONCLUSION

Learning to use theory in practice, or integrating thought with action, has plagued and frustrated mental health professionals for a long time (Argyris and Schon, 1980:3). Theory is something that has always been used by interventionist professions to organize explanations of how they intervene as well as to disguise their failures at intervention. In social work, the mixing of theoretical orientations with action techniques has too often resulted in confusion. The best place to begin to deal with this concern is supervision. This chapter has identified basic coping mechanisms for supervisors and practitioners to use in this effort.

Case Exercise:
The Case of Jerry

Jerry is a sixteen-year-old adopted child who was placed in a state mental facility eighteen months ago after he became angry with a classmate who called him a "son of a bitch." Jerry "destroyed" a classroom by throwing furniture, books, and other objects around the room. Jerry was in the residential facility for one month and was discharged to a small group home (eleven beds). He has been placed at the group home for the past seventeen months. He had a change of therapists in July of this year. It is now October. Jerry was placed in the group home in April of the previous year. This chronology is explained here because it has temporal aspects that become important in understanding Jerry's behavior.

Jerry's adoptive mother died of cancer when Jerry was six years old. Nothing is known about Jerry's biological parents. Jerry's adoptive mother was a high school teacher; she taught music and foreign languages. Jerry's adoptive mother died a painful and debilitating death over a one-year period. Jerry witnessed much of his adoptive mother's painful process, though he was not told that she was dying. Jerry's father married one year after the adoptive mother died. The stepmother attended the same church that Jerry and his parents attended. The stepmother was a religious, but not affectionate or expressive person. She and Jerry's father removed all traces of Jerry's dead mother from their lives. They moved into a new house with new furniture, and all pictures and other objects associated with Jerry's adoptive mother were removed. At the time of admission to the group home, Jerry explained to his therapists that he "hated" his adoptive mother for dying and "leaving me," and that he hates his father and his adoptive mother for "not telling me she was dying." Jerry hates his adoptive father and stepmother for "removing all traces of my mother." Jerry does not think about his adoptive mother anymore. He continues to resent his father for "being a wimp." He explained by stating that he wishes his father would "stand up to" the stepmother, and he wishes his father "would have the strength to discipline me when I act up."

After six months at the group home, Jerry was allowed to go home for weekend visits, but the visits were discontinued after several months because of Jerry's behavior. Jerry would dress in black, refuse to attend religious services with his parents, ridiculed his parents' religion, and professed to be an atheist.

Jerry would listen to music that was objectionable to the father and stepmother. A violent argument erupted when the parents destroyed all of Jerry's CDs and removed his CD player from his room. Jerry threatened his parents and they terminated the visit by driving him back to the group home on Saturday night. This incident precipitated the termination of all visits because the stepmother expressed fear for her safety in his presence.

Jerry continued to be depressed and would use dissociation to avoid dealing with people. Jerry explained this by saying that when he did not want to listen to people, he would focus on the junction of the wall and ceiling in the room and think about the words of his favorite song. The therapist would try to engage Jerry in discussion about his mother and his relationship with her, but Jerry would resist and dissociate. The therapist, Karen, expressed frustration to the supervisor that "nothing seems to work with Jerry" and that she "could not get through to him." She expressed, "I have tried everything with him." The supervisor helped Karen develop a strategy of shifting from discussing Jerry's feelings about his mother's death to discussion of the struggles that people have after losing a parent. A plan was devised in which Karen would use a video of a television documentary the supervisor had purchased in which famous musicians discussed the struggles that they had with the death of parents, children, and band members. The video contained the stories of a number of famous musicians, some of whom Jerry idolized. This strategy had limited success with Jerry at the time.

In April, as Jerry was completing his first year at the group home, a nationally televised broadcast report on a school shooting in which children were killed and wounded. Jerry became agitated about these events and made veiled threats about hurting others. The staff became concerned about Jerry and complained to Karen, who discussed the case with her supervisor. The supervisor recommended an outside therapist at the local mental health clinic in addition to the therapy with Karen. Karen questioned the need for an outside therapist and viewed this as a lack of confidence in her skills, even though the supervisor explained that she had recommended an outside therapist because Jerry may be having thoughts of harming staff and residents of the group home and would most likely not discuss that with an in-house therapist for fear of being stopped, punished, or discharged. The supervisor reasoned that Jerry would be more likely to share his thoughts about such actions with an outside therapist, and if he declared intent to do harm, the outside therapist would have to alert the facility because the state has a specific duty-to-warn statute. If this occurred, then the facility therapists would not have been the ones to report Jerry and the relationship could be maintained. The supervisor told Karen to continue to have therapy with Jerry even though an outside therapist would be assigned. The supervisor had to explain her reasoning for the request to get authorization from the group home administrator, who wanted to know why the in-house therapist could not work with Jerry. After explaining her reasoning to the agency director, the request was approved. Jerry was never assigned an outside therapist, however, because the group home had difficulty getting authorization for treatment through the MCO that administered the state Medicaid program.

In July, Karen left the group home to take a job with a local department of social services doing foster care planning. Jerry was assigned another therapist, Jane, who had worked at the group home for several years and had a style of intervention much different from Karen's. Jerry had a strong negative reaction initially to the change of therapists. Jane's style, by her own description, was "more matter of fact and more task oriented than Karen's style." No thought was given to this at the time because there was also a change of supervisors when this new therapist was assigned to work with Jerry. Later it was postulated that the change of therapists caused Jerry to symbolically relive his prior experience of the death of his mother and the replacement by a different mother.

Jerry began to act out in August. In September, soon after the new school year began, Jerry had to be removed from school because he was threatening to harm other students. The group home had Jerry hospitalized. He was discharged from the psychiatric hospital after five days with a slight change in his medication, and the recommendation that the group home seek an outside therapist for Jerry (the psychiatric hospital staff were not aware that Karen's supervisor had made the same recommendation). Soon after leaving the psychiatric hospital, Jerry threatened staff and residents and was returned to the state hospital for three weeks. The state hospital was in Jerry's hometown and was the same hospital he had been sent to after he became violent at school and "destroyed" the classroom. Jerry's parents began regular visits with him at the hospital and had several family therapy sessions. After three weeks, Jerry was discharged because the staff felt Jerry was "starting to feel too comfortable here." It was not clear what the staff meant by this statement, but the hospital social worker told Jane that Jerry was not responding to therapy and was starting to manipulate and control other patients on the adolescent unit.

When Jerry returned to the group home, his behavior got worse but took a different turn. Jerry would have brief angry outbursts, but at other times he would cry profusely for no apparent reason. Jane stated to the supervisor that she did not "know what to do about Jerry, especially around the crying spells," and that she "now really understood Karen's frustration with Jerry." The supervisor suggested that Jane use a simple strategy with Jerry. She should take Jerry into her office when he had a crying spell, allow him some time to become calm, and then simply ask Jerry, "Can you tell me what is making you cry?" Jane did not feel that this would be helpful; it seemed too simplistic and would probably provoke an "I don't know" response from Jerry. The supervisor encouraged her to try it since it could not do any harm and Jerry may be able to connect the crying with some emotion. Jane tried the strategy, and she was surprised at Jerry's response. He stated, "I have been thinking about my mother and I have feelings of guilt and sadness whenever I think of her, and this is what causes me to cry. I do not know why I am crying like this, but it always comes when I think about my mother, and I guess I never let it come out like this before."

You are the supervisor. (1) How would you help Jane understand this case in historical, clinical, and theoretical contexts? (2) What would you recommend regarding the assignment of an additional therapist outside the agency? (3) What would you recommend Jane do next?

SUGGESTED READINGS

Argyris, C. and Schon, D. A. (1980). *Theory in Practice: Increasing Professional Effectiveness.* San Francisco: Jossey-Bass.

An excellent discussion of the practical aspects of theory in use in professions. This book was the source for some of the material in this chapter. It includes discussion of the issues of theory and professional education.

Bailey, J. (1980). *Ideas and Intervention: Social Theory for Practice.* London: Routledge and Kegan Paul.
This book is an advanced treatment of sociological theory. The discussion is somewhat abstract but stimulating. One chapter is devoted to social work and social theory.

Corsini, R. I. (ed.) (1986). *Current Psychotherapies.* Itasca, IL: Peacock.
Coverage of thirteen major theories of psychotherapy. This book is helpful to the supervisor working to help practitioners apply espoused academic theories of psychotherapy.

Ericsson, K. A. and Simon, H. A. (1993). *Protocol Analysis: Verbal Reports As Data.* Cambridge, MA: The MIT Press.
Analysis of verbal reports in research that can provide insights about the type of reporting clients do in therapy.

Kaplan, A. (1964). *The Conduct of Inquiry: Methodology for Behavioral Science.* San Francisco: Chandler.
A classic discussion of the scientific method. The explanation of "logic in use" and "reconstructed logic" has much practical relevance to the use of theory in practice. This book is basic reading for the serious student of the scientific method in the behavioral sciences.

Kazan, A. E. (ed.) (1992). *Methodological Issues and Strategies in Clinical Research.* Washington, DC: American Psychological Association.
Basic overview of research methods relevant to clinical practice.

Lastrucci, C. L. (1967). *The Scientific Approach: Basic Principles of the Scientific Method.* Cambridge, MA: Schenkman.
A basic and thorough introduction to the scientific method.

Pine, F. (1990). *Drive, Ego, Object, and Self.* New York: Basic Books.
Survey of the different schools of psychoanalytic theory.

Robson, C. (1993). *Real World Research: A Resource for Social Scientists and Practitioner-Researchers.* Oxford, UK: Blackwell.
Research from a practitioner perspective. Highly compatible with the theory/research focus in this chapter.

Rosenbaum, M. and Ronen, T. (1998). "Clinical Supervision from the Standpoint of Cognitive-Behavior Therapy," *Psychotherapy,* 35(2), pp. 220-230.
Discussion of cognitive and behavioral therapy (CBT) applied to clinical practice and clinical supervision.

Turner, F. J. (ed.) (1996). *Social Work Treatment: Interlocking Theoretical Perspectives,* Fourth Edition. New York: The Free Press.
A comprehensive and consistent comparison of twenty-seven theories of intervention used in social work practice.

> The study of inspired error should not
> engender a homily about the sin of pride;
> it should lead us to a recognition that the
> capacity for great insight and great error
> are opposite sides of the same coin—and
> that the currency of both is brilliance.
>
> Stephen Jay Gould
> *The Panda's Thumb*

Chapter 9

Evaluation of Practice

The emphasis in this chapter is on evaluation from the perspective of enhancing learning about practice. This form of evaluation is discussed separately from evaluations done in an administrative sense for promotions, salary increments, annual performance reviews, or letters of reference. Practice learning evaluation is illustrated in a simple, four-cell conception derived from a research study of therapy session outcome. The importance of and methods for dealing with practice errors are explained in connection with evaluation. The role of the supervisor in giving criticism and the role of the supervisee in receiving it are explored from an educational, evaluative perspective. Lists of specific suggestions for handling criticism are given for both the supervisor and supervisee. A self-assessment format is explicated that can be used to place a portion of the responsibility for the evaluation on the supervisee to promote a more positive outcome. The roles of research, practice, and note taking from an evaluative perspective are covered. Legal liability of supervisors in connection with evaluation is documented. The relationship between educational and administrative evaluation is articulated. The legal and ethical responsibilities of the supervisor in conducting and directing practice research as evaluation are explained.

INTRODUCTION

A teacher of a group of preschool children asked them, "If you could ask your parents one question that you don't know the answer to, what would it be?" Ninety percent of the children said their question would be, "Do you love me?" (Wiseman, 1979). This seems quite amazing in this age of communication and expression of feelings, but it seems to be a perennial question. Decades ago, Bertha Capen Reynolds wrote, "What are the questions that press in upon everyone who has to get used to living on this planet? Most primary of all for the young child is probably: Am I loved?" (Reynolds, 1965/1942:14). Reynolds held that as the child grows the questions evolve to, "Am I able to do what anybody else my size can do?" and "Can I hold my own with others?"

After hearing about the teacher of preschoolers and reading Reynolds' observations, the author asked the research question of supervisees, "If you could ask your supervisor one question he or she has not answered for you, what would it be?" Almost all of the supervisees were intrigued by the question and gave it a great deal of thought. The overwhelming majority of the answers were variations on the reply, "How do you think I am doing in my work?" This illustrates that people need to know if they are "holding their own."

The answer given by so many supervisees was unexpected, but apparently they are not getting this much-needed feedback from their supervisors. In questioning the supervisees further, it became clear that more attention needs to be given to evaluation and feedback in supervision. The following practitioner response summarizes the attitude of many practitioners:

> I got along with my supervisor. She is a nice person. But there was something about her I couldn't understand. We were on a different wavelength. I think she is smart and knows what she is doing, but she didn't share much of it with me. During the four months she supervised me, we had only two individual sessions together, and each session was about twenty minutes long. I feel badly about that. She really didn't teach me anything. I really regret that. I can't blame her though; she is a very busy person. The hospital expects too much of her, but I can't do anything about that.
>
> I thought we would spend more time together. Aren't you supposed to meet at least once a week? I guess part of it is my problem, though. I never brought any of this up when I met with her. Even when we had our evaluation conference at the end, I didn't say anything about my problems. You see, my evaluation wasn't too good.
>
> I had a lot of personal problems during the past four months, and they affected my work, but I didn't share any of this with her. I never told her about it, so I guess I can't blame her. I wish we would have

been able to talk about it, but it's too late now.

Your question is a hard one to answer, but if I could ask her one question, it would be, What do you see as my major deficiencies?

EVALUATION OF LEARNING

In exploring evaluation in supervision, the term is being used here in a different sense than is commonly thought. It is not used to mean judging the outcome or effectiveness of the treatment. Nor is the evaluation done for administrative purposes, such as promotions, annual reviews of performance, or reference letters. Evaluation as used here is related to the supervisor and practitioner jointly evaluating the supervisee's practice to enhance learning and, therefore, effectiveness in practice. The assumption is that if learning is increased, effectiveness is increased. Practitioners at times should be asked to rate their effectiveness before the evaluation begins. Through using this strategy, the supervisor has a baseline assessment of the supervisee's perception to use in gauging the accuracy of the supervisee's current self-perception, and it can be used in performing a developmental evaluation in six to twelve months. If the supervisor does not establish an initial baseline assessment of the supervisee's level of functioning, the subsequent evaluation has no comparative value.

Evaluation for learning must be separated from measurement of effectiveness to remove opportunities for defensiveness as much as possible. If either the supervisor or the practitioner becomes defensive, the learning ceases. The best way to avoid defensiveness in supervision is to

1. openly admit that defensiveness is waiting in the wings during all discussions and can take up center stage without much provocation;
2. agree to evaluate at any given point in the supervision that defensiveness has possibly emerged and explore ways of eliminating it; and
3. remove at the outset any potential methods that could lead to defensiveness, such as annual performance evaluations, promotion reviews, or comparison to other practitioners.

Where all external evaluation processes are removed from learning-oriented supervision (i.e., when the practitioner is required to undergo such administrative evaluation only at other times), defensiveness tends to be greatly decreased. Practice at nondefensive evaluative learning can aid in developing non defensive styles in administrative evaluation that are effectiveness oriented. This type of evaluation can be referred to as *error acceptance learning;* that is, errors in practice are expected and known to occur, and the supervision process will be a search for such errors without punitive action for the errors discovered. This is similar to the Airline Pilot Association's policy of encouraging pilots to report near misses and other pilot errors without penalty so they can be studied and ways found to remedy them. This mode of evaluation is aimed more at helping the client than it is at judging the practitioner.

SIMPLICITY

Evaluation of learning in supervision must be kept simple to be applied effectively. The structure for discovering errors and promoting learning is simple, but the discussion of discovered errors can be quite complex. When complicated evaluative schemes are devised, error is rarely discovered because much energy and defensiveness go into mastering the scheme, and the process becomes tedious and is often abandoned. This is why it is important to separate research studies and their instruments from evaluation instruments used in supervision.

Simple evaluative instruments and structures can be derived from sophisticated research studies. For example, a study of the therapist's experiences in psychotherapy by Orlinsky and Howard (Gurman and Razin, 1977:566-589) resulted in a number of complex variables being reported in a four-cell conception that is presented in Visual 9.1. Based on thirty-two therapists' perceptions, their effectiveness and the degree of patient distress were tabulated for five sessions each (total of 160 sessions). The questions used to measure these two variables were then scored on a scale of 0 to 20 and divided into low (0-10) and high (11-20). This resulted in the four cells of Type A, B, C, and D that were labeled "smooth sailing," "heavy going," "foundering," and "coasting," based on the practitioner's perception of high and low effectiveness and high and low patient distress during the session. Those interested in the details of the study can refer to the citation given previously, but here we are interested in how this can be reduced to a simple instrument that can be used in supervision to structure the initiation of discussion of the practitioner's response to a given session.

Visual 9.2 is a simplification of the four-cell table. The practitioner can be shown this simple diagram and asked to identify the cell that best fits how he or she perceived the session selected for evaluation. Once a cell is selected, the supervision can be focused on identifying the ways in which the practitioner saw himself or herself as being low or high in effectiveness, and on discussing patient behaviors that indicated low or high distress. After the session is discussed, supervisor input and insight gained by the practitioner can result in the cell selection being changed. Regardless of the initial cell selection, there is ample basis for discussion even if the cell selected is "smooth sailing." A "smooth sailing" selection can be used to elicit from

VISUAL 9.1 Practitioner's Perception of Sessions

Sessions in Which Therapist Was Warmly
Involved, Empathic, or Effective

		Low (0-10)	High (11-20)
Sessions in Which Patient Was Distressed or Anxiously Depressed	Low (0-10) (N = 127; 79.4%)	Type D: Coasting 17 (10.6%)	Type A: Smooth Sailing 110 (68.8%)
	High (11-20) (N = 33; 20.6%)	Type C: Foundering 6 (3.8%)	Type B: Heavy Going 27 (16.9%)
	Total (N = 160; 100%)	23 (14.4%)	137 (85.6%)

Source: Adapted from David E. Orlinsky and Kenneth L. Howard. "The Therapist's Experience of Psychotherapy," in Alan Gurman and Andrew M. Razin (eds.), *Effective Psychotherapy: A Handbook of Research.* White Plains, NY: Pergamon Press, pp. 566-589.

VISUAL 9.2. Practitioner Perception of a Session

Patient Distress	Practitioner Effectiveness	
	Low	High
Low	Coasting	Smooth Sailing
High	Foundering	Heavy Going

practitioners what techniques and behaviors they see as being effective so that these behaviors and techniques can be reinforced and anchored in their practice style. This type of discussion is important because practitioners will often perceive sessions as being highly effective and powerfully therapeutic without giving much thought to what produced the positive outcome. If the specific effective strategies can be identified, the worker can have more control over positive experiences, rather than having the sense that such sessions are arcane and rare occurrences that happen without explanation, which is the orientation many practitioners have toward powerful treatment sessions.

When the practitioner selects the "heavy going" cell, the supervisor should support the worker and provide encouragement because some practitioners have slight depressive reactions to sessions in which much effort is required. Even though they perceive themselves as effective, practitioners will frequently respond in terms of whether the effort they must make is worth the outcome.

When the categories of "coasting" and "foundering" are selected, error selection begins. The practitioner needs to focus on session activity that led to low effectiveness. It is better if workers can identify the specific actions that detracted from their being effective, and the supervisor must guide them in the search for alternative techniques and behaviors that will help them avoid these outcomes in future sessions.

The diagram can be used from session to session so that, when there are cell changes, supervision can be focused on what brought about the change. This four-cell conception is just one illustration of how supervisors can simplify conceptualizations from complicated research studies to meet their supervisory needs. To do this, supervisors need to read research literature from a dual perspective. First, they need to read from the point of view of how the outcomes of the research are useful in practice. Second, they need to ask how the research methodology can be reconceptualized in such a way as to promote learning in supervision.

PRACTICE ERRORS

It is helpful to orient the practitioner to the fact that everyone makes mistakes in treatment. Mistakes can be devastating; at best, they are hard to admit. Mistakes do happen, and more often than is realized. Mistakes and errors in technique are important to supervision because the more closely work is scrutinized, the more mistakes that are uncovered. In orienting practitioners to identifying and rectifying mistakes and errors, it is valuable to point out that skilled practitioners make mistakes. It is helpful to point out that even Freud was subject to errors and "blind spots." This can be done by referring to Langs' analysis of Freud's treatment of Dora. Langs' analysis, based on Freud's writings, resulted in the conclusion that there was "misalliance with his patient and [it] contributed to the premature termination of her analysis. There was evidence that his modifications in the frame reflected specific countertransference difficulties in his relationship with Dora and contributed to his blind spots regarding her communications and their interaction" (Langs, 1976:393-394). For a general discussion of Freud's errors, the reader is referred to Sartre's study of the young Sigmund Freud, "when his ideas had led him into hopeless error" (Sartre, 1976:129-132). Calling attention to errors by renowned therapists can do a great deal to relieve supervisees from self-imposed expectations that they need to be perfect in their practice.

A number of commercially produced videotapes show renowned practitioners at work, and, in some instances, they are not at their best therapeutically. Viewing such tapes can help practitioners to develop a positive attitude toward openness to admitting error.

Practitioners will naturally avoid the issue of errors and never directly admit mistakes or confusion about how to proceed with difficult cases. In such instances, practitioners will introduce complexity into the case and point to the client's lack of clarity and resistance, rather than focusing on how and where they, as practitioners, erred or could have been more effective. It is the supervisors' role to help practitioners overcome their avoidance of viewing the therapeutic relationship realistically. Supervisors can take pressure off the workers by identifying ways they themselves would have been confused or would have made mistakes in the same aspects of the treatment had they been the practitioners. This makes it easier for supervisees to begin identifying their weaknesses. Relating to the practitioners in this way is one of the situations in which it is appropriate for supervisors to use *philosophical abstraction* related to case discussion, but it should be followed by use of *technical strategy* (see Chapter 4).

At times practitioners will perceive themselves to be making errors or not making progress in a difficult case. At such times they tend to criticize themselves and occasionally to question their competence. The supervisor can help the practitioner by pointing out that the case is an extremely difficult one and that the difficulty does not rest with the worker's lack of skills. However, the supervisor must be prepared to pinpoint the problem areas in the case and offer the supervisee assistance in how to deal with them. This strategy can lead to difficulty when the supervisor recognizes that a clinical problem does arise from a practitioner's lack of skill or knowledge, and rather than dealing directly with the supervisee's shortcomings, the supervisor will attribute the difficulty to the complexity of the case. To support failures in practice in this manner is an unprofessional act on the part of the supervisor and is actually a process of sanctioning poor practice. Although supervisors periodically make such errors, to do this as a pattern is to reward bad practice, perpetuate incompetence, and expose clients to undue risks.

FOLLOW-UP AND EVALUATION

Follow-up and evaluation of a case are related but separate functions. Evaluation deals with the progress and effectiveness during a course of treatment; follow-up relates to gathering information about the client's functioning at a given interval or at several intervals after treatment is completed. The expectation and importance of follow-up should be made clear as a part of termination to avoid client feelings of remote dependency on the worker. Follow-up can be informal—through a telephone call or letter from the client or worker—or formal—through a brief, mailed questionnaire to the client. Regardless of the method used, the nature and form of the follow-up should be made clear at the time of termination.

CRITICISM OF CLINICAL MATERIAL

To help practitioners learn and grow, supervisors will have to be critical of their work from time to time. This is a basic, inherent part of the supervisory role. In American society, criticism is disliked and having to give it or receive it is avoided. Criticism is avoided if at all possible in clinical practice and supervision. This avoidance cannot be afforded in supervision.

Learning to offer criticism effectively takes much practice and skill. Weisinger and Lobsenz (1981) have written a book devoted entirely to how to give criticism effectively. Some of their general principles can be adapted to supervision of clinical practice. The following points will be helpful to the supervisor in offering criticism:

1. Criticism is a tool used to promote personal growth and enhance relationships.
2. To criticize is to communicate information to practitioners in ways that enable them to use it to their advantage and benefit.
3. Criticism can be delivered in a nonnegative manner.
4. To be helpful, criticism must draw a distinction between the behavior criticized and the individual involved.
5. Criticism is destructive when words and phrases are used that indicate or imply that the behavior in question was done deliberately.
6. The criticism must be specific if the practitioner is expected to act on the basis of it or change as a result of it.
7. Ensure that the practitioner understands the criticism. This is the only way that an exchange of information and learning can result from the criticism. It helps to ask whether the practitioner agrees or disagrees with the criticism.
8. Personal feelings or emotional aspects of the supervisor's relationship with the practitioner are to be separated from criticism given the practitioner. The supervisor needs to consider, Am I aware of my feelings about the practitioner? Are my feelings positive or negative?
9. When offering criticism, avoid such words as should and shouldn't.
10. Criticism must be offered at a time when the practitioner is ready to deal with it, and sufficient time should be allowed to discuss the criticism. State the criticism clearly and concisely, and then get feedback.

11. Criticism is offered without threats or ultimatums.
12. Criticism is offered without being in the context of "I told you so."
13. Criticism is helpful when it is not stated as an accusatory question.
14. When offering criticism, consider in advance, What behavior do I want to criticize?
15. Before offering criticism, consider, Can the behavior to be criticized be changed?
16. Consider in advance, How can the criticism help the practitioner?
17. Consider how the criticism will generate new approaches to the issue.
18. Criticism is best focused on the positive (i.e., What can be done? rather than What was not done?).
19. Offer criticism as an opinion, not as a fact.
20. When offering criticism, consider, Am I expressing my criticism in a manner that conveys that I understand how the practitioner feels and thinks?

REACTIONS TO CRITICISM

The nature of supervision necessitates that the supervisor evaluate the practitioner's work critically, and this evaluation must involve exploration of actual case material. It is possible to think of euphemisms for the word *criticism* in an effort to make it easier for the supervisee, but the fact remains that it is criticism, and the supervisee will perceive it as such. The supervisor can make every effort to be constructive and supportive when offering criticism. This can be accomplished without too much difficulty.

What the supervisor has no control over is the supervisee's response to criticism. When criticism is viewed negatively and is resisted, the supervision process becomes tense, anger on both sides increases, and learning ceases. Educational programs do not emphasize how to deal with being evaluated. Educational programs place emphasis on doing evaluation or being in the role of evaluator. Most beginning practitioners have no preparation for being evaluated. Some practitioners have a fear of any criticism of their performance (Munson, 1979b).

One way to help avoid these problems is to explain the role of criticism in supervision at the beginning and provide the supervisee with guidelines for constructively accepting criticism of their clinical material (Munson, 1980c). These guidelines also apply to the supervisor when the worker offers criticism, a practice that should be encouraged by supervisors to improve their effectiveness. These guidelines can also be used in treatment with clients who have difficulty accepting criticism. The following guidelines (in part adapted from Weinberg, 1978) should be offered to practitioners to aid them in dealing with criticism:

1. Listen to the criticism in detail. Avoid rushing to defend yourself or your position.
2. Evaluate in your mind the validity of the criticism. If the criticism is fair, formulate ways in your mind that you could change your performance.
3. Try to gain more understanding by asking for detailed information about the criticism. If the criticism is general, as it often is, ask the supervisor to be specific. Ask how the activity could have been done differently or better.
4. Avoid implying that the supervisor has a personal motive. Keep the criticism on a professional level and always relate it to professional performance.
5. Avoid getting angry with the supervisor and losing self-control. This accomplishes nothing.
6. Avoid attempting to shift the responsibility to someone else.
7. Avoid attributing the criticism to personal weakness, and avoid presenting yourself as a total failure.
8. Avoid trying to shut off the criticism by saying that you cannot deal with negative comments.
9. Avoid changing the subject to avoid any direct discussion of the criticism.
10. Avoid repeatedly admitting that you were wrong, and refrain from continually questioning the supervisor as to what you can do to make up for the criticism.
11. Avoid focusing the conversation on giving justifications and excuses for what you did.
12. Refrain shifting responsibility onto the supervisor by saying that the supervisor is overreacting or is just looking for something to criticize.
13. Avoid turning the criticism into a joke or verbal one-upmanship.
14. Clarify for yourself, or ask the supervisor, how your behavior was inadequate. If the supervisor cannot offer an explanation, then assess whether the criticism is valid.
15. Regardless of whether you accept or question the criticism, let the supervisor know that you heard and understand the criticism.
16. If you accept the criticism, acknowledge it and either offer an alternative for the future or ask your supervisor for possible alternative behavior.

17. Remember that criticism is not a threat to you personally or professionally. It is a way of gaining new information about different and perhaps better ways of performing.

This list of ways to deal with criticism should be discussed openly with the practitioner at the point of initiating the supervisory process. If the expectations are made clear, the supervisee can avoid becoming defensive when the supervisor must be critical of the supervisee's work. The supervisor may choose to review the supervisee's work through audiotapes, videotapes, process recordings, or after-the-fact discussion, but to be effective, the supervision must involve open exploration of the treatment process. When supervision has been structured on the basis of positive expectations regarding criticism, the outcome is more objective for both the supervisor and the supervisee.

EVALUATION AND SELF-ASSESSMENT

The supervisee must be an active participant in the supervision for it to be effective and internalized. One way this can be done is to have the supervisee select the treatment material that will be used in the supervision and to prepare a self-assessment of the material prior to the supervision session. The author has devised and used a self-assessment form based on the following:

1. How long did the interview last?
2. Do you feel the interview was too short, too long, or just about right? Explain what factors contributed to the interview's being too short or too long. Who contributed most to this? What could have been done to overcome this?
3. Did the interview have a focus? If yes, what was the focus? If no, what prevented a focus from being developed? What could have been done to focus the interview more?
4. Do you feel that the client got what he or she came for? If yes, what did he or she get? If no, what prevented him or her from getting what was expected?
5. Did the session have a flow of interaction or continuity? If yes, describe this characteristic and how it was achieved. If no, what prevented it?
6. Describe how you felt prior to the session.
7. Describe how you felt during the session.
8. Describe how you felt after the session.
9. Describe your behaviors during the session that were positive.

10. Describe client behaviors during the session that were positive.
11. Describe your behaviors during the session that you felt were not effective.
12. Were there client gestures or behaviors that enhanced the communication process?
13. Describe client behaviors during the session that you felt were distracting or disturbing.
14. Are you aware of any gestures or behaviors by you that enhanced the communication process?
15. Are you aware of any gestures or behaviors on your part that detracted from the communication process?
16. Are there any problems associated with this session with which you would like help?
17. What would you do differently if you could do the interview again?
18. Based on what you know now, what are your plans for the next interview?
19. What were the primary and secondary therapeutic outcomes of this session? If there were no therapeutic outcomes, what prevented any from occurring?
20. What are the specific questions you want ask in supervision about this session or about the client?

These questions are presented in questionnaire format in Appendix VI and can be reproduced for use in supervision. This form can be used routinely in educationally focused supervision, or it can be used to identify a specific problem in a specific case. Having practitioners write out the answers prior to supervision for a specific problem promotes a reflection process that leads supervisees to awareness of what the problem is before they get to supervision. It is rewarding when this happens because this is genuine self-teaching and learning. The self-assessment format advocated here promotes efficient use of supervisory time and is helpful when time available for supervision is limited. The trend toward self-assessment seen in the literature is associated with the recent emphasis on autonomous practice (Wallace, 1981).

RESEARCH AND PRACTICE

Learning in supervision has been vaguely defined in relation to evaluation of and research in practice. The research on psychotherapy can help with the distinction that needs to be made. During the 1950s and 1960s, a distinction was made between process and outcome research. Process research deals with *how* changes take place in a given interchange between client and practitioner; outcome research is concerned with *what* changes take place as a result of treatment (Hersen and Barlow, 1976:20). During the early days of such studies, there was a flight into process that led to an increase in process research. Methodological problems later led to a decline in process research. This distinction between outcome and process research led to a dichotomy between the two approaches that hampered measurement of effectiveness of psychotherapy. Although these were technical considerations in psychotherapy's pure research circles, the dichotomy has implications for learning in supervision because research attention later turned to the relationship between process and outcome, and this relationship is important to learning in supervision and to evaluation of practice in supervision.

There has been much speculation about, and a limited amount of questionable empirical research on, the negative effects of psychotherapy. The major source of information about negative effects in psychotherapy has been client reports. Such reports are subject to distortions, inaccuracies, and varied perceptions. Strupp and colleagues (1977) argue that more reliable sources of such effects are supervisors' observations of practitioners in training. The empirical research on the "deterioration hypothesis" does not provide compelling evidence that negative effects are widespread. Even with increased, sound empirical research on psychotherapy outcome, "it is doubtful that scientific evidence alone will suffice" (Strupp et al., 1977:23). Psychotherapy is an extremely complicated process that involves many personality variables, moral and philosophical issues, and diverse perceptions. Just as it can be argued that recovery occurs spontaneously in spite of therapeutic intervention, it can be postulated that deterioration occurs in spite of therapeutic intervention. We are a long way from attributing causation of improvement or deterioration to therapeutic intervention. For the time being, making associations between events is the best that can be done. It is to be hoped that with courage and self-confidence improvement and negative effects will be reported and that the positives will outnumber the negatives. Good supervision is the best way to ensure the integrity and accuracy of positive and negative observations. Since the world contains so many unknowns, supervision can help monitor therapeutic efforts and offer assessment of what to do and what not to do in treatment.

Practitioners have little concern for or patience with sophisticated research in their practice. It is difficult enough to deal with clinical dynamics from a therapeutic standpoint without adding the complex thinking and procedures required for research, especially since most clinicians have little or no training in research skills. This scientist/researcher split is epitomized by Matarazzo, who observed:

> Even after 15 years, few of my research findings affect my practice. Psychological science per se doesn't guide me one bit. I still read avidly but this is of little direct practical help. My clinical experience is the only thing that has helped me in my practice to date. (quoted in Bergin and Strupp, 1972:340)

Carl Rogers, a leading clinical researcher, "as early as the 1958 APM conference on psychotherapy noted that research had no impact on his clinical practice and by 1969 advocated abandoning formal research in psychotherapy altogether" (Bergin and Strupp, 1972:313). These views continue to prevail among a large number of psychotherapists but are difficult to maintain in the modern environment of research that has direct application to clinical practice.

The antiresearch attitude does not mean that research concepts cannot be applied to clinical material, especially in supervision. For example, process material and outcome measures can be applied to specific case material. The desired outcomes in a case can be related to the therapeutic processes to be used in achieving these outcomes. The supervisor and practitioner can first identify the outcomes and the processes that have the most potential to achieve the outcomes, and the case can be monitored for progress in reaching the identified outcomes. Specific cases can become the focus in supervision, with the objective that this procedure of analysis becomes a routine thought-and-action pattern for the practitioner in all cases.

The key to a research orientation in supervision and practice is that the research focus must remain simple, understandable, and connected to clinical material. Other evaluative tools that have a simplified research orientation are the self-assessment form developed (see Appendix VI) for this book and the four-cell conception of research discussed earlier in this chapter. These formats can be used by supervisors when they encounter a problem in a case. When evaluation is approached from this perspective, practitioners are less likely to resist a research-in-practice focus when they recognize a problem in a case and perceive themselves as needing help.

There has been an expansion of research focused on specific clinical populations, and this research should be used to inform supervisory practice. Such population-based research can be helpful in treatment planning done as part of the supervision process. For example, research on domestic violence has demonstrated that when a woman is in an abusive relationship, her children are at significant risk of being abused by the person who is abusing the mother (Margolin, 1998). In cases involving domestic violence, the supervisor and practitioner should assess the risk to the children in the family even if they are not the focus of the treatment. It is important that the supervisor and the practitioner keep up to date on research focused on the population that is primarily served as part of the clinician's practice. If the clinician treats a case that involves a rare disorder, the supervisor and practitioner should review the literature for research on the topic and self-help groups that may be available to aid the client. The Internet is a good resource for upgrading knowledge of practice research, locating self-help organizations, and finding referral resources. Morrison and Stamps (1998) have developed a good guide for mental health information Internet resources. Although this type of information and research does not directly relate to evaluation and outcome measures of practice and evaluation of the practitioner, it can be used to inform the criteria for evaluation of the individual practitioner.

NOTE TAKING

Much controversy surrounds note taking during treatment sessions. It can be viewed as a distraction for both the practitioner and the client. This is a matter of style. It is difficult to do a diagnostic interview without taking notes, especially in a complex case and when case information will be shared with colleagues. When note taking is a part of the treatment from the outset, it rarely becomes an issue. For many clinicians, taking brief notes in treatment is not a distraction. Note taking can help clinicians remain alert and focused. A train of thought can be reestablished through notes, patterns of behavior can be clearly documented, and notes can aid in preparing for future sessions. Some clinicians find note taking to be a distraction. The function of treatment note taking should be explored in supervision as a style issue. If a clinician does not take notes in treatment sessions and has difficulty recalling details of the case in supervision, the supervisor may have to work more closely with the practitioner to establish a way to improve the practitioner's clinical recall. The practitioner may need to develop a way to take notes during sessions or be required to dictate or write notes immediately after sessions.

Although note taking is a matter of style in treatment, it is a necessity in supervision for both the practitioner and the supervisor. Notes are important to case planning and follow-up. Notes are important for the worker since much time may elapse between supervision sessions and subsequent client interviews. Notes are important in settings in which periodic evaluations of the practitioner's work are required. Where disagreements occur in supervision, notes can aid in clarifying issues and determining what position each participant held in a given case or series of cases. The best time to prepare for a supervisory session is just after the previous one. Notes can be helpful in organizing and reflecting upon what has just taken place in a session and in documenting material that should be followed up in a subsequent session.

In brief, treatment note taking is essential since the practitioner does not have the luxury of asking the client to recall and re-present forgotten material. In addition, good notes are important to learning in treatment and are essential to research and evaluation of treatment (Lewin, 1970:58-59).

RECORD KEEPING

Organizational procedure affects supervision directly in the learning process through record-keeping procedures. The supervisor must ensure that the supervisee is keeping records that conform to agency procedures to facilitate flow of information and to meet mandatory external regulations. Record keeping has taken on increased significance because in most modern agencies record keeping is tied to funding. Much funding is dependent on providing accurate, detailed, and current records to payers. In addition, it has been estimated that approximately 30 percent of practitioner time is devoted to record keeping. The supervisor who does not assist supervisees at becoming proficient in this area could be neglecting an important and significant part of the practitioner's work.

It is the supervisor's function to orient the newly employed practitioner to record-keeping requirements. When the supervisor is performing an educational role exclusively, the decision must be made regarding what form of record keeping will be required for learning purposes. Some supervisors rely on the basic mandatory records as a basis for teaching and on discussions surrounding these basic records. Others view mandatory records as minor activities that must be dealt with and tolerated so that the larger task of teaching and learning can be pursued. Some supervisors require additional record keeping, such as process recording and process summaries, that is used exclusively for learning purposes and does not become part of the agency's formal records.

Regardless of the style of record keeping required by the agency or the supervisor, the methods and procedures should be made clear to the supervisee at the outset of supervision. Some supervisors avoid this because they view record keeping as a minor irritation that they would rather not deal with at all. The reality is that record keeping is important to the ongoing functioning of the agency as an organization, to sustaining a record of the client's contact with and service received from the agency over time, and to organizational life. If the supervisee, supervisor, or agency becomes involved in a legal action, the records can be a crucial defense against allegations. An adage in legal circles related to professional liability states, "If it is not written, it did not happen." In situations in which the allegations involve failure of professionals to take action or intervene, often the only proof of what took place is the written record.

When the details of record keeping are not attended to, they can interfere with the teaching activity in supervision. This is illustrated by the following case:

> A psychotherapist would avoid dictation for months and never encouraged his supervisees to be current with their dictation. When recertification evaluations would be scheduled, this practitioner would have to cancel all of his therapy sessions for an entire week to bring his records up to date, resulting in a disruption of treatment for his clients and placing an additional burden upon other practitioners, who would have to assume his intake cases during the time he was literally locked in his office dictating. He also created problems for the records department, which had to locate and pull all his charts, as well as type all the dictation.
>
> This psychotherapist spent much time having disagreements with his supervisees about records and record-keeping procedures because of his resistance to performing these tasks. Precious supervisory time was spent discussing these problems. His lack of clarity in this area led to many lost hours in supervision when confrontations would occur. This was unfortunate because this supervisor was an excellent teacher, and he failed to see that his abhorrence of record keeping led to its taking up more, rather than less, time in supervision, which distracted from what he did best—teaching psychotherapy.

Agencies have varying requirements for record keeping. The variation in record keeping is often associated with federal and state regulatory bodies as well as service and contract payers. Beyond the agency requirements, supervisors and practitioners should consider records from two perspectives: legal liability and personal use. In the past, keeping separate agency and legal or personal records was a common practice. Such separation had professional sanction and legal recognition (Schutz, 1982:52). Under current standards, keeping dual or separate sets of records is not recommended, and if separate records are kept they can be subject to subpoena. If separate records are kept for the purpose of avoiding disclosure to courts or attorneys, and this practice is discovered, the clinician or agency may be found in contempt (Melton et al., 1997:112).

A good record should contain the following:

1. Signed informed consents for all treatment
2. Signed informed consents for all transmission of confidential information
3. Any treatment contracts
4. Notation of all treatment contacts and significant information and actions regarding the contact (including face-to-face contacts with clients, client relatives, and others, and telephone contacts)

5. Notations of failed or cancelled appointments
6. Notations of supervision and consultation contacts
7. All correspondence and record of contacts with other professionals
8. A complete social history or initial database, including past and present evaluations and treatment, a medical history, and record of a current physical examination
9. A diagnostic assessment or statement, which should be reviewed, revised, and documented periodically
10. A list of all medications the person is currently taking
11. A record of the practitioner's basis for the assessment made and the treatment provided
12. Notations of suggestions, instructions, referrals, or directives made to the client and whether they were followed
13. The practitioner's informal notes, including such items as
    a. speculation about client dynamics,
    b. impressions about the course of treatment,
    c. problems resolved,
    d. problems being worked on,
    e. problems to be worked on in the future,
    f. projections about termination, and
    g. summary of perceptions of significant treatment session dynamics
14. A treatment plan that is updated every ninety days, including
    a. client problems,
    b. short- and long-term goals (stated in observable and measurable form),
    c. notation of dates of achievement of goals, and
    d. signatures of client, therapist, and supervisor

In many respects, the supervisory records are integrated with the client records, and for legal purposes, significant supervisory contacts should be a part of the client record. The legal status of separate supervisor records is less clear than the requirements for client records. Agency requirements vary for supervisory record keeping, and individual supervisors' preferences vary. Supervisory records should include, at least,

1. the supervisory contract, if used or required by the agency;
2. a brief statement of supervisee experience, training, and learning needs;
3. a summary of all performance evaluations;
4. notation of all supervisory sessions;
5. cancelled or missed sessions;
6. notation of cases discussed and significant decisions; and
7. significant problems encountered in the supervision and how they were resolved, or whether they remain unresolved and why.

A recommended supervisory session form is included in Appendix X.

It is important that the supervisor keep good records on each supervisee. When supervision of a practitioner begins, it is not known what the outcome will be. It could end on a positive note several years later when the supervisee becomes a supervisor or moves to another position, or it could end in an agency or professional grievance hearing. Some supervisory relationships reach such a point, and it is difficult for the supervisor who is unable to document in a grievance how a supervisee's performance was unsatisfactory. The supervisor's memory and speculative recounting of the problems are insufficient. Supervisors who rely on their memory are open to manipulation by difficult supervisees. If a grievance should result in a legal action, the courts often use the standard "If it is not written, then it did not happen" (Koocher, Norcross, and Hill, 1998). For this reason, thorough supervisory and treatment recording are important professional and legal safeguards.

The supervisory record should be a tool for promoting ongoing growth and development of the practitioner. Under the best conditions, it aids the supervisor in fostering professional growth of the practitioner. In difficult adversarial situations, the record is a documented defense against unrecognized and unaccepted practitioner failure in performance.

ADMINISTRATIVE EVALUATION

An annual performance evaluation should be taken seriously and not viewed as a routine form that is filled out hastily so that the supervisor and supervisee can get on with the work of the agency. This attitude and pattern of behavior are easy to assume in agencies that focus on doing therapy, and in which routine forms are viewed as a necessary evil. If the supervisor has been working regularly with the supervisee using the techniques discussed in this chapter and previous chapters, the administrative evaluation will not come as a surprise and will meet with minimal resistance.

The point of this chapter has been to note the distinction between administrative evaluation and the evaluation of practice as part of the supervisory process. Clearly, the two are related, but they often involve different procedures. For example, practice evaluation can involve discussion of many minute practice actions that are changed immediately by the practitioner and reevaluated in a week, and any such change is the result of the supervisor and the supervisee negotiating a shared solution. Administrative evaluation is general and may not be reevaluated for some time. Practice evaluation is usually confined to the supervisory relationship. Although content of the administrative evaluation is agreed upon by the supervisor and supervisee, it can result in actions taken by others outside the supervisory relationship that can directly affect the supervisee, such as the amount of a salary increase or action regarding a promotion. Practice evaluation is specific, continuous, and basically self-contained, and administrative evaluation is general, periodic, and external to the supervisory relationship.

Although administratively mandated evaluations can vary greatly in their frequency, form, and content, the supervisor should work with the higher-level administration to ensure that administrative evaluation procedures are fair, objective, and open, so that administrative evaluation does not hinder the supervisory relationship. Basic guidelines for administrative evaluation of clinicians that supervisors should strive for are listed here:

1. Administrative evaluation policy should be established at a higher level in the organization, implemented at a lower level, and reviewed at the higher level. All levels of the organization should have input in the development of evaluation policy, including structure, content, and process of evaluation.
2. The supervisee should be informed of the format, content, and procedures of the evaluation at the beginning of the evaluation period.
3. The same evaluation instrument should be used over time. This is the only way change in performance can be identified.
4. The individuals to be evaluated who make up the organizational unit should participate in development of the evaluation instrument.
5. Evaluate the position and the performance, and avoid evaluating the person.
6. Avoid evaluating any function or task the supervisor has not been designated to evaluate.
7. Refrain from evaluating someone who performs a function about which the supervisor knows little or nothing.
8. Evaluation assumes that the supervisor knows what the process and outcome of the performance should be.
9. If the evaluation instrument is quantified, the person evaluated must be able to determine how the composite score was calculated.
10. Evaluate the supervisee only for the time period that the supervisee was subject to the supervisor's direction.
11. Evaluation begins long before the forms are to be filled out. Evaluation is an ongoing process, and the supervisee should be aware of the policies and procedures from the beginning of the evaluation period.

PRACTICE RESEARCH AND SUPERVISION

In a study by Rosenblatt, a sample of social workers rated supervision and consultation as significantly more helpful to them in practice than research findings (1968:55). Rosenblatt found that research was of limited value to practitioners, and that it was not viewed as highly relevant to or integrated with what takes place in supervision. The researcher, practitioner, and supervisor were described as separate specialists performing different functions; the researcher was portrayed as a "threat" to the practitioner and the supervisor (Rosenblatt, 1968:58). Although Rosenblatt's study has not been replicated, other research has produced similar results. A study by Kirk and Fischer (1976:69) suggests that social workers show a propensity to avoid using research in an objective manner when it is identified as potentially useful to them in their practice. Other studies have found that despite the significant increase in emphasis on research in social work education, little empirical research relates directly to practice (Munson, 1996d, 1996e).

One trend was to deal with the problems of research and practice by attempting to integrate the two areas. Rather than approaching integration by encouraging researchers and practitioners to join forces, the effort focused on combining the two roles in one person by training practitioners-researchers (Grinnell, 1981; Jayaratne and Levy, 1979; Wodarski, 1981; Hudson, 1982). This orientation to research focused on single-subject designs, which incorporate research procedures as an integral part of practice intervention. These designs emphasize observations and analyses of the effects of interventions on specific behaviors rather than proof of hypotheses, as is the case in group research designs (Grinnell, 1981:373-375). None of these approaches mentions the role of supervision in promoting and regulating research in practice. The combined researcher-practitioner approach has had moderate success but has not resulted in an increase in practice research (Munson, 1996d, 1996e), and indications are that little progress has been made in overcoming social work practitioner and supervisor resistance to research since the research of Rosenblatt.

Much debate still centers around how best to apply research principles in practice (see Geismar and Wood, 1982; Ruckdeschel and Farris, 1982). Single-subject designs have been compared and contrasted with good process records. The debate about and use of the two approaches will undoubtedly continue. What seems to be agreed upon by those on both sides of the debate is that any research in practice must be based on an analysis of specific interactional exchanges between client and practitioner. As long as this basic principle is adhered to by the supervisor and supervisee, the chances of error in evaluating practice will be reduced.

There has to be a rational alternative to the old model of the two-person research-practice combination and the current model of a single person doing both research and practice. Although research and practice involve similar procedures, as writers on the topic have pointed out, they are not the same activity. Each area has discrete goals and objectives. When research is combined with practice, it must be done with caution, and the purposes must be made clear. The research must be compatible with the practice and care must be taken to avoid letting it detract from, impede, or confuse the goals of the treatment. The factors just mentioned must be monitored by the supervisor to ensure that client rights are being protected and that treatment efforts are not being superseded by research interests. If they are going to be helpful to this new type of practitioner, supervisors need to be trained in the research procedures being used and must be experienced at doing research.

The role of the supervisor in monitoring and evaluating the ethics of practitioner research is vague and unclear. This is in part because government regulation of research activity did not begin in earnest until 1974, after the public disclosure of the Tuskegee Study, which involved research for forty years on over 400 black men, some of whom had syphilis (see Jones, 1981). An interesting aside about this study is that a social worker was the first person to raise questions concerning the ethics of the research, and he was responsible for setting in motion the events that halted the experiment (Jones, 1981:188- 205).

Most institutions that receive government funds and do research now have institutional review boards that review research protocols to protect human subjects. Supervisors who work in such settings have a moral and quasi-legal responsibility to be familiar with requirements for institutional review of research conducted by their supervisees. The term *quasi-legal* has been used in relation to research in practice because it is unclear what the precise responsibility of the supervisor is in this area.

What is clear is that under the legal doctrine of *respondent superior* (let the superior give answer), the supervisor is not absolved from responsibility for actions of supervisees. Schutz has pointed out:

> While therapists are not guarantors of cure or improvement, extensive treatment without results could legally be considered to have injured the patient; in specific, the injury would be the loss of money and time, and the preclusion of other treatments that might have been more successful. To justify a prolonged holding action at a plateau, the therapist would have to show that this was maintaining a condition against a significant and likely deterioration. (1982:47)

Under these circumstances, if research is a component of treatment in a situation in which there is no improvement, the practitioner and supervisor are open to the accusation that the treatment was only a subterfuge to carry out the research. In such cases, the professionals involved will undoubtedly be required to demonstrate how the research was designed to enhance the effectiveness of the treatment and to show that the client was informed about and consented to the research procedures. In light of the recent developments in practice research discussed earlier, legal and ethical issues will continue to emerge in this area, and supervisors will need to keep abreast of developments in the judicial and professional arenas regarding research and responsibility for practice outcomes. It is possible that legal action from outside the profession will bring about practice and supervision reforms that have not taken place within the social work profession during its almost 100 years of existence.

Without regard to research in practice, legal liability of the supervisor for the actions of the practitioner is changing. In the 1950s, when the social work profession was attempting to decrease the use of supervision in the quest for autonomy and professionalism (see Chapters 1 and 2), Fizdale viewed supervision of the established professional as "potentially detrimental." She went on to argue that the caseworker is fully and independently responsible for intake decisions, referrals, techniques used, and termination decisions (Munson, 1979c:122-127). Scherz held a similar view by advocating that supervisors cannot make social workers competent by injecting knowledge into them (Munson, 1979c:73). From a professional point of view, this trend continued to evolve in the 1950s, but from a legal perspective, the standard has shifted to the supervisor and clinician sharing responsibility for clinical outcome (Knapp and Vandecreek, 1997). Supervisors must be consider this:

> When one undertakes to supervise the work of another practitioner, one also assumes a legal liability not only for one's acts but for those of the supervisee. Legal liability rests on the de facto or de jure (actual or mandated by law) control the supervisor has over the therapy process to coordinate, direct, and inspect the actions of the treating practitioner. (Schutz, 1982:47)

Under current conditions, the supervisor and supervisee have a mutual responsibility to make every effort to ensure that all major decisions about treatment have been reviewed in supervision (Schutz, 1982:47-52).

SUGGESTED READINGS

Calsyn, R. J. et al. (1999). "Evaluating Team Leaders and Peers in Group Supervision," *The Clinical Supervisor,* 18(2), pp. 203-210.
Empirical research results of a scale used to evaluate supervisors.

Weinberg, G. (1978). *Self-Creation.* New York: St. Martin's.
This book was used to develop the material in this chapter on how to deal with criticism. It is recommended for the supervisee who wants to develop more knowledge and ability to deal with criticism and on self-development.

Weisinger, H and Lobsenz, N. M. (1981). *Nobody's Perfect: How to Give Criticism and Get Results.* Los Angeles: Stratford.
An excellent, readable guide to giving and getting criticism. This book is highly recommended and was used to develop some of the guidelines in this chapter.

> We social case workers are asking
> why others should have too much
> leisure and we too little. Are we trying
> to sweep back the sea with our little
> brooms, when we ought to be building
> solid dikes against misery?
>
> Bertha Capen Reynolds
> *Between Client and Community*

Chapter 10

Stress Reactions

This chapter defines stress and identifies its manifestations as well as its causes and cures. The research on stress among social workers is reviewed along with the conflicting results of the research. Supervision and stress are explored, as are demands that can lead to this stress. The chapter includes excerpts from research interviews with workers making observations about their experiences with stress that illustrate the conceptual material. The supervisor's role in helping practitioners prevent and overcome stress is explained. Specific pointers and pitfalls of aiding workers are covered. Special attention is given to helping beginning professionals deal with stress since the research shows that, perhaps unexpectedly, stress is highest among this group. The points for combating stress can be applied to work with supervisees but also can be useful for supervisors in dealing with their own propensity to burn out.

INTRODUCTION

The idea of distress associated with the helping-oriented professions was identified almost a century ago:

> He who carries self-regard far enough to keep himself in good health and high spirits, in the first place, thereby becomes an immediate source of happiness to those around, and, in the second place, maintains the ability to increase their happiness by altruistic actions. But one whose bodily vigor and mental health are undermined by self-sacrifice carried too far, in the first place becomes to those around a cause of depression, and, in the second place, renders himself incapable, or less capable, of actively furthering their welfare. (Spencer, 1902:223)

So much for the idea that stress is a recent phenomenon. In modern terms, Hans Selye, the famous stress researcher, stated, "My own code is based on the view that to achieve peace of mind and fulfillment through self-expression, most . . . need a commitment to work in the service of some cause that they can respect" (Selye, 1974:4). Before reading the literature that exists on the concept of stress, supervisors and supervisees should read Selye's little book *Stress Without Distress.* Selye is considered the earliest scientist to develop a perspective on stress from a biological viewpoint while taking into account its psychological ramifications. Selye's work is important because he identifies the overall origins of stress, its manifestations, and ways of combating it in a general sense.

RESEARCH ON STRESS AMONG SOCIAL WORKERS

The empirical research on distress among social workers is in the early stages of development and has been given sporadic attention in the literature. After the early accounts of stress just cited little attention was paid to stress issues until the 1980s, when a series of studies examined stress related to social workers, but this research declined in the 1990s. For this reason, most of the research and theoretical writings cited in this chapter come from this earlier era. The earlier writing on stress is relevant since reactions to stress do not change over time (Munson, 1992), but what is not known is whether the amount of stress has increased over the past twenty years or whether practitioners have developed more effective strategies to cope with stress.

The content of this chapter is not intended as a substitute for medical treatment of physical or psychological symptoms. When such symptoms occur, medical advice should be sought.

The few data-based studies of stress have produced interesting, but sometimes confusing, results. Reiter (1980), in a study of clinical social workers, found that 46 percent would not choose social work as a career if they had it to do over. This is interesting in light of the view that jobs and professions in society have always been sex-typed, and social work has traditionally been considered a woman's profession (82 percent of the respondents in Reiter's study were women). Since socialization processes prepare people for these roles in conscious and unconscious ways (Pogrebin, 1980: 535), the consciousness raising of the feminist movement could be the source of this regretted career choice, or it could be the result of unfulfilled expectations and job-related distress. Further research should provide answers to such questions. Regardless of these issues, Reiter raises an important question that is significant for supervision and practice distress:

> [S]ocial workers who have responsibility for . . . training . . . other workers are regretful of their . . . career choice. Whether . . . that regret translates into negative feelings of professional identity that are transmitted to the supervisee is a matter for speculation. . . . [T]hese feelings . . . emerge in ways that could hinder not only the supervisory process but the professional identity of the less experienced worker. (1980:204)

Reiter did not study distress among practitioners directly, but a study by Bissell and colleagues (1980) did. Data were collected from fifty alcoholic social workers who had been free of alcohol abuse for at least a year. The researchers reported that in spite of a combined incidence of 63 arrests, 120 inpatient admissions, 13 suicide attempts, and reported addiction to alcohol and other drugs, colleagues, supervisors, and therapists who treated them were "extremely reluctant" to confront the alcoholism. Some participants reported that they did not approach their supervisors because the supervisors were denying that a problem existed. The social workers reported suicide attempts at twice the rate that physicians did, but at slightly lower rate than that reported by nurses. This could be a reflection of the gender difference in the professions and that, in the total population, more females attempt suicide than males (although males are three times more successful at it) (Pogrebin, 1980:75).

What is disturbing about this study is the failure of the supervisors and colleagues to assist these professionals who were giving clear indications that they needed help. Perhaps these people represent the hardest ones to reach, but there is need for open discussion about how to address these forms of impaired functioning when they become apparent. Supervisors cannot afford to overlook such problems.

The question remains, How widespread are these problems of distress in the profession? Two studies offer perspective on the extent of stress. Streepy

(1981) surveyed 108 practitioners in twelve family service agencies. Over 75 percent of the respondents found job satisfactions greater than the frustrations, and few workers were considering a job change. Stress as manifested through physical and psychological symptoms was at a low level. The findings revealed that stress was higher when family income was low, education level was low, attitudes toward the profession were negative, and work experience was minimal. Stress showed no correlation with type of experience, sex, or job satisfaction. It was the inexperienced, poorly trained workers who experienced the highest levels of distress, but, overall, stress was not widespread among these workers.

A study of 180 practitioners and supervisors in a public welfare setting (Munson, 1982b) revealed that 72 percent reported having experienced stress, and almost all reported going through cycles of stress. Physical symptoms such as headaches, persistent colds, and gastrointestinal upsets were reported by 43 percent of the group, and 37 percent reported psychological symptoms such as anxiety, depression, and inability to sleep. Even though these high levels of cycles of stress were reported, 86 percent of the participants stated that they were satisfied with their jobs and the agency. That money is not the total solution to stress is reflected in the fact that the overwhelming majority of people who leave high-risk, successful careers do so to enter low-paying service occupations. A commitment to help others and to make a contribution to society is an important factor in life satisfaction that rarely gets discussed openly. It could be that such psychological needs account for the fact that many people have high levels of distress in their jobs but at the same time feel their agency is a good place to work. Writers have pointed out that child welfare service workers and supervisors are highly stressed (Daley, 1979; Harrison, 1980; Zischka, 1981), research indicates that child welfare workers do not have significantly higher levels of stress than other professionals (Munson, Study D).

Schor (1991) found that stress has increased because of more demands on time, resulting in 30 percent of adults complaining of stress. On an average daily basis, people are getting sixty to ninety minutes less sleep than is needed for optimal performance. Marriages are conflicted due to family and work obligations competing for people's time. Schor found that in 1987 people were working 163 hours more a year than in 1969. Women were working 305 hours more, and men ninety-eight hours more.

STUDENTS AND STRESS

Stress among professional social workers has been a focus of increased concern during the past several years, but there has been no parallel study of stress among graduate social work students. In one of the first attempts to study stress among students, a seventy-five item questionnaire was administered to a random sample of eighty-two first- and second-year graduate students in a large, urban university (Munson, Study E). The variables under study were clustered in the areas of demographics, physical symptoms, psychological symptoms, field placement satisfaction, and supervisory satisfaction.

The findings revealed that physical and psychological stress were at low levels for the total group. Respondents did identify that they experienced more physical and psychological stress associated with classroom work than with fieldwork. No major differences were found in stress symptoms for men and women, for first- and second-year students, or on the basis of marital status. In general, satisfaction with supervision did not produce any significant correlations with physical or psychological stress, but specific supervisory interaction variables (friendliness, openness, and putting the student at ease) did produce moderately significant correlations with certain physical symptoms (frequency of colds, headaches, and gastrointestinal [GI] upset). Number of years of social work experience prior to entering graduate school showed no significant correlations with physical symptoms. In general, the respondents were satisfied with their supervision and their agency placements. These supervisory and agency satisfaction levels appear to contribute to low levels of stress among students and to help prevent depersonalization of clients. The study lends support to the notion that supervision is important to preventing burnout.

As this brief survey of the research reveals, there are many unanswered questions and mixed findings about practitioner distress. The supervisor's responsibility is to know the manifestations, help workers recognize their reactions, and support them in dealing with them. Although the research findings vary regarding the extent of distress, the supervisor should look upon each practitioner as unique and be ready to assist him or her at the earliest signs of stress.

SUPERVISION AND STRESS

Supervision can work for or against practitioners in dealing with stress. Many workers identify supervisors as offering little help for distress, and in many cases supervisors contribute to intensifying it (Edelwich and Brodsky, 1980). At the same time, workers involved in my research have identified good, supportive supervisors as the main source of help in dealing with stress. Given this information, it is surprising how little most supervisors know about distress, its causes, its manifestations, its cures. Without serious study of distress, supervisors become instant experts with instant advice, and when such quickly devised, simplistic solutions do not work, workers can become more distressed. In the worst possible situation, the worker can be assigned a formerly distressed worker as a supervisor.

Distress or burnout is not always a gradual, downhill process. Research has shown that burnout occurs in cyclical patterns in the majority of workers (Munson, Studies D and E). Little is known about how these cycles occur, their duration, or what causes them to subside. Also, the research demonstrates that practitioners experience distress differently. Some complain almost exclusively of physical symptoms, others experience mainly psychological reactions, and still others undergo a combination of the two.

It is not known what causes different workers to gravitate to one pattern of reaction. It could be preexisting personality or physical variables; it could be something specific to the work setting itself. For example, in medical settings, some workers develop imaginary illnesses that mimic diseases treated in the setting (e.g., cancer, depression, heart disease). It could also be a reaction to comments the supervisor makes or to behavior the supervisor manifests. As discussed in Chapter 5, practitioners form reactions to their supervisors, and if workers are exposed to supervisors who are manifesting distress, it is easy for the supervisees to follow the same pattern.

SUPERVISOR STRESS

Supervisors who are in distress have a responsibility to seek help for it, but they should avoid seeking relief through their supervisees, and they have a responsibility to avoid exposing supervisees to their own burnout. Just as practitioners should not seek solace from their clients, supervisors should not seek solace from their supervisees. Just as supervisees can become overly involved with their clients, supervisors can become overly involved with their supervisees. Supervisors can become too close personally and socially with their supervisees, so that their authority and competence are eroded. Supervisors can become overly involved professionally with their supervisees and overly directive of their cases to the point that they are perceived as meddling, which results in conflict and frustration. The supervisor must be alert to the potential for such overinvolvement, and this is most likely to occur where the supervisor has no equal or consultant with whom to share supervisory concerns. The supervisor should recognize that supervisees need a differential role model to whom to relate. The supervisor is best perceived as a more experienced, more skilled, more knowledgeable source of assistance.

Concern has emerged about the importance of providing support groups for supervisors (Hamlin and Timberlake, 1982). As practice becomes more sophisticated and practice demands become more complex, more consideration will have to be given to providing such supports for supervisors. Supervisors will need to be alert to their own potential for distress if they are to be effective in assisting the practitioners they supervise. Supervisors are often placed in the same bind with supervisees as the supervisees are with their clients. Supervisors are often called upon to take unpopular stands with their supervisees in order to help them. For example, Wolman pointed out:

> Quite often, younger colleagues came to me for supervisory sessions with a glowing feeling of success because their patients expressed love and admiration for them. The beginning practitioners often take the expression of transference love as a sign of therapeutic success. (1976:16)

Under these circumstances, to be helpful, the supervisor must dissuade the practitioner regarding such illusions of power. This can result in the supervisor's being accused of trying to turn affection into cynicism, but to genuinely enhance the treatment, the supervisor must aid the supervisee in being more realistic about the therapeutic interaction. The supervisor should face this issue at the onset so the supervisee avoids being set up for frustration and a sense of failure when the client eventually becomes angry and resentful. It is difficult for the supervisor to be the carrier of such news, but it is often the basis of helpful supervision. When supervisors fail to recognize the importance of this aspect of their role, it can gradually lead to supervisor distress and alienation from supervisees.

THE ROLE OF SUPPORT

The passage of time in the same demanding practice position and a heavy workload are bound to catch up with the worker and can result in distress. Recognition of this basic combination of factors by the supervisor can be one of the chief safeguards against being overwhelmed by distress in practice. A practitioner who is struggling to combat distress can progress into a full-blown episode of distress if support is unavailable. A client who commits suicide, a family that is liked by the practitioner but that angrily withdraws from treatment and blames the worker, or an alcoholic who returns to a bout of heavy drinking are examples of such distress-precipitating events. Supervisors must be alert to such events and provide a supportive environment that gives practitioners the opportunity to articulate and work through their anger, frustration, guilt, sense of failure, or other strong reactions they may have to perceived responsibility for unsuccessful outcomes.

The word *burnout* has gained popular usage as a global phrase, but it is not descriptive of what most people undergo. Burnout implies a final state, something that has been reduced to ashes, rubble. Research (Munson, Studies D and E) shows that workers' responses to pressure are cyclical. The question is, Is there life after burnout for supervisors and supervisees? The answer to this question is, Yes, there is life after burnout, and often it is a more realistic and effective existence if the stress is recognized and dealt with appropriately. The following sections can be used by both supervisors and supervisees in understanding and combating burnout.

GENERAL PRINCIPLES

Selye (1974) makes a distinction between stress and distress.* Stress "is the nonspecific response of the body to any demand made upon it" (Selye 1974:14), it can be pleasant or unpleasant, and it is not necessarily something to be avoided. Physical activity produces stress, but it is not necessarily damaging. Damaging or unpleasant stress is distress. Stress is not a unitary entity; it is composed of a set of stressors that can be of various types and origins. When stress is cumulative or the number of stressors is too great, the result eventually is distress. When the stressors are withdrawn, the more normal biological and psychological state is reestablished.

Selye has identified a process of reacting to stress that he has labeled the general adaptation syndrome (GAS), which has three stages:

1. Alarm reaction
2. Stage of resistance
3. Stage of exhaustion

The first stage involves recognition that something is wrong, and in the second stage, the person offers resistance to the stressor. If the stressor is continually applied and not withdrawn, the person will eventually reach a stage of exhaustion. It is this stage with which the term *burnout* is associated. From this it can be seen that burnout, as normally viewed, is only one part of a three-stage process. Distress usually occurs during times of psychological and physiological vulnerability. Selye's conception has been advanced through research showing that the stages of stress are repeated and that the symptoms of stress become more intense with each recurring cycle.

Job-related distress is considered quite common, and few workers are viewed as immune to it. There is no unified definition for "burnout" or job distress. Generally, it can be defined as "to deplete oneself, to exhaust one's physical and mental resources, to wear oneself out by excessively striving to reach some very high expectations" (Freudenberger, 1977:90).

Source of Expectations

High and unrealistic expectations of self and clients are held to be a primary source of distress. Unrealistic expectations are believed to take two forms: internal and external. Clinical practitioners are more susceptible to

---

*Selye's basic formulations about stress and distress are the foundation of much of the content of this chapter.

internal, or self-imposed, unrealistic expectations, and social service workers are more susceptible to external—societally or bureaucratically imposed—unrealistic expectations. Research on child welfare workers revealed that they suffered from internal forms of burnout as much as from external ones (Munson, Study D). It is an open question regarding what form of stress certain groups undergo or whether different practice settings produce a mixture of the two forms.

To illustrate this point, the following excerpt from an interview with a child welfare worker who experienced burnout is fairly typical:

RESEARCHER: Some of the research that has been done on burnout identifies the sources of stress as being in some cases internal—that is, the person places too many demands on herself—as opposed to external—where not enough resources are available to complete the job. Which type of burnout do you think you predominantly had, or did you have both?

WORKER: I think I definitely predominantly had the internal form of burnout because I think I did put a lot of demands on myself, and I think that was probably my biggest problem—that I wasn't able to separate emotionally enough from my clients. I got too involved and felt responsible for their whole lives, which is impossible to do and really be effective. I think you have to be able to shut off your work life at the end of your day and go home and have something else to do. I think I really carried the burden, felt real responsible for everybody, which is really not good.

RESEARCHER: Do you think you have a different attitude about that now?

WORKER: I think I do. I think right now I am able to separate it more. I think it is just something you have to realize. You have to still be compassionate and get involved with the problems, but you have to know that a lot of it is dependent on the client. They are responsible for their own lives. You can only go so far.

Excessively high, unrealistic expectations, internal or external, are most likely to occur as a result of values and beliefs professionals adopt based on a belief in hard work, doing good for others, and the importance of being dedicated to a task.

Process of Stress Reactions

Because of the belief systems they adopt, clinicians resist admitting that distress occurs. In the work setting, this would be the practical equivalent to Selye's stage of resistance (Selye, 1974). The practitioner is unable or unwilling to admit that a problem with his or her functioning exists. This is a gradual process that can come and go over a long period of time. In the first stage the person recognizes that something is wrong but does not know what it is. Selye's alarm reaction manifests as anxiety, anger, aggression, and depression, which is usually focused on events or other people.

The development of distress is not always as clear as the literature would have people believe, and this gradualness of distress makes the supervisor's job more difficult. The comment of one worker illustrates this point:

> Now that I look back on it, I went through several periods of burnout, but I didn't realize it at the time. In the past twenty years, I have had three prolonged periods of burnout. At the height of each one I changed jobs. I thought at the time that I was doing it to get ahead. Now I know there were other factors of boredom involved. It took three to four years for it to develop. At times I would tell myself that it was nothing. It was a natural reaction. I was just a little depressed. I can't tell you any point . . . where it started or when it first began to show. I just know that the result was that I was miserable for a long time, and I thought it was something that somebody was doing to me.
>
> The breakthrough came when I realized I was doing it to myself. I did all the other things you are supposed to do—jogging, diet, attitude change, etc.—until I came to the realization that I could control this, and I was not being controlled by others. To explain what I have been through and to explain the solution to someone else is very, very difficult to do.

Selye's third stage is exhaustion. In this stage the practitioner continues to function but coping mechanisms are depleted. The person undergoes disorganization to the point that even though he or she might work harder, the person actually accomplishes less. The person feels no sense of reward from work, and cynicism toward clients is common. The worker can become immobilized and develop disillusionment to the point that he or she feels the whole world is dysfunctional. The worker goes through the motions of working with clients without any commitment to the belief that intervention will do any good. This attitude becomes self-defeating and self-fulfilling because clients can sense the practitioner's sense of hopelessness. A research interview with a former child welfare worker illustrates this point:

RESEARCHER: How did you know you were burned out?

WORKER: I think that probably it was just the feeling of being emotionally exhausted and actually not wanting to see the problems rather than delving into them and looking for them, wanting to gloss over things. Actually, just feeling exhausted, feeling like you have given all of your emotions up, and drained.

RESEARCHER: So when you would come home from work at the end of the day, how would you feel?

WORKER: I think child welfare really messes up your private life. I think your whole life becomes child welfare, or it did for me anyway, for a while. You sort of lose your perspective on things, like that is your whole world. You come home, and you're exhausted, and you don't have a lot to give other people, friends, and family.

RESEARCHER: How about in other workers? Could you see burnout in them?

WORKER: I think people that I saw generally became cynical, and I think it is just from the pressures of the job, of seeing so much, and feeling also inadequate to deal with a lot of it. You could see the problems, but you didn't know how to help them. A lot of times it was impossible to really make any changes, and so I think it varies from person to person because I think there are ways of dealing with it, and I even think there are probably people that go through periods of burnout and then maybe are effective again.

I don't think it is necessarily a continuous thing, but I would think that after a couple of years that that is when most people start to burn out. I think people come in, and they are very idealistic, and they really feel good about their job, and they feel they are doing things, and gradually they see that a lot of their clients just don't cooperate. I think they start feeling like maybe they aren't making as many changes as they thought they would. They sort of lose their positiveness about the job, and that is when they start burning out, just maybe doing enough to get by.

And, also, I don't know if it is really all the clients, but a lot of it, I think, is administrative problems within the agency, since it is such a large organization. A lot of it does depend on the supervisor. But one supervisor in particular that I had, her whole attitude was, "If you don't like it, get out," which doesn't create real positive feelings, doesn't make you feel real good about how worthwhile you are, how good the job is, when, if you have a problem you can't discuss it—you are just told if you don't like it, leave. And that was just her general attitude with everyone.

Sources, Structures, and Targets of Stressors

One way to think about all that has been stated about stress to this point in this chapter is that stressors have a structure that you can visualize. Individual stressors are short-term in nature and do not endure for long periods of time. Short-term stressors occur, for example, when your bus breaks down and you are late for work. When you get to work you discover that you left your wallet and agency identification badge at home. If there is a new security guard at the entrance to the agency, you become even more late while you are being cleared for access. You are thirty minutes late for your first appointment, and your client is angry about having to wait. This is a brief example of how stressors can be cumulative and occur with increased frequency with small periods of relief between the occurrence of the stressors. The key factor is not that a person experiences multiple stressors, but the length of period of relief between stressors. If stressors take place in rapid succession and without relief, they become cumulative and begin to merge or pile up. This pattern of stressors is illustrated in Visual 10.1. Pattern A illustrates regularly occurring stressors with recurring periods of relief. Pattern B illustrates cumulative stressors without periods of relief, and it is this pattern that leads to distress and Selye's eventual stage of exhaustion discussed earlier. For example, a single difficult case may last for several days, weeks, or months, but usually the case is resolved, either positively or negatively. People undergo multiple single stressors in the normal course of life and can recover if there are periods of relief.

Also, it helps to view yourself as a target of stressors. Stressors are always seeking a target. If you view yourself as a target of stressors from multiple sources, such as personal events, clients, colleagues, supervisors, and internal sources as well as unidentified sources, then you can visualize these events mounting around you. The visualization of stressor sources is important to decreasing or eliminating stressors. If a person does not know where a stressor is originating from, methods cannot be found to cope with it. A person cannot not know the sources of all stressors, but to manage stress, he or she must know the origin of the majority of stressors. This is illustrated in Visual 10.1 as Stressor Sources. Using this visual to conceptualize your stressors is the first step in managing and mastering stress. Try to refrain from using the global term *stress* ("I am under a lot of stress" or "I can't deal with all this stress"). Think and speak in terms of specific stressors ("My key stressors right now are getting this report done, finding a good day care provider, and deciding if I really have time to take on this new consulting job").

Behavioral Indicators

The supervisor must recognize that each practitioner will have a unique way of dealing with stress. In assessing burnout, the behavior gauge should not be comparing a given practitioner to other practitioners, but comparing the worker to his or her own past performance record. Since distress is a result of stages, the worker's previous performance will be the best indicator of changes in functioning. To compare the worker to others can increase the worker's distress.

Behavioral indicators usually take three forms: interactional, psychological, and physical.

Interactional

The earliest signs occur in relation to clients but are not easily observable by the supervisor because the supervisor has little contact with the practitioner in this area. This is one of the reasons it is important that the supervisor observe and participate in the worker's practice periodically.

VISUAL 10.1. Sources, Structures, and Targets of Stressors

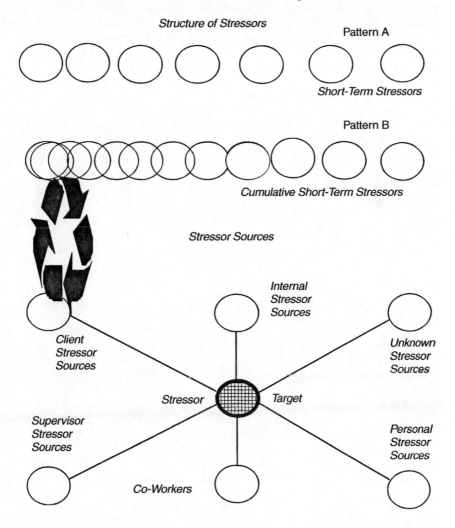

Structure of Stressors

Pattern A

Short-Term Stressors

Pattern B

Cumulative Short-Term Stressors

Stressor Sources

Internal
Stressor
Sources

Unknown
Stressor
Sources

Client
Stressor
Sources

Stressor   Target

Supervisor
Stressor
Sources

Personal
Stressor
Sources

Co-Workers

When dealing with clients, the worker's interactional indicators are loss of interest, inattentiveness, forgetfulness, cutting off exploration with clients, and cutting sessions short. The worker shows a tendency to become impatient with clients and to become angry when they do not respond in ways the practitioner desires.

The more apparent interactional elements occur in relation to co-workers, supervisors, and administrators. A normally pleasant, sociable worker becomes withdrawn, and stops responding to phone messages, written messages, letters, and memos. The quiet, retiring practitioner can become argumentative and obstinate. The worker avoids the supervisor or frequently challenges the supervisor's authority and actions. When such changes in the practitioner's relationships with others occur, the supervisor has a key indicator that a stress reaction is taking place. Co-workers will often comment to the supervisor about changes in the practitioner.

The worker's interaction with others outside the work setting is usually altered. Friends and relatives detect changes, but the supervisor is not usually aware of these changes. Marital problems can develop, and some have attributed divorce to work-related stress, but this is speculation, since no reliable information is available to determine whether, in fact, the divorce rate is higher in the helping professions than it is in the population as a whole.

Psychological

Depression and anger are common reactions (Rippere and Williams, 1985). Such work-related psychological changes are hard to distinguish from reactions originating from personal problems. General depression can be confused with work distress (Bramhall and Ezell, 1981b:23; Bramhall and Ezell, 1981a, 1981c). When depression is a factor in the practitioner's functioning, the supervisor must explore the origins with the person. The worker can develop cynical attitudes toward clients and become callous about clients and their motivations. Supervision can come to be viewed as harassment rather than a source of help. Negative attitudes toward administrators emerge.

Some workers manifest rapid mood changes. Suspiciousness and feelings of isolation are accompanied by a loss of sense of humor. The practitioner questions his or her ability to help others and talks of regret about his or her career choice. The worker tends to lose interest in others and to express a sense of uncaring attitudes on the part of others. He or she may be less willing to assume new roles and express feelings of hopelessness and futility about agency functioning.

Physical

Physical symptoms can be quite diverse and are caused by various factors. As with psychological symptoms, the supervisor and the practitioner should be cautious about attributing physical symptoms to job-related stress. When physical symptoms due to organic causes are blamed on job stress, the person might be engaging in denial that could result in damage to physical health. When the practitioner raises the issue of physical symptoms in supervision, the supervisor should encourage the person to see a physician.

While almost all writers on stress provide long lists of physical symptoms that can be associated with job stress, studies carried out in several settings reveal that fairly low levels of physical symptoms were reported overall, with a low incidence rate of attributing these symptoms to job-related stress (Munson, Study D).

Given these findings, it is suggested that the supervisor consider the interactional patterns and psychological reactions primarily in assessing the worker's behavior and performance over time to detect reactions to job stress. Although physical symptoms might be identified, the supervisor's role should be limited to suggesting medical evaluation. In reviewing worker behavior, the supervisor should remember that individuals will respond differently to the same amount of stress. Burnout can be manifested in a variety of forms. Each individual needs to identify the ways in which he or she reacts to stress. Also, if a person has just a few of these reactions, but the reactions are exaggerated and affect functioning, an assessment should be done to determine if the worker is experiencing distress. Once stress reactions are identified, one can begin to deal with them.

Another excerpt from the interview with the former child welfare worker will illustrate the points that have just been made:

RESEARCHER: How did you actually behave in relation to burning out? What were the kinds of things you felt, the kind of things that actually happened to you behaviorally?

WORKER: On the job or personally?

RESEARCHER: Both, because I don't think we can separate the two, can we?

WORKER: Well, I know I felt burned out. I think I just really wasn't as effective. I think I did what I had to get by, and just really didn't feel good about the job I was doing—about myself, maybe.

RESEARCHER: How did you feel when you came home at the end of the day?

WORKER: Pretty exhausted. I think most of the time I was pretty exhausted, maybe even more so in the beginning, because I was more involved with my clients, and so when you came home, you were just exhausted and felt your whole life was your work, and towards the end maybe I was putting less into it, so in some ways my personal life improved, but my professional life wasn't real good. [Pause.]

I think there is a real high divorce rate. All the people I knew, most of them were single, a lot of them were divorced. I think that is a real hazard of the occupation.

RESEARCHER: How about drinking? Do people turn to alcohol or drugs?

WORKER: Definitely there is an active happy hour group—every agency that I worked in.

RESEARCHER: But yet that didn't seem to relieve the tension even though it was maybe designed for that?

WORKER: Actually in some ways I am sure it did relieve it because we were able to sit and complain about things and work out some feelings—but that only goes so far. I think there are a lot of other things that attribute to your feelings of stress, and I think a lot of it is probably, or some of it anyway, is the administrative attitude that—there is a general feeling sometimes—that if you stay too long in maybe any agency in one position, you're probably not an effective person, that you've stagnated. So I just think there is an overall feeling that unless you are constantly moving that you're not really a great worker, and you start taking some of those feelings in about yourself and your job, and you lose some of your effectiveness.

CONTRIBUTING FACTORS

The interview segments illustrate that burnout is a reaction to job-related stress that can result in high rates of turnover and decreased effectiveness. Job-related stress is not caused by a simple, single stimulus, but rather by objects, emotions, and personal interactions that make up a series of contributing factors. Daley (1979) identified four sources of stress that can be contributing factors to distress: barriers to achieving goals, poor and uncomfortable working conditions, incompatible demands, and ambiguous role expectations. For example, those seeking social work careers place value on working with people. However, Daley reported that workers in protective services spend as little as 25 percent of their time in direct contact with clients. Time is spent instead transporting clients, completing forms, keeping case records, and attending staff meetings (Daley, 1979:377). Other contributing factors are large caseloads, arbitrary deadlines, and workers being prevented from seeing a case through to completion.

In many settings the worker is attacked by the community regardless of whether he or she takes action. Workers are frequently not given support by supervisors and administrators for decisions they make. Practitioners are often criticized by their clients if they side with certain family members on an issue, while at the same time if they refuse to take a stand, they are criticized for being unconcerned and uncaring. Even the professional literature is contradictory about what to do in many of these situations. Practitioners frequently see their behavior patterns reflected in clients. Many clients present problems for which practitioners have no clear intervention strategies designed to deal with them. These and other factors can accumulate for the practitioner, resulting in the manifestations of distress.

DEALING WITH STRESS

Ultimately, the practitioner is the only person who can overcome stress reactions. The external contributing factors mentioned earlier will not change. Many organizational problems and high caseload demands are persistent factors. The critical variable is how the practitioner perceives and adapts to these conditions. The following suggestions are based on the literature and on practitioners' observations from the author's studies on stress.

Insight. The practitioner, with support from the supervisor, must gain insight into his or her own behavior and how he or she handles stress. It is easy for the practitioner to give up on himself or herself, to say, "I'm not worthy; I can't cope; why bother to try." Until the person finds that such an attitude is not healthy, little can be done to change the situation. The practitioner has to develop self-confidence, make a commitment to doing the best job he or she can, and accept the limitations within himself or herself, his or her clients, and the organization. Self-awareness and insight are only a beginning. The practitioner has to work hard at maintaining a positive attitude. Minor setbacks should be accepted and not allowed to trigger a pervasive fatalistic view. Workers have commented that this form of mental self-regulation is essential to combating a cycle of stress.

Exploration. The practitioner needs to discuss his or her feelings and reactions with others, especially the supervisor. Withdrawal and internalizing feelings only increase distress.

Defining the situation. Exploration with others should not be focused exclusively on complaints. The discussion needs to be aimed at how to overcome the problems or how to adjust to the situation. The problems should be viewed as situational and not ingrained in personalities. The concern should be how to alter or manipulate this situation to produce a positive outcome. It is important to recognize that practitioners need to work within the parameters of the organization. They need to accept the givens in the situation and concentrate on the factors that can be changed. Organizations cannot be expected to be rational, and the worker should not attempt to make the organization rational. Instead, the practitioner should accept responsibility for only what he or she can control.

The environment. The work setting in many agencies leaves much to be desired. Practitioners can take action to create the best possible environment for themselves and their clients. The addition of plants, pictures on the wall, lamps, and small radios can improve office appearance. Workers can request that the walls be painted, and that bookshelves and rugs be added to improve office appearance.

Education. The worker should seek education and training. The practitioner should identify areas of his or her work that cause difficulty and request training that will help him or her overcome these problems. Self-confidence can be greatly enhanced when the worker successfully helps a client using some technique or method learned in a training seminar. If the worker desires to advance in the agency, he or she should learn what education is needed to achieve this goal and work toward it. The worker who has long-range goals has little time to engage in self-pity and despair.

Developing outside interests. The worker needs to develop boundaries on work time and use his or her own time to develop outside interests. Work diversions such as drug use, heavy drinking, and gambling merely add to the worker's problem. Hobbies, recreation, physical exercise, and various other activities can serve as healthy outlets. Such activities do not have to be limited to nights and weekends. A lunch period can be used to pursue interests. Vacations can be planned in advance, and the activities associated with planning a vacation can be a wholesome diversion from work.

Any activity that keeps the worker focused on future goals and activities decreases the opportunity to dwell on present problems and past failures. In selecting outside activities, the worker needs to be careful to avoid activities that can increase stress. For a detailed discussion on how to select helpful activities, the reader should see the section Distress and Recreation in this chapter.

Career reorientation. If the worker suffers prolonged job stress, and all corrective efforts fail, consideration should be given to a career change. Such decisions should not be made hastily, but continuation in an unrewarding career can result in long-term frustrations that can influence all aspects of a person's life. During such discussions, the supervisor should put aside practical interests in order to aid the supervisee. For example, a supervisor should not avoid discussing career goals with a supervisee out of fear that the supervisee will leave the agency and the supervisor will need to recruit a replacement.

Although it is sometimes good for some people to change careers, it is tragic when practitioners with potential leave the profession because of their association with severely distressed supervisors. One practitioner's decision is reflected in her comments:

> Another major obstacle is my supervisor, who is experiencing burnout. My supervisor has gone through all the stages of burnout, and he is stuck in the exhaustion stage. I don't know if he sees it and knows it, but I do. He is in a double bind. On one hand, he enjoys his work with the patients, but on the other hand, he is frustrated by low pay, low status, and the agency system. The result of my supervisor's negative feelings toward himself, his job, and his role as a social worker has affected the quality of my supervision and my perception of the social work profession. My desire to continue to work in the field of social work has decreased. I have accepted a job outside the field of social work. It

is a job in industry doing personnel work. I decided to take this job because of the pay, learning experience, and the opportunity for growth.

THE SUPERVISOR'S ROLE

All of the self-corrective efforts for the supervisee mentioned in the previous section can be supported by the supervisor. The supervisor should work to create the conditions that facilitate the worker's efforts. If the supervisor does not assume a supportive role, he or she becomes another contributing factor to the practitioner's distress. The supervisor can follow other general principles in assisting supervisees.

Facilitating insight. Although the practitioner is the only person who can achieve insight into his or her burnout and its control, the supervisor can foster development of insight through encouraging discussion of the problem. This can be done in individual supervision as well as through group sessions in which feelings and attitudes are explored openly. Such discussions should not be allowed to become quasi-therapy for the practitioners or mere gripe sessions, which tend to increase frustration.

The supervisor has a responsibility to keep the discussion focused on job-related issues and on defining the work situation. The supervisor should listen and make suggestions that will help practitioners to gain insight and to find their own solutions. When the supervisor gives direct advice or tells workers what to do, anger on the part of the workers is likely to result. The supervisees should be approached in a nonthreatening manner to avoid alienating them or producing feelings of guilt and failure. The practice of telling supervisees how the supervisor solved his or her own burnout should be used with caution, since what worked for the supervisor may not necessarily be the solution for the workers.

The environment. The supervisor should work to create the best possible work environment for practitioners. When supervisees make requests for office equipment and decorations, the supervisor has a responsibility to support reasonable requests. When supervisors fail to take such requests seriously and fail to follow through with them, they lose credibility in the eyes of the workers. It is not valid to expect that all requests will be approved, but the supervisor has an obligation to present reasonable requests to administrators who control and plan budgets.

Education. The supervisor has a key role in promoting education and training for supervisees. The importance of education and training should not be underestimated because research indicates that the more highly trained the practitioner, the less likely he or she is to experience stress (Streepy, 1981). The supervisor has a responsibility to monitor training to ensure that workers are getting the type of training they need. Workers who are subjected to mandatory training or even voluntary training that does not help them cope with their work become frustrated and resentful.

An educational plan should be developed for each worker, and the supervisor should evaluate with the worker each seminar or course he or she attends. The supervisor should encourage the worker to discuss career goals and what education and training he or she needs to achieve these goals. The supervisor should survey the worker's educational needs and advocate training that meets these needs.

Role model. One of the best ways the supervisor can help supervisees deal with job distress is to serve as an effective role model. Practitioners develop many of their attitudes and behaviors from the relationship they have with their supervisors. Through positive attitudes and demonstration of effective work habits, the supervisor can indirectly convey to workers many strategies for combating stress. The practices advocated in this book are designed to foster positive performance by the supervisor.

UNANSWERED QUESTIONS

Many unanswered issues about stress remain. For example, why is it a serious problem? Why was it not identified as a problem earlier? There is evidence that caseworkers at the turn of the century underwent stress, so this is not a new phenomenon, but it is coming to attention more.

What about society generates so much stress? It could be such things as high mobility, rapid change, urbanization, affluence, increased bureaucracy, increased mechanization, and professionalization of charity. For many practitioners, burnout could be the result of stress associated with conflicting moral demands in practice rather than overwhelming workloads or inadequate resources.

Some feel that stress could be a positive indicator, reflecting the fact that society is working harder to solve its ills. The real challenge is not stress, they say, but the societal ills that promote it—poverty, crime, drug addiction, juvenile delinquency, mental illness, alcoholism, child abuse, aging, terminal illness, to mention just a few of a long list of factors (Chance, 1981:94-95).

Keep in mind that the best practitioners may experience stress at different times in their careers. What really counts is how they deal with it.

DISTRESS AND RECREATION

It has been a common practice to encourage workers to deal with distress by engaging in recreational activities. This general advice can be counterproductive. For example, people who burn out have been identified as hard-working, committed, high achievers. When such people are encouraged to take up recreational sports, they often select high-activity, heavily competitive sports such as tennis, racquetball, basketball, and handball. When people engage in these activities for recreation, more distress can result as they strive to be the best. If workers select sports activities for which they are not suited, instead of becoming a source of relaxation, the activity can be the cause of additional stress. High achievers tend to turn everything into work, so that a highly stressed worker who turns to a sport and takes it too seriously could be compounding his or her problems.

Supervisors should assist workers with choosing recreational activities because many workers are not aware of the harm they can do to themselves by selecting the wrong activity. For example, watching television or attending movies for relaxation can in fact increase tension. Much television and film content today focuses on social commentary and social problems; even comedy and variety shows have become problem focused (Lichter et al., 1991; Miller, 1988). Stress is even portrayed as entertainment on many television shows. Many documentary television shows highlight content that can intensify feelings of burnout. The individual is portrayed as helpless, a pawn, a victim in mass society controlled by giant, impersonal, unchecked institutions. Little is known about people's responses to prolonged exposure to such television content.

Research evidence suggests that people do have immediate mood changes associated with watching distressing news programming (Munson, 1974), but we do not know the long-term effects of such television content. The dynamics of contagion associated with stress reactions can be identified among staff in agencies, but the contagion effect through television, movies, magazines, and books remains unexplored. Practitioners who use such media as relaxation can be in for another barrage of the problems they see and hear about in their work all day. In many psychotherapy education programs (Fritz and Poe, 1979), and in schools of social work, cinema and literature are increasingly being used to train practitioners. This can lead the practitioner unconsciously to analyze movies and books from a professional point of view rather than seeing them as entertainment.

Leisure Activity Guidelines

Given this information, can one gain any relaxation and relief from television, movies, sports, or books? Yes, but one should answer the following questions to ensure that one is engaging in leisure activities for the purpose of leisure:

1. Am I doing this because I want to do it? For example, am I playing tennis because I want to or because it is the fad in the neighborhood? Am I going to this movie because I want to or because a friend wants to

go? Am I reading this book because I want to or because I want to appear informed at the book club meeting?

2. Am I physically and psychologically suited to the leisure activity I have selected? For example, sports such as tennis and basketball require good eye-hand coordination, mental anticipation of your opponent, and physical stamina. Chess, on the other hand, requires much mental anticipation of your opponent without the physical requirements of tennis. Baseball involves one in a team effort that is much different from a single-opponent sport.

3. Does this activity truly give me pleasure while I am doing it? If you play on a baseball team for leisure, and you are constantly angered by the errors and failures of your teammates, you are probably not getting much relaxation.

4. When I complete the activity, do I feel good? If you play backgammon for leisure and you pick a partner who constantly defeats you and, after a series of games, you are planning how to get even, the goal of the leisure activity has been defeated.

5. Has the activity become a chore for me? If you find yourself relieved because the tennis match has been cancelled because of rain, there is a good chance that your recreation has become work.

6. Am I investing too much time in one form of leisure activity? If a recreational activity is consuming too much of your time and taking away from other pursuits, it is no longer leisure. The person addicted to jogging is an example of this. Leisure researchers recommend that, for the best results, one should engage in several leisure activities rather then focusing on one.

SUPERVISOR TRAINING

Supervisors should be well educated about stress since it has been identified as having such a high risk potential in many agencies (Wallace and Brinkerhoff, 1991). Training programs for supervisors should include content that assists them in identifying stress and in helping practitioners deal with it. When training is not provided to supervisors, they should take it upon themselves to learn about stress. The suggested readings at the end of this chapter are a good starting point.

A key conceptualization the supervisor should keep in mind is that stress, practice demands, and coping strategies are interrelated. Practitioners who have a large number of coping strategies to use in relation to practice demands will experience less stress. It is the supervisor's job to help the worker develop as many coping strategies as possible and to work to keep the practice demands in reasonable relationship with the coping strategies.

This is illustrated in Visual 10.2 through depiction of the desired and unde-
sired states when considering these three factors. Most of the content of this
book is designed to increase the coping strategies of both the practitioner
and the supervisor.

DESPAIR AND ISOLATION

The chief function of the supervisor is to aid the supervisee in translating
activity into practice, but another important function is to prevent the isolation of the practitioner. This covert function has been practiced but unrecognized for decades. To avoid being overwhelmed, becoming frustrated, undergoing moderate chronic depression, and becoming callous toward clients,
the practitioner should maintain a wholesome contact with colleagues.

The demands placed on practitioners in their role with clients can be devastating and produce gradual, chronic, and sometimes permanent changes
in therapeutic activity and personality of the practitioners. Practitioners
themselves are usually the last to recognize or admit these changes. The
more serious the mental illnesses with which the practitioner works in treatment, the greater the potential for therapeutic despair. Farber has identified
this phenomenon in work with schizophrenic patients as the peculiar and

VISUAL 10.2. Coping Strategies, Practice Demands, and Stress

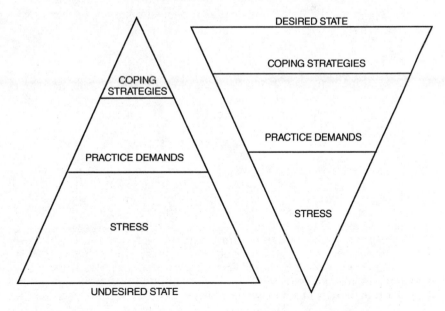

painful nature of therapeutic life that produces "emptiness, meaningless-ness, lack of confirmation—in short the circumstances that lead to a particular despair on the part of the therapist and that may subsequently evoke in the patient a response of pity for his doctor's plight." It is Farber's contention that this despair "is more or less intrinsic to the therapeutic life with schizophrenia and that such despair, moreover, if acknowledged rather than disowned, if contended with rather than evaded, *might* (the word is important) have a salutary effect on therapy" (Boyers, 1971:90).

Skillful recognition and articulation by the supervisor are required for such practitioner reactions to be managed positively for the benefit of the practitioner and the therapy. The supervisor must help the worker recognize what is taking place and aid in developing ways to manage and use despair in the treatment to assist the client. In exploring this process with practitioners, supervisors can gain insight into their own practice and use their experience to help the practitioners. In dealing with such material, the supervisor can combine the supervisory styles of *philosophical abstractions* and *technical strategies.* Philosophical abstractions are useful in identifying the process, and technical strategies are helpful in designing means of capitalizing on practitioner despair to assist in the client recovery process.

There are degrees and varying forms of practitioner despair, depending on the types of clients with whom the practitioner works. The supervisor needs to be alert to particular patterns of client problems that occur repeatedly in the worker's practice and give rise to a constellation of despair-producing symptoms. The following practitioner summary of a supervisory session illustrates the point that is being made here:

> I was doing this group therapy with eight outpatients from a state mental hospital. The group seemed to be making little progress as a group or as individuals. On several occasions in the group I experienced this wave of feeling of despair. It is hard to describe. I would withdraw into myself in the group. I was aware of what was being said, but it was like I wasn't there at the same time. It mildly scared me, and I was reluctant to talk about it with colleagues or my supervisor.
>
> On two occasions I felt like adjourning the group by telling them I couldn't help them, and it was pointless to continue meeting. These two instances occurred at times when feelings of depression were at high levels of expression in the group. During a supervisory session, my supervisor asked how the group was going. I don't know if he detected something was bothering me or not, but he commented that such groups could be demanding and made reference to having a similar group at one time in which he would experience feelings of being lonely without being alone. This paradox troubled him to the point that he shared it with colleagues who admitted to similar feelings. I felt relieved and shared my experiences. This became the focus of sev-

eral supervisory sessions and resulted in exploration of ways I could interpret these feelings for the group as an observation of concern for the failure to make progress in the group. This helped me focus the feelings and relate them to the group task and my role as therapist. This helped me stay with the group interaction.

After my interpretation to the group, they expressed frustration about their progress and began to share problems and feelings that provided rich therapeutic material. The group genuinely moved to a new level of therapeutic endeavor.

Supervisors must foster the kind of relationship that promotes sharing of the practitioners' deepest fears and concerns about their feelings and attitudes that they perceive as irrational or unprofessional. Only in a trusting and accepting supervisory relationship will practitioners share these deepseated fears. To deal with such content confidently, supervisors must be well prepared, experienced, and supported themselves. Wolman (1976) has argued that three ingredients make a good therapist: aptitude, training, and experience. The same three ingredients are essential to good supervision. Good practitioners must function at a level different from that of their patients (Wolman, 1976:15), and good supervisors must function at a level different from that of their supervisees if they are to be helpful to them.

THE BEGINNING PROFESSIONAL

Much has been written about stress in occupations, and especially in the helping professions, but little attention has been devoted to stress that occurs before actually entering a career. The assumption is that burnout originates on the job. It could be that many professionals are well on the road to burnout before they enter their chosen profession. For many, this process begins during their academic training. Social work is a good example of this attempt to track the origins of stress. A key indicator is the observation of many graduate social work educators that first-year students are motivated, interested, and excited about social work, but as they progress to the second year of training, they become bitter, hostile, withdrawn, and cynical. These attitudes and behaviors are commonly identified as being associated with stress, but, ironically, when they are observed in graduate students, such responses are rarely attributed to stress.

One survey lends support to the notion that some students undergo high degrees of stress (Munson, Study E). In addition to the sixteen hours a week spent in course work and the twenty hours a week in field placements, the survey found that 50 percent of the students spent an average of twenty-six hours per week employed. In addition, the majority of social work students are married women with an average of two children. With such a profile and the added hours required for study and library work, the average social work student is under a great deal of stress. Class meetings, field experience, work, and study add up to an average work week of seventy hours for many students.

Unrealistic expectations have been identified as a factor in the process of burnout. Social work students are more fortunate than students of other professions in that the reliance on field placements throughout undergraduate and graduate education introduces them early to the conditions and limitations they will face as practitioners. However, field experiences are limited, and often students are protected from extreme cases and agency problems by their field instructors. Large numbers of students want to enter clinical practice in private settings. Their view is one of working in plush offices in the suburbs, with a psychiatrist for backup support, with middle-class clients who have emotional and family problems. Few will enter this small, highly competitive area of social work practice. The reality for many will be large caseloads of poor, disabled clients who need services and resources that the agency is hard-pressed to provide. Offices are dingy, cramped, shared with others, and poorly equipped. Managed cost organizations have gradually decreased reimbursement rates for private practitioners and have forced many clinical social workers into large group practices.

Schools have placed increased emphasis on autonomy to promote professionalism. This conception proves unrealistic as new workers discover that many agencies allow little independent practice, and that much of their work is controlled, evaluated, and dictated by supervisors, administrators, managed cost organizations, courts, and community pressures.

Beginning practitioners often have little preparation for the stresses of practice. The small caseloads, frequent holidays, breaks, and supportive supervision of student training are an unrealistic preparation for long workdays, heavy caseloads, and sporadic supervision in the world of full-time practice. Education programs teach little about stress, and agency orientation programs rarely mention it.

Practitioners interviewed in one study of stress indicated that they received no advance preparation for the demands of practice (Munson, Study D). At the same time, many indicated that if they had been alerted in advance, they could have avoided many of their negative reactions, withdrawal, and persistence against overwhelming odds. These workers reported that since they were not warned in advance, they tended to perceive the stress as personal and to internalize it rather than to view it as inherent in the position. Another significant finding of this study was that practitioners felt regular, supportive supervision was the most effective aid in combating stress.

CONCLUSION: STRESS AND IDEALISM

Stress has always been an issue for clinicians. Descriptions of stress reactions in the literature date back almost 100 years. Perhaps what is occurring now is no different from what took place in the past. A key question is whether things are really different now or whether the same old problems have a technological "Teflon coating" that makes them seem new.

One aspect of the stresses that practitioners now face makes the situation different from the past. In the 1950s and 1960s, we experienced an era of abundance and dramatic expansion of helping services that we believed would never cease. Supervisors and practitioners trained in the 1960s and early 1970s were part of the constant growth mentality. The retrenchment and changes that are now occurring cause those of us who "grew up professionally in the good times" to make adjustments that can be anger provoking or depressive, or both. Job loss, additional work without compensation, and eliminated or decreased benefits have distressing effects.

Supervisors are in the middle between the organization that demands more work and clinicians who say they cannot possibly do any more. Supervisors handle this in different ways. Some "tough it out" and engage in strategies to keep the organization "at bay" while they try to protect practitioners. Some engage in conflict with their own supervisors as they try to justify and document that increasing workloads are having negative consequences. Some become harsh, demanding, and insistent with practitioners that they do more. These strategies lead to conflict and increased stress for the supervisors. There is no good solution for supervisors in relation to what is happening in the work setting. Plenty of trainers are willing to offer supervisors quick-fix solutions for the stresses they face, but this leads to more stress and frustration when the supervisors realize there are no good quick or extended fixes.

Another difference from the past that affects supervisors is that many of the younger practitioners never experienced the "golden age of growth." Their careers have been witness to the gradual decline of services that is the reverse equivalent to the gradual increases the older supervisors experienced. Many younger practitioners have a perspective and an inherent cynicism about "the system" that older supervisors cannot completely understand or relate to. These younger practitioners cannot appreciate the older supervisors' simultaneous anger, hope, and belief that the situation will eventually change for the better, if one holds on long enough. The old idea that the supervisor must instill a sense of optimism and promote hopefulness in supervisees is considered unrealistic by many supervisors in the current environment. The supervisee cannot appreciate grand expectations and the supervisor can no longer embrace this view, given the steadily increasing work demands placed on the professional and the supervisor's memories of the "golden age" workloads.

It is possible that the new era of social service delivery will place increasing and differing demands on practitioners and unique pressures on supervisors to enforce the new and increased expectations of workers. Little understanding of the new model exists, and the results of the increased expectations of practitioners cannot be anticipated.

In the supervisory situation, a first step in dealing with this new era is for the supervisor and supervisee to work at developing a mutual understanding of the current situation, as well as an understanding of each other's "professional mentality" and "philosophy of practice."

Another change that produces stress for the practitioner is the demand for more highly specialized skills that require more education for practitioners. Agencies and employers are shifting responsibility for continuing education to the professional person. Professional groups have unwittingly contributed to this through licensing mandates for continuing education. Since this responsibility has been placed exclusively on the professional, agencies and employers have retreated from paying for education and have eliminated release time for attendance at continuing education programs. As a result, professionals are required to use weekends and vacation time to increase professional knowledge. This is a direct manifestation of Schor's (1991) observation that the amount of leisure time has been steadily decreasing for the past thirty years.

Even while requiring practitioners to take on new specialized responsibilities, employers are aware that the organizations are under no obligation to provide training to perform the new functions. This becomes a problem because services increasingly are highly specialized and educational programs resist preparing graduates for specialization. Public agencies are moving to adopt a private-practice model of viewing the practitioner as autonomous when it comes to responsibility but as an employee when it comes to function. This is an ideal model from the perspective of employers driven predominantly by profit, and this is the case with private employers as well as public agencies. Many public-sector agencies now operate as quasi-private facilities. These public agencies often collect "fees" and make "profits" from other agencies that make referrals and "compete" with private service providers to collect for third-party reimbursement.

Although agencies and employers have been reluctant to support continuing education for staff, many have been eager to sponsor such programs because of the revenue-generating potential. This is part of the new model that contributes to practitioner cynicism about employers. Professions in the current economic environment seem powerless to provide protection against these abuses, and there are indications that they even support such practices. Some professional organizations have come to resemble profit-driven employers, with every policy or position based on what it will mean for the organization, not on what best serves the interests of the membership or the public. This is the reason that major professional organizations are not protesting the repressive policies of the government and the private sector. Witnessing such actions by professional organizations is another source of cynicism and frustration for practitioners.

Practitioners can come to resent and mistrust higher-level administrators in such an environment, especially when practitioners are told to do more with less but witness increases in perks and supports for higher-level administration. Practitioners have difficulty understanding how even small benefits are denied them in light of expenditures and resource allocations for administration. For example, one practitioner observed that the director of an agency, after much urging from the staff, purchased a computer system. However, the only computer software the administrator purchased was for billing and accounting. The system is used exclusively for administrative purposes to support billing, increase collections, and make practitioners more accountable for how time is used. The administrator has refused to purchase a relatively inexpensive clinical software package that would assist the practitioners in documentation and record keeping. In such situations, clinicians need to organize and present to administrators in a persuasive manner needs for supports and resources.

In addition to being disillusioned by the actions of employers and professional organizations, practitioners are increasingly frustrated by the actions of clients. Clients are more frequently failing to pay fees, missing appointments, and becoming angry at the practitioner for matters that the practitioner does not control. Much of the violence committed against practitioners is aimed at agency-created regressive policies rather than the actions of the individual practitioners. Growing numbers of practitioners resent being the front line of defense for agencies. The practitioners' anger and frustration are increased when the agencies do not take seriously practitioners' expressions of concern about safety and fail to provide adequate security measures.

It is difficult to raise these issues, and some would disagree as well as argue that the negative aspects of employer-employee relations (it is fitting that in the current environment professionals are referred to in the context of employer and employee) should be ignored. Downplaying the negative aspects of practice, however, can create the stresses practitioners experience. These problems must be recognized and addressed if working conditions for professionals are to improve. In addition, in this current environment, supervisors are forced to spend less time in supervision on clinical issues directly and to deal more with organizational issues, time management, professional self-preservation, and career planning. Supervisors can avoid such discussion by focusing exclusively on clinical issues, but this may not be in the supervisees' best interests.

The tendency has been to view burnout as the end stage of distress, but it appears to be one stage in a process that is not yet completely understood. Practitioners have reached a new stage that goes beyond burnout. Workers in this stage develop cynicism and paranoia about other staff, supervisors, and administrators that go beyond what we have seen in the past. They develop a mistrust of clients and even achieve some cynical glee from the clients' plight. They have a sense of loss regarding the good old days of practice, whether they lived in those days or read or heard about them from others. This stage can be labeled "sense of betrayal," derived from the work of Peter Homans (1989), in which he describes "de-idealization" in relation to personal development:

> In the most obvious sense de-idealization refers to the pre-oedipal line of development. . . . It is an inner psychological sequence of states, characteristics of adult life, with a beginning, middle, and end . . . it begins with conscious and unconscious idealizations and an enhanced sense of self-esteem, accompanied by feelings of loyalty, merger, and fusion with other objects—persons, ideas, ideals, groups, even a social and intellectual tradition. Since history rarely optimally facilitates psychological development, such mergers are eventually challenged by interpersonal, social, and historical circumstances. As a result, the idealizations lose their firmness and may even crumble, leading to a weakened sense of self, *a sense of betrayal* [italics added], a conviction that an important value has been lost, moments of rage at the object (subsequently perceived as having failed the self in some way or other), and a consequent general sense of inner disorganization and paralysis. The final disposition of the de-idealization experience usually takes one of three directions: (1) it may move toward new knowledge of self, new ideals, and consequent new ideas, or (2) the paralysis can persist, leading to apathy, cynicism, and chronic discontent, or (3) one may disavow the experience entirely and instead attack, often fiercely and rebelliously, the events or persons producing the de-idealization. The first and desired outcome is usually supported by a fresh mandate for introspection, an invitation to self-healing through the building of psychological structure, and the capacity to entertain what could be called "new structures of appreciation" or new values. To some extent, every outcome is a mixture of all three. (pp. 24-25)

Homans has described vividly in the personal context what takes place in the professional context. The personal self is preexisting and is intertwined with the professional self. The organization and its representatives, the supervisors, the administrators, and even the clients become the "objects" of the professional self. Homans' description of the three reactions to de-idealization is parallel to the reactions of the professional to the "losses" explored here.

The sense of betrayal stage can be characterized by relationships with clients in which the therapist views the client as enduring less pain than the therapist. This can lead to the therapist having intrusive thoughts during treatment, such as, "Why is this client telling me and why am I listening to this trivial material over and over? I have a headache. Why can't this client say something new or interesting so that I can stop thinking about this headache?"

This sense of betrayal can intensify when the client gets better and treatment is terminated or when the client drops out of treatment. The client moves on, but the therapist remains to repeat the process over and over. Winnicott (1986) described this in the health field as "reduplicated and repetitive mourning" (p. 118). The therapist in the full-blown betrayal stage will commit less to the relationship with each new client. Clients begin to see the therapist as aloof, uncaring, and withdrawn. This leads to a self-fulfilling prophesy in which the therapist sees therapy as useless because, in the therapist's view, the client is not committed to the treatment.

Good supervision can detect these responses and help the practitioner begin the steps to recovery, but impaired practitioners can mask these responses from the supervisor and develop the same attitude toward the supervisor as exists toward clients.

In the sense of betrayal stage, the practitioner takes little or no pride in his or her identity as part of the helping professions; professional self-image is diminished because the practitioner experiences society as abandoning clients. The practitioner's withdrawal and misuse of supports and resources reinforces the client's perception of self and eventually is reflected in the self-image of the practitioner. An appropriate supervisory protocol has not been developed for assisting practitioners in working through these perceptions and the other stresses raised in the sense of betrayal stage. New realistic, nonidealistic supervisory protocols must be developed that integrate clinical and organizational concerns if clinical social work is to survive individually and collectively.

Case Exercise:
The Case of Mark

Mark is one of your supervisees. You work in a child protective services unit. You supervise four social workers. Each social worker carries thirty-five cases. Mark has been working at DSS for eight years. He is a good worker and relates well to the children and their families. He told you in his monthly supervisory conference today that he feels stressed out and overwhelmed. He and his wife are having marital problems, but he does not believe this is causing his stress. He believes he has become traumatized himself through working with this population of children for so long. He told you he has been experiencing symptoms of inability to concentrate, a sense of numbing, loss of his sense of humor, and overconcern with some of the children with whom he works. He also stated, "There are some other things I don't want to talk about." He reported that in client sessions he sometimes loses track of the conversation, and in staff meetings, he daydreams about other things.

You are surprised to learn of Mark's difficulties; had no idea of the stress he was experiencing. You are concerned about losing Mark as a staff member. The county office is undergoing major restructuring to accommodate legislatively mandated reorganization of the state office. You are about to assume new administrative responsibilities, and you were going to recommend that Mark assume your supervisory position.

(1) How would you respond to what Mark has told you? (2) What would you do to assist Mark? (3) Would you tell Mark of your plans to recommend him for a supervisory position?

SUGGESTED READINGS

Edelwich, J. and Brodsky, A. (1980). *Burnout: Stages of Disillusionment in the Helping Professions.* New York: Human Sciences.
    Identifies causes, manifestations, and ways to deal with job-related distress based on interviews with distressed people in several professions.

Freudenberger, H. J. and Richelson, G. (1980). *Burn-Out: The High Cost of High Achievement.* New York: Anchor.
    General discussion of distress from a personality perspective.

Munson, C. E. (1992). "Editorial: The Ideal of Stress Revisited," *The Clinical Supervisor,* 10(2), pp. 1-8.
    Overview of stress reactions and how they can be related to idealization.

Olshevski, J. I., Katz, A. D., and Knight, B. G. (1999). *Stress Reduction for Caregivers*. Philadelphia: Brunner/Mazel.
    Guide to understanding and reducing stress in family caregivers of older relatives.

Selye, H. (1974). *Stress Without Distress.* New York: New American Library.
    This is a highly readable account of the biological and psychological basis of stress and distress. It is recommended that all supervisors read this book.

Streepy, J. (1981). "Direct-Service Providers and Burnout." *Social Casework,* 62(June), pp. 352-361.
    Research study that can give supervisors ideas of areas on which to focus to reveal indicators of worker distress.

Wolgein, C. S. and Coady, N. F. (1997). "Good Therapists' Beliefs About the Development of Their Helping Ability: The Wounded Healer Paradigm Revisited," *The Clinical Supervisor,* 15(2), pp.19-34.
    Overview of stress reactions.

> Obsessive personality features in top leadership are found quite frequently. On the positive side, the focus on orderliness, precision, clarity, and control may foster stable delegation of authority and clarity in the decision-making process. . . . On the negative side, some dangers are the leader's excessive need for order and precision, . . . need to be in control, and the expression of the sadistic components that often go with an obsessive personality.
>
> Otto Kernberg
> "Regression in Organizational Leadership"
> in M. F. R. Kets de Vries,
> *The Irrational Executive*

Chapter 11

Administrative Activities

The supervisor must attend to certain administrative tasks and functions that are beyond the normally defined administrative duties. This chapter covers topics that the supervisor often overlooks, but that can be important to the practitioner. Some of the topics covered are general record-keeping guides, legal issues in practice, duty-to-warn rules, ensuring practitioner safety, and credentialing requirements. The last section covers administrator styles that can be helpful to supervisors in dealing with their own supervisors and administrative leaders.

INTRODUCTION

It is rare that a clinical supervisor has the opportunity to exclusively do clinical supervision. It is impossible to do any clinical supervision without it having some administrative component. Most supervisors in public or private practice do administration as part of supervisory functioning. Some supervisors actually do more administration than clinical supervision. Growing evidence suggests that practitioners are increasingly required to do administrative tasks as a part of their clinical work. For example, there are estimates that 30 percent of clinicians' time is spent on record keeping. Others have estimated that much client information is recorded as many as eight times in the record. This is indicative of the increased time the supervisor must spend doing administration and teaching supervisees about how to perform administrative functions.

Practitioner administrative tasks and supervisor tasks are often connected. For example, treatment plans must be developed in many settings, and methods for doing this must be taught by supervisors. Initial and review treatment plans done by practitioners must be reviewed and signed by supervisors. Increasingly, method of payment for services requires practitioners to complete numerous forms and submit various measures of client progress that the supervisor must approve and sign. These examples illustrate the joint nature of administrative and clinical supervisory functioning. The old view of administration in supervision as something the supervisor did to or for the supervisee has shifted, and administration is now viewed as a task the supervisor performs in conjunction with the supervisee.

PRACTICE PROTOCOLS

In the current environment of individual and agency accountability for all aspects of practice activity, supervisors are being called upon to use standardized protocols or procedural guidelines to justify interventions. Accrediting organizations, private payers, and courts are requiring practice protocols for specific areas of practice. Each agency should have practice protocols established by supervisors, practitioners, and agency administrators. These should be expressed as protocols for intervention. In the absence of standardized protocols or practice standards, supervisors are often called upon to establish practice protocols. Even when agency or program administrators do not require practice protocols, the supervisor should design such protocols for the areas of practice they are responsible for in their setting. Supervisor-established protocols can be an effective defense against allegations of malpractice, incompetence, and ethical violations. To assist supervisors who are faced with developing practice protocols, the following guidelines are provided for what can be referred to as practice protocol plans (PPPs):

A. A protocol is simply a written description of how intervention and routine procedures are conducted. For example, a unit of a child therapy practice that does evaluations of sexually abused children should have a written protocol for how evaluations will be conducted with children and caregivers.

B. The expectation is that clinicians performing these procedures will follow the written protocol as closely as possible, and when deviations are necessary justification can be provided. For example, if an evaluation of an abused child needs to be done and the child has elective mutism and will not talk to the evaluator, then it would be permissible for the caregiver to be in the consulting room and for the child to whisper answers to the caregiver, who would then speak the answers to the evaluator.

C. The protocol items can vary based on the nature of the agency practice. The following ten criteria are considered basic to any PPP:

   1. What is the population served by the agency/group/practitioner?
   2. What are the primary and secondary problems presented by the population served?
   3. What are the demographics of the population served? This can include factors that are characteristic of the symptom/problem presentation:
      a. Age of onset
      b. Gender factors
      c. Family factors
      d. Social factors
      e. Occupational/educational factors
      f. Health factors
      g. Course of symptoms/problems
      h. Prior treatment pattern
      i. Substance/alcohol factors
      j. Criminal justice factors
   4. What are the general strengths of the client in dealing with the symptoms/problems?
   5. What are the limitations in dealing with the symptoms/problems? (Can refer to item list in #3).
   6. What training and capabilities do staff have to meet the needs of the client? How would the agency determine whether it is capable of meeting the client's needs?
   7. How can the agency measure the effectiveness of staff in meeting the client's needs?

8. If the agency is unable to meet the client's needs, how would the agency deal with the limitation (e.g., improve staff capabilities or make referrals)?
9. What supports are provided to staff to meet client needs?
10. What supervisory/administrative action is necessary to reconcile gaps in client need and practitioner effectiveness?

Practice protocols are different from practice guidelines (also referred to as practice parameters and best practices), standards of practice, and standards of care. These terms are often confused and used interchangeably inappropriately.

Practice guidelines are a set of client care strategies and methods to aid practitioners in making clinical decisions (for more details about and examples of practice guidelines, see APA, 2000b).

Standards of practice are general guidelines set by professional organizations to guide practitioners in day-to-day professional activities in relation to clients. These standards usually have sanction in legal and ethical matters. Reamer (1995) defines standard of care as the way an ordinary, reasonable, and prudent professional would like under similar circumstances. This is an outdated view of standards of practice; most current practice standards go far beyond Reamer's view. Reamer's view of reasonableness is from an earlier era when professions did not have the sophisticated knowledge and interventions that are available today. Although social work does not have the same level of sophistication in intervention knowledge as other professions, the social work profession is being held to the same general principles of practice standards as other professions. Standards of practice used in resolving disputes are based on the principle of professional expectations; that is, the acts of the professional are judged on the basis of the question, Did the act of a given professional, in given situation, conform to expectations of practice as defined by general consensus of professionals working in that area of practice? Practice standards of professional organizations have five general uses:

1. To monitor members through adjudication of grievances
2. To guide licensure boards in resolving grievances
3. To guide courts of law in resolving legal questions
4. To guide agencies in setting internal standards of practice and care
5. To guide supervisors in directing and evaluating the work of supervisees

Standards of care refer to activities related to the delivery of service to a specific population or a specific individual for a specific disorder or problem. Standards of care are based on available clinical data and are subject to change as research and knowledge advances (APA, 2000a). Standards of care are established by professional organizations or advocacy groups.

The social work profession is far behind other professions in establishing practice protocols, practice guidelines, standards of practice, and standards of care. Psychiatry, psychology, nursing, and education have made much progress in these areas in the past decade, but the social work profession rarely uses any of these methods to ensure high-quality practice. The dramatic increase in research and knowledge about mental and social problems that social workers treat has not led the profession to codify this information, as other professions have done, to offer the best possible treatment for clients and patients. The NASW Code of Ethics is often considered a substitute for the various forms of practice guides, but it is too general to be considered a substitute for protocols, guidelines, practice standards, or standards of care. If social workers are to meet the increasing challenges to their practice methods, then the profession will have to develop precise practice guidelines based on the "professional expectation" principle mentioned earlier.

RECORD KEEPING

Many times agency accreditation can depend on the degree of completion of the complex array of forms and required documentation. A new worker, experienced or inexperienced, can be overwhelmed by the incredible detail that must be mastered to have a record be current and up to date. It is recommended that the supervisor devise a flow chart or visual of the forms that are required for each record and distribute it to supervisees. Visuals 11.1 and 11.2 illustrate the flow chart and record keeping in a typical mental health setting. No two agencies have the same record-keeping procedures, but the concepts involved are usually quite similar. The supervisor should go over these illustrations several times with new supervisees and review them with supervisees who fall behind in record keeping. It is helpful with beginning practitioners to provide them with visuals similar to Visuals 11.1 and 11.2 that are based on the agency's form requirements. Such visualization can decrease the time it takes to master the forms process.

Most clinical agencies require an initial database, an initial treatment plan, progress notes done usually every thirty days (it is preferable to do a contact note for each client contact), and a review treatment plan normally every ninety days. It is important that the practitioner develop an understanding that clinical record keeping is a process designed to document the progression of the treatment. In Visuals 11.1 and 11.2 the term *progress note* has been replaced with *contact note*. This change was made because in legal

VISUAL 11.1. Typical Clinical Forms

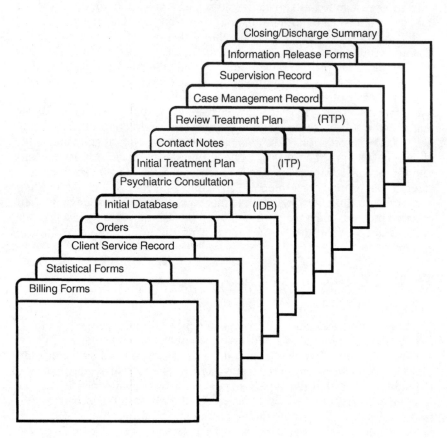

proceedings the term *progress note* implies improvement in the client's functioning, and this has been challenged when there is no evidence that the client has made "progress" or gained improvement in functioning, or when the client has gotten worse while in treatment. When a practitioner testifies that a client is unchanged or has deteriorated during treatment, use of the term *progress* cannot be justified.

Frequently clinicians view record keeping as an unnecessary chore that exists only for administrators to keep track of them and evaluate them. The job of the supervisor is to teach not only the importance of documentation and how to do it but also how to use documentation to benefit the client.

VISUAL 11.2. Diagram of the Typical Treatment Process

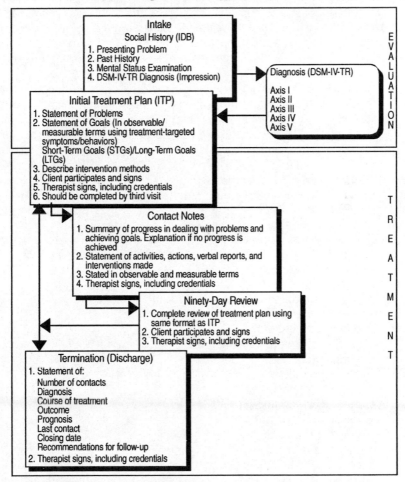

Documentation takes much of the practitioner's time. The supervisor has a responsibility to teach how to do documentation as efficiently as possible. Supervisors often overlook several common problems:

1. Practitioners often have not been taught how to use dictation equipment.
2. Frequently clinicians do not know how to summarize material or how to present the most salient features in a case or a session, and instead they will dictate lengthy details that give few clues to the patterns in the case.

3. Practitioners need help in organizing their time. For example, many practitioners are unaware that certain documentation can be done in treatment sessions. In fact, treatment plans should be done in the session since the person is expected to be an active participant in the treatment planning and, in many settings, is required to sign the treatment plan.
4. Practitioners often have limited understanding of the connection that should exist between the initial database, the treatment plan, the contact notes, and the closing summary. These items should be an integrated whole. To develop this view takes training and practice and the supervisor plays a key role in aiding the worker in this area.

Practitioners should view documentation as a reflection of the significant activity in a case so that a person unfamiliar with the case could read the record and have a basic understanding of the case.

Treatment records that follow guidelines established by the National Committee on Quality Assurance (NCQA) can be helpful to supervisors and administrators who are having difficulty with record-keeping policies. The following is a summary of the NCQA guidelines:

1. Each page in the treatment record should contain
   • client name and
   • client ID number.
2. Each record should contain
   • client address,
   • employer/school,
   • home/work telephone,
   • emergency contacts,
   • marital/legal status,
   • consent forms, and
   • guardianship information, if applicable.
3. All entries made in the treatment record should include the responsible clinician's name, professional degree, and ID number, if relevant, and all entries should be dated.
4. The record must be legible.
5. Relevant medical conditions should be listed, identified, and updated.
6. Presenting problems and relevant psychological and social conditions affecting the client's medical and psychiatric status should be documented.
7. Special status situations, such as imminent risk of harm, suicidal ideation, or elopement potential, should be prominently noted, documented, and updated in compliance with written protocols.

8. Each record should indicate what medications have been prescribed, dosages, and dates of initial prescriptions.
9. Allergies and adverse reactions should be clearly documented.
10. A lack of known allergies and sensitivities to medications and other substances should be prominently noted.
11. Past medical and psychiatric history should be documented, including previous treatment dates, provider identification, therapeutic interventions and responses, sources of clinical data, relevant family information, results of laboratory tests, and consultation reports.
12. For children and adolescents, prenatal and perinatal events and a complete developmental history (physical, psychological, social, intellectual, and academic) should be documented.
13. For clients age twelve and older, documentation should include record of past/present use of cigarettes, alcohol, and illicit, prescribed, and over-the-counter drugs.
14. A mental status evaluation should be included that documents the patient's affect, speech, mood, thought content, judgment, insight, attention/concentration, memory, and impulse control/risk management.
15. A DSM-IV-TR diagnosis should be documented, consistent with presenting problems, history, mental status examination, and/or other assessment data.
16. A treatment plan should be included that is consistent with the diagnosis given and that has objective, measurable goals with estimated time frames for goal attainment or problem resolution.
17. The focus of treatment interventions should be consistent with the treatment plan goals and objectives.
18. An informed consent for medications and client's understanding of the treatment plan should be documented.
19. Progress notes should describe client strengths and limitations in achieving the treatment plan goals and objectives.
20. Clients who become homicidal, suicidal, or unable to conduct activities of daily living should be promptly referred to the appropriate level of care, and any actions taken should be documented.
21. The treatment record should contain documentation of preventive services provided, such as relapse prevention, stress management, wellness programs, lifestyle changes, and referrals to community resources.
22. The treatment record should reflect continuity and coordination of care between the primary clinician, consultants, ancillary providers, and health care institutions.
23. The treatment record should include documentation of follow-up appointments and/or a discharge plan.

LEGAL ISSUES

The supervisor has an administrative responsibility to ensure that the clinician is aware of legal safeguards that must be observed in relation to clients and colleagues. The legal rights have become so complex and extensive in the past three decades that it is impossible to discuss in detail here the specific issues involved. It will be necessary instead to focus on general principles.

It has been reported that 90 percent of all malpractice suits against helping professionals were filed in the past thirty years (Meyer et al., 1988:11). Although the threat of lawsuits against mental health professions has not been extensive, most agencies and practitioners dread the thought of possible lawsuits to the extent that it impedes practice. For example, one clinician who feared lawsuits would not interview a child alone. When he had a mother and daughter in the office he would not close the door, and he never touched any clients. All of this was done in the belief that such actions would protect him against accusations. His actions afforded little protection, but they certainly altered the nature of the treatment. Ironically, his action of not closing the office door exposed him to possible legal liability due to breach of confidence/privacy, which ranks fifth in liability actions (Meyer et al., 1988:21)

Some of the defensive actions that agencies take are based on real threats, and some are imagined and based on erroneous beliefs about what the laws are regarding certain acts. The supervisor has a responsibility to be knowledgeable about client rights and legal developments regarding practice activity and agency obligations. This can be a significant task, but the supervisor should make a concerted effort to be aware of the legal requirements. Both agency-based and private practitioners should periodically consult with a knowledgeable attorney about legal concerns. Many excellent seminars offered by lawyers can be helpful to the supervisor. It is important that the supervisor be able to demonstrate that reasonable steps have been taken to help people and to avoid harm.

Supervisors and practitioners can take an absolute view of the law and believe that if certain specific acts are taken, no legal problems will occur. The law is not that simple. The legal system views acts as sequences. A good example of this is confidentiality. Supervisors can think that confidentiality is merely protecting the chart or not revealing information the client has shared. Confidentiality has become complex and is not a simple action (Wilson, 1978). Protecting the client's confidentiality is relative and not absolute. The supervisor and practitioner must take reasonable measures to protect the client's confidentiality and privacy through a series of acts. The practitioner should make clear to the client the limits and exceptions to confidentiality. It is not sufficient simply to tell the client that everything he or she tells the therapist is absolutely confidential. The therapist must take reasonable care to guard confidentiality, but many situations in the modern world make it difficult for the therapist to maintain this confidence.

One simple illustration of this is the dilemma presented by a telephone answering machine and leaving a recorded message for the client. The therapist has no control over who hears the message, and identifying oneself could be detrimental to the client if the message is heard by others. The technology of caller ID is problematic for clinicians because the practitioner does not have to leave a message to be identified. Once a call is placed to a client, the caller's number is recorded by the caller ID device unless the clinician has a device or service installed on the office telephone that blocks identification of the calling number. If a blocking device is not used by the clinician, then any person having access to the telephone of a client who has caller ID will know that the clinician telephoned the client.

Society has become so complex that when a person is treated, many people can become aware of the treatment and aspects of it without the therapist sharing information. In addition to the therapist, some of the people who can be aware of the treatment are secretaries, receptionists, bookkeepers, insurance company staff, employers, custodians, other therapists, other clients, and school officials. This small list of the people who can come to have knowledge of treatment illustrates that confidentiality cannot be totally guaranteed or controlled by the therapist.

When considering the legal implications of supervision, the following general principles should be kept in mind.

Supervisor Liability

1. Supervision is generally defined as a legal, ethical, contractual relationship in which the supervisor is responsible for and controls the supervisee's work.
2. Consultation is defined as a professional relationship with ethical requirements, but there are no legal standards for responsibility when a consultant renders advice that a consultee can accept or reject.
3. Supervisors can be held liable for unethical conduct and inadequate services provided by supervisees, but liability is less clear in consultant relationships.

Supervisor Negligence

This is usually dependent upon the following:

1. A professional relationship exists between the supervisor and the supervisee.

2. The supervisee's actions are below what are considered community standards for the profession.
3. The client was in some way injured.
4. The injury to the client was a direct result of substandard care.
5. Supervisors can be held liable if trainees fail to meet accepted standards of practice. Lack of adequate training can be a failure to meet standards of practice, and this standard applies equally to probationary workers, interns, and field placements.

Supervisor Expertise

How a supervisor's expertise was obtained is a source of determining liability. Key questions raised in relation to supervisor liability are as follows:

1. How did the supervisor learn to conduct supervision?
2. How did the supervisor acquire knowledge of the legal aspects of supervision?
3. Has the supervisor taken graduate-level courses in supervision?
4. Does the professional organization to which the supervisor subscribes have standards for practice and supervision?

Professional and Agency Practices

Supervisor liability can be related to professional and agency practices. Relevant questions at this level are as follows:

1. Do professional organizations take an active role in training supervisors?
2. Does the state licensing board set standards for practice and supervision?
3. Does the state licensing board conduct supervisory training?
4. Does the employing agency have standards for practice and supervision?
5. Does the agency require formal training for supervisors?
6. Does the agency require documentation of supervision activity?

Types of Liability

1. *Direct liability* involves injury caused by the supervisor through incorrect acts or omissions or supervisor failure to follow licensure board or professional association established guidelines.
2. *Vicarious liability* involves incorrect acts or omissions committed by supervisees, based on *respondent superior* (let the master respond) in contract law, in which an employer has authority over the worker and can profit from the employee's actions. Three conditions must be met:

a. Supervisee has agreed to work under the direction of the supervisor in ways that benefit the supervisor regardless of financial gain.
b. Supervisor has the authority to control the supervisee.
c. Supervisee's activities are within the scope of agreed-upon activities.

Guidelines for Effective Supervision

The following guidelines are designed to minimize supervisor liability:
1. The supervisor and agency should ensure that client services are above minimum standards.
2. There should be thorough documentation of supervision activity.
3. All clients should be informed of the supervisor's name, address, and telephone, and the clients should be notified when there is a change of supervisors.
4. Supervisory relationships should be appropriately terminated.
5. Clients should be informed about confidentiality policy related to supervision of the practitioner.
6. There should be documentation of the conditions of the supervisory relationship, including frequency of sessions, duration of sessions, documentation of sessions, and financial components.
7. All payment and insurance forms should be completed accurately and thoroughly. Changes should be updated routinely.
8. The supervisor should document the supervisee's job qualifications.
9. The supervisor should monitor the supervisee's functioning routinely.
10. The supervisor should assist supervisees in adhering to legal, ethical, and professional responsibilities.
11. The agency should ensure that the supervisor has adequate training and experience to provide the required supervision.

Every agency and every supervisor should review these principles and make every effort to comply with them in order to avoid allegations of substandard practices. If allegations of below-standard practices are made against a practitioner, supervisor, or agency, the principles summarized here will most likely be used to establish whether the allegations made are justified.

Case Exercise:
The Case of Will DePart

Will DePart worked for a public mental health center as a clinical social worker. The agency was privatized, and Will decided to accept the employment package offered as part of the privatization process. After one year Will decided to resign from the private agency because he could not accept some of its practices. He departed and opened his own private practice. When Will left the agency, several of his clients also left the agency to continue with Will in his private practice.

Three months later Will received a letter from an attorney who was acting for the executive director, who had a degree in professional counseling, of the privatized agency. The letter indicated that Will had violated ethical practices by taking clients of the agency with him when he entered private practice. The attorney indicated that the agency was filing a lawsuit against Will since he signed a contract with the agency agreeing not to take agency clients. The attorney demanded the names of the clients Will had transferred to his practice from the agency, and that Will pay $1,500 for lost fees. Will countered by stating that before he signed the contract he had added a handwritten clause stating that he would abide by the contract within the bounds of the NASW Code of Ethics, and Will believed he had not committed any ethical violations. He refused to release the names of his clients. The attorney notified Will that the lawsuit was going forward. Several other MSW social workers had also signed a similar contract and added the NASW ethics clause.

You have been providing consultation to Will since he has been in private practice. Will told you about this situation and would like your advice on how to deal with the situation. (1) What would you recommend Will do? (2) Do you believe Will violated the NASW Code of Ethics? (3) Do you believe that Will is obligated to release the names of the clients?

Case Exercise:
The Case of Barry

Barry, age fourteen, had been living with his mother in Florida following his parents' divorce. The mother began using drugs and had a drug dealer move into her home and traded sex for drugs. The drug dealer physically and sexually abused Barry. The father learned of the abuse and sought custody. The father moved to Pennsylvania two years later and entered family therapy with his new wife and Barry. The therapy was initiated because of acting out by Barry. He refused to attend school and was aggressive toward the stepmother. The therapist, Bee M. Pathy, a clinical social worker, was able to resolve some of the family relationship issues, but Barry refused to discuss any aspect of the physical and sexual abuse. In addition to the family therapy, the therapist saw Barry for individual therapy. Barry improved and the case was closed after six months of therapy. Several months later Barry developed a major depressive disorder and was hospitalized. Upon release from the hospital Barry began to act out again. He threatened his stepmother with a knife and she called the police. When the police arrived, Barry accused his father of sexually abusing him for six years. The father was charged with sexual abuse after an investigation by the department of social services. The father's attorney contacted Bee about release of her records regarding the family therapy. The attorney wanted to document that the father had tried to help Barry. The attorney said he would subpoena Bee to testify in court if she did not make her records available.

You are Bee's consultant to her private practice. What would you recommend she do?

In addition to the previous guidelines for assessing supervisor liability, guidelines established by the National Committee on Quality Assurance (NCQA) regarding general agency practice procedures can be helpful in decreasing liability. The following is a summary of the NCQA guidelines.

Practice Procedures

- Provide prompt telephone communications.
- Have a system to record telephone communications.
- Process referrals promptly.
- Have a clear, efficient intake procedure and process.
- Record all appointment cancellations.
- Have an appointment cancellation policy.
- Protect records from public view (including computer screens).
- Keep confidential records secured.
- Have a confidentiality policy in place for *all* staff.
- Have a reliable emergency on-call policy.
- Have policies and procedures for on-site emergencies.
- Have policies and procedures for on-site safety of staff/clients.
- Display the payment policy.
- Have procedures to measure client satisfaction and outcome.
- Have a policy to cover client requests to view records.
- Have a policy on managed care and brief therapy.
- Make educational/informational materials available to clients.
- Display and distribute qualifications/credentials of staff.

Facility Safety and Accessibility

- Ensure adequate security of the building.
- Provide adequate internal lighting.
- Provide a clean, orderly waiting area.
- Keep comfort station facilities (rest rooms) clean.
- Enforce smoking restrictions.
- Provide accessibility for disabled individuals.
- Provide access to public transportation.
- Ensure that fire exits and emergency evacuation plans are posted.
- Ensure that fire extinguishers are available and working.
- Have clearly marked exits.
- Provide separate entrances and exits.
- Have a written safety plan for emergencies in effect.

RISK MANAGEMENT

Introduction

Risk management is discussed in this chapter on administration because, if the supervisor's role is one of oversight, then risk management is an administrative function. Risk management refers to identification and minimization of risks to reduce liability (Feldman and Fitzpatrick, 1992). Risk management is discussed in this chapter from two perspectives. The first perspective involves the client or others alleging that the practitioner did not take reasonable therapeutic action or took action that caused harm to the patient. The second perspective involves situations in which the practitioner is placed at risk of danger or harm. The supervisor has a responsibility to monitor all aspects of the factors that are discussed in this chapter.

Liability Insurance

The supervisor should be familiar with liability insurance for clinical practice and review the standard policies with supervisees. Social workers tend to assume that if they purchase a liability policy they are thoroughly covered against all risks. Liability insurance has become more complex in the past several years, and it is essential to discuss with an insurance company representative exactly what insurance a person has. Companies now make distinctions between "occurrence coverage" and claims-made or "extended liability" coverage. It is important for a practitioner to know which coverage he or she has and the extent of the coverage. For example, usually occurrence coverage applies only to the current period of the policy, while claims-made coverage pertains to longer periods of time. Such distinctions are important because claims can be made against a therapist for activities as far back as twenty years ago. How one calculates the coverage period can be quite complex and requires the insured person to ask the insurance representative questions about such terms as *extended reporting period, extended discovery period, date of discovery requirements,* and *statute of limitations of liability.* If the practitioner and supervisor are in a group practice in which other persons or other disciplines are covered under the same policy, the insured should inquire about the degree of liability in connection with others covered under the policy. Having good, comprehensive, extensive liability insurance and thoroughly understanding the insurance coverage are the first steps in effective risk management.

Reasonable Action

To ensure that clients receive the best possible care, the practitioner and supervisor must begin the process of risk management before the client enters the door of the agency or practice. When a client telephones for an appointment, a referral form should be completed that gives basic background information. The form is used to record the reason the person is seeking intervention. A brief summary of all behaviors and symptoms should be documented on this form. The person handling the telephone call should record what directions were given the client and what actions the practitioner said he or she would take. If this includes giving the client an appointment, the date and time of the appointment should be recorded as part of the form. This form should be made part of the record. The client should complete prior to or at the time of the first interview a form that includes a checklist of past medical history and past mental health treatment information. This form should also be made part of the record. If the person alleges at a later time that certain symptoms or experiences were explained to the practitioner at intake, the intake screening instrument can be a valuable source of reported information, helping to rule out the client accusing the practitioner of forgetting the information. Many agencies use standardized instruments for such screening. For agencies and practices with no such instruments in place, the following can be used as a guide for creating an intake screening instrument:

Name of person providing information:_____
Name of identified client:_____

❑   Has been in a state mental hospital or residential treatment facility
❑   Is court ordered to come to treatment
❑   Hears voices or sees things that are not there
❑   Appears dazed most of the time
❑   Says strange or weird things
❑   Threatened to harm self or others
❑   Is in a serious state of depression most of the time
❑   Has severe mood swings (occurring within hours)
❑   Refuses to talk or communicate with others
❑   Has injuries due to physical or sexual abuse (within the past thirty days)
❑   Has serious physical symptoms, such as
    ❑   vomiting
    ❑   diarrhea
    ❑   insomnia
    ❑   loss of appetite
Presenting problem:_____
Initial onset:_____
Precipitating factors:_____

❑ Suicidal threats/gestures
❑ Drug/alcohol abuse
❑ Sexually active
❑ Violence or sexual abuse in the past
   (indicate if reported or not)_____
❑ Exposure to traumatic events
   (list)_____
❑ Previous treatment
   Therapist's name:_____
   Relationship with therapist:_____
   Length, diagnosis, and outcome:_____
Other self-corrective measures:_____
Major illnesses and hospitalizations:_____
Family history of illness:_____
Date of most recent physical exam/physician's name:_____
Medication history:_____
Legal custody (if child):_____

The following supplemental information can be included as part of the initial screening or database:

- Activity level (catatonia, coordination, sexual acts, psychomotor agitation/retardation)
- Anxiety (avoidance, compulsions, derealization, social anxiety, obsessions, panic, worry)
- Appearance (sad, crying, sexually seductive, untidy)
- Behavior (rage, apathy, antisocial behavior, identity disturbance, disorganization, lies, recklessness, drug use, suicidal tendencies)
- Cognition/memory/attention (aphasia, distractibility, impaired thinking/poor judgment, lack of concentration, indecisiveness, memory loss)
- Eating habits (binges, appetite loss/gain, induced vomiting, weight gain/loss)
- Energy level (decreased energy, fatigue, hyperactivity)
- Thought/speech patterns (speech pressured/slurred, idea flight, incoherence, racing thoughts)
- Mood/affect (anger, apathy, blunted affect, depression, elevated mood, grandiosity, hopelessness, irritability, mood swings)
- Occupational/social functioning (lack of recreational interests, impaired work/school functioning, limited socializing)

- Perception (body distortion, hallucinations, illusions)
- Personality (interpersonal conflict, poor relationships, overwork, perfectionism, procrastination)
- Physical symptoms (dizziness, dry mouth, flushing, chills, sweating, tachycardia, diarrhea, blurred vision, gait, headache, numbness, nystagmus, paralysis, tremor, pain)
- Sleep disturbance (hypersomnia, insomnia)
- Thought content (delusions of grandeur, body image issues, guilt, persecution, somatic complaints, gender confusion, paranoia)

Limits of Practice

It is important that the practitioner and the supervisor establish the limits of the expertise and knowledge of the practice being conducted. If the practitioner specializes, this should be made clear on stationery and other materials that are circulated to clients. Specialty areas should be explained to clients, and referrals should be promptly made when clients present problems that are outside the range of the practitioner's expertise.

Documentation

Documentation has become a critical part of risk management. A thorough paper trail should be established from the minute the client initiates contact or is contacted. The practitioner should take care to complete all required agency or managed care forms in a timely fashion. Record keeping should reflect the flow of treatment activity from diagnosis and assessment. Treatment plans should show a direct connection to the diagnosis and should be monitored on a regular basis and updated every ninety days (the time frame for updates can vary from setting to setting). It is recommended that the term *contact notes* be used instead of *progress notes* and that such notes be updated after every contact. In some settings, practitioners may be required to update contact notes only periodically (usually monthly), but this is not recommended. Important information can be forgotten when periodic-updating strategies are used.

Contact or treatment notes should have summaries of all critical activities inside and outside the treatment, including telephone contact with the client as well as any contact with collateral sources. It is recommended that treatment notes have sections that are labeled statements, observations, and interpretations. Statements refer to any vital comments made by the client or practitioner and should be recorded verbatim. This does not mean that lengthy quotes should be transcribed, but key phrases should be quoted and placed in the record. Any observations the practitioner makes about the client's statements and any interpretations of the client's behavior or statements should be recorded.

Informed Consent

Providing the client with as much information as possible before treatment begins is an important aspect of risk management. Written informed consent should cover the following basic items (some agencies and practices may include additional items):

- What will be done in treatment
- What cannot be done in the treatment by the client or the therapist
- What methods will be used and whether they are standard or unconventional methods
- Sharing of clinical information, including diagnosis
- Potential negative outcomes of treatment
- Identification of indicators that reflect improvement
- What the cost will be and payment requirements
- Duration of treatment and how termination will be decided
- How confidentiality of communications and records will be managed
- How the therapist can be reached in an emergency
- What to do if the person is not satisfied with the therapy or the therapist
- What to do should the client have concerns or questions about the therapy
- Statement of the therapist's credentials and experience

These items should be part of an informed consent brochure, and most of the items should be included in a written treatment contract that the practitioner and client sign. The client should be given a copy of the contract. Some managed cost companies have informed consent forms and contracts that clients must sign before the practitioner can be paid. It is recommended that the practitioner have a form for individual use in addition to any forms signed to meet managed cost requirements.

Boundary Issues

Practitioners who violate boundaries with clients and supervisors who violate boundaries with supervisees run the risk of professional sanctions. Physical contact under any circumstances should be avoided. Personal contact or relationships should not be encouraged. Legal and ethical requirements in this area are often vague and contradictory. Caution is the best policy when guidelines for conduct are not clear. The following guidelines should be adhered to strictly:

- No sexual contact with current or former clients
- No personal relationships with current or former clients

- No business relationships with current or former clients
- No giving or receiving of gifts
- No physical contact

Boundary issues relate to authority and power. Therapists have significant control and power because clients are usually vulnerable and do not know what to expect from practitioners. It is incumbent on the practitioner and the supervisor to act responsibly in any situation. Even if the client seeks personal or physical contact, the therapist should decline. The best strategy to avoid such interaction is to have a written statement regarding these areas and to give a copy to the client at the beginning of treatment. The policy should be reviewed with the client. This can help the practitioner or supervisor avoid potentially embarrassing situations later in the treatment.

Boundary issues for the therapist include practicing within the limits of training, experience, and expertise. A practitioner should not agree to treat clients with problems that are not within the practitioner's range of knowledge and training. Referrals should be made when a client presents with problems that are outside the therapist's expertise, even if the client resists referral. The client could continue with the therapist for problems within the therapist's expertise and be referred for the other problems. For example, if a client who presents with depression reveals a drug dependency problem, the person can be referred for drug treatment but remain with the therapist for treatment of the mood disorder.

Transference/Countertransference

It is not uncommon for clients to experience strong transference reactions to the therapist (Luborsky and Crits-Christoph, 1990). Transference and countertransference are complex and highly interrelated (Tosone, 1998). Transference can be positive or negative. The positive form of transference can put the practitioner at most risk. If the client seeks more than a professional relationship, the therapist can gently guide the client through this phase of the treatment and be candid with the client about transference. It is not recommended that therapists alert clients to transference factors, but when a therapist observes indicators of transference, such as glowing and caring remarks about the therapist, or the client reports dreaming about the therapist, this should be acknowledged and handled in an objective, professional manner. The supervisor should review with supervisees the client situations in which transference is likely to occur.

Therapist countertransference is common, but many practitioners tend to deny strong positive attraction to clients. Feelings for clients are bound to occur if one is a caring, committed therapist. What one does with those feelings is the core of an appropriate response. The supervisor is the first line of defense when the practitioner experiences countertransference feelings.

The supervisor can help the practitioner acknowledge such feelings and find ways to deal with them. The supervisor can alert the practitioner to indicators of impending countertransference, for example, if the therapist begins discussing or sharing with the client personal information about himself or herself that is not relevant to the treatment; if the therapist begins sharing personal concerns or other issues with the client; if the therapist spends time outside the therapy wondering about what the client is doing or where he or she might be at a given time; or if the therapist is dreaming about the client or talks a lot with others about the client outside the therapy. If such feelings are not acknowledged and openly discussed, the practitioner can subtlety act them out in the therapy and add momentum to the client's transference reaction. Marshall and Marshall (1988) have defined eight forms of countertransference that can be useful in exploring this aspect of intervention in supervision.

Negative transference and countertransference can also presents risks for the practitioner. If the client is angry, combative, confrontive, and abusive, the therapist can be provoked into actions that can be harmful to the client and set off a counterreaction on the part of the client. The supervisor can be helpful to the supervisee in working out negative countertransference. Negative countertransference is usually more apparent than positive countertransference, but it is also easily subject to denial because clinicians are taught to believe that they can control and master most situations. Admitting to positive or negative countertransference can cause practitioners to feel that they have not been effective therapists. The supervisor should help the practitioner see that transference and countertransference are a natural part of the work. Firefighters can be overcome by smoke, but that does not mean they are inferior firefighters. Dealing with smoke is part of the job and sometimes it can overcome the firefighter. The same is true of clinical work. Transference and countertransference are always in the air and can overcome clinicians and supervisors at times. Supervision can be an effective breathing apparatus that helps clinicians reenter the therapy without being overcome by the smoke of transference and countertransference.

Hypnosis

Hypnosis should be used only by practitioners fully and thoroughly trained in the technique. It is best performed at the client's request rather than at the practitioner's insistence or suggestion. Before using hypnosis, the practitioner should administer relevant measurement scales to establish a baseline of functioning. For example, it is common for hypnosis to be used with clients who were traumatized as children, but some risk is involved. In some cases, in which therapists used hypnosis as part of the treatment, clients later alleged that the use of hypnosis led to repeated, involuntary childhood regression.

Unintended Harm

Practitioners can be at risk of exposure to harm or diseases in situations in which the client is unaware of the potential harm, particularly with certain communicable diseases or in high-risk relationships. For example, a social worker who agreed to do marriage counseling with a couple discovered during the intake evaluation that the husband was extremely angry at the wife for having an affair. The wife revealed during the session that she was still seeing the other man. The husband bolted out of the room. The wife informed the practitioner that the husband was most likely going to his truck to get a rifle and would be back to shoot her and the therapist. Fortunately, the therapist worked in a setting where safety issues had been discussed and the practitioner was able to implement a plan that included preventing the man from reentering the building, alerting other staff, and moving the wife to a safe room. Practitioners increasingly find themselves put at risk by their proximity to their clients. For details on how to deal with this form of risk, see the section Violence and Safety in this chapter.

Inadvertent exposure to diseases and disorders can be a risk for practitioners. In some settings practitioners may be required to undergo medical screening for tuberculosis and blood-borne pathogens. In some hospital settings and other potentially high-exposure settings, the policy on screening is not always clear or definitive. It is the supervisor's responsibility to work to clarify such policies as much as possible.

Confidentiality

Confidentiality is a risk management issue, even though social workers do not generally view it as a risk because it is so essential to social work's basic orientation. Confidentiality must be considered in the broader context of society. Confidentiality is a professional issue and privacy is a societal issue. Some societies have little or no privacy, as it is conceptualized in the United States. The terms *privacy, confidentiality,* and *privilege* must be distinguished:

- *Privacy* is the freedom of clients to determine sharing of behavior, beliefs, and opinions.
- *Confidentiality* is professional understanding that nothing about an individual will be revealed except under agreed-upon circumstances.
- *Privilege,* or privileged communication, is a legal term used to maintain confidentiality in a legal proceeding.

Confidentiality is affected by integration of services, consolidation of services, and specialization of practice. It has been estimated that when a mental health claim is filed, at least seventeen people have knowledge of the treatment. It has been partially in jest observed that confidentiality can be ensured only by paying cash and using a false name.

Confidentiality is no longer general or sweeping. It varies from discipline to discipline, situation to situation, client to client (child versus parent). Contradictory and confusing lawmaking has produced conflicts and misunderstanding about confidentiality. The supervisor should review all state laws relevant to confidentiality to ensure compliance with the laws and to show that a good-faith effort has been made to be in compliance. General guidelines are provided later in this section, but these guidelines should not be used as a substitute for becoming familiar with relevant specific state or jurisdiction laws regarding confidentiality. These principles are especially relevant to child sexual abuse, physical abuse, and neglect cases.

A supervisor in an agency that uses fee collection services should review with the agency administrator the collection agency policy regarding confidentiality as well as the practices followed in attempting collection. An issue of confidentiality arises in regard to the laws on sexual abuse and the use of fee collection agencies. Some of these agencies use extreme and threatening tactics to collect fees. Increasingly, mental health agencies are using collection services, and it is possible that if a practitioner treats cases involving abuse or neglect, he or she could violate state laws regarding confidentiality by using such services.

Review of the Concept

The law makes distinctions about confidentiality, legal, ethical, and moral issues. It helps to view confidentiality as a client issue, not the therapist's issue. The privilege is the client's; it belongs to the client. Confidentiality is dependent on who controls the information. Technology has made confidentiality more complex because control of the information is so much harder to maintain. Once a practitioner places a report about a client in a fax machine, he or she has no real control over where it ultimately goes. The fax number could be wrong, an error could be made in dialing the number, or someone other than the intended receiver could pick up the report. Telephone answering machines present the same problems of control as fax machines. It is recommended that supervisors instruct practitioners never to leave messages for clients on answering machines. This includes not leaving a name or a number for the person to call. Most telephone answering machine messages can be accessed by simply randomly dialing digits to find the correct replay code.

Legal Aspects of Privilege and Confidentiality

Psychiatrists and psychologists have "general privilege," meaning that in judicial, legislative, or administrative proceedings, a patient or his or her authorized representative has the privilege to refuse to disclose, and to prevent a witness from disclosing, communications relating to diagnosis or treatment of the patient's mental or emotional disorder. Social workers once had a slight variation on the psychiatric general privilege, but clinical social work communications were placed on equal footing with psychiatrist and psychologist privilege in the *Jaffee, v. Special Administrator for Allen, Deceased v. Redmond et al.,* 1996, case that was decided by the U.S. Supreme Court. The opinion of the Supreme Court should be read by every clinical social worker and by every clinical supervisor. This case has had significant impact on the clinical social work profession, and the Supreme Court made highly positive statements about clinical social work in its written opinion. For these reasons, a summary of the court's opinion is included here.

United States Supreme Court
Jaffee, v. Special Administrator for Allen,
Deceased v. Redmond et al., 1996
Case Summary

Case Facts

Redmond, an on-duty police officer, killed Jaffe. Jaffe's family filed suit. The Court rejected the view that psychotherapist-patient privilege existed in this case and ordered the therapy notes of Karen Beyer, a clinical social worker who counseled Redmond after the shooting, to be given to attorneys. The jury found in favor of Jaffe after the judge instructed the jury to assume the notes contained information damaging to Redmond. The appeals court reversed the finding under Federal Rule of Evidence 501. The case was then appealed to the Supreme Court, which held that conversations between Redmond and her therapist and the notes taken during counseling sessions are protected from compelled disclosure under Rule 501.

Key Quotes from the Majority Opinion

The majority opinion was delivered by Stevens, who was joined by O'Conner, Kennedy, Souter, Thomas, Ginsburg, and Breyer.

- The federal privilege, which clearly applies to psychiatrists and psychologists, also extends to confidential communications made to licensed social workers in the course of psychotherapy. The reasons for recognizing the privilege for treatment by psychiatrists and psychologists apply with equal force to clinical social workers, and the vast majority of States explicitly extend a testimonial privilege to them.

- The question . . . is whether a privilege protecting confidential communications between a psychotherapist and her patient promotes sufficiently important interests to outweigh the need for probative evidence. . . . Both reason and experience persuade us that it does.

- Like the spousal and attorney client privileges, the psychotherapist patient privilege is rooted in the imperative need for confidence and trust. Treatment by a physician for physical ailments can often proceed successfully on the basis of a physical examination, objective information supplied by the patient, and the results of diagnostic tests. Effective psychotherapy, by contrast, depends upon an atmosphere of confidence and trust in which the patient is willing to make a frank and complete disclosure of facts, emotions, memories, and fears. Because of the sensitive nature of the problems for which individuals consult psychotherapists, disclosure of confidential communications made during counseling sessions may cause embarrassment or disgrace. For this reason, the mere possibility of disclosure may impede development of the confidential relationship necessary for successful treatment.

- The psychotherapist privilege serves the public interest by facilitating the provision of appropriate treatment for individuals suffering the effects of a mental or emotional problem. The mental health of our citizenry, no less than the physical health of our citizenry, is a public good of transcendent importance.

- In contrast to the significant public and private interests supporting recognition of the privilege, the likely evidentiary benefit that would result from the denial of the privilege is modest. If the privilege were rejected, confidential conversations between psychotherapists and their patients would surely be chilled, particularly when it is obvious that the circumstances that give rise to the need for treatment will probably result in litigation.

- Because . . . a psychotherapist patient privilege will serve a public good transcending the normally predominant principle of utilizing all rational means for ascertaining truth, we hold that confidential communications between a licensed psychotherapist and her patients in the course of diagnosis or treatment are protected from compelled disclosure under Rule 501 of the Federal Rules of Evidence.

- . . . psychotherapist privilege covers confidential communications made to licensed psychiatrists and psychologists. We have no hesitation in concluding in this case that the federal privilege should also extend to confidential communications made to licensed social workers in the course of psychotherapy. The reasons for recognizing a privilege for treatment by psychiatrists and psychologists apply with equal force to treatment by a clinical social worker such as Karen Beyer. Today, social workers provide a significant amount of mental health treatment. Their clients often include the poor and those of modest means who could not afford the assistance of a psychiatrist or psychologist, but whose counseling sessions serve the same public goals. Perhaps in recognition of these circumstances, the vast majority of States explicitly extend a testimonial privilege to licensed social workers. We therefore agree with the Court of Appeals that drawing a distinction between the counseling provided by costly psychotherapists and the counseling provided by more readily accessible social workers serves no discernible public purpose.

Dissenting Opinion

The dissenting opinion was filed by Scalia, who was joined by Rehnquist.

- . . . privilege analogous to the one asserted here—the lawyer client privilege—is not identified by the broad area of advice giving practiced by the person to whom the privileged communication is given, but rather by the professional status of that person. That is the illusion the Court has produced here: It first frames an overly general question (Should there be a psychotherapist privilege?) that can be answered in the negative only by excluding from protection office consultations with professional psychiatrists (i.e., doctors) and clinical psychologists. And then, having answered that in the affirmative, it comes to the only question that the facts of this case present (Should there be a social worker client privilege with regard to psychotherapeutic counseling?) with the answer seemingly a foregone conclusion. At that point, to conclude against the privilege one must subscribe to the difficult proposition, Yes, there is a psychotherapist privilege, but not if the psychotherapist is a social worker.

* ... the Court treat the Proposed Federal Rules of Evidence developed in 1972 by the Judicial Conference Advisory Committee as strong support for its holding, whereas they in fact counsel clearly and directly against it. The Committee did indeed recommend a psychotherapist privilege of sorts, but more precisely, and more relevantly, it recommended a privilege for psychotherapy conducted by a person authorized to practice medicine or a person licensed or certified as a psychologist.

* ... the Court's very methodology—giving serious consideration only to the more general, and much easier, question—is in violation of our duty to proceed cautiously when erecting barriers between us and the truth.

* Effective psychotherapy undoubtedly is beneficial to individuals with mental problems, and surely serves some larger social interest in maintaining a mentally stable society. But merely mentioning these values does not answer the critical question: are they of such importance, and is the contribution of psychotherapy to them so distinctive, and is the application of normal evidentiary rules so destructive to psychotherapy, as to justify making our federal courts occasional instruments of injustice?

* When is it ... that the psychotherapist came to play such an indispensable role in the maintenance of the citizenry's mental health? For most of history, men and women have worked out their difficulties by talking to, inter alios, parents, siblings, best friends and bartenders—none of whom was awarded a privilege against testifying in court. Ask the average citizen: Would your mental health be more significantly impaired by preventing you from seeing a psychotherapist, or by preventing you from getting advice from your mom? I have little doubt what the answer would be. Yet there is no mother child privilege.

* The Court confidently asserts that not much truth finding capacity would be destroyed by the privilege anyway, since without a privilege, much of the desirable evidence to which litigants such as petitioner seek access ... is unlikely to come into being. If that is so, how come psychotherapy got to be a thriving practice before the psychotherapist privilege was invented? Were the patients paying money to lie to their analysts all those years? Of course the evidence generating effect of the privilege (if any) depends entirely upon its scope, which the Court steadfastly declines to consider. And even if one assumes that scope to be the broadest possible, is it really true that most, or even many, of those who seek psychological counseling have the worry of litigation in the back of their minds? I doubt that, and the Court provides no evidence to support it.

* The Court suggests one last policy justification: since psychotherapist privilege statutes exist in all the States, the failure to recognize a privilege in federal courts would frustrate the purposes of the state legislation that was enacted to foster these confidential communications. This is a novel argument indeed. A sort of inverse pre-emption: the truth seeking functions of federal courts must be adjusted so as not to conflict with the policies of the States.

- The Court's failure to put forward a convincing justification of its own could perhaps be excused if it were relying upon the unanimous conclusion of state courts in the reasoned development of their common law. It cannot do that, since no State has such a privilege apart from legislation. What it relies upon, instead, is the fact that all 50 States and the District of Columbia have [1] *enacted into law* some form of psychotherapist privilege. Let us consider both the verb and its object: The fact that all 50 States have enacted this privilege argues not for, but against, our adopting the privilege judicially. At best it suggests that the matter has been found not to lend itself to judicial treatment—perhaps because the pros and cons of adopting the privilege, or of giving it one or another shape, are not that clear; or perhaps because the rapidly evolving uses of psychotherapy demand a flexibility that only legislation can provide. At worst it suggests that the privilege commends itself only to decision-making bodies in which reason is tempered, so to speak, by political pressure from organized interest groups (such as psychologists and social workers), and decision-making bodies that are not overwhelmingly concerned (as courts of law are and should be) with justice.

- . . . this brief analysis . . . contains no explanation of why the psychotherapy provided by social workers is a public good of such transcendent importance as to be purchased at the price of occasional injustice. Moreover, it considers only the respects in which social workers providing therapeutic services are similar to licensed psychiatrists and psychologists; not a word about the respects in which they are different. A licensed psychiatrist or psychologist is an expert in psychotherapy—and that may suffice (though I think it not so clear that this Court should make the judgment) to justify the use of extraordinary means to encourage counseling with him, as opposed to counseling with one's rabbi, minister, family or friends. One must presume that a social worker does not bring this greatly 'heightened degree of skill to bear, which is alone a reason for not encouraging that consultation as generously. Does a social worker bring to bear at least a significantly heightened degree of skill—more than a minister or rabbi, for example? I have no idea, and neither does the Court. The social worker in the present case, Karen Beyer, was a licensed clinical social worker in Illinois, a job title whose training requirements consist of a master's degree in social work from an approved program, and 3,000 hours of satisfactory, supervised clinical professional experience. It is not clear that the degree in social work requires any training in psychotherapy. The clinical professional experience apparently will impart some such training, but only of the vaguest sort, judging from the Illinois Code's definition of clinical social work practice, viz., the providing of mental health services for the evaluation, treatment, and prevention of mental and emotional disorders in individuals, families and groups based on knowledge and theory of psychosocial development, behavior, psychopathology, unconscious motivation, interpersonal relationships, and environmental stress. But the rule the Court announces today . . . is not limited to licensed clinical social workers, but includes all licensed social workers. Licensed social workers may also provide mental health services . . . so long as it is done under supervision of a licensed clinical social worker. And the training requirement for a "licensed social worker" consists of either (a) "a degree from a graduate program of social work" approved by the State, or (b) "a degree in social work from an undergraduate program" approved by the State, plus 3 years of supervised professional experience. . . . it does not seem to me that any of this training is comparable in its rigor (or indeed in the precision of its subject) to the training of the other experts (lawyers) to whom this Court has accorded a privilege, or even of the experts (psychiatrists and psychologists) to whom the Advisory Committee and this Court proposed extension of a privilege in 1972. Other States, for all we know, may be even less demanding. Indeed, I am not even sure there is a nationally accepted definition of social worker, as there is of psychiatrist and psychologist. It seems to me quite irresponsible to extend the so-called psychotherapist privilege to all licensed social workers, nationwide without exploring these issues.

- Another critical distinction between psychiatrists and psychologists, on the one hand, and social workers, on the other, is that the former professionals, in their consultations with patients, do nothing but psychotherapy. Social workers, on the other hand, interview people for a multitude of reasons. The Illinois definition of licensed social worker, for example, is as follows: Licensed social worker means a person who holds a license authorizing the practice of social work, which includes social services to individuals, groups or communities in any one or more of the fields of social casework, social group work, community organization for social welfare, social work research, social welfare administration or social work education.

- Thus, in applying the social worker variant of the psychotherapist privilege, it will be necessary to determine whether the information provided to the social worker was provided to him in his capacity as a psychotherapist, or in his capacity a an administrator of social welfare, a community organizer, etc. Worse still, if the privilege is to have its desired effect (and is not to mislead the client), it will presumably be necessary for the social caseworker to advise, as the conversation with his welfare client proceeds, which portions are privileged and which are not.

- In Oklahoma, for example, the social worker privilege statute prohibits a licensed social worker from disclosing, or being compelled to disclose, any information acquired from persons consulting the licensed social worker in his or her professional capacity (with certain exceptions . . .). The social worker's professional capacity is expansive, for the practice of social work in Oklahoma is defined as: The professional activity of helping individuals, groups, or communities enhance or restore their capacity for physical, social and economic functioning and the professional application of social work values, principles and techniques in areas such as clinical social work, social service administration, social planning, social work consultation and social work research to one or more of the following ends: Helping people obtain tangible services; counseling with individuals families and groups; helping communities or groups provide or improve social and health services; and participating in relevant social action. The practice of social work requires knowledge of human development and behavior; of social economic and cultural institutions and forces; and of the interaction of all of these factors. Social work practice includes the teaching of relevant subject matter and of conducting research into problems of human behavior and conflict.

- Thus, in Oklahoma, as in most other States having a social worker privilege, it is not a subpart or even a derivative of the psychotherapist privilege, but rather a piece of special legislation similar to that achieved by many other groups, from accountants, to private detectives. These social worker statutes give no support, therefore, to the theory (importance of psychotherapy) upon which the Court rests its disposition.

- Thus, although the Court is technically correct that the vast majority of States explicitly extend a testimonial privilege to licensed social workers, that uniformity exists only at the most superficial level. No State has adopted the privilege without restriction . . . and 10 States, I reiterate, effectively reject the privilege entirely. It is fair to say that there is scant national consensus even as to the propriety of a social worker psychotherapist privilege, and none whatever as to its appropriate scope. In other words, the state laws to which the Court appeals for support demonstrate most convincingly that adoption of a social worker psychotherapist privilege is a job for Congress.

In judicial or administrative proceedings, a client has the privilege to refuse to disclose, and to prevent a witness from disclosing, communications made while the client was receiving counseling.

Generally the following definitions are used in relation to confidentiality and privilege laws:

- *Client:* person who communicates to or receives services from a clinical social worker regarding mental or emotional condition; other person participating directly with the clinical social worker.
- *Clincal social worker:* person licensed under the laws of the state.
- *Witness:* clinical social worker or other person participating directly with the clinical social worker; a person rendering services or consultation under direct supervision of the clinical social worker.
- *Privilege:* in judicial or administrative proceedings, the client's right to refuse to disclose or to prevent a witness from disclosing communications while receiving counseling.
- *Exceptions:* disclosure for purpose of placing person in facility for mental illness; court-ordered examinations; civil or criminal proceeding; client introduces mental condition as claim or defense; after client's death in defense or claim; client makes malpractice claim against the clinical social worker; client waives for suit or claim on policy of insurance on life, health, or physical condition.
- *Exemptions:* administrative or judicial nondelinquent juvenile proceedings; guardianship or adoption proceedings for the disabled; criminal or delinquency proceedings involving child abuse/neglect.

Confidentiality of Records

The confidentiality of records can vary, and not much clarity exists about records in general. Each agency should have a written policy regarding confidentiality of records and oral communications. Zuckerman (1997), in the book *The Paper Office,* created a number of standard forms that can be used to inform clients about confidentiality. This book is recommended for supervisors and agency administrators.

Most jurisdictions have clear confidentiality standards regarding abuse and neglect cases. The following are some general rules:

1. All child abuse and neglect records are confidential.
2. Unauthorized disclosure can be a criminal offense.
3. Child abuse and neglect records can be disclosed
   - under court order;
   - to social service officials, law enforcement, state's attorneys, and members of multidisciplinary case consultation teams who are investigating reports of abuse and neglect;
   - to local or state officials with child administration functions;
   - to an alleged child abuser;
   - to a licensed practitioner, agency, or institution providing treatment or care to the child;
   - to the parent or caregiver; and
   - to the school superintendent when a school employee is a suspect.
4. Confidentiality of records should not be construed to prohibit
   - publication of research statistics or data without identifiers, or
   - social service agencies obtaining financial records to establish public assistance eligibility.
5. State social service agencies usually are charged by law with issuing regulations governing access to and use of confidential information.

The supervisor should consult with all relevant agencies and governing bodies to ensure that accurate and up-to-date information is used in providing written and oral instructions to supervisees regarding appropriate actions and precautions to take. The supervisor must aid practitioners in avoiding becoming immobilized by the fear that any action can involve risk. The best protection against this is good information and clear policies and procedures. If one gets involved in allegations of misconduct, the best protection is the ability to demonstrate that reasonable and responsible action was taken by the practitioner and supervisor.

Child Abuse Reporting Requirements

Practitioners are required to report any known or suspected child physical abuse, sexual abuse, or neglect. The practitioner can be at risk of legal sanction if there is a failure to report. Many assumptions are made about reporting, and the supervisor has a responsibility to ensure that practitioners act appropriately in child abuse situations. The supervisor should consult relevant statutes, attorneys, and agencies to make sure that he or she is accurately informed and up to date on laws governing reporting. The general rules regarding reporting of the areas of child abuse and neglect are outlined here:

1. *Child* is usually defined as any individual under the age of eighteen years.
2. *Abuse* is generally defined as the "physical injury" or "sexual abuse" of a child by the child's caretakers.
3. *Sexual abuse* is generally defined as any act that involves sexual molestation or exploitation of a child by a parent or other person who has permanent or temporary care or custody or responsibility for supervision of a child, or by any household or family member.
4. *Neglect* is generally defined as leaving a child unattended or other failure to give proper care and attention to a child by the child's parents, guardian, or custodian under circumstances that indicate that the child's health or welfare is significantly harmed or placed at risk of significant harm.
5. Those who report are normally granted immunity from civil liability or criminal penalty for doing so in good faith.
6. Generally there are no legal or privileged communications exceptions (except for attorneys).
7. Any report made is confidential, may be disclosed only under the limited circumstances specified by statutes, and cannot be disseminated to the public at large.
8. Social workers acting in a professional capacity who have reason to believe that the child has been subjected to abuse or neglect must notify the designated social service agency or the appropriate law enforcement agency.
9. If acting as a staff member of a hospital, agency, child care institution, juvenile detention center, school, or similar institution, the social worker should immediately notify and give information to the person who is the director of the institution.
10. An oral report should be made as soon as possible. The practitioner should notify his or her supervisor and the agency director before notifying the designated agency or the police.
11. Written reports are usually required within forty-eight hours of learning the information. Oral reports are not sufficient. The written report should contain
    - name, age, and home address of the child;
    - name and home address of the child's parent or the person responsible for the child's care;
    - whereabouts of the child;
    - nature and extent of the abuse/neglect of child;

- evidence or information available to the reporter concerning possible previous instances of abuse or neglect; and
- any information that would help determine the cause of abuse/neglect and the identity of the person responsible for the abuse/neglect.
12. Normally within twenty-four hours of a report of suspected abuse, and within five days of a report of suspected neglect, the designated investigatory agency or the appropriate law enforcement agency should
   - interview the child;
   - attempt to have an on-site interview with the child's caretaker; and
   - decide on the safety of the child, and of other children in the household.
13. Usually all records and reports concerning child abuse or neglect are confidential, and their unauthorized disclosure can be considered a criminal offense.
14. Information in reports or records concerning child abuse and neglect can be disclosed under the following circumstances:
   - To meet the conditions of a court order
   - To personnel of local or state departments of social services, law enforcement personnel, and members of multidisciplinary case consultation teams who are investigating a report of known or suspected child abuse/neglect or who are providing services to a child or family who is the subject of the report
   - To local or state officials responsible for the administration of the child protective services necessary to carry out their official functions
   - To the person who is the alleged child abuser or who is suspected of child neglect, if that person is responsible for the child's welfare and provisions are made for the protection of the identify of the reporter or any other person whose life or safety is likely to be endangered by disclosing the information
   - To a licensed practitioner, or an agency, institution, or program that is providing treatment or care to a child who is the subject of child abuse or neglect
   - To a parent or other person who has permanent or temporary care and custody of a child if provisions are made for the protection of the identify of the reporter or any other person whose life or safety is likely endangered by disclosing the information

In some jurisdictions, it is required to report when there is reason to believe that child abuse or neglect occurred in the past, even if the alleged victim is an adult when the incident is discovered. The fact that the victim is now an adult should be part of the report, and this fact may be taken into account by the authorities who receive the report when they determine the actions to take in response to the report. In Maryland, even if the alleged abuser is believed to be deceased, a report must be made. Information that the alleged abuser is deceased should be included in the report, and the authorities receiving the report may take appropriate account of that circumstance.

DUTY TO WARN

Duty to warn, also referred to as "failure to warn" and "Tarasoff rule," is closely related to the confidentiality issues, and the concept has caused much concern and controversy in the helping professions.The essence of this issue is that if a therapist learns that a client intends to do harm to others, the therapist has a duty to inform the people who have been threatened. The courts in several cases have established that therapists have a duty to warn people who have been the focus of threats made in therapy by clients, and some states have enacted duty-to-warn laws. In addition, the courts have held that if a client makes threats to destroy the property of others, the practitioner has a duty to warn the owner of the property. For example, if a client threatens to set fire to someone's home, the therapist has a duty to warn. Much vagueness surrounds duty to warn regarding property, and therapists have no clear guidelines to follow in determining how far the property threat extends.

The supervisor has a responsibility to ensure that practitioners understand the concept of duty to warn and to offer guidelines for therapists to follow. Some states have passed laws that include guidelines for therapist actions in such situations. The supervisor or therapist should inquire of the state in which he or she practices whether it has a law and what steps she or he must follow to meet its requirements. In the absence of a law, the supervisor or therapist should seek agency or group practice-approved procedures for duty to warn. The following general set of guidelines are to aid practitioners in the absence of state laws and agency policy; these guidelines (which are in part based on a Maryland duty-to-warn law) should not be considered rules for a specific situation or setting:

1. Duty to warn rests with licensed health care providers and administrators of some institutions under certain circumstances.
2. A duty to warn exists when the practitioner has direct knowledge of potential harm to an individual, group, or property. Direct knowledge consists of three elements: (a) the client has a propensity to commit violence, (b) the client intends to inflict physical injury, and (c) the cli-

ent has named a specific person or group of persons who are to be the victims.

3. Duty to warn includes reasonable and timely efforts to (a) seek commitment of the client, (b) take treatment action designed to eliminate the carrying out of the threat, or (c) inform the police and the identified victim.
4. The warning given to the identified victim should include (a) description of the threat, (b) identification of the person making the threat, and (c) identification of the intended victim or victims.
5. Duty to warn usually is exempt from confidentiality for the therapist.

Even when the agency establishes guidelines, the practitioner will confront many situations that are ambiguous and will react to threats in different ways, given the circumstances. For example, it is easier for therapists to make a decision to warn when threats are made by clients with whom they have had a difficult relationship than when made by clients with whom they have had a positive relationship. Clients the practitioner has seen for a long time will be more difficult to report about than a client seen for the first time. Some therapists will deal with the duty-to-warn requirement by avoiding content in the treatment that could lead to threatening remarks, but this strategy does not always work, since some clients make impulsive threats after becoming agitated.

The supervisor can help the supervisee by discussing the duty-to-warn requirements in detail. This includes helping the supervisee understand that a threat does not mean the therapist must immediately warn the potential victim. The practitioner can discuss the threat with the client and suggest measures to prevent the client from acting on the threat, such as encouraging the client to agree to voluntary hospitalization or seeking the client's permission to warn the intended victim. The supervisor should be a resource for the practitioner to use in developing and considering the range of strategies to deal with the client and the threat.

VIOLENCE AND SAFETY

Social Worker Stabbed to Death in Mental Health Agency
Worker Beaten to Death with Baseball Bat During Home Visit
Workers and Patients Taken Hostage in Hospital
Worker Making Home Visit Injured When Nearby Drug Deal Goes Bad
Social Worker Shot to Death at Children's Treatment Center
Social Worker Stabbed to Death by Man Who Was Denied Service
Man Denied Services by Agency Kills Social Worker

All of these headlines are associated with incidents of violence against social workers. Our society is extremely violent, and many statistics grimly document this. Although it is unclear whether our society is more or less violent than in the past, it is known that our society is quite violent and becoming more so each year. Violence against social workers is on the increase.

No organization is currently gathering data on violent acts against social workers. The author has been gathering data informally for more than a decade, and the previous headlines are from actual cases that occurred in that time period. In exploring these cases, some significant patterns became evident. First, the violence is not random. The person committing the violent act has some complaint against the agency, real or imagined, that provoked the individual. In one case in which the social worker was stabbed to death, the person was a client of the mental health center where the social worker was employed and had recently been terminated from service because of funding cuts. Second, the precipitating incident is fairly recent and not long-standing. Third, a minor incident often precedes the serious violent incident; for example, the person gets in an argument with someone at the agency or telephones and becomes argumentative. Fourth, the violent incident occurs when the agency does something outside the established practices of the agency. For example, in the hospital case, the social worker agreed to interview the client in the waiting room, even though this was not normally done, because the client had become belligerent after entering the hospital. After shooting the social worker, the client held other people who were in the waiting room hostage for several hours. If normal procedures had been followed, it is possible that the tragedy could have been avoided, or that the number of people involved could have been much smaller. Fifth, in most violent incidents, the person returns to the agency soon after having been in an altercation, argument, or disagreement with a staff member. Based on research conducted by the author, it is recommended when a client returns to an agency or office soon after a violent confrontation with a staff member, precautions should be taken to protect staff because the return visit is usually to commit a violent act.

Supervisors and administrators have a tendency to minimize the potential for violence in clients and inadvertently put workers at risk. One violent incident can have significant impact on staff, even when no serious physical harm occurs. When staff are held hostage, they suffer psychological and emotional stress for quite some time. Some people never completely recover from witnessing or being a part of a violent incident.

The supervisor has a responsibility to prepare practitioners by orienting them to the signs of potential violence in a client. Signs of agitation, such as heavy breathing, trembling, raising of the voice, trembling in the voice, glaring at the worker, sudden use of profanity, pacing, and clenched fists, are primary indicators of possible impending violence (for more details, see

Shea, 1998:183-187). Clients do not always give indications that they are going to be violent, and unsuspecting items can become weapons. In one situation an adolescent, schizophrenic client, without provocation, threw a clipboard at a clinician during an interview. The clipboard hit the practitioner in the mouth and caused a three-inch cut on his chin. The client's mother was in the room but made no attempt to control her son. The clinician was dazed but able to recover as the client went to pick up the clipboard. The clinician placed his foot on the clipboard so the client could not retrieve it. Fortunately, the client returned to his chair when the practitioner prevented him from getting the clipboard, launching into a long explanation about why he needed the clipboard. The practitioner explained that the clipboard would not be returned to him until after the session ended. The clinician was able to recover and continue with the session, but he experienced heightened sensitivity to unprovoked aggression and weapons of opportunity for several months after this incident.

The supervisor has a responsibility to take precautions to protect the safety of supervisees. If the agency does not have a policy on safety, the supervisor should take the lead in organizing the staff to develop a policy. A basic safety policy should include the following elements.

1. *Office arrangement.* Offices should be arranged so that workers are next to the door. The workers should avoid placing the client between them and the door. All sharp objects or those which can be easily thrown at workers should be removed. Any object in the office that could become a potential weapon should be removed if possible, for example, letter openers, glass ashtrays, lamps, etc. Where possible, the doors should have small, elongated windows with blinds. The blinds can be opened when workers are interviewing clients who cause them to be concerned about violence; the windows can be a deterrent to the client taking action. Clients should never be interviewed in an office that does not contain a phone.

2. *"Buddy system."* The staff should discuss in advance a system for warning one another if they are attacked or trapped in an office by a client. A general policy should be in place, and an individualized policy for when the workers know in advance that an interview is likely to be problematic. On the day that a troublesome client is to be interviewed, colleagues and supervisors should be alerted and specific strategies devised. The supervisor should reinforce with practitioners that it is not a weakness to express concern and fears associated with interviewing certain clients. Talking in advance can offer much support and comfort to the practitioners because they can enter the session reassured and clear about what to do if the interview situation escalates.

If staff are working late at night or on weekends, when few people are in the building, they should take special care. It is not a good idea to give clients the impression that you are in the building alone. Leaving buildings after dark and late at night can be hazardous. Workers should arrange to leave in groups. It is at these times that workers are most vulnerable, but the least likely to take measures to ensure safety.

3. *Warning devices.* In settings where the potential for violence is high, the staff should consider installing devices in each office that allow the practitioners to unobtrusively alert someone outside the interview room that help is needed, for example, a buzzer switch mounted on top or under the desk. If the agency will not provide an electronic system, the workers can keep whistles in their desks or pockets to use for alerting others that they are experiencing difficulty.

4. *Proximity.* When clients become agitated, practitioners can be unsure of how to deal with the anger. This is because our society is conflicted about expressions of anger and families offer few developmental coping patterns for dealing with such expressions. This is why society wavers between passivity and silence and explosive, violent behavior. Practitioners need to be trained in advance in how to behave when a client begins to escalate. Workers left to their own strategies will draw on the traditional ways of dealing with anger, which is to move toward the client and try to give support, often by touching. From experience it is known that this is more likely to increase the client's anger. The preferred strategy is for the practitioner to move slightly away from the client, remain seated, or return to his or her seat. The practitioner should avoid the position of towering over the client that is created by the practitioner standing while the client is seated. The worker should speak in a low voice and reassure the client that he or she heard the communication, and, if possible, agree with the client. It can be helpful for practitioners to role-play such situations so that they have advance experience in general procedures to follow in very frightening situations. Strategies that have only been discussed in supervision can all too easily be forgotten.

5. *Restraint.* The agency should have a policy outlining conditions under which clients will be restrained and how they will be restrained. The supervisor needs to take the lead in this area if the agency has no policy. It is the supervisor's responsibility to insist that one be developed. At times clients have to be restrained from doing harm to themselves, to others in the room, or to the practitioner. When the client takes action against another person, the agency needs to have a policy and a plan for restraint. This will always require more than one staff member. It has been documented that untrained staff are more likely to be the victims of violence (Davis, 1991:587). The staff should receive specific training in restraining clients in a way that minimizes the possibility of hurting the client. If staff are not trained and in-

jure a client in the process of restraint, the agency could be the object of legal action brought by the client. Improperly applied restraint procedures can also increase the possibility of violence. Under these circumstances a policy and plan for restraint is of much value to the agency in demonstrating that reasonable and prudent caution was taken. The primary reason for a restraint policy is to minimize the possibility that anyone would be physically injured in a clinical setting. In many locations, the police department will offer such training for staff. Some private organizations offer training seminars and continuing education seminars are available as well. All staff should be thoroughly trained in restraint techniques.

CREDENTIALS AND EXAMINATIONS

The credentialing process has been expanding in all professions, and social work has not been an exception. Membership organizations and credentials abound today. Most states have licensing or certification at one or more levels. The National Association of Social Workers (NASW) has the longstanding, but broadly defined, Academy of Certified Social Workers (ACSW), as well as the newer clinical credentials of Diplomate in Clinical Social Work (DCSW), Qualified Clinical Social Worker (QCSW), and School Social Work Specialist (SSWS). The American Board of Examiners in Social Work (ABE) has an advanced credential, the Diplomate (BCD). The American Association of Marriage and Family Therapists (AAMFT) certifies practitioners and supervisors. Practitioners who work with children can receive certification as a Registered Play Therapist (RPT) and a Registered Play Therapist Supervisor (RPT-S). There are also certification bodies for drug and alcohol counselors, and groups that certify sex counselors. The credentialing situation could become more complex, as some of these bodies are considering multiple levels of credentialing as well as specialty credentials. See Appendix III for a visual presentation of the array of credentialing bodies. Although credentialing bodies and credentials have expanded, the primary payers for mental health services, such as managed cost organizations, require only the highest level of state licensure for reimbursement.

All of these credentials can be confusing for practitioners. The supervisor has a responsibility to be thoroughly familiar with the various credentials in social work and to assist supervisees in what credentials are essential for practice, as well as what credentials may be important to career plans (see American Association of State Social Work Boards, 1998). For example, a practitioner in a public mental health clinic may need only a state license to practice, but if that person desires to develop a private practice, he or she should consider working toward diplomate status and certification in AAMFT. Career planning should include credential planning as well. The supervisor can be helpful to the supervisee in doing career planning in relation to credentials.

Part of credential planning and awareness should include information about how to take examinations. Most credentials require an examination, and the most common is a several-hundred-item, multiple-choice examination during a time-limited (usually three hours) period. Unfortunately, more study guides are available for preparing for the New York City sanitation workers examination than for all the social work examinations. Because of this the supervisor may be called upon to assist supervisees in how to study for the examination and how to prepare for the actual taking of the examination.

Studying for the examination and preparing for the examination are two different processes. Studying deals with reviewing content for the examination and takes place for months prior to the examination. Content review is much more difficult today because the examinations no longer deal with factual information exclusively; they consist primarily of questions that require the person to use logic and reasoning processes to arrive at an answer. Preparation deals with the way the person approaches taking the examination, covering several days before the examination to the administration of the examination. The supervisor can provide the supervisee with many hints and suggestions that will decrease anxiety. Manuals and workshops are available for mastering content and dealing with examination anxiety. The supervisor is the best resource for the supervisee who is preparing for an examination because the supervisor is available to the practitioner on a regular basis and can monitor and support study and preparation for the examination.

Examination anxiety is experienced by most people and can significantly influence scores. Social work schools do not rely on examinations as much as other professional educational programs, and supervisees will often have limited experience in taking examinations, which can further increase examination anxiety. Office gossip about the difficulty of an examination can also increase anxiety. The supervisor who is working with practitioners preparing for a credentialing examination should devote a portion of supervisory time to the practitioner's progress and should be supportive of the worker during this difficult process of competence measurement.

Social Work Licensing Examinations

The following list provides basic information that supervisors can use to inform supervisees about licensure:

1. Examinations have four levels: basic, intermediate, advanced, and clinical. The applicant should inquire of the licensing board in his or

her state what examination to take. The examination taken varies by state and level of licensure for which the person is applying.

2. In many states the examination is administered by computer. Accommodations can be made for disabilities.
3. Questions are prepared by social work practitioners who are trained to write questions. A task analysis is performed to group questions and to select questions for inclusion in the examinations.
4. Examinations are administered at designated sites by appointment on designated days. The applicant should contact the state licensing board about scheduling.
5. Four hours are allowed to complete the examination.
6. The examination consists of 170 multiple-choice questions that include twenty pretest questions that do not count in the scoring.
7. The examination covers the DSM-IV-TR diagnostic and statistical manual of the American Psychiatric Association (2000a).
8. The examination content areas and percentage of questions in each area for each examination are as follows (*Note:* The percentages and categories provided are estimates, and the actual percentages and grouping of questions on each examination could vary from the information provided):

Content Area	Estimated Percentage of Questions			
	Basic	Intermediate	Advanced	Clinical
Practice	29	32	32	33
Assessment and diagnosis in social work	19	20	20	20
Human development and behavior	19	16	16	15
Social work administration	07	07	07	06
Supervision in social work	06	06	06	06
Professional worker-client relationship	04	04	04	07
Professional values and ethics	03	04	04	03
Interpersonal communication	03	03	03	00
Practice evaluation and use of research	05	03	03	04
Policies and procedures in service delivery	03	03	03	04
Culture/race/ethnicity/sexual orientation/gender	02	02	02	02

9. Examinations are prepared under the direction of the American Association of State Social Work Boards (AASSWB).
10. Study guides for each level of the examination are sold by the Association of Social Work Boards:

Association of Social Work Boards
400 South Ridge Parkway, Suite B
Culpeper, Virginia 22701
Telephone: 800-225-6880
            540-829-6880
FAX: 540-829-0142
Web page: http://www.aaswb.org

The following are strategies supervisors can share with supervisees who are preparing to take a licensing examination:

1. Buy a legitimate study guide. Do not study from photocopied material from an unknown source. This type of material may contain misleading and inaccurate information.
2. Be positive, not negative, about the examination. Use positive attack skills in studying for the examination and when answering questions.
3. Remember that the examination is difficult for everyone.
4. Do not be self-critical. Research shows that self-criticism lowers test scores.
5. Focus on choosing the *best* answer, not necessarily the correct answer.
6. Long-range study is best—approximately one to three months prior to examination.
7. Study in small units of time—one to two hours or less. Do not vary length of study times. This strategy enhances retention.
8. Study at a regular time. This increases retention. Do not study when tired or distracted. This reduces retention.
9. Study different topics in different locations. Research shows this increases retention through association.
10. Periodically retrace memories of material studied. That is, try to recall information at times when written study materials are not available.
11. Do not use unnecessary items (e.g., multicolored markers, Post-Its, etc.) to highlight study materials.
12. Do not study with the radio or the television on.

13. Form study groups, but do not rely totally on this method. Use diverse study methods.
14. The day before the examination
    - do a quick review of the contents,
    - review the instructions,
    - get a good night's sleep.
15. The day of the examination, do the following:
    - Eat a nutritious breakfast. Research shows that this increases short-term performance.
    - Wear layers of clothes, regardless of season. They can then be removed to adjust to room conditions.
    - Arrive at the test site early.
    - Carefully follow the instructions given by the proctor.
    - Relax. Do deep breathing, stretching, neck rolls, clasp and pull hands, do in-seat exercises.
    - Use a small clock to monitor time. You have an average of 1.4 minutes per question.
    - Inform the proctor of distractions. If the test is administered by computer and there are problems with the equipment, call the proctor. If you have major hardware or software problems, write down what happened.
    - *Read each question carefully before answering.*
    - Use the POE technique—process of elimination. Eliminate incorrect answers to arrive at correct answers. This increases the probability of getting the correct answer when guessing at answers is necessary. Eliminating one response improves the odds from 25 to 33 percent, and eliminating two responses improves odds to 50 percent.
    - If it is allowed, use scratch paper to work out difficult questions.
    - Answer questions on the basis of literature and the premise, not on what you think is the best practice strategy.
    - Concentrate. Be quiet. Practice focusing on questions and blocking external stimuli.
    - Mark difficult questions and return to them. Guess if necessary.

DEALING WITH THE ADMINISTRATOR

The supervisor also has a boss, but little has been written for supervisors on how to deal with this boss. Several popular books deal with bosses in general, but nothing in them relates to the helping profession supervisor. In an effort to deal with this, the author conducted a study of practitioners' and supervisors' perceptions of supervisors or administrators they had to deal with directly. What follows is a description of these bosses and strategies for dealing with them. The models have been tested in numerous seminars and workshops, and the responses have confirmed the accuracy of these descriptions.

Administrators have been described in stylistic categories because the theme of this book is interactional styles of supervision. By staying with this format, it is easier for the supervisor to relate to the types that have been observed. Each type has been given an acronym to aid in identification and utilization of the types. It is recognized that there are good administrators who are effective, efficient, sensitive, open, and democratic in carrying out their duties. Supervisors can deal with good administrators and have little difficulty in relating to them. It is the chronically problematic administrator with whom supervisors struggle. Often the strategies devised by the supervisor are of limited value and make the problem worse. The purpose of devising these six categories from the research was to offer the supervisor ways to identify certain types of administrative styles and to offer strategies for promoting better relationships with these administrators.

The six styles that have been classified are: Benevolent, Affable Democrat (BAD); Cool, Aloof Decider (CAD); Sophisticated, Learned, Informed Commander (SLIC); Sadistic, Authoritarian Divider (SAD); Jovial, Outgoing Klutz (JOK); and Worried, Anxious Determinist (WAD). Each type is discussed in reference to five areas: communication patterns, forms of interaction, problem-solving methods, decision making, and supervisor response strategy. No administrator will conform completely to a particular categorical style, and some will manifest characteristics from all of the types. The purpose is to provide a crude classification system so that supervisors have a way to begin to organize strategies for dealing with specific actions and behaviors of administrators they perceive as problematic for them. Visual 11.3 gives details of the styles presented here along with strategies for dealing with administrators.

Administrator Styles

Benevolent, Affable Democrat (BAD)

Communication patterns. The administrator who fits this style engages in communication that is always pleasant, but infrequent. In problem-solving activity and communication, this type of administrator makes the same promises to different people. The motivation for most communication is to get the person initiating the communication to go away. These administrators will rarely initiate communication, and staff must approach them. When duplicate promises are discovered by the parties the promises were made to, the administrator tries to get the people to share in the promises through dividing them up or working together. If this strategy does not work, the administrator will simply make a new round of promises to one of

VISUAL 11.3. Administrator Styles

Style	Communication	Interaction	Problem Solving	Decision Making	Response
Benevolent Affable Democrat	Same promises to different people Noncommittal Forgets Infrequent	Avoids evaluations Enjoys gossip Hates conflict Nonconfronting Denies/forgets	Approves requests/ even opposites Single-minded Forgets actions Denies/forgets	Delegates freely Never questions Avoidance/delay Nonconfronting Questions others	Personalize No judgments Cooperate Limit memos Socialize
Jovial Outgoing Klutz	Flood of memos Distributes everything Inconsistent	Friendly Humorous Hysterical Extensive	Impulsive Outrageous Loses focus Inconsistent	Brash Unrealistic Embarrassing blunders	Insist on rules Joke No memos
Sophisticated Learned Informed Commander	Lengthy memos Expects loyalty Formal Regular	Brief/pointed Secret favorites Formal Pleasant gibes	Analytic Efficient Orderly Sporadic	Rational Quick Limited input Global	Be clear Be brief Be loyal Be rational
Cool Aloof Decider	Reveals when forced to Brief memos Delayed response Guarded	Pleasant when needs you Controlling Angry when challenged	Calculates Gives answers Solo Inconsistent Logical	Makes decisions/ does not inform Instant reactions Frequently changes	Use reason Be kind Praise Limit contact
Worried Anxious Determinist	Promise/deny No memos Forgetful	Verbal detail Question/challenge Conceals motivation	Simplistic Secretive/solo Consults others	Contradictory Talks fast Inequitable	Limit sharing No memos Avoid logic
Sadistic Authoritarian Divider	Terse, demanding memos Ignores good performance Associates with weak staff Confrontive	Anxious Cliquish Untruthful Formal Targets people Avoids staff Masks anger	Plots Issues policies Combative Impulsive Takes all credit Denial Shallow	Solitary Sloppy Inconsistent Embarrassing blunders Covers up mistakes	Document Be silent Be calm Good reports Accept tasks Be present Be pleasant

the parties involved. Although these administrators make promises, they are noncommittal regarding resources or making specific decisions.

Forms of interaction. This type of administrator will minimize and limit interaction. They detest conflict and will terminate interaction when conflict emerges. These people prefer to hear gossip and will eagerly engage in discussions about the failures, shortcomings, and problems of others if another person initiates such interaction. They will inquire about others in order to give the person an opening to discuss someone, but the administrators do not initiate or share gossip.

They will avoid doing any task that has the potential for disagreement or conflict, such as doing performance evaluations or allocating salary increases. These administrators will delegate these tasks to others, and if delegation is not possible, they will not do the tasks unless forced to do them. When they do perform tasks that have the potential for conflict, they will do so in the absence of the parties involved and will avoid contact with them about the tasks. When confronted with their failure to perform tasks, they will deny they forgot and blame the error on other people or events.

Problem-solving methods. This type of administrator is friendly and likable. The problem is that this administrator has difficulty saying no. This leads to approval of all requests, even when the people have opposite requests. The person who benefits from this behavior is the supervisor who is last to present a request to the administrator.

The approach to problem solving is single-minded and reduced to its simplest form. In the process of defining the problem this person will take extensive notes, but it is not clear what is done with these notes, which may never be seen again. In subsequent meetings during which the same problems are discussed, old notes are not used, and the person continues to take new notes. This administrator's office is neat and the desk is cleared at the end of the day. Simple problems are resolved quickly. By the end of the day, complex problems that require time to be solved are delegated to others or ignored.

Decision making. The BAD hates to make decisions and will go to great lengths to avoid making even the simplest ones. The strategy is avoidance and delay, which causes frustration for supervisors and staff. The delays are often so prolonged that the administrator forgets the decision that must be made and needs to be briefed to be brought up to date. This administrator will often respond by treating this as a new problem and attempt to delay the decision again. This causes the staff to spend much time repeating explanations of problems requiring action to the point that demoralization sets in. This type of administrator will delegate decision making and likes to have subordinates who take charge and make decisions in bold and swift fashion.

Supervisor response strategy. It is good to socialize with this type of administrator. Always be pleasant and engage in small talk. If you have information about the organization and colleagues, share it with this administrator but always be careful to avoid negative and unprofessional interaction. Offer much support and general praise, and console the administrator when he or she discusses with you how difficult it is to be an administrator. Volunteer to do projects and tasks, especially those you care about and want to see implemented. The administrator will gladly delegate them. It is unproductive to become argumentative and to avoid this type of administrator. If you avoid him or her, you will be on the outside and others will gain control. Avoid confronting this administrator or pushing him or her about decisions. If you must discuss problems or decisions, it is always a good idea to have a proposed solution in mind before you approach this type of administrator. Remember that instead of looking for a solution, he or she will always be looking for a way out of making a decision. This is the primary orientation of a BAD, and the supervisor can develop a strategy that will fit this style of administration.

Jovial, Outgoing Klutz (JOK)

Communication patterns. A JOK style administrator communicates everything. Every memo received by the JOK is circulated to all staff. The JOK writes frequent memos and describes items in great detail. There is much joking in memos and often the focus is lost in written communication.

Forms of interaction. This person is friendly and enjoyable to be around. JOKs make a joke of every item or issue and they are constantly in motion. Individual sessions are brief and disorganized. Group meetings are slightly chaotic, and communication is pleasant and enjoyable, but confused.

Problem-solving methods. This administrator is the most impulsive in problem solving. Decisions are made immediately. The desk is cleared at the end of each day. If this cannot be accomplished, the briefcase goes home full and the work is finished by the next morning. In the process of problem solving, this person is so anxious to arrive at a solution that often the decision is made with such haste that it is not even connected to the problem.

Decision making. Decisions are made in a brash, authoritative manner with an attitude that the JOK has keen insight into most situations. Announcements of decisions contain quips and quotes that are designed to bolster the effectiveness of the solution. Staff have trouble making the connection between the solution and the quips. Most decisions are unrealistic and go beyond the bounds of what staff can accomplish because they are so grandiose. Staff become frustrated and simply do not act on many of the decisions because they are unreasonable. JOKs become angry and depressed because they cannot comprehend why so few of their decisons get implemented. When they are implemented, they frequently result in embarrassment for the staff and the organization. JOKs handle this by making a joke about the blunder and associate it with some philosophical comment about the ups and downs of life.

Supervisor response strategy. The supervisor in this situation should insist on following rules and procedures. This will help keep the JOK in reasonable limits. Discussions should be highly structured and based on specific, written materials that require a response. Memos sent to a JOK administrator should be brief and specific. A good approach is to propose a solution to the problem, rather than allowing the JOK to grapple with a problem and attempt to find a solution. It is not a good idea to make jokes or quips in your communication. This should be left to the JOK to do. It could be viewed as a challenge or as sarcasm when the supervisor engages in it. When outrageous solutions are proposed by a JOK, the supervisor should be prepared to indicate reasons the solution cannot be implemented but avoid saying it will not work. This strategy avoids personalizing the efforts of the JOK administrator.

Sophisticated, Learned, Informed Commander (SLIC)

Communication patterns. Communication is formal, but upbeat, and promotes confidence even when it is not warranted. SLIC administrators conduct lengthy planning meetings and issue memos explaining policy in great detail. These administrators expect strict compliance with rules and regulations and become upset when they discover someone has not observed the rules. They will issue memos that demand compliance with the rules. They will use the rules to avoid establishing a policy they do not like. Although SLICs see "the big picture," most communication will focus on particular aspects of policies and procedures.

Forms of interaction. Interaction with SLICs is brief and to the point. They are usually preoccupied and eager to move on to the next meeting or task. Supervisors feel they can never capture a SLIC's attention long enough to make their point. SLICs have secret favorites and will use them to get information about what is taking place in the staff. These secret staff favorites receive special perks for their information and loyalty. Loyalty is a key concept for these administrators, and any act of disloyalty will result in permanent banishment from significant interaction with SLICs.

Problem-solving methods. This type of administrator is organized, orderly, analytic, and efficient. Relational database computer programs, automated file systems, or any system for tracking work and people are hallmarks of the SLIC administrator. The SLIC administrator will approach every problem from an analytic perspective. Unlike the CAD, who appears to be burdened by administration, the SLIC appears to see administration as a challenge and moves directly to deal with problems in a style similar to the military commander who is confident of impending victory.

Decision making. This type of administrator makes decisions quickly, uses logic, and presents a rational justification for decisions. SLICs make comprehensive, global decisions and leave the details to subordinates to develop and implement. If others do not do what the SLIC thinks is effective implementation, a SLIC will become involved in the details of the implementation process.

Supervisor response strategy. When dealing with this type of administrator, the supervisor should follow the SLIC's decision-making schedule and be prepared to implement decisions quickly and effectively. The supervisor should avoid having to offer justification and excuses for not having implemented a decision that a SLIC has made. The best way to avoid having all control taken out of the supervisor's hands is to be on top of tasks and responsibilities as they are issued. Responses to a SLIC should be brief, logical, and organized. It is best to discuss matters with the SLIC and follow up with written summaries of the decisions, policies, and procedures that are agreed upon in meetings.

The supervisor should seek feedback from this type of administrator. SLICs will usually be honest and direct in sharing impressions and doing evaluations. It is important to remain loyal to SLICs and to use low-key strategies to express loyalty. It is good to discover discreetly who the "secret favorites" are and try to have open and frequent communication with them. They will often provide clues about what the SLIC is thinking or planning, or the supervisor can suggest ideas to them indirectly that they will then communicate to the SLIC. Do not expect to get credit for these ideas. If you are a "secret favorite," you are blessed, but you must be careful not to take advantage of this status or flaunt it with other staff. In communication with the SLIC, you should be discreet and careful not to be unprofessional. The SLIC will not expect this of you, but should it happen, it could lead to difficulty. A SLIC will expect you to be logical and rational in discussions, and objectivity and factual observations should be the basis of discussions with a SLIC.

Cool, Aloof Decider (CAD)

Communication patterns. Communications from this type of administrator are rare. Memos are brief and to the point. Written and verbal communication occur only when the CAD is compelled to do so. Communications that the CAD receives but decides not to act on will go unanswered. This can result in frustration for the supervisor. This type of administrator does not telephone staff, invite staff members to talk to him or her, and never just "drops in" staff offices to talk.

Forms of interaction. The CAD interacts with staff when it is necessary, and the interaction is pleasant unless something is proposed with which the CAD disagrees. CADs are usually calm and soft-spoken but will raise their voice and show slight anger or sarcasm when they do not get their way or when challenged. The CAD prefers one-on-one interaction and is quite verbal in this format. The larger the group the less the CAD will say. Interaction is always planned in the form of structured meetings, with little informal, spontaneous interaction. Although CADs can become angered if put on the spot, they do not hold grudges, and staff are relieved and amazed when they are rewarded in some way after an unpleasant exchange with a CAD administrator.

Problem-solving methods. This administrator calculates and plans most acts, usually in secret. The staff only know about actions when they are announced. Program changes, staff reorganization, and hiring of new staff are a few examples of actions that are simply announced, and no staff input is sought. The CAD sits quietly in meetings and rarely says anything. It is difficult to determine what the person is feeling or thinking. Staff are usually uncomfortable in this administrator's presence and guarded in comments, since guardedness is the style of the administrator. This is ironic because the CAD appears to use information presented in meetings to make decisions, but if the staff are reluctant to voice opinions, the administrator is denied information important to devising solutions. The CAD is logical in thinking, and most times attempts to be fair. The CAD approach to problems is logical, but the solutions are inconsistent. When inconsistencies are glaring, the staff will fail to raise the issues because of the guardedness in relation to the CAD. The CAD gives the impression of being a lonely person and limits social contact with staff. The CAD is seen as a person who is a "solo" operator. She or he is reliable and calm most of the time, but it appears to the staff as if administration is a burden for the CAD.

Decision making. This person makes decisions in isolation and notifies staff or has others notify the staff. Some decisions are simply made and implemented without notifying staff. People find out about policies when they fail to observe them and are then told what the policies are. The CAD makes the decisions but attempts to distance himself or herself from the decision, if possible. CADs will accept responsibility for decisions if necessary and are bold in coming to the staff with decisions when they feel the situation requires it. When a CAD administrator feels pressured, decisions are made instantly to resolve the situation. Instant decisions occur in staff meetings, a situation the CAD finds uncomfortable. A CAD will frequently change decisions if he or she is not getting the desired results.

Supervisor response strategy. It is important to be pleasant toward CADs and to praise them occasionally for the good decisions they make. The supervisor should be slow to propose invitations to socialize with a CAD administrator. Some prefer an occasional lunch meeting, but it is best to limit such meetings unless the CAD gives indications that he or she enjoys and prefers this type of contact. The more formal, regularly scheduled meeting is the preferred model of the CAD. The best strategy is to ask questions and to develop unobtrusive methods for ensuring that you learn about policies that may have been implemented without being announced.

Efforts to change bad decisions of a CAD are best done in staff meetings where staff support can be stated, even if it is guarded support. Preparation for the attempt to change the decision can best be done by meeting with the CAD individually and casually mentioning the problem, but offering no solutions. Staff who offer solutions are viewed by CADs as trying to usurp their power, and CADs will do the opposite of what is being suggested to assert and make clear who has authority.

When new policies are implemented, it is best not to express surprise but to find out as much about the policy as possible. In other words, ask questions about the policy rather than questioning the policy. Try to base observations on logic, and focus on the organization and the meaning of the policy for clients and staff instead of attempting to identify the policy as coming from the administrator personally. Only for situations about which staff members feel very strongly should the issue of failure to get staff input before making the decision be raised with the CAD administrator. This will have to be done periodically because CADs do not change their style significantly; they do not evolve into participatory decision makers even after being repeatedly confronted about the lack of staff input. This type of administrator will ignore agency policies and legally mandated requirements related to decision making in such matters as hiring, retention, and dismissal of staff. Because of this characteristic, the CAD is vulnerable to grievances and legal action.

Worried, Anxious Determinist (WAD)

Communication patterns. The WAD is friendly but can be blunt and abrasive when working to get his or her way on an issue. These people do not send memos; they send handwritten notes. Communication is sudden, intense, and often vague and brief.

Forms of interaction. WADs are constantly in motion; they go from task to task, rarely completing a task or forgetting what task they were in the process of completing. They are quite forgetful and will deny they have forgotten. When you confront forgetfulness, they become defensive and accuse you of having misunderstood. WADs often make promises that they forget and later will deny that they made any promises. They describe everything in great detail and treat staff like children who are learning for the first time. Presentations are often confusing, and the essence of tasks get lost in the enormous detail. WADs ask many questions and challenge the statements of others, but there is no logic in this, and the motivation for the WADs' combative stance is puzzling to the staff. WADs often complain of being overworked, and they are constantly in crises.

Problem-solving methods. This type of administrator engages in solo, secretive, and simplistic problem solving. All problems are reduced to simple black-and-white, right-and-wrong conceptions. This person will consult others by asking questions but does not reveal why the questions are being asked. Only later do staff realize the questions were used to get information to make decisions, but since the questions were not presented in this context, the staff feel duped. This pattern leads eventually to the staff being guarded about any responses given to questions asked by a WAD.

Decision making. WAD administrators make decisions rapidly and before sufficient information has been gathered to make the decisions. WAD decisions are often contradictory. A contagion effect occurs among staff when WADs feel the urgency to make decisions. The smallest decisions often take on the quality of emergencies for WADs. WADs consume much energy in this process and will reverse themselves and say there is no hurry to complete the task when they feel intimidated by the process. This is related to depletion of the WADs' energy, so the problem is no longer an emergency. In such an environment, staff become distraught and withdrawn.

WADs feel they have to make decisions on everything that comes before them. If a supervisor comes in just to talk, the WAD becomes anxious early in the conversation and turns the content of the discussion into a major problem that must be solved. By the end of the conversation, the supervisor regrets having brought up the subject or even going to talk to the WAD. If the supervisor withdraws and does not come to talk, the WAD projects that into being a problem, so the supervisor has the feeling of being in a no-win situation.

Supervisor response strategy. WADs can be demanding and difficult to deal with. The supervisor must balance communication and contact with the WAD so that he or she can avoid the no-win situation just described. It is best to discuss with the WAD only items that involve him or her directly. Items that require speculation or new ideas are best explored with other staff. It is recommended that memos be sent to a WAD only when absolutely necessary. It is important to keep good notes and to document discussions and phone conversations.

Trying to use logic with these administrators does not work because they will see it as a challenge and create a new logic based on their own perceptions, which can be even more confusing. The better strategy is to try to determine what the WAD wants and to ask questions that will help to make clear what he or she is trying to get done. WADs are usually in a mode of trying to get something done but are confused about what to do. The WAD will not admit to this confusion or the need for help, so the supervisor must study the WAD's comments to determine what the WAD wants from an exchange.

Sadistic, Authoritarian Divider (SAD)

Communication patterns. SADs communicate through terse, demanding memos. Written communication is issued as an order to do something or to stop doing something. SADs are not available for individual meetings with staff, and when one does get in to see them, the meetings are brief and non-committal. The key factor to remember about SADs is that they desire to make decisions alone and perceive communication to be important only in one direction—from themselves to the staff.

SADs will have staff discussions of problems, but they devalue this input and ignore it. Their view is that the only requirement is that the staff be allowed to express views, but these views should not in any way influence SAD's right to make decisions unilaterally.

SADs do communicate with the few people whom they take into their confidence. These people have much hidden power in that they influence decisions, and many times their recommendations are based on personal animosities.

Forms of interaction. These administrators proclaim harmony and desire smooth operations, but they act very differently. They are constantly in conflict with staff, and they target individual staff to be recipients of punitive actions. They avoid people and communicate through memos. When confronted they become anxious and angry. They will mislead people and distort situations and conversations to achieve their goals. These people are unpleasant to work for and can become impossible to relate to if you become the target of punitive actions. They usually target only one person at a time, and if a designated target transfers or quits, a new target will be found. There are brief lapses between the time one person is the target and another person becomes the target. During these periods the supervisor should keep a low profile.

Problem-solving methods. Problem solving is done in a secretive and devious manner by this type of administrator. Problems are approached as challenges that require a plot to be solved. The SAD tends to use the plot to punish and harass people. This punitive strategy has no behavioral basis but seems to be part of the person's personality.

SADs solve problems alone or on the advice of one other person who has been temporarily taken into confidence. SADs constantly rely on two or three people to be their advisors. These administrators have much anxiety and act on impulse to solve problems. Acting on impulse, they make mistakes and unjustly accuse staff of making mistakes or acting inappropriately. This leads to much conflict and frustration. When challenged, SADs become angry and upset. This occurs in private as well as group meetings. Although they try to contain the anger, it is obvious to all that they are irritated. After such encounters, this administrator will take action that results in punitive measures for all or some staff.

Decision making. Decisions are made in solitude and occasionally after consulting a key staff person. Decisions are made hastily and result in embarrassment for the administrator and the organization. Many times decisions are in direct conflict with earlier decisions that this administrator made. Logic and consistency are not important to this type of administrator. Decisions that become blunders are handled by blaming staff for the failures. If decisions go well, the SAD will take personal credit and not acknowledge the work of staff.

Supervisor response strategy. The best strategy with a SAD administrator is to be laid back and to do your assigned tasks. Accept requests to perform special projects and assignments without complaint. Avoid confronting a SAD if your report is later distributed with the SAD's name on it. To confront such issues will make you a potential target. If a targeted person has recently departed, it is best to lay low for several months and not approach the SAD because you are vulnerable during this time to becoming the new target. The supervisor should keep a low profile in relation to a SAD, but be present and in frequent communication with other staff. Withdrawal is not a good strategy with a SAD because this results in isolation that could make you a target. It is a good idea to befriend all staff, especially the two or three people who are the confidants of the SAD. You should share ideas you would like to see developed with these people because they will most likely share them with the SAD. It is a good idea to be quiet in meetings and to retain documentation of all important actions and activities of your work. It is not a good idea to confront these administrators or to send memos to them unless absolutely necessary.

Case Exercise:
The Case of Kurt

Kurt is a child protective services worker in a suburban DSS office. He loves his work with families and children, but he also requested to be a supervisor. He was assigned to supervise two social workers and a volunteer. Kurt reports to a female program director who in turn reports to the male agency director.

Kurt has had difficulty supervising David from the beginning. David is a recent hire who is on six months' probation that is scheduled to end in three weeks. David is distant and not communicative. He responds to questions but volunteers no information. David is always late with paperwork, and some requests from Kurt he has ignored. Kurt requested that David give him a list of all his cases and a brief summary of each client's progress. He has asked David for this three times. David on one occasion responded to the request by asking Kurt why he wants to check up on him and why he does not trust his professional competence. David has resisted any discussion of what he is doing therapeutically with his cases.

Kurt has tried repeatedly to discuss David's client contact activities with him without much success.

Another staff member reported to Kurt that David did the intake on a case and ignored the referring physician's written request that the child be referred for mental health treatment. The case involved a suicidal fourteen-year-old boy who was depressed over abuse by a minister.

Kurt was concerned about what to do since David's probation period was over in three weeks and he would then become a permanent employee. Kurt discussed the situation with the program director, who discussed the situation with the agency director. The director indicated that Kurt should give David a written dismissal notice to be effective in two weeks. Kurt did this, and David protested to the agency director, who rescinded the notice on the basis that not enough notification time had been given.

Kurt feels betrayed and wounded by this action. He is frustrated and angry. He is having trouble sleeping and feels he is not doing a good job with his clients because of the problems he is having supervising David.

You are the program director. (1) What would you do as Kurt's immediate supervisor? (2) How would you handle this situation with the agency director? (3) How would you explain your role in this matter to Kurt?

Case Exercise:
The Case of Jane

Jane is a secretary in a state-run social services department. She has been employed by the state for nineteen years. She is the primary secretary with a child protective services unit. The director assigned her to this unit because she has been "a thorn in my side for a long time." This unit is located at a site distant from the main offices (across town), and the director felt you could perhaps deal with her because you are such a skilled supervisor. Jane accepted the distant assignment readily because she is a loner and has had trouble getting along with other staff for many years. Jane is condescending toward clients, and clients have complained to workers about her. She is a good typist and handles all the administrative details of the unit with much efficiency, but she prefers to work alone and alienates other secretaries temporarily assigned to assist the unit. The typing of reports and staff dictation has piled up, with a backlog of six weeks.

(1) How would you, as the unit supervisor, deal with this situation? (2) What would you say or do about Jane's rudeness to clients? (3) What would you say, if anything, to the director about Jane?

ADMINISTRATIVE TRANSITIONS

As part of their administrative responsibilities, supervisors are often required to manage program transitions and modifications. Departments and programs can be altered, restructured, and merged. Programmatic changes are occurring more frequently because of privatization, dissatisfaction with program outcomes, and funding cuts. Any organizational change can cause anxiety, confusion, and resistance in workers who have to undergo the transition. Supervisors can underestimate the impact of the slightest change on workers' functioning. This can be illustrated by an experience the author had when providing clinical consultation to a small group home staff:

> The employee parking had to be moved from the east side of the staff building to the west side because of construction of a new building for an educational program. The parking lot was relocated only by about 200 feet. The staff became upset in subtle ways and started complaining to one another. They complained of having to walk farther in the rain and snow to enter the building and that they would have to walk out into the hot western sun at the end of the workday. Complaints arose that there would not be an adequate walkway to the building from the new parking lot and that there would be less lighting at night. Some staff felt that the education staff were being shown preference by the administration and that the parking lot was being taken over by the "educators." The complaints continued to increase, and the staff investment in complaining was affecting their work performance.

None of these complaints were valid. There were no real differences in the exposure to weather or walking distance or in the adequacy of the walks and lighting. The complaints reflected staff resistance to the change. The administration had not recognized the importance of providing a transition process for this smallest of change. Imagine the intensity of the resistance if this had been a major change in location or function.

Bridges (1991) has argued that failure to recognize the impact of change and to plan a process for implementing organizational change will cause the change to fail. Bridges' model for implementing change was developed in the business world but has much relevance for clinical agencies. Bridges holds that "[i]t isn't the changes that do you in, it's the transitions." Change is not the same as transitions, and supervisors who have to implement changes should take this difference into account. Change is situational and is a physical, objective event. Transition is a psychological process that people go through to deal with the new situation. For Bridges, change is external to the individual and transition is internal. The process of successful change and transition is viewed differently in this model than is customary for clinical social workers. Social work training focuses on the therapy process as sequencing from beginning to middle to end. Social workers tend to apply this line of thinking to other aspects of functioning, as most people do. Bridges holds that change transitions cannot use this process. For a new beginning to be successful, the ending of the old methods must be followed by a "neutral zone" period in which the old methods are gone and the new procedures are not yet comfortably in place. The neutral zone is where the staff work through the difficult process of changing from the old to the new methods. That the staff are in this stage needs to be acknowledged and their difficulties recognized. After the staff have moved beyond the ending and the neutral zone they can effectively implement the "new beginning." Explaining this three-stage process and allowing staff to go through it can be helpful to any agency or unit experiencing large or small changes. The process does not have to take a long time, but the more significant the change, the longer the transition will take. Bridges' model of managing change is highly recommended to supervisors who must oversee agency or program changes. His book *Managing Transitions* (1991) is easy to read and apply. A summary of the model is presented in Visual 11.4 and can be used to plan change efforts.

SUGGESTED READINGS

American Association of State Social Work Boards (1998). *Social Work Laws and Board Regulations: A Comparison Guide.* Culpeper, VA: American Association of State Social Work Boards.
   Provides a detailed comparison of social work regulatory boards and statutory requirements for the practice of social work throughout the United States. A comprehensive reference volume for supervisors.

Bridges, W. (1991). *Managing Transitions: Making the Most of Change.* Reading, MA: Addison-Wesley.
   Guide to planning organizational change. This model was briefly explained in this chapter.

Davis, S. (1991). "Violence by Psychiatric Inpatients: A Review." *Hospital and Community Psychiatry* 42(June), pp. 585-589.
   A review of the literature on violence by patients and helpful information on violent clients.

Flach, F. (1998). *A Comprehensive Guide to Malpractice Risk Management in Psychiatry.* New York: Hatherleigh.
   Although written for psychiatrists, this book has extensive information about malpractice risk that is relevant to all mental health professionals.

Kets de Vries, M. F. R. (1984). *The Irrational Executive: Psychoanalytic Studies in Management.* Madison, WI: International Universities Press.
   A conceptual discussion of leaders in organizations from a psychoanalytic perspective. Much of the information can be applied to clinical settings and associated with the styles described in this chapter.

Kets de Vries, M. F. R. and Miller, D. (1984). *The Neurotic Organization: Diagnosing and Revitalizing Unhealthy Companies.* New York: Harper Business.
   A conceptual discussion of organizations from a management perspective. Much of the information can be applied to clinical settings.

Lowe, J. I. and Austin, M. J. (1997). "Using Direct Practice Skills in Administration." *The Clinical Supervisor* 15(2), pp. 129-145.
   Relates direct practice and administration.

Moline, M. E. et. al. (1998). *Documenting Psychotherapy: Essentials for Mental Health Practitioners*. Thousand Oaks, CA: Sage.
Comprehensive presentation of mental health records methods aimed at current standards of care.

Morgan, N. (1995). *How to Interview Sexual Abuse Victims*. Thousand Oaks, CA: Sage.
Guide for practitioners and supervisors who deal with sexual abuse cases.

Munson, C. E. (1996). *Clinical Supervision Curriculum Guide: Training Curriculum for Supervisors of Social Workers Seeking Licensure as Licensed Clinical Social Workers (LCSW's) by the Virginia Board of Social Work*. Culpeper, VA: Virginia Board of Social Work and American Association of Social Work Boards of Examiners.
Information on how to address many of the issues discussed in this chapter.

Shea, S. (1998). *Psychiatric Interviewing: The Art of Understanding*. Philadelphia: W. B. Saunders.
Includes good information on safety issues and how to deal with potentially violent clients.

Tosone, C. (1998). "Countertransference and Clinical Social Work Supervision: Contributions and Considerations." *The Clinical Supervisor* 16(2), pp. 17-32.
Review of countertransference in clinical social work supervision.

Zuckerman, E. L. (1997). *The Paper Office: Forms, Guidelines and Resources,* Second Edition. New York: Guilford.
Includes an array of commonly used mental health practice forms as well as a computer disk that allows reproduction of the forms.

VISUAL 11.4. William Bridges' Process Model of Change

Ending

Transition starts with an ending

- Identify what is ending and what is being lost
- Describe changes in detail
- What are the secondary changes
- What is over for everyone?
- Overreaction from past losses causes transition deficit
- Acknowledge losses openly
- Recognize signs of grieving:
  1. Denial
  2. Anger
  3. Bargaining
  4. Anxiety
  5. Sadness
  6. Disorientation
  7. Depression
- Define what is over and what is not
- Mark endings
- Treat past with respect
- Retain some aspects of the past
- Show how endings ensure continuity

Neutral Zone

Limbo between old and new

- Dangers in NZ:
  1. Anxiety rises and movitation decreases
  2. More absenteeism
  3. Old weaknesses reemerge
  4. Staff are overloaded, in flux, and confused so unreliability can emerge
  5. Polarization of old and new ways
  6. Vulnerable to threats from outside and within
- Normalize the NZ
- Redefine the change ("sinking ship" versus "new voyage")
- Create temporary systems
  1. Protect people
  2. Review policies and procedures
  3. What new structures need to be created?
  4. Establish outcome checkpoints
  5. Do not expect high productivity in NZ
  6. Provide training for staff
- Strengthen intragroup connections
- Use Transition Monitoring Team (TMT) made up of cross-section of staff
- Encourage creativity
- Engage in reflection
- Encourage experimentation
- View losses and setbacks as challenges
- Do not give premature closure to the past

New Beginning

Old is gone, new not yet comfortable

- Frightening because:
  1. Reactivate old anxieties
  2. Represent a gamble
  3. Trigger old memories of failures
  4. Destroys fun of NZ
- Approach to NBs:
  1. Explain purpose
  2. Draw outcome picture
  3. Make a plan
  4. Give each person a part
- To reinforce the NB:
  1. Be consistent
  2. Ensure quick successes
  3. Symbolize the new identity
  4. Celebrate success

Source: Adapted from Bridges, W. (1991). *Managing Transitions: Making the Most of Change.* Reading. MA: Addison-Wesley.

Chapter 12

Audiovisual and Action Techniques

In this chapter, audiovisual and action techniques used to promote learning in supervision are discussed. Society has experienced rapid advances in electronic technology, but few guidelines have been developed for use of this technology in learning about practice, and most supervisors and supervisees approach this material as they approach electronic media—as entertainment. The use of television (videotape) and audiotape are explained, along with specific guidelines for sequencing and manipulating such material to enhance learning. Ethical and nonintrusive uses of electronic devices by supervisors are covered.

Role-play has become a popular educational technique. Specific techniques for role-play are explored along with role-play procedures organized around (1) planning, (2) monitoring, (3) evaluation, (4) debriefing, and (5) physical setting. The use of live supervision is explained. The concepts of privacy and confidentiality are discussed in relation to the use of electronic devices and action techniques.

TELEVISION (VIDEOTAPE)

Most practitioners and supervisors have grown up with television as an essential and extensive component of their lives. The pervasive impact of television on practitioners, supervisors, and clients is illustrated by compelling statistics (Finn, 1980:473-474; Famighetti, 1999:188; Wright, 1999:406):

1. Ninety-eight percent of homes have at least one television. Forty percent have three or more television sets, and 34 percent have two televisions. Eighty-five percent of homes have a videocassette recorder (VCR).
2. The average television is on more than seven hours a day.
3. Children between two and seventeen years of age watch television an average of three hours a day.
4. By age eighteen, the average person will have spent the equivalent of 2.5 years watching television—45 percent more time than is spent in classroom education.
5. By age sixty-five, the average American will have spent nine full years watching television.

Given these statistics, it is ironic that most practitioners have not been exposed to audiovisual methods in practice and supervision. When such materials are used, it is with little training or critical application. In this section, common techniques for using television in supervision and training are covered.

Matisse observed that the invention of the camera relieved artists of the need to copy objects. In a similar sense, television applied to practice is not used to permit practitioners to copy the styles of others but is a means of enhancing the use of imagination and creativity in developing their own styles.

Knowledge Gap

The advance in audiovisual technological knowledge and mechanical application has far exceeded the development of knowledge regarding its utilization in the behavioral sciences in general, and in the field of social work in particular (Munson, 1988). Little research or theoretical speculation has focused on the use of audiovisual technology in supervision.

In a study by Nelson (1978), social work trainees showed greater preference for verbal descriptions of therapy content over videotaping of treatment for use in supervision or supervisory observation than did psychiatry and psychology trainees. Although the reasons for these differences are not known, the study does illustrate that social work trainees are more likely to resist, avoid, or fear videotaping and action techniques. The supervisor needs to be aware of this reluctance and to approach the use of such techniques with sensitivity.

Nelson's findings were confirmed in a study in which a "clinical exposure index" was developed as a special case of interaction between the practitioner and supervisor (Munson, Study J). The scale measured the extent to which workers and supervisors shared with one another their practice methods through direct observation, videotapes, audiotapes, and process recordings. The scale ranged from 5 (never) to 20 (regularly). The mean score was 6, indicating that virtually no sharing of clinical material was taking place. Process recording accounted for most of the activity. Kadushin had similar findings in another study, and he concluded that "no use is made of modern technology to obtain data of on-the-job performance" (Kadushin, 1974:295).

The failure to use electronic devices to promote learning is not understandable given the current availability of videotape equipment. The most basic system for videotaping now costs less than $500, and even fairly sophisticated systems are available for under $2,000. Availability of the equipment does not seem to be the barrier because, as one study showed, almost all of the agencies reported having videotape equipment available (Munson, Study J). Perhaps other psychological resistances are at work. The material in this section is designed to help in overcoming these resistances.

Television As Entertainment

People have been oriented to watching television for entertainment. When television is used for educational purposes, the participants must develop a new perspective for viewing the material, especially clinical material. The size of the problem of overcoming television as entertainment is reflected in the estimate that the average person will spend over 16,000 hours during childhood watching television. Each visual image will last 3.5 seconds for programming and 2.5 seconds per commercial. This adds up to 1,200 visual images per hour. People watch television; they do not read it, write it, and, more important, think about or analyze it.

Television is a purely visual medium that is based on rapidity of visual images. It is not cognitively stimulating. All of this must be understood in the context that the three major activities of children are sleeping, watching television, and going to school. Television is being used more in school, and educational viewing added to personal viewing makes television the number one educational tool in the United States.

Supervisees will comment after viewing a videotaped interview, "That was so boring. Couldn't it be more lively?" Statements of this nature are an indication that the practitioners are viewing the tape from an entertainment perspective. Car chases and crashes, people falling off mountains, or scuba diving do not occur in videotapes of practitioners doing treatment. Good treatment is not always exciting or emotionally charged. Supervisees have to be prepared in advance for learning-oriented television. The supervisor must specify what to watch for but must not pinpoint too much detail in advance. One strategy for dealing with this in supervision is to use brief segments of video- or audiotape to highlight specific ideas.

Television As Measurement

One of the chief ways television can be used in supervision is to watch practitioners change, grow, and develop. Emphasis in supervision is placed upon growth and development, but good measures are rarely used to highlight or evaluate growth. Videotapes and audiotapes made of beginning students and practitioners that are preserved and reviewed a year or two later can provide valuable documentation of growth. They can be used to reinforce growth and to specify the changes that have occurred in the practitioners' style, comfort level, skill, and utilization of techniques. Practitioners and supervisors who are serious about evaluating growth will need to have such records to gauge their performance over time.

It is not sufficient to base an evaluation solely on verbally reflecting and recalling changes over time. When verbal recall is all that is used, much of what is learned is forgotten with time and, therefore, is not available for reinforcement at the assessment points. For the supervisee to say, "Well, I learned a lot this past year," is not helpful. The verbal recall method can be manipulated by both the supervisor and supervisee to avoid dealing with sensitive, but important, issues. A comment of one supervisee illustrates this point: "I am sensitive to criticism, so I set it up so that I don't get it, but when you are on tape, you can't avoid it." Also, verbal recall by the supervisor is limited even when giving the practitioner positive feedback. Another supervisee comment illustrates this: "My supervisor said, 'You really had poise in that first interview,' but I have trouble accepting his positive feedback." If the supervisee could have seen herself being poised, it would have been easier for her to accept the praise. In this case, the old saying is true—"Seeing is believing."

The use of electronic records works in favor of the supervisee. Watching a videotape of past work highlights all areas of a person's change—knowledge, skill, flexibility, confidence. It is not unusual for supervisees to say, "I forgot I did that" or "It's been a long time since I made that mistake." Such responses allow the supervisor and practitioner to get specific about the change that has taken place. Once supervisees are exposed to learning and evaluation based on electronic records, they find it stimulating and helpful. Little information is available for the supervisor to use in deciding when, how, and where to use audio or video technology in treatment and supervision. Many questions remain unanswered: When should supervisors ask practitioners to bring audiotapes of their treatment to supervision sessions? When should videotaped material be used instead of audiotaped material? When using videotape, should split-screen techniques (one camera on the client and one camera on the practitioner) be used? Should the supervisory process itself be subjected to audiovisual techniques? These are just a few of the basic questions that arise regarding such methods. The following material offers suggestions in dealing with these basic questions as well as others.

TAPING THE THERAPY TO BE SUPERVISED

Practitioners who have not used electronic devices in their therapy are intimidated by such activities and will resist their use on the grounds that they are too threatening to the client. Repeated, unplanned, and unskillful use of electronic devices in treatment reveals that the practitioner has more difficulty in dealing with it than the client. Kagan first observed this when using videotaped material to develop the strategy of Interpersonal Process Recall (IPR) (Berger, 1978:72). Kagan found that in using videotaping for learning, the tasks had to be ordered in a progression from least threatening to most threatening. Means of accomplishing this are discussed here.

Even though most practitioners have been reared in an era of widespread exposure to television, they remain shy of appearing on television. This is easily observed in stores where video equipment is set up for display purposes. People will be startled at seeing themselves on the monitor. They will look at themselves briefly, quickly move out of range of the camera, and then dart back for a second, brief look. People are torn between wanting to see themselves and being fearful of how they will look. The same phenomenon occurs when videotape is used in treatment. Practitioners and clients report that initially they are fearful of how they will look, and then they are fearful of how they will perform and how their performance will be judged. At the same time, they want to view how they look. While watching a videotape of a session the client will say, "I don't want to watch this," while watching the monitor intently. The evaluation of the performance is more acute for the practitioner than the client. It is the practitioner who is on the spot and knows that the performance will be judged and evaluated. In dealing with such fears, familiarity breeds comfort.

It is best to introduce the practitioner to electronic devices by moving from the simple to the complex. Audiotapes of treatment sessions should be used before videotapes. The practitioner should be supported by the supervisor in advance regarding the difficulty in risking such exposure. The supervisor should explain in advance how the audiotaped material will be used in supervision. The supervisor can share his or her own taped material in advance to illustrate how the practitioner's tape will be used. The supervisor should discuss with the worker procedures for getting the client's permission to do the taping.

After the initial taping, the practitioner should be encouraged to listen to the tape alone before it is used in supervision. The practitioner should be requested to make notes about the tape regarding his or her feelings about its impact on the treatment, areas of concern to be discussed in the supervision, and plans for subsequent sessions. When the initial tape is used, the supervisor should allow the supervisee the opportunity to identify problems, mistakes, unrecognized dynamics, and successful interventions before the supervisor makes any comments, interpretations, or suggestions.

When videotaping is used, to achieve maximum performance, the person in charge of the taping needs to be aware that some of the most significant material regarding the participants occurs prior to the beginning of the taping and just after the conclusion of the taping. The director (practitioner) of the videotaping must ensure that all participants (clients) are clear about their roles and put them at ease. At the conclusion of the taping, the participants are usually relieved, relaxed, and jovial. This is a good opportunity for the director to explore with the participants their feelings and thoughts about the session. While the material is still fresh, the participants are often quick to point out errors or what they consider as alternatives to actions they took. They also will share what was going through their minds when they took an action or failed to do something they wanted to do.

One taping is not sufficient to develop skill in the use of electronic recording devices. One taping session can lead to familiarity in most cases, but subsequent sessions are needed to develop comfort and skill.

The supervisor and practitioner should not be videotaped too often. The amount of videotaping will vary with the person and the circumstances, but once a month during periods of intensive learning is adequate. Workers being taped need time to apply what they learn from seeing themselves. If time to integrate visualization of self in action is not permitted, the person will become too self-conscious and learning, as well as performance, can be hampered.

To learn from videotapes of some forms of therapy, especially family therapy, the session should be viewed twice. When viewing long tapes, the supervisor should attempt to get the practitioner to develop a comprehensive understanding of the interaction and dynamics. This can be accomplished by asking such questions as, What process is taking place? What are the unified dynamics of the session? What is the common or persistent theme? What is the thread that holds the interview together?

Videotaping the practitioner's treatment is not the exclusive means of using this medium in supervision. The supervision itself can and should be taped. Videotaping supervision sessions prevents the supervisee from developing the sense that he or she alone is being evaluated. The supervisor is subject to evaluation when supervisory sessions are videotaped, and the supervisor as well as the practitioner will be taking risks and be under scrutiny. Taping of the therapy session and of the subsequent supervision of that session can add continuity and deeper meaning to the taping.

Using split-screen techniques in individual interviews makes it easier to evaluate the interaction process because the worker and client are facing each other. When the supervisor wants to focus on the actions of the client or the practitioner exclusively, he or she can reverse the images so the participants appear on screen positioned back to back. This requires advance planning and special equipment (two cameras and a special effects generator), but it is one of the real advantages of television—reality can be manipulated for learning purposes without disturbing the actual therapy situation.

Listening to or watching portions of tapes can be helpful when specific techniques or problems are being addressed. Thematic, theoretical, or conceptual learning is more comprehensive and requires reviewing tapes of whole sessions. Portions of tapes are not helpful with comprehensive learning; they cloud the significance of prolonged silence, resistance to interventions, dissolving of resistances, dysfunctional patterns of relating, shifts in roles, interactional themes, and focusing on one person or one problem at the expense of others. A good rule to follow is to use whole-session tapes with inexperienced practitioners and to use portions of tapes with more experienced practitioners. It is good to begin the supervisory process with whole-session tapes and, as the supervision advances, to progress to segmental tapes once the supervisor is confident that the supervisee has an appreciation for the comprehensive nature of therapy. These are general rules, and there are always exceptions. It should be remembered that whatever approach the supervisor uses should be based on an assessment of the practitioner's learning needs.

Some supervisors and workers resist videotaping because they have only "old black-and-white equipment." This attitude is another product of advanced technology and daily exposure to commercial television. It is true that much of the equipment available to most practitioners and their supervisors is crude when compared to commercial television. However, research indicates that black-and-white television is better for practice training because there are fewer extraneous distractions (Berger, 1978:52). All that is needed is a good-quality picture, free of distracting distortions. Only the extremes of picture quality should be avoided. Poor-quality images and high-quality images are distracting. A balance between technical sophistication and simplicity must be maintained, as well as a clear and consistent focus on the treatment interaction recorded.

Rewards and Problems

It should be pointed out that television in training and therapy can be a devastating experience for some. Television has been used in treatment historically and has been highly acclaimed by those using it, but not much independent research has documented its negative or positive impacts. Some practitioners have reported highly negative outcomes when videotape was used in therapy. In one study of nine married couples, chosen by random sampling, in a therapy setting in which video feedback was used, six of the couples suffered "casualties" in the form of emotional crises, breakdowns, and suicide attempts. At the same time, forty-one other couples treated by the same practitioners without video feedback experienced only seven casualties, and none were suicides. Although the outcomes could not be directly attributed to the use of video feedback, this is sufficient reason to approach the use of television with caution and to encourage more extensive research on the method (Brandt, 1980:81-82).

There are limited outcome studies of the use of television in training, and it could be that some clients and practitioners in training are being put at risk without sufficient safeguards. A study by Howe (1989) found that family therapy clients resented the use of video in the therapy. This could be due to the way the video was presented and used rather than due to the technique of using video. In many training programs, students are expected to engage in video self-confrontation, to videotape family of origin groups, and to be videotaped in group supervision sessions. Many of these sessions delve into highly personal material. In some instances, no supervisor is present and no supervisor even reviews the tapes with the trainees. The unskilled trainees are expected to review one another's personal thoughts and experiences in the name of personal growth, professional growth, and professional development of self-awareness, without a specific purpose and without supervisory guidance. Such exploration should be avoided as a part of supervision.

Such groups have been used to give the trainees practice at developing techniques and skills in exploring feelings. It is questionable whether such exercises accomplish anything. Students who undergo these experiences are rarely able to connect them with learning tangible aspects of therapeutic technique. Some supervisees have become uncomfortable in these groups and find the videotaping a source of increased discomfort. They become slightly distrustful of their fellow students and their teachers for placing them in vulnerable situations in which little control is exercised over the limits of the material that becomes the basis for exploration.

These students say that they withdraw and withhold information to protect themselves. They can be criticized by teachers, supervisors, and fellow students for being unable to be open about themselves, which calls into question their potential as practitioners. The students readily admit and understand that their learning has been limited in these situations, but they attribute this to the misguided focus of the learning rather than to a genuine inability to share feelings on their part. Any videotaping sessions should be well planned and supervised to guard as much as possible against negative outcomes.

AUDIOTAPING

The advantages of audiotaping are that it is inexpensive, requires little technical skill, and is not distracting in the treatment sessions. Small cassette tape recorders with built-in microphones and several tapes can be purchased for less than $50. Tapes can be easily edited for teaching purposes. For example, audiotaping was used as part of the supervision of a young practitioner who had a tendency to use "uh-huh" to the point of distraction and to ask questions as a consistent way of responding to the client, without much effect. The practitioner was asked to tape a session, and the tape was reviewed with her. She had difficulty hearing the distracting speech pattern, so the tape was edited, with the client's talk removed from the tape, leaving only the practitioner's dialogue. Review of a fifteen-minute segment of the tape revealed that the practitioner had said "uh-huh" fifty-seven times and had asked twenty-four questions. She was amazed upon recognizing this pattern and began working to change it. Subsequent tapes showed a change in her part of the dialogue and an improvement in the course of the treatment.

Linguistic analysis of case material is growing in importance (Grinder and Bandler, 1976; Efran, Lukens, and Lukens, 1990; Kennedy-Moore and Watson, 1999). When doing linguistic analysis of case material with a practitioner who is an active or action-oriented person and/or a client who is very verbal, it is better to use audiotaping in supervision than videotaping. It is possible to miss the linguistic elements of a videotape completely since the video aspects can be so overpowering.

AUDIO-VIDEO SEPARATION

Videotapes can be manipulated so that only the audio or video portions of the tape can be played back. Many supervisors do not realize that the audio and video elements are separate components that are merged to make a videotape and that either part can be used separately. Separation of audio and video portions of tapes in supervision can be effective in clinical interactional hypothesis testing. By only listening to the audio portion of the tape, the supervisor and practitioner can speculate about nonverbal gestures. Later the audio and video portions can be played back in unison to confirm or refute the hypotheses.

More emphasis must be placed on coordinating the use of auditory and visual material in teaching in supervision for effective learning. This is supported by research indicating that people remember 15 percent of what they see, 25 percent of what they hear, but 50 percent of what they see and hear at the same time (Bagg, 1980:35).

ROLE-PLAY

Role-play in training, educating, and supervising social workers has increased, yet there has been little systematic evaluation of or empirical research on its value, effectiveness, or effect on the participants. Role-play is used widely in practice and supervision, and supervisors and practitioners need to learn more about its application (see Etcheverry et al., 1980). This section attempts to offer guidelines on the use of role-play for nontherapeutic purposes.

The growth of role-play in education and supervision has paralleled the increased popularity of psychodrama in therapy. Also, increased use of role-play has paralleled the modern rise of anti-intellectualism in theory of therapeutic technique. The search for nontraditional and nonacademic modes of learning in part gave rise to the development of role-play and, for some, led to playing at learning rather than traditional academic effort.

Role-play is of limited value in education and supervision. It should be used as a last resort and only after other techniques have been explored and found to be ineffective, unavailable, or inapplicable. Live interviews, videotapes, films, audiotapes, and, in some instances, lectures and discussions are preferable.

Role-play exercises limit the depth of feelings that can be expressed, especially when the participants have limited experience with the type of material under exploration. In training programs, this can result in students developing the belief that therapy is mainly information gathering, and that complex and sensitive material is easier to deal with than is actually the case. When student practitioners are required to role-play material related to serious illness, death, depression, divorce, etc., of which they may have had little direct experience or knowledge, it can result in distorted views of the therapeutic skills and techniques required to deal with such material.

Videotaping of role-play of therapy should not be required of student practitioners before they have been given some other form of training in how to handle the material being explored. Role-play should not be used when the learner has not had any clinical experience in the case area that is to be the subject of the role-play. To videotape role-play with the objective that students will learn from the activity itself sets students up to fail, puts them in a vulnerable position, and can give rise to anxiety that inhibits learning. In formal courses and training programs, videotaping of sessions and role-plays should take place near the end of the course or the training program. In addition, role-play should take place only when a skilled supervisor or teacher is present, and the students playing the roles should have prior experience with the material being covered and/or be thoroughly rehearsed in the material before the role-play is attempted. The decision to use role-play should be linked to the purpose and process of the learning to be accomplished. Any decisions made in the process of the role-play activity should be made in the context of what is to be taught and learned.

Role-Play Procedures

Most teachers or supervisors who attempt role-play in the classroom do so without any formal training in the technique. At best, a teacher has read something about the procedure, has attended a demonstration, or has participated in a role-play session. Such experiences provide little of the needed information to lead role-play activities successfully. Role-play demonstration or participation rarely includes instruction on techniques being used by the leader to conduct a successful role-play. This can cause the potential role-play leader to be deceived into thinking that successful role-playing is easy. The teacher or supervisor who wants to do role-play should get training in the method before attempting its use, but if training is unavailable, the following procedures should be followed.

The process that the teacher or supervisor must go through in utilizing role-play can be understood as having four distinct, sequential components: planning, monitoring, evaluating, and debriefing. Each component is discussed separately.

Planning

Any role-play activity should be planned in advance. The leader should know in advance what is to be illustrated, demonstrated, and acted out. The leader should know in advance exactly what is to be portrayed. Portrayal takes several forms, such as covering life experiences with which the participants are unfamiliar, bringing out into the open material that the practitioner is resisting, or rehearsing for dealing with a problem the practitioner has expressed inability to handle.

People with whom the leader thinks the person could best identify should be selected in advance to play roles. The leader should know or learn the capabilities of each participant to perform certain roles. Some people are actors, and some people are not. The leader should discuss the role-play in advance with each participant. This can be done before the group assembles or in the presence of all group members. None of the group members should be assigned to or coaxed into a role-play (Etcheverry et al., 1980:8-10).

When practitioners are asked to participate in a minimally specific role-play, the pressure of performing can cause personal material to surface that the practitioners, under other conditions, most likely would not share. In educational settings in which the role-play participants are unskilled students, such personal material is poorly handled, often unacknowledged as important and sensitive, and rarely given closure. In some educational programs, unskilled students are required to role-play for videotaping when no skilled supervisor or teacher is present. Educational programs and supervisors should give serious consideration to the appropriateness of putting student practitioners in such uncontrolled situations.

A case example illustrates this point:

> A group of student practitioners was required to role-play for video-taping without the teacher present. The teacher's logic for not being present was that she did not want to inhibit the students' performances, and she would view the tapes privately at a later time. Three students and a technician were present in the audiovisual laboratory for one of the taping sessions. The role-play was set up to be about a woman who came to a mental health center for an initial interview because of unspecified depression, and the learning goal was to develop the ability to do an intake interview. The practitioner was role-played by a male student. The student playing the woman client eased into the role, and as the interview progressed, the source of the depression focused on the client's having a sister who was dying of cancer. The student practitioner, wanting to perform well, gratefully focused on the client's feelings about her sister. The role-play client became visibly upset as the interview progressed and was near tears at the conclusion of the session. When the role-play was concluded, the technician asked the woman student if she in reality had a sister who was dying of cancer, and she indicated that she did. The students discussed this briefly, and the woman uncomfortably shared more information about her sister before leaving the laboratory in an agitated state.

The actual client who was the focus of the role-play did not have a sister who had cancer. The role-play unintentionally gravitated to a problem the student was experiencing. If the teacher had been present, this situation, which was uncomfortable for the student and the class, could have been avoided.

This example illustrates how significant personal material can surface and not be given closure. The student performing the client's role was led into the personal material by accident, and feelings she had not acknowledged before were tapped. At the close of the session, she was left with the feelings, and no skilled practitioner or supervisor was present to help her understand, accept, or work through these feelings and make recommendations for her to get help with the problem, if she desired it. In addition, the videotape was played back for the entire therapy class, causing the student to experience the feelings again and leaving her classmates to speculate about whether the situation was real.

The student's confidentiality was violated. Several students asked her about the situation, which she ultimately resented. Although she felt supported by some of her fellow students, she did not like so much attention being focused on her, and she grew weary of explaining the situation to interested fellow students. She wanted to cut off the querying but, at the same time, did not want to appear rude to her student colleagues. If the supervisor had planned sufficiently, this woman could have avoided exposure of this family trauma. If she had desired help with this, she could have been assisted privately by the supervisor. The learning goal of developing skill at intake interviewing was not achieved because of the discomfort that the participants experienced. The focus shifted from the client under review to the role-playing student's personal life, which had no relevance to the learning goal and task.

Before starting the role-play, the leader should explain each role again and allow a few minutes for each person to warm up to his or her role. Asking participants how they feel about playing their roles helps to ease people into the role-play. Such activity can help the leader identify which persons might have difficulty getting in touch with aspects of the roles, and the leader can then directly or indirectly be of assistance to those persons.

The leader should explain to the group before beginning the role-play that role-play for educational purposes is similar to, but different from, role-play in the therapeutic situation and that it requires a different focus and approach on the part of the leader. The role-play audience should be instructed to take notes to use in the post-role-play discussion. If specific points are to be observed and recorded, they should be mentioned by the leader before the role-play begins. Also, the leader should mention briefly before beginning that the role-play might have to be terminated if it moves away from the intended purpose.

Whenever possible, videotape or audiotape the role-play. If the role-play is successful, it can be used with subsequent groups with much less preparation. Consistent role-plays are difficult to re-create even with the same actors. If the role-play is recorded, written permission of the participants should be obtained.

Monitoring

Monitoring relates to directing and controlling the role-play. It is the leader's responsibility to ensure that the role-play remains focused and related to its intended purpose. Two ways of managing control are based on the level of involvement of the leader. The first is for the leader to be one of the actors. In this method it can help if a coleader is available as a nonactor, but this is not always possible. The second method is for the leader to direct the role-play as a nonactor participant. The method used will depend on the style and preferences of the leader and on the nature of the role-play to be performed.

The role-play should be of short duration. If it takes a great deal of time to set up the situation, most likely the role-play is focused on too much or too complex material. The set-up time should be no more than five minutes, and the actual role-play no more than fifteen to twenty minutes. It is better to break complex material into two or three separate role-plays and to use discussion time to integrate the material. Role-play is one of many techniques the supervisor has available, and more consideration should be given to using a short role-play in conjunction with such other techniques as lecture, discussion, written assignments, and audiotaped and videotaped case material.

If any or all of the actors are having difficulty getting into the roles, it is better to abandon the role-play after several brief assists from the leader rather than to persist with the effort. This is an important part of the leader's monitoring role. The leader can salvage aspects of a bad role-play by discussing with the actors and the audience why the role-play was difficult to enact. In some instances the barriers and blocks can be sufficiently identified to resume the role-play.

In some instances it might be necessary to shift the roles of certain actors to overcome problems and resistances. Some people lack the experience, knowledge, or will to assume certain "as if" stances of particular roles. A sensitive leader will be able to identify such difficulties and make the necessary adjustments. If the role-play is unsuccessful, and if the leader feels it is not a good idea to persist further with this method to deal with the material, the leader should not attempt to justify or explain away an unsuccessful role-play. Another strategy is to have several members of the group interview the client or to have participants take turns at being the client. This increases participation and gives more people the opportunity to experience the action of the role-play.

The author developed the concept of *role-play deviance* to describe situations in which role-plays diverge in any way from the supervisor's original purpose or direction. When a supervisor makes the mistake of conducting a spontaneous role-play without a specific focus, role-play deviance will not occur. This does not mean that difficulty cannot result; it means that when difficulty does develop, the supervisor has no basis for terminating or reorienting the role-play.

Role-play deviance occurs when the interaction moves away from the intended focus or when an actor becomes upset by the content of the role-play. When the interaction moves away from the intended focus, the supervisor has the responsibility to intervene and redirect the focus or terminate the session. To redirect the focus to the original purpose takes more skill than is apparent. The supervisor must follow the interaction closely and ask questions and make comments or suggestions without distracting the actors from their roles. In a real sense, the supervisor has to be there without being there. This can be accomplished by kneeling behind the actors and making comments or whispering commands to nonactive actors, when the leader is not directly involved in the role-play. When the leader is involved in the role-play, he or she can use the role to refocus the interaction.

Evaluation

At the conclusion of the role-play, the leader should discuss the content of the role-play and emphasize the points that were to be illustrated as well as any material that emerged as a result of the role-play. Observations of both the actors and the audience about certain points should be explored, since actors and audiences can develop differing perspectives of the role-play. The leader should attempt to integrate these differing perspectives to maximize learning. It is helpful in this regard to focus on what the audience observed about a certain role and on what the actors felt as they performed these roles. Often a person in a role does not perceive events in the same manner as those observing the roles, and the leader should relate these two perspectives to the practice setting.

One problem of role-play is that the leader has no control over wrong, weak, or inappropriate responses by actors during the role-play. During the follow-up discussion, the leader should pick up on such responses and help the group find different ways of handling the situation. This can be approached by exploring with the actors how they felt about the adequacy of their responses. Frequently actors readily recognize and admit weakness and inadequacy in their responses.

Debriefing

After evaluating and discussing the role-play, the leader should debrief the actors and the audience. Actors' feelings about the roles they played should be discussed. Connections between feelings identified in the "as if" situation and the real-life role should be explored. Insights that have been gained should be identified. Incongruent ideas and conflicts in feelings and thoughts that emerge should be kept open for discussion within the group, privately with the leader, or with other appropriate professional or personal contacts. The debriefing should include the leader explaining that role-play techniques used by the participants are not always obvious, and the parts of the performance that were not obvious should be illustrated by the director. In explaining techniques, the leader should make a distinction between doing a role-play to help professionals learn something about therapy and doing a role-play to teach them how to use role-play in the therapy situation.

Participants should be encouraged to incorporate material from the role-play in their practice, but the leader should caution participants that there is no guarantee that components of the "as if" situation of the role-play will emerge in the reality of practice.

Physical Setting

Good role-play conditions require equipment. The average classroom, group therapy room, and office are not conducive to good role-play. The supervisor who is serious about role-play should be aware of this. Role-play can best be performed on a stage where lighting can be controlled. Where this is not possible, two or three floodlights or stage lights mounted on tripods will suffice. The room should be darkened as much as possible, and the spotlights should be placed between the audience and actors and focused on the actors.

This will assist greatly in preventing the actors from seeing the audience. Actors should be positioned in a way that will give the leader freedom of movement to assist in or direct the action. When the leader is a role-play participant, he or she should be centrally positioned to see as much of the action as possible.

LIVE SUPERVISION

Live supervision, in which the supervisor actually participates in the treatment by being present during the treatment session or by observing the treatment through a one-way viewing mirror or on a television monitor in another room, is one of the most effective ways to do supervision. In situations in which the supervisor is not present in the therapy room, it is a common practice to use a telephone or phone device for the supervisor to have direct contact with the practitioner.

This is an effective method of conducting supervision, but it does have limitations. This form of supervision is fast moving and leaves little time for integration and reflection. It is a much better method for teaching techniques and mastering process in treatment than it is for applying theory, developing a philosophical orientation, or planning a course of treatment. Live supervision can be used effectively, and can come closer to bridging the gap between a technical orientation and theoretical abstractions, when there are follow-up sessions to the live supervision in which speculation, reflection, and contemplation are allowed. The follow-up meeting and its relation to what took place in the treatment session are extremely important because, in live supervision, both the supervisor and supervisee tend to let important points go unnoted, since they believe the points will be covered in the follow-up supervision. Often the material is forgotten or not discussed as more pressing issues arise.

It has been argued that the concept of parallel process that has been developed in practice theory also carries over to supervision (Kahn, 1979). The parallel process that develops between practitioner and client can pass through to the relationship the practitioner has with the supervisor. In live supervision, the potential for such double-parallel process is increased because both the practitioner and supervisor are directly influenced by the client. If this is not recognized and clearly identified, it can lead to supervisory conflict—the origins of which neither the supervisor nor the supervisee will be able to identify.

Live supervision is more than supervision—it is teamwork that requires much role flexibility, role acceptance, and role confidence on the part of the supervisor. When live supervision is used, the supervisor has to be more responsible and aware than is the case in other forms of supervision. If television is being used, the supervisor must be sensitive to comfort levels of the practitioners and clients. The supervisor must be responsible for minimizing distractions, such as bright lights, movement by television technicians, and talking by the supervisors and others observing behind a one-way mirror. If the supervisor overuses a telephone or earphone device to communicate with the practitioner, this can be a distraction for both the practitioner and client.

When a supervisor works behind a one-way mirror and other supervisees are allowed to observe, the supervisor must be careful of what is said about the supervisee doing the treatment. The simplest and most innocuous remarks, repeated to the performing supervisee by the observing supervisees, can be misinterpreted. When members of a group of supervisees take turns at performing live supervision and observing, the sense of competition can become greatly increased if it is not defused by the supervisor. A case example illustrates this:

> A supervisee got upset when voices could be heard from the viewing room while she was interviewing. The supervisee became distracted and did not perform a good interview. In the follow-up session, she cried and accused her fellow trainees of trying to sabotage her treatment.

The supervisor has an absolute responsibility to prevent such situations from occurring. Silence behind the mirror is the best policy. The supervisor and observers should take notes and save the discussion for the follow-up session. A viewing room is for viewing. When people are talking, they are not observing, even if they are talking about the treatment session in progress. The supervisor should make these conditions clear to supervisees and colleagues when observing the live work of others.

Many problems can occur in the various forms of live supervision. The supervisor may have to make split-second decisions. In such situations, the client's comfort and well-being must be the first consideration. In some situations, if a technical problem occurs, it is better to let the treatment continue and allow the live supervision to lapse. In other situations, it is better to stop the treatment if the live supervision is too distressing for the client. To avoid abrupt distraction of the practitioner, the supervisor should give thorough information about the live supervision and how it works in advance. It helps to let the supervisee experience the room and the setup of the equipment before the live session begins. If an earphone device is used, the supervisor and clinician should practice with it before the live interview. Supervisees should be alerted to common problems that can occur and instructed on how to handle them in advance. It is a good idea to have practitioners observe live supervision before they participate in it. In live supervision, the supervisor has a responsibility to be alert to the rights of and amount of discomfort experienced by both the practitioner and the client. For this reason, in live supervision, it is important to place emphasis on the evaluation of the supervision as well as on evaluation of the treatment.

Live supervision done in a sensitive, positive manner is effective in promoting confidence and eventual autonomy in the practitioner. When live supervision is applied in an authoritarian or punitive manner, it results in the practitioner's trying to copy the supervisor's therapy style in order to lessen the supervisory demands. This inhibits the practitioner from developing his or her own style and decreases the potential for confidence and creativity.

INTRUSION OF PRIVACY

It has been argued that any audiovisual device used in the treatment or any observation of the treatment is an intrusion and affects the client-practitioner relationship, especially its confidentiality (Langs, 1979:25-26). If the logic of the confidentiality argument is consistently applied, supervision would not exist because any discussion of the therapy outside of the therapy threatens confidentiality. At least when audiovisual devices are used, the client has complete control over what is revealed or not revealed. The use of audiovisual material in supervision provides assurance that the client and the problem will be presented more accurately than when the practitioner attempts to portray or explain the client to the supervisor.

In addition, much concern has been raised about the quality of psychotherapy as the number and type of psychotherapists increase. Clients have limited means of knowing whether they are receiving good or bad treatment. The more a practitioner's work is exposed to other professionals through supervision, the less the risk to the client of undergoing poor or unethical treatment. It is appropriate to share with the client the notion that use of audiovisual devices is designed to enhance the quality of the treatment he or she receives without destroying the client's confidence in the practitioner.

With respect to confidentiality, it should be kept in mind that the supervisor operates within the same ethical standards as the practitioner. It is true that gaining benefits from relationships involves taking risks. Some protection is given up when audiovisual devices are introduced into the treatment, but something can be gained in the form of new insights, more effective treatment, and more rapid resolution of problems.

RANKING OF TECHNIQUES

This chapter has covered the major audiovisual devices and action techniques used in treatment supervision. As a quick reference for the supervisor, these devices and techniques have been ranked on the basis of their effectiveness and efficiency. They are ranked from 1 to 10, with 1 being the most useful and 10 being the least useful.

1. Live joint interviews
2. In-ear listening devices
3. One-way mirror observation
4. Videotapes—live material
5. Videotapes—commercially produced
6. Audiotapes—live material
7. Audiotapes—commercially produced
8. Discussion of case material
9. Process recordings
10. Role-play

Therapy and the training to perform it, as with many aspects of society, have become a technological game, so that for many people, one-way mirrors, in-ear listening devices, videotaping and audiotaping, and role-play have emerged as therapeutic gimmicks that become ends rather than means. Any technological devices used in treatment or supervision must be planned and implemented as a supplement and focused on how they enhance the improvement of the client.

SUGGESTED READINGS

Berger, M. M. (ed.) (1978). *Videotape Techniques in Psychiatric Training and Treatment*. New York: Brunner/Mazel.
   This book covers the history, theory, and techniques of applying videotaping to practice and training. Basic technological material is included that is helpful to the supervisor who wants to get started in videotaping.

Gallant, J. P. and Thyer, B. (1989). "The 'Bug-in-the-Ear' in Clinical Supervision: A Review." *The Clinical Supervisor* 7(Fall/Winter), pp. 43-58.
   Literature review and summary of the use of electronic feedback devices in practice.

Urdang, E. (1999). "The Video Lab: Mirroring Reflections of Self and the Other." *The Clinical Supervisor* 18(2), pp. 143-164.
    Strategies for using video recording to teach practice skills.

Utz, P. (1980). *Video User's Handbook.* Englewood Cliffs, NJ: Prentice-Hall.
    Guide for the supervisor who wants to learn the basics of videotape and audiotape operation.

In my own day-to-day attempt to provide
a meaningful psychotherapy, I find myself
increasingly thwarted by the reality
outside the therapy, by the social and
material culture of the patient and the
therapist, the ambience, the setting, the
milieu in which the therapy takes place.

Fred Bloom
"Psychotherapy and Moral Culture"
in T. J. Cottle and P. Whitten
Psychotherapy: Current Perspectives

Chapter 13

Supervision in Different Settings

This chapter covers supervisory practice in different settings. All of the various settings in which social workers are employed cannot be covered, and the specialized practice settings have increased significantly. Specialization has advantages but can present challenges for the practitioner. The chapter begins with a list of eight characteristics that can be used to explore supervisory practice in any agency that is considered unique or specialized. Issues of several different settings are explored, including medical settings, geriatric settings, criminal justice settings, and rural practice.

INTRODUCTION

Historically there has been a gradual expansion of the number and type of settings in which social workers function. This expansion has also led to specialization of practice that provides advantages and challenges (Earle and Barnes, 1999). The proliferation of practice settings is advantageous as far as job opportunities for social work practitioners and supervisors are concerned, but it makes it difficult for an author to cover all the possibilities within the space limitations of a book chapter. Even in practice settings that offer "identical" services in a number of agencies, each agency will have a unique set of characteristics that the practitioner and supervisor will need to take into account. To make such a complex topic manageable, only general principles and common settings and situations are covered here. The following list of general characteristics should be considered in aiding supervisees in a given setting:

1. Social, economic, and cultural characteristics of clients
2. Psychological characteristics of clients and their families
3. Interactional patterns of clients
4. Interactional patterns of staff
5. Structural dynamics of the agency
6. Organizational dynamics of the agency
7. Geographical location of the setting (e.g., urban, suburban, rural)
8. Locale of the agency (e.g., the neighborhood or medical complex of which the agency is a part)

MEDICAL SETTINGS

Knowledge Base

In medical settings the supervisor must be aware of and sensitive to several special areas. Practitioners in medical settings and specialized medical service areas must master what often seems to be a whole new knowledge base. In order to assist patients and their families, practitioners must learn the etiology of the disease being treated, the terminology associated with the disease, the process of the disease, and the problems associated with the course of treatment.

Organizational Structure

The organizational structure of medical settings often is more complex and more diverse than the structures with which many practitioners are accustomed to dealing. The multidisciplinary setting in which teamwork is advocated, but may or may not be a reality, must be mastered and adapted to by the practitioner. The power of the medical and nursing professions in many settings must be understood, as well as how to relate to less highly trained staff, who often have the most and closest contact with patients (see Krause, 1977:33-67). The supervisor has an important role to play in aiding the practitioner to adjust to and to influence these other disciplines in order to help the patients and their families. The nature of the supervisor's approach will vary according to the size and nature of the facility. The supervisor, who has spent years dealing with the complexities of the organization, will sometimes assume that the practitioner also possesses such knowledge and will fail to spend adequate time helping the practitioner in this area.

Terminal Illness

In some medical settings, dealing with death and terminal illness is a common experience. For example, large cancer wards commonly have an average of one or two deaths per day. Many times, when patients are discharged, the professional staff know that death is imminent for these patients. Practitioners must be helped to deal with reactions to death and its onset. Many times the most sensitive and committed practitioners have the strongest reactions. The realities of death are especially distressing for practitioners and supervisors who work in medical settings that care for infants and children. In such settings support groups that engage in group processing of emotions are important. Supervisors must be prepared to help practitioners work through their reactions.

Psychological Reactions

Upon entering certain medical practice areas, practitioners may have psychological reactions to intense exposure to some diseases. Cancer, kidney disease, and heart disease are a few examples of some of the diseases that can cause reactions in workers. Workers can develop responses that mimic the symptoms of the disease being treated. The supervisor must be alert and prepared to help practitioners with such reactions.

Practitioners may have reactions to the trauma and disfigurement they witness in some medical settings. New as well as experienced workers can have reactions to such situations, and supervision is an arena for dealing with these reactions. Trauma debriefings are helpful but are only the beginning of the healing process. There must be follow-up to such debriefings. Debriefings are usually general and done in large groups. Such generalized debriefing can expose the practitioner to new stresses through content brought up by participants from other services that can actually add to the practitioner's stress. The supervisor must be available to deal with these secondary reactions.

Death and Dying

In dealing with dying patients, the practitioner needs help relating to the patient, the patient's family, and other staff. Patient needs are often viewed as immediate. New practitioners have some difficulty accepting the fact that their own lives and work schedules go on when patients are near death. As one practitioner commented in her supervision, "Here I am planning to go sailing this weekend, and this patient is dying." Practitioners must come to accept that they do as much as they can for the patient, but that there must be limits.

Practitioners have reported that they "get more depressed" when their supervisors are away from the agency for vacations or other matters. Practitioners also become more depressed when a patient gets worse or deteriorates, and they are more affected when the dying patient is younger. Practitioners report frustration when patients are unable to accomplish things they wanted to before they became incapacitated. Practitioners have difficulty accepting that they cannot control the situation. The comments of one practitioner summarize this concern: "People go downhill so fast. People die in spite of how they feel and in spite of their feelings, and you can't control the process; nothing you do will stop it."

Interestingly, supervisees also report being more depressed immediately after supervision sessions in which difficult cases are discussed. At the same time the supervision is considered as helpful and worthwhile because supervisees are able to express and explore feelings that under other circumstances "just get bottled up," which can be more harmful than the temporary depression associated with sharing real feelings with the supervisor.

Practitioners in such settings can at times talk about extraneous matters and deal with a series of related and unrelated issues that are not connected with the real issue of the patient's dying. As one supervisee said, "Hospitals are full of denial." The supervisor needs to be alert to this kind of rambling, confusing discussion and bring up the real issue of the dying patient.

In working with families of the dying patient, special problems can develop. Some families engage in massive denial and attempt to cut the patient off from needed communication. In some families relatives will refuse to visit the patient, leaving the patient with many doubts and concerns. Other families will go to great lengths to protect the patient from knowledge of the condition. Some family members react with anger. Some patients also react with anger, and they may remain angry until death and not "die in peace," as the practitioner prefers. Families need help in dealing with the patients' unyielding anger. Some practitioners show a tendency to move psychologically and interactionally ahead of where the family is emotionally, pressuring them to deal with what it will be like after the patient dies before the family is ready to handle this content. Some patients and their families lose time orientation in the stressful period before death, and practitioners need to be prepared to help them with this confusion. The patient and family members can have justified and unjustified anger at the hospital staff. The supervisor needs to aid the clinician in balancing his or her position as staff member with the need to support the client and family. With medical illness, what clients often need most is information about the illness and about quality of life and life expectancy to assist in planning for care, living arrangements, or death. Such information can be essential for the client to have as much control as possible. Social workers often are not trained in information provision, especially with respect to medical conditions, and can become conflicted as the family communicates independently with medical staff and social work staff. Team effort and integrated care are essential under these circumstances, and one of the supervisor's roles is to work to assist in making integrated functioning a reality.

Other staff who are less trained in human behavior can have adverse reactions to the dying patients and their families and focus their lack of understanding on social workers as they try to intervene. Staff also try to protect the patients and families from the realities of the illness. When social workers attempt to intervene and promote openness about the situation, they may be accused of meddling, interfering, and upsetting the patient. Such criticism, overt and covert, can be upsetting and disheartening to the social worker. The supervisor must be prepared to support and help the practitioner with such staff reactions.

The supervisor in geriatric and/or medical settings must be able to help supervisees deal with issues of death and dying confronted by patients and their families. In many instances supervisees will need to be sensitized to these issues, especially the younger workers. Weisman (1972:157) has developed a set of seven questions the supervisor can explore with supervisees to help them become more empathic in this area:

1. If you faced death in the near future, what would matter most?
2. If you were very old, what would your most crucial problems be?
3. If death were inevitable, what circumstances would make it acceptable?
4. If you were very old, how might you live most effectively and with least damage to your ideals and standards?
5. What can anyone do to prepare for his or her death, or for that of someone close?
6. What conditions and events might make you feel that you were better off dead? When would you take steps to die?
7. In old age, everyone must rely upon others. When this point arrives, what kind of people would you like to deal with?

Hospice Settings

Medical social work in hospice settings is a developing speciality. The concept of hospice care for the terminally ill and their families is relatively new in the United States but is increasing. Hospice settings in the United States now include those within nursing homes and hospitals as well as free-standing hospices. The hospice concept is organized around the idea of a team effort involving physician, nurse, social worker, clergy, patient care coordinator, volunteers, the client, and the family of the client (Ajemian and Mount, 1980:65-93). A hospice offering inpatient and outpatient care is usually viewed as a small agency by its staff, even when it is part of a larger facility. The social work department usually consists of two or three social workers plus a supervisor.

The supervisor in a hospice has a unique responsibility because all of the supervisees are members of an interdisciplinary care team. Frequently, social workers, as well as other staff, have little experience functioning as a part of such teams. Supervision of the social worker participating in such teams requires a strong sense of professional independence and autonomy based on knowledge and skill. The supervisor's role is made more complex because, in many hospices, volunteers engage directly in bereavement counseling, which can lead to confusion about accountability, evaluation of intervention, and exercise of authority.

Team membership involves conflict, negotiation, compromise, participative decision making, and flexibility. The social worker and supervisor must be confident about the practitioner's independent professional competence, while not be threatened when concessions must be made to the team. Lack of professional competence can bring the practitioner into conflict with other team members because authority is diminished on the team. This model of team functioning promotes individual team members' giving way to enabling roles and leadership shared among team members at appropriate points in the treatment process (Rossman, 1977:107).

Because hospice care is a newer form of practice, ground rules and clear procedures are not always available. Participants are free to experiment with new methods and procedures, but, at the same time, fear of the unknown and untried strategies can promote insecurity and undue caution in practitioners. This situation creates new challenges and opportunities for the social work supervisor.

GERIATRICS AND GERONTOLOGY SETTINGS

Supervising the practitioner in geriatrics (diseases of aging) and gerontology (science of aging) settings can impose special problems for the supervisor. The most salient concern of the supervisor should be the negative stereotypic notions that the young practitioner might have about the aged, which Butler (1969) has identified as "ageism." Research indicates that such stereotyping is a problem among children (Seefeldt et al., 1977) and students in training for the helping professions (Geiger, 1978). Social work and medical students have been found to be significantly lacking in information and knowledge about the elderly, to fail to perceive accurately problems that the elderly are likely to identify, and to show no preferences for working with the elderly. Practitioners in training, as well as practicing therapists, have few opportunities to work with healthy and active older people, and their work with the frail elderly can reinforce the impression that aging is associated with impaired functioning, decreased activity, and gradual or sudden disengagement. This can result in certain assumptions in relating to the elderly person seeking treatment that can promote dependency and disengagement. Although there have been some limited attempts to sensitize professional students to the elderly (Birenbaum et al., 1979), the majority of young practitioners have limited experience with such programs, and their attitudes and behaviors need to be monitored for stereotypes that can distort treatment efforts. Although social work has been present in medical settings for most of this century, social workers are relative newcomers to geriatric settings.

Social work in aging has been focused on three areas: curing, preventing, and enhancing (Lowy, 1979). Interventive efforts on the part of social workers have occurred through the three practice methods of casework, group work, and community organization. Casework has centered on, but has not been limited to, the curative and enhancing functions through work with individuals and their families. Group work has centered on these same two functions in relation to small groups, while community organization has related more to the preventive function through work with large groups.

Social work education has been reactive to practice developments regarding social problems and groups to be served. Social work practice historically has lacked widespread application in the field of aging (Lowy, 1979). This is not to imply that there is no history of social work in aging or societal concern with the elderly.

In general, social workers have had limited desire to work in the field of aging because of societal and personal lack of interest in the elderly, because of low professional status associated with this area of practice, and because of low salaries. This has been the case in both community-based and institutional programs, but these factors have been especially important

Portions of Geriatrics and Gerontology Settings are reprinted from Carlton E. Munson, "Social Work in Aging," *Gerontology and Geriatrics Education,* 1(1) (Fall 1980), pp. 17-23, and Carlton E. Munson, "Social Work Educational Consultation in Church-Related Nursing Homes," *Gerontology and Geriatrics Education,* 1(3) (Spring 1981), pp. 175-180. Reprinted by permission of the University of Texas Press.

with respect to the institutionalized elderly. The entry of social workers into geriatric settings has been due to federal and state regulatory mandates implemented in the nursing home field. At the same time there has been reluctance on the part of both the nursing home field and the social work profession to establish social work services for the institutionalized elderly.

Statistical information about manpower in various practice specializations is more highly developed in other professions than in social work. The NASW has no reliable statistics on its membership, which makes it difficult to speculate with any accuracy about the number or characteristics of trained social workers, historically or currently, with respect to practice activity in aging in comparison with other practice areas. Also, accurate statistics for social work education for geriatric practice are not available. Although the Council on Social Work Education (CSWE) compiles annual statistics on the total number of students, faculty, and accredited educational programs, no statistics exist for student or faculty specialization in various practice areas or for the number of programs offering degree specializations. In order for sound manpower and educational planning to occur, the practice and educational components of the profession—through the two national organizations (NASW and CSWE)—must make a concerted effort to gather and analyze such information (Munson, 1980b:17-18; Munson, 1996e).

Motivation and learning needs of practitioners in aging have received limited attention from social work educators or supervisors. Some practitioners select aging because of an emotional experience with an elderly relative or because of the promise of good job opportunities, without having a realistic perception of the demands that can be placed on them. Many are quite young and have little understanding of or appreciation for the functioning or problems of the elderly. Supervisors need to be alert to ways of sensitizing practitioners to the elderly. In accomplishing this, models for teachers and supervisors need to be developed that will appropriately orient practitioners to effective ways to intervene with the elderly. Currently, the literature is limited in this area.

Long-Term Care Facilities

Work in nursing homes or long-term care facilities (LTCFs) poses unique problems for the social work supervisor, and special attention is given to the supervisory role in such settings. Social workers find the nursing home field alien because proprietary and nonprofit facilities operate from a free-enterprise perspective and use business management strategies. The pattern has been for most LTCFs to contract with professional social workers to serve as fee-for-service providers on a part-time basis. Such social workers are frequently—but it seems to me inappropriately—referred to as consultants. When social services are provided by outsiders, there is little motivation to develop services within the facility, and regular staff tend to shy away from direct helping activities for fear of intruding on the work of the outside service providers. This section presents a different view of the role of the social worker in LTCFs. An interpersonal role model of the social worker is presented that focuses on integrative functions as well as provision of clinical services. From this perspective the practitioner engages in enhancing the helping skills of regular staff, interpreting and integrating roles of various disciplines in relation to social services, and developing service programs.

In role theory, roles have been distinguished as conventional and interpersonal (Hewitt, 1976:144-146). Conventional roles are based on routine responses to human situations and regularized structures. Interpersonal roles develop out of unique interactive situations, and repeated interaction leads to creative role performance and expectation. When one accepts the position of practitioner in an LTCF, both the practitioner and the facility staff—and especially the administrator—draw on conventional role models. The administrator hires a social worker from the perception that the social worker will function structurally much as the physician; that is, he or she will be a part-time professional service provider who relates to residents' basic needs and addresses special problems as they arise. Social workers readily accept this model because, conventionally, they have been trained to work, and have worked, in agencies in which they provide casework and group work services directly to clients. Residents accept this model because they have rarely had any contact with social workers prior to admission, and this is a new role experience for them. When the social worker assumes this conventional role model, the facility has little incentive to develop a fully integrated social work program.

With the assistance of the supervisor, the social worker needs to assume an interpersonal role model in which the practitioner works directly with all staff, including the facility administrator. The focus of the supervisor should be on defining the role of social services in relation to other disciplines and departments. The functions of the supervisor from this perspective are

1. to establish a social service policy;
2. to define who will deliver the social services;
3. to develop job descriptions and guide recruitment efforts;
4. to provide in-service training for social service staff and other disciplines regarding the role of social work;
5. to establish admission procedures;
6. to develop treatment strategies, including goal-setting and recording procedures; and
7. to interpret regulations regarding social services.

The extent to which the supervisor focuses on specific functions depends on the nature of the individual facility. Some facilities have MSW staff; others have full-time employees with little or no training who serve as social service designees. Some facilities have thorough admissions procedures; others have none at all. Some facilities have adequate recording procedures; others have haphazard and inconsistent methods. Some facilities master social service regulations without difficulty; others respond with frustration and confusion.

Role Differentiation

In LTCFs, the social worker often experiences difficulty with the administrator and nursing staff, especially the director of nursing. The supervisor must work to help differentiate the roles of social workers, nurses, and administrators. In religiously affiliated facilities, the administrator usually has a religious background. When administrators have not been trained to distinguish between the role of administrator and clergy, role strain can develop. When a social worker is brought into this situation, role confusion often develops, resulting in conflict, frustration, and isolation. Administrators who view their residents as a congregation to be ministered to unconsciously view themselves as *all-inclusive* administrators. They run the facility much as they performed their former clergy duties. They handle all the administrative tasks as well as counseling residents and their families. They are used to dealing with death, grief, guilt, and tragedy, and often they prefer these challenging tasks to mundane administrative tasks, which they are sometimes ill prepared to perform. A social worker operating in the shadow of such an administrator feels discounted and becomes frustrated and isolated in the organization. It is easy for an administrator to bypass a social worker at any level of education, experience, and skill. For example, the *all-inclusive* administrator can admit patients without involving any other staff, can counsel a dying patient on wills and burial arrangements, or can deal directly with the family of a dying patient (Munson, 1980b).

This problem can be dealt with by the supervisor through role differentiation on a potential and actual basis by conducting joint sessions with both the administrator and the social worker. These sessions should not be based on abstract explanations of organizational roles but should instead deal with specific case material that is problem oriented. In the process of discussing the case material, specific responsibilities should be delineated and agreed upon. Such cases should be discussed more than once and should be followed for several months until the problems are resolved. A secondary outcome of this process is that the administrator and social worker get a perspective on what happens to residents over time. This allows them to recognize indicators of change in functioning and adjustment of residents. The ongoing sessions also reinforce the role differentiation and prevent the administrator from falling back into the all-inclusive pattern. On certain occasions, it may be determined that the administrator should have more, rather than less, involvement with some residents. For example, the majority of LTCF residents, and the majority of social workers, are women. Male residents often feel isolated, and if a male administrator is present, informal involvement with the male residents can be helpful.

Regulations

Social work services in LTCFs are much needed, poorly developed, and little understood. They are the least-regulated service, and the meager regulations are marginally enforced. Enforcement of state and federal regulations varies from state to state, and although federal regulations mandate minimal standards, supplemental state regulations vary substantially. In addition, the qualifications of evaluators and surveyors differ from state to state. In some states evaluation is done by nurses, physicians, or social workers. Where social workers are employed or contracted with to serve on evaluation teams, they usually have little or no experience in LTCFs. This can be problematic because the evaluators have limited understanding of the role of the social worker in LTCFs, and they have even less understanding of the role of the supervisor. This is compounded when evaluators lack clarity about the regulations or how to evaluate their implementation.

Special attention is given to regulation because the supervisor is often expected to help the facility with the regulations and the regulators. It is easy for the neophyte supervisor to be overwhelmed by this staff concern and to devote a substantial portion of time to this subject. At the same time, the supervisor who refuses to discuss meeting regulations with the staff, because he or she views the supervisor's role as dealing with only practice problems, will not be viewed as helpful by the staff. Also, supervisor efforts to improve staff service delivery will have marginal effectiveness when dealing with a group perpetually concerned with meeting regulations.

Instead of being overwhelmed by or ignoring regulations, the supervisor should use regulations as a means of focusing content about organizing and delivering services. To do this, the supervisor must become thoroughly familiar with federal and state regulations and the guidelines used to implement the regulations. Usually, social service regulations are minimal and general enough to allow development of alternative styles of service delivery.

It is also helpful for the supervisor actually to participate in an evaluation of the facility to learn how evaluation reports are formulated and to assist staff at interpreting social services for the evaluators. The supervisor can assist survey team members to understand the role of social work in LTCFs and to evaluate the effectiveness of social work services. For example, in one survey an evaluator came to the conclusion that the social worker was not involved with the residents. When questioned about this, the surveyor admitted that the judgment was based solely on having asked several residents what the social worker's name was. It was explained by the staff that such a technique was not a reliable measure when dealing with a population that is known to have substantial short-term memory loss for various reasons. The staff explained and documented for the evaluator the amount and variety of contact and activity engaged in with the residents. Such information, which can be provided by only social work staff, can do much to add balance to an evaluation. To achieve such interaction, the staff must be trained to be active participants in the evaluation process, rather than passive recipients of judgments made by evaluators that are based on resident records and simple, but not necessarily relevant, questions asked of residents. Surveyors welcome such input from the staff; they have admitted possessing little knowledge, little guidance, and few skills at implementing social service regulations (Munson, 1981a).

Regulations can be used to train staff to work with residents. For example, regulations deal with documentation of social history data, treatment plans, and long-term and short-term goal setting. The supervisor can use documentation in any of these areas to establish how to gather data, what data to gather, how to determine priority of needs, how to establish goals, what goals to establish, and how to interrelate long-term and short-term goals. For example, social history data about the childhood development of a seventy-year-old resident is secondary to knowing what family members are available as a resource to the resident. In setting goals, workers and evaluators tend to think in global and total-recovery terms. Such thinking can divert the practitioner from understanding the real needs of old and incapacitated residents. Goals need to be thought of in basic and simple terms: getting a resident to sit up, to eat in the dining room, to talk. Regulations are geared more to when and where to document, and the role of the supervisor must be related to what and how to document. An entire training program for staff can be built around this basic premise.

Role Support

To carry out the role of the supervisor as defined here, the supervisor must have support at the highest level of the organization. For administrators, nurses, physicians, and other departments to cooperate, the supervisor must be perceived as understood, accepted, and supported by those who operate the facility. The supervisor must have access to the decision makers and must be viewed as working in conjunction with them. A supervisor who is expected simply to satisfy regulatory requirements has no basis on which to build an effective social work program.

The effective supervisor becomes a strong support for the social work staff as they carry out their jobs in a demanding setting. As other departments that do not have a similar type of supervisor see social workers gaining further training and education, having a forum for identifying and solving problems, and having assistance in dealing with regulations, they become envious and, at times, threatened. The social work supervisor can be of further assistance to the total functioning of the facility by advocating that others, such as nurses, administrators, physicians, and activities staff, be provided with supervisors, consultants, or parallel support systems (Munson, 1981a).

CRIMINAL JUSTICE SETTINGS

The main unique feature of criminal justice settings—for probation, parole, or incarceration—is the authority invested in the practitioner. Most young, inexperienced practitioners entering such settings have had little or no experience with the power and authority granted to courts and their representatives. Often they have not experienced court proceedings and do not understand the intricacies of the legal system. Also, practitioners are sometimes overwhelmed by the degree of pain and suffering inflicted on others by those who become their clients. Practitioners are often in the position of working with people who have radically different values from their own, and they react to these differences.

The supervisory role is similar in parole, probation, and institutional settings, especially with respect to authority issues. In institutional settings, the role of the family in relation to the adult offender should be given consideration in supervision of the practitioner. For the inmate, the role of family is sometimes forgotten, and the offender can be viewed by the staff exclusively in the context of institutional life. Tobin has pointed out that the practitioner can lose sight of the role of the inmate's family in promoting motivation for the offender to change through therapeutic intervention (Mishne, 1980:278). The supervisor should monitor the practitioner to ensure that this important aspect of the rehabilitation process is not neglected.

Group Home Settings

The role of the supervisor regarding child and adolescent offenders is discussed here in the context of group home settings, but the points can be applied to other criminal justice settings.

The trend has been toward shifting rehabilitation efforts for acting-out children and adolescents from large institutional settings to small group homes. Such group homes employ staff with varying degrees of training in clinical work with children and adolescents (Handler, 1975). Efforts have been made to identify the functions of the supervisor in these settings in relation to untrained staff. This section focuses on one aspect of that role, in which the staff and residents are viewed as a small group and the dynamics of staff interaction are reflected in resident behavior. The staff and resident group process is analyzed by exploring

1. achieving honest and clear communication,
2. accepting and using authority,
3. dealing with staff anxiety in threatening situations, and
4. developing appropriate levels of genuineness and self-awareness.

The discussion that follows is based on historic and current models of group home facilities that involve the following situations:

1. The director of the group home functions both as an administrator and as a frontline staff member.
2. All staff members are predominantly paraprofessionals who have little formal training in therapeutic relationships.
3. Staff and residents participate in regularly scheduled "house" meetings.
4. There are regularly scheduled staff meetings.
5. The program is based on a therapeutic model in which the staff are engaged in change efforts.

A cohesive, unified staff built on this model can be effective, regardless of the philosophic or theoretical basis on which the group home operates.

Before any change efforts can be effectively attempted, conditions must be created for honest and clear communication. This is basic in situations in which residents are accustomed to dealing with the world through manipulation, and staff are expected to accomplish a great deal with little training. Decision making is the basis of much interaction between staff and residents. The staff exist as a group, and the residents exist as a group. Individual behavior by a member of either group is often interpreted in a group context rather than on an individual basis. Behavior in this context is based on what Redl and Wineman (1952:20) identified in one of the earliest group home experiments as "social reality." Often the two groups are polarized around issues and problems, which results in no resolution and continuing frustration. When staff use group manipulation to deal with perceived resident manipulation, communication breaks down. This is epitomized in one resident's comment in a house meeting: "We ain't going to play the staff's games, so we don't expect you to play ours." This comment occurred after an incident in which the staff attempted to decrease "horseplay" in the house by increasing fines for such activity and notifying residents after the fact. Staff felt a need to make immediate decisions to maintain order in the house, but residents viewed this as a change in the rules without their input. The staff could have contained the horseplay more effectively by assessing repeated violations at the agreed-upon rates rather than increasing the amount for the sake of expediency. Rules are effectively applied only when they are carried out according to previously agreed-upon decisions that involved both the staff and resident groups.

Given the opportunity, residents as a *group* can develop self-regulation that removes the pressure from staff and allows them to intervene only when self-regulation fails. This allows the staff to avoid the "game-playing" stance, but it is difficult to achieve when staff live with the constant fear that interpersonal conflict will escalate out of control. This fear is real in an unstructured situation in which the staff group is smaller in number and often physically weaker than a resident group that has limited self-control under stress. Less control is not being recommended here, but control should be exercised as agreed upon. Residents will not adhere to rules when the staff are perceived as not observing them. It is recognized that unique situations develop that require immediate decision making. In situations of this type, it is important that the staff group subsequently communicates to the resident group why such decisions were made. When feedback is not provided, such staff decisions will be viewed by the resident group as arbitrary and punitive.

Individual residents use the group to negate individual deviance, as one resident's comment illustrates: "I was drinking in the house. So what? Everybody drinks in the house." The resident group will also focus on individual behavior to avoid group issues. This is illustrated when a group of residents dislikes a particular resident and reports the resident for various infractions, to which the disliked resident responds, "You just want to see me kicked out of the house." The staff must be trained to recognize this variable use of the individual and the group to avoid communication of the real issues. Both of the examples given demonstrate dysfunctional behavior that must be exploited for clinical purposes through use of what has been identified as "influence and interference techniques" (Redl and Wineman, 1951:41-46).

Use of authority comes with difficulty in any circumstance, and appropriate use of authority is even more difficult to attain. Young, untrained staff recognize the need for authority but at the same time question its use, since no exercise of authority goes unchallenged by the resident group. First, variations of authority within the staff group must be identified. The individual staff member's authority varies when on duty and off duty. In small, informal group homes with a milieu orientation, staff are frequently in the house when off duty. Residents often attempt to negate the authority of staff at such times. This can be handled by making clear that staff are invested with their authority at all times.

Staff are more likely to use authority when angry. Thus, residents see them exercise authority inconsistently. Staff often knowingly, in full view of residents, overlook infractions of the rules when activity in the house is calm and on a positive note, but the same infractions can result in the entire house being put on restriction when matters are going badly. The supervisor must help the staff to develop skill at exercising authority when they are not angry and to avoid using their authority excessively when angry. This balancing of power use can help the staff avoid the staff-resident standoffs that are so common in group homes. As one resident commented, after the staff had placed the entire house on warning in an angry display of authority, "You staff are idiots; with everybody on warning there are just going to be more fights in the house." What the resident was saying epitomizes the standoff situation: when staff put residents on warning in anger, the residents respond by putting staff on warning through their behavior.

There is space here only to make the generalization that authority must always be available for use, but it must be applied consistently and based on rational, rather than emotional, responses. There are many other authority issues, and the supervisor will find that the resolution of specific authority problems is endemic and must be dealt with regularly in staff meetings and house meetings.

The director exercises authority at another level. This can become problematic, conflictive, and confusing when the director also carries the role of frontline staff member because, when in the directorial role, he or she can use more sweeping authority in a resident encounter than a regular staff member can. The director must be helped to recognize this difference and encouraged to use the directorial authority sparingly when functioning as a staff member. The director who does not make this distinction will become isolated from residents, their feelings, and their behavior. The director is by nature in a difficult position and "is always the last one to know" about deviant behavior in the house. The power of the director is inherently recognized by the residents and other staff; by making the distinction just described, the difficulties of the position can be minimized, though certainly not overcome completely.

The supervisor has the most dubious authority. Supervisors can exercise much authority if they allow the staff to view them as experts and become dependent on them for decisions, or they can function solely as facilitators who allow the staff to work out all problems within the staff group. The most appropriate role for the supervisor is somewhere between these two extremes. The staff should rely on resident self-regulation as much as possible; the supervisor should rely on staff self-regulation to an even greater extent. To achieve this, the supervisor needs to meet regularly with the staff, and the focus of these meetings should be improved staff intervention through discussion of problem-solving efforts in the house. The supervisor is often the only source of support for individual staff members and the staff group. Staff have many conflicts and confrontations with residents that can be the focus of these sessions, but staff also have conflicts, disagreements, and occasional confrontations with one another that must be handled. Staff are more willing to discuss their conflicts with residents than their conflicts with one another, but staff conflict must be explored to promote more unified and healthy staff functioning. Residents are keen observers of weaknesses in staff relationships, and they will manipulate staff conflict. Frequently, the supervisor will learn about staff conflict from the residents before it is even identified by the staff.

Residents have authority that often is not recognized as such by the staff. Often residents are assigned duties related to the operation of the house that require supervision of other residents. Daily cleanup details and meal preparation are examples. Staff must be careful that assignment of such authority does not put some residents in a difficult position or give residents the opportunity to take advantage of a position of power. For example, it is appropriate to put a resident in charge of a cleanup detail, but the evaluation of the cleanup should be done by a staff member. Any authority granted to residents requires supervision by a staff member to avoid abuse, as well as to prevent the resident in authority from being subjected to what Redl and Wineman have defined as "social death" within the resident group as a result of being perceived as allied with the staff (Redl and Wineman, 1952:20).

The group home situation is sufficient to create anxiety in the most skilled practitioner. From the moment residents enter the home, their symptomatic behavior can overwhelm the staff with intensity and great velocity (Redl and Wineman, 1951:46). In the face of such behavior, untrained staff impose external controls rather than using the behavior for therapeutic purposes. This is only natural given the staff's coping mechanisms. External controls do not necessarily result in therapeutic change. Anxiety emerges from insufficient techniques for dealing with behavior, and when the few techniques available to the staff do not work, anxiety becomes more intense. The main strategy for the supervisor to use in decreasing staff anxiety is to help them develop nonthreatening interventive skills. The emphasis should be on using external controls only as a last resort. Staff need to be exposed to interventive techniques that encourage residents to develop internal control mechanisms. Anxiety can be lowered by removing some interaction from the resident group.

Staff should be supported and trained in doing individual counseling with residents. Issues such as drug use, sexual activity, and school performance can produce much less anxiety for a staff member and a resident when discussed in an individual relationship. The opposite is also true. At times sensitive issues cannot be articulated on an individual basis, and a group approach in which no individual is singled out allows exploration without provoking severe anxiety among residents or staff.

No amount of training or support will relieve all anxiety. Staff get anxious for the same reasons that residents do: lack of coping mechanisms (see Pearlin and Schooler, 1978). The more coping mechanisms the staff develop, the more coping mechanisms they can pass along to the residents. This is the essence of the therapeutic process in a group home. An anxiety-ridden staff will only increase anxiety among residents. It is in this area that the supervisor can contribute the most to the therapeutic program of the group home.

The helping professions have long been concerned with the importance of self-awareness in therapeutic relationships without much study of how much and what kind of self-awareness is appropriate. The concepts of genuineness and self-awareness are important for the staff who work in a highly unstructured environment in which roles are not well differentiated. Genuineness refers to sharing *how* one feels; self-awareness refers to knowing *what* one feels. Staff often engage in work activities, recreational activities, and leisure time directly with the residents as well as "living in" the house while on duty. Genuineness is more appropriately discussed in conjunction with staff-resident relationships, and self-awareness, in connection with staff relationships. Genuineness involves sharing with a resident *how* it makes you feel when a staff member is the object of a barrage of profanity, and self-awareness relates to discussing in a staff meeting why one responds personally to such an attack of profanity. In a threatening and anxiety-producing encounter with a resident, it is not always good to share fear and anxiety, but in a staff meeting, this can be discussed to develop self-awareness about what in the situation was threatening and anxiety producing, and how new and alternative coping mechanisms can be developed.

Self-awareness can be used in encounters with residents just as genuineness can be discussed in staff meetings. For example, during a house meeting, after genuinely sharing his feelings about how he deals with anger, the director was helped by residents and staff to develop the self-awareness that often, when he is angry, he responds inappropriately by placing restrictions on the entire resident group. As another example, in a staff meeting, the staff shared their feelings that a house meeting held earlier that day was "lousy." With help from the supervisor, they were able to be more genuine and share that what they really felt was discomfort because the meeting involved some intense, negative exchanges between staff and residents. They went on to discover that they rated meetings on the basis of control and that they associated comfort and good meetings with controlled sessions in which little genuine feeling was shared. Staff have a propensity to be more genuine when angry or frustrated, which can result in inappropriate sharing of feelings. The supervisor must work to help staff be genuine when they are in control, rather than being genuine only when they are out of control.

Genuineness and self-awareness discussed in the context of the work setting help staff develop cohesiveness, resulting in a positive, supportive work group. The supervisor has a responsibility to prevent such sharing from becoming therapeutically oriented and focused on the personalities of the individual staff members. When this type of sharing is the focus of the supervisor, the staff can become disillusioned, frustrated, and immobilized. Instead of concentrating on the motives of the staff for their behavior, the supervisor should function as a role model for positive therapeutic intervention with residents. To do this, the supervisor must have a well-articulated repertoire of interventive strategies and coping mechanisms, including appropriate levels of genuineness and self-awareness, specifically when working with aggressive, manipulative, and poorly socialized adolescents. The timid and insecure supervisor will quickly lose the respect of residents and staff and will increase anxiety, especially in the staff group.

Supervisors in the group home setting should monitor staff work with the community. Staff deal with a range of community-based professionals, including schools, courts, police, social services, therapists, and mental health practitioners. The supervisor should work to ensure that contact with community resources is frequent, communication is clear, and relationships are positive in nature. Group homes depend on community support, and good community relationships with professionals and agencies are essential.

RURAL PRACTICE SETTINGS

Are rural social work practitioners different? When reading the literature on rural practice, this question repeatedly emerges as a central theme. It is understandable that this is a common question, since social work has always been, and remains, substantially an urban phenomenon (Munson, 1980d). Articulation of rural practice has emerged in the shadow of urban practice. Conceptualization of rural practice cannot be effectively accomplished in comparison or contrast to urban practice. Too much time and effort have been devoted to differentiation of rural and urban practices that rarely goes beyond descriptions of clients, communities, and educational programs.

Supervision is an appropriate arena in which to begin to define and document rural practice. Much practice wisdom has been developed through the years around supervision, but only small portions of that wisdom have been preserved and transmitted in the literature.

Although rural social work practice is generic—the rural practitioner being a generalist—it should be kept in mind that rural practice is conducted in service-limited agencies (those having specific services to deliver and specific functions to perform). The terms *generic* and *generalist* have been used to perpetuate vagueness, uncertainty, and inconsistency about what is done in rural practice. The fact remains that in rural areas, clients come to social services departments, courts, family service agencies, nursing homes, and mental health centers for services that are specific to the agency. Networks of agencies in rural areas offer good, coordinated services, but at the same time, "generalist" supervisors and workers will refer clients to other agencies because they have a "family problem" or an "emotional problem."

With more trained workers being employed in rural areas, supervision needs to relate more to the capabilities and limitations of the workers. Many BSW-level workers have been trained in interventive skills that go unused because they are encouraged to rely on the generalist practices of referral and coordination of services that often exist only on paper. It is essential that the MSW-level professional reach out to the BSW worker to offer parallel services to some clients. In this context, it might be good to revive the former practice of having a mental health worker, at the insistence of a supervisor, contact a BSW social worker and his or her supervisor in public social services or corrections to coordinate service delivery. Distance and travel are compounding factors in rural areas, but coordination of home visits and agency visits for this purpose can be accomplished. Often social service caseworkers or probation workers transport clients to a mental health centers, sit in the waiting room during the visit, and never have any contact with the mental health staff. In rural areas, one overlooked function of the supervisor is that of helping the supervisee effectively utilize services and information provided by other professionals. The MSW worker needs to reach out to other professionals, but often this does not happen. Workers need to be assisted by supervisors in providing information and intervention when it is not requested. Passivity among timid workers contributes to ineffective practice and is an appropriate issue for supervision.

Self-Reliance

It has been held that supervision is hard to find in rural practice (Ginsberg, 1976) and, therefore, that the worker must be self-reliant. In many instances, supervision is unsolicited rather than unavailable. Generalist workers can be subjected to the subtle suggestion that they are not being "good generalists" if they need help with cases—that they are not being self-reliant. It is easy for supervisors to convey this message to the worker unwittingly, since the self-reliant worker makes few or no demands on the supervisor. If worker dependency is suspected, this can be addressed in the supervision process. When personal and professional performance intermingle in supervision, supervisors have the responsibility to ensure that they supervise the position and not the person (Munson, 1976).

Self-reliance is not synonymous with good practice. Many self-reliant workers are inefficient and ineffective, and their self-reliance allows them to avoid being accountable. To ensure that self-reliance is genuine and appropriate requires periodic evaluation of the worker's practice, and evaluation is best achieved within sound, sensitive supervision. Evaluation must be carried out within a larger context of supervision that is oriented toward promoting growth and development of the worker. Supervision carried out exclusively for the purpose of evaluation becomes merely "checking up," which can lead to worker and supervisor resentment. Evaluation should be periodic, expected, scheduled, consistent, goal oriented, and verbal as well as written. It should provide continuity and contain input from both parties. Further, evaluation should deal only with worker activity of which the supervisor has direct knowledge. Evaluation based on speculation about behavior is to be avoided.

Self-reliance and autonomy are not synonymous with self-monitoring. Self-monitoring involves a deliberate process in which the worker evaluates his or her practice and decisions made in practice. Self-reliance relates to the power to make decisions in the midst of a practice situation, since autonomy is oriented to the present. Self-monitoring involves after-the-fact evaluation of decision making. The granting of autonomy to the worker should be on the basis of trust in the worker's decision-making ability in his or her practice, and not because the supervisor has little time to deal with problems. Too often workers perceive their autonomy as deriving from supervisor default rather than from a design to promote autonomy. The case example that follows illustrates these points:

A social worker in a rural nursing home appealed to her supervisor, the facility administrator, for help with an eighty-three-year-old man who had been a resident for a year. He was depicted as gradually getting worse. The patient was described as "depressed," "having hallucinations," and "paranoid." He reported seeing strange objects and former family members in his room at night, especially his deceased wife. The patient was nervous, confused at times, and hinted at suicide. This created mixed feelings among the staff, since they were not certain whether the patient was capable of committing suicide. He would fight off staff and other residents when they attempted to get him out of his room. The facility physician recommended a psychiatric evaluation. The social worker had observed that the patient's deviant behavior followed a cyclical pattern as his medication was altered. Rather than discussing the mechanics of the referral, the administrator merely approved the referral and indicated that funds were available to pay for the psychiatric evaluation. The worker had never done a referral to a mental health center, and this is what she really was asking for help with, but the administrator was not prepared to provide supervision in this area. The worker, left on her own, made the following decisions: the patient was not told of the referral until the day of the psychiatric visit, resulting in an increase in his paranoia, hostility, and depression; an aide was assigned to transport the patient the twenty-four miles to the mental health center; and no list of questions, social history, or description of symptoms and behavior was prepared for the psychiatrist. This resulted in the patient's appearing normal and rational to the psychiatrist, and the written evaluation was of little value to the social worker or the nursing home staff because the report was mostly a new version of the patient's social history already in the facility's records.

With social work supervision provided after the fact, the worker was able to see that the patient should have been prepared for the referral in advance, that the social worker should have accompanied the patient to the mental health center, that a special list of questions should have been prepared for the psychiatrist (especially questions about the role of medication and suicidal threats), and that the worker should have met with the psychiatrist to formulate recommendations and a treatment plan to be implemented with the patient in the facility. These steps could have been the basis for future case evaluation and planning of additional treatment goals.

This is one example of how self-reliance does not always result in good practice. Good supervision could have avoided this waste of time and the resulting sense on the part of the LTCF staff that psychiatrists can be of little assistance in dealing with the institutionalized elderly. Another problem that developed from the worker's random autonomy and limited intuitive self-reliance in this case was that the patient's family was not notified of the psychiatric evaluation. When family members later learned of the referral, they demanded a meeting with the social worker to express their anger about the facility staff's seeing their relative as "crazy." The family members were concerned, and justifiably, about the intervention of a psychiatrist since no member of their family had ever been considered mentally ill.

Defining Need

The agency should make every effort to provide supervision for the worker, and the worker should actively seek supervision. When supervision is demanded and the need for it well articulated, agency administrators will normally make every effort to see that it is provided. When supervision cannot be effectively provided, an acceptable alternative is to bring a qualified consultant to the agency or to have the worker go to another agency in the community for consultation. When nonagency consultants are sought, workers must ensure that the consultation meets their specific needs and must be assertive about their needs when they are not being met. Another case example illustrates this point:

A rural social services department hired an MSW consultant from the local mental health clinic for its protective service workers. The consultant came to the agency once a week and held individual consultation sessions with the three workers. The consultant was considered sensitive and helpful. One worker had been assigned a case in which a young couple had appeared in court several times for neglect of their four children. The father had recently been laid off from his seasonal orchard work. The family was suffering increased economic deprivation, and the worker's home visits led her to believe the youngest child was being abused. A court hearing was held, and the child was ordered removed from the home and placed in temporary foster care. The worker brought this case to the consultant for discussion, and the consultant offered advice on how to approach the family. The worker hesitated to act and continued to raise questions about the case. The consultant listened in a sensitive manner but failed to pick up on the worker's real concern. Finally, the worker raised the issue. The worker was afraid to go to the home alone to remove the child. After the court hearing, the father told the worker that he would take whatever steps were necessary to prevent removal of the child, including violence. The father's history indicated that he was quite capable of acting on his threats, and during past visits the worker had observed several rifles in the home. The consultant supported the worker and recommended to the director of the social services department that arrangements be made to have the state police accompany the worker to the home for the removal of the child. The director agreed to this arrangement, the child was removed without incident, and the worker was greatly relieved.

Workers in rural areas are sometimes placed in threatening situations that are not recognized or taken seriously by administrators and supervisors. Workers often report being threatened with firearms, physical assault, and attack by animals (mainly dogs). Consultants and supervisors should be sensitive to such threatening situations, and when they are not, the workers should not hesitate to share their feelings.

Use of Relationship

It has been argued that relationship is a key concept in rural social work practice (Davies, 1974). The use of relationship is not unique to rural practice and is an essential component of all forms of social work practice, regardless of where the practice is carried out. The informality of relationship has been carried to the extreme in much of rural practice, as is illustrated by this statement: "The most destructive professional in the rural area is the one who maintains a 'clinical' objective involvement with those he serves, this defense driving him further from rapport" (Davies, 1974:511). Such statements need qualification.

Research shows that clients relate better to workers they perceive as different from themselves (Munson and Balgopal, 1978). A client, regardless of his station in life or geographic location, desires a worker who has knowledge and is trained to perform in an objective manner. All theorists who have described the professional relationship view it as unique and as requiring a delicate balance between empathic objectivity and "disciplined subjectivity" (Kadushin, 1972: 58). It requires of the worker a certain degree of emotional and social distance—a greater degree of authority and control, self-awareness, and self-discipline than is expected of the client (Siporin, 1975:205). To conduct an interview, a social worker must engage in more than a "folksy" conversation with the client (Kadushin, 1972:8-11). In rural areas, "who you know is as valuable as what you know" (Davies, 1974:510), but the worker must know a substantial amount about services and practice principles to be effective.

The supervisor can be especially helpful to the worker in maintaining an appropriate balance between objectivity and subjectivity in professional relationships. The concepts of primary and secondary relationships can serve as a guide to supervisors. Primary relationships involve an atmosphere in which the participants exchange intimate knowledge, act and react with some degree of spontaneity, and provide realistic conceptions of themselves and of what others expect of them. Secondary relationships are based on a necessity for cooperation that exists for the fulfillment of aims or goals of interaction of short duration with little emotional or personal involvement. Social workers engage in both types of relationships. Depending upon the setting and how the situation is defined, some workers engage exclusively in primary or secondary relationships, and other practitioners alternate between the two forms. A paraprofessional food stamp interviewer in a social services department engages exclusively in secondary relationships with clients; a practitioner in private practice is more likely to develop only primary relationships with clients. A caseworker in a social services department or a mental health clinic uses both types, depending upon the situation.

Workers who have only brief contact with clients mistakenly minimize the importance of relationship, and those who interact with clients over long periods of time tend to overemphasize the importance of relationship. Primary social work relationships can be associated more with psychotherapeutic efforts to change personality and patterns of social relations; secondary relationships deal more with provision of concrete, tangible services. Both types involve varying emotional, temporal, and structural elements. If there is to be conscious use of relationship by the worker to promote change in the client, the worker must offer the client a differential model for identification at given points in the relationship. A young, African-American, BSW social worker who was the only African-American worker in a rural mental health clinic made the following observation, which illustrates this point:

> When I went to work here at the clinic, my supervisor decided to start me off by giving me all black clients since, as she put it, "I could identify the problems more easily and accomplish more in less time since I was black and could readily identify with black clients." I agreed and really thought it would be so easy for me, and I was relieved that I didn't have a lot of white clients to start out with. Well, it was terrible. It was a mistake. Since I was black, the clients felt they didn't have to explain anything. They would get angry because I didn't know exactly what they were talking about. I even had one client tell me I was dumb. After a while, my supervisor realized the problem and gave me a mixed caseload; but in the meantime, I was so frustrated I almost quit.

If the supervisor had recognized the importance of differentiation in relationship, a great deal of frustration on the part of the worker, the clients, and the supervisor could have been avoided.

The worker should refrain from engaging in a cold, calculated objectivity that creates a distance between the worker and the client, and the practitioner should engage in a sensitive, empathic objectivity that enhances relationship and rapport, rather than decreases it. The tendency among rural practitioners is to abandon theory and put in its place "down home" philosophy when conceptualizing practice (Munson, 1979d). This could explain why social workers are not called upon to contribute to efforts to confront rural problems (Coppedge and Davis, 1977).

SUBSTANCE ABUSE TREATMENT

The direct and indirect costs of substance use in the United States are more than $300 billion annually, and substance use is a major health problem (APA, 2000b). The diagnosis and treatment of substance and alcohol problems is complex and can be confusing. The term *addiction* has been criticized and abandoned by the APA in its diagnostic manual. The term *addiction* is used here as a generic term and is not intended to have any precise technical meaning. It is used to refer to persons who frequently use drugs and spend much time focused on using drugs, obtaining drugs, or talking about drugs (Ray and Ksir, 1996).

Supervision in settings that address issues of substance and alcohol use and abuse has become more complex as the knowledge of the effects of substances and alcohol has increased. Diagnosis, assessment, and treatment have become more complex as well. The largest section in the DSM-IV-TR covers the substance-related disorders, representing 15.6 percent of the manual (Munson, 2000b).

The supervisor must ensure that practitioners in this area have thorough knowledge of the diagnostic criteria for specific substance disorders and the ability to do differential diagnosis. Since substances and alcohol are often used in self-medication, other mental disorders can be masked. Disorders such as depression, anxiety, and dissociation can coexist with numerous other mental disorders, and the practitioner must be aware of the dual nature of these disorders. The diagnostic distinctions between substance use, dependence, intoxication, and withdrawal must be understood. The clinician must know the criteria for full and partial remission.

The supervisor should ensure that practitioners know the importance of thorough assessment and are able to administer and interpret standardized measures and scales related to addiction. Practitioners who enter the field of substance and alcohol problems after working in more general areas of practice will have difficulty understanding the importance of the more technical and precise nature of documenting the person's history and current use of substances and alcohol. Such practitioners may not be attuned to the propensity of substance/alcohol users to manipulate, charm, and lie to the therapist in order to continue their habit. Practitioners who have not been trained in the characteristics of persons with addictions can become frustrated and disillusioned when clients take advantage of their good intentions.

The treatment of addictive disorders also requires special understanding by the supervisor and practitioner. Treatment protocols for addicts are more precise than in many other mental health settings. The decision to use drug-free intervention or substitution can be a difficult and challenging one, but, fortunately, it is usually not made by individual practitioners. The physical risk of substance and alcohol abuse must be taken into account as part of treatment planning. Client pregnancy or physical disorders can complicate intervention. The treatment activity often requires the practitioner to have many collateral contacts in order to be of maximum assistance to clients, and this level of activity can be frustrating to some practitioners. Clients who violate the law to support their habits can bring the practitioner into contact with law enforcement and criminal justice professionals, and some practitioners may not want to work with authority figures. Treatment activity can be much more diverse than in other practice areas. Treatment of cocaine, alcohol, cannabis, and polysubstance abuse can require very different treatment approaches.

The complex and demanding nature of addictions work coupled with the chronic nature of substance use disorders can lead to worker stress. The supervisor in addictions settings needs to be constantly alert to the potential for stress-related problems.

The difficult nature of practice and supervision in the addictions field has been addressed in an overlapping, four-foci model of supervision developed by Powell and Brodsky (1993). This model views supervisor functions as administrative, evaluative, clinical, and supportive. The four areas are used to provide direction for the supervisor and the practitioner in addressing the addictions practice areas covered here.

DOMESTIC VIOLENCE PROGRAMS

Domestic violence has only recently been recognized as a major national problem. The concern for domestic violence has been slowly emerging since the 1970s as an outgrowth of the modern women's movement. By the mid-1990s, the incidence rate had reached 4 million cases per year. In one study, 35 percent of victims had been assaulted daily, 45 percent had been assaulted during pregnancy, and 75 percent of the assailants spent less than eighteen hours in jail (Berry, 1998). Each year millions of women are wounded, crippled, disfigured, and traumatized by male partners. Annually 1,500 women are killed by current or former male companions. In 90 percent of the killings, there was at least one prior report of abuse. The average number of police contacts prior to a domestic homicide is eight. Domestic violence contributes to 24 percent of female suicide attempts. One of every three women (or 1 million women) treated in hospital emergency rooms are the victims of domestic violence. Medical expenses for treating victims of domestic violence average $3 billion to $5 billion annually. Women make up 95 percent of the total victims of domestic violence. Of men who abuse female partners, 50 to 70 percent also abuse children and pets in the home. If four or more children are in the home, the incidence rate climbs to 90 percent (Berry, 1998).

These extensive statistics, which are only the highlights of many more disturbing statistics, are presented to illustrate how difficult and complex this area of practice can be. Practitioners and supervisors who work in batterers programs, women's counselling programs, and shelter programs for women and children deal with a daily caseload of pain, suffering, fear, harm, poverty, anxiety, depression, and numerous other mental problems that clients present. The supervisor in such settings needs to assist beginning workers with the density of the despair present in these settings. Female workers can develop anger at males, and male workers can begin to experience guilt. Supervisors cannot overlook the personal responses of practitioners to work in domestic violence settings. Anger at law enforcement and the courts can arise from the feeling that little is being done to protect clients. The immediacy of many interventions, such as providing emergency care for a fleeing mother and her children, can take a toll on the most resilient of practitioners.

The process of assessing past history to predict the potential for future violence in a relationship is difficult. Some crude measures do exist (see Visual 6.1, Domestic Violence Rapid Assessment Scale, in Chapter 6). The assessment of violence potential should be done only for treatment planning and should not be used to assess risk for women who are planning to return to live with their abusers. Clinicians should be cautious and always alert to the risks associated with a woman's returning to an untreated abuser, and they should not reassure the woman about the possibility of less risk of violence upon return.

The sense of desperation that can occur when a family must leave a shelter after a mandated limit of stay, even though the family has no safe place to go, can dishearten clinicians. If a family leaves a shelter to return to living with the perpetrator, practitioners can feel that they have failed. The treatment process can be difficult when the woman takes the stance that her behavior caused the abuse or that she can change the abuser. These reactions can result in the worker experiencing the same feelings of powerlessness that the woman has expressed in making her decisions. The parallel process that emerges in domestic violence work is always present. Supervisors need to give much support and encouragement to workers in domestic violence settings.

Research shows that most women make several false starts before finally leaving a batterer, but once the decision is made, the lives of women change significantly. This does not mean that departure is the solution to all problems. Research has documented that after departure stalking can occur, threats can increase, financial problems can get worse, the need for mental health treatment can arise, and available housing may be substandard, but the passage of time usually brings improved functioning and mental health (Jacobson and Gottman, 1998). Supervisors need to help clinicians develop patience and a willingness not to be assertive and demanding with women as they go through the struggle of leaving a relationship.

Practitioners need to learn the dynamics and histories of batterers and their mates. Certain dynamics are usually present in men and women who become involved in these complex relationships, and practitioners must have a thorough grounding in understanding the problems faced by these clients. Both the men and women come from backgrounds that often involve violence and control issues (Dutton, 1998; Jacobson and Gottman, 1998).

Violent men have impact on not only their mates and children. These men encounter difficulty in relation to other extended family members, employers, law enforcement, and courts. They intimidate numerous people and often cause others to withdraw from them out of fear, leaving them to continue to abuse. The intimidation and fear that abusers generate extend to the clinicians who are involved with the families as well as supervisors and agency directors. When a batterer threatens a client, all levels of agency staff can become intimidated if they do not know how to react or what to do for fear of making the situation worse. This results in a process that can cause individual clinicians and supervisors to enter a helpless state that can lead to a thought process that parallels the clients' thinking. Practitioners and supervisors can develop denial ("I cannot imagine he would do it; he is all talk"), disbelief ("She is exaggerating"), avoidance ("Just keep quiet and this will perhaps all blow over and settle down"), or wishful thinking ("Maybe he will leave town") (see Visual 13.1). Because of the possibility of such a dynamic, agencies should use staffing sessions employing a team approach in which there is multiple input regarding how to deal with known threats of violence against a client. Only through a team approach can the parallel process response of the individual practitioner be avoided. The supervisor should have a key role in coordinating the teaming of global intimidation.

CHILD AND ADOLESCENT THERAPY

Supervision of child treatment presents challenges to the supervisor. The field of child treatment is much more complex today than it was in the 1950s and 1970s, when the primary reason for children entering treatment was sib-

VISUAL 13.1. Domestic Violence and Parallel Process in Supervision

ling rivalry and hyperactivity. Today the majority of children enter treatment because of physical and sexual abuse, neglect, witnessing traumatic events, or loss associated with parental abandonment or separation. These children have a range of mental disorders, but most often oppositional defiant disorder, conduct disorder, major depressive disorder, dysthymia, or an anxiety disorder (Munson, 2000b). The incidence of physical and sexual abuse of children has increased from 10,000 reported cases in 1962 to 2.9 million cases by the mid-1990s. Some estimates suggest that the actual number of cases is much higher (Wells, 1995).

Although most schools of social work do not teach child intervention, and there are no books or articles on supervision of child and adolescent therapy, a significant amount of research does focus on diagnosis and assessment of children beginning in the early 1990s. This research was slow in developing and gradually emerged after the 1960s' research on the "battered child syndrome" (Trickett and Schellenbach, 1998). So much research is available now on various child and adolescent disorders that one of the roles of supervisors in this area of practice is to ensure that clinicians are up to date on the latest knowledge. The research about diagnosis and assessment of children far exceeds the research on treatment. A number of books and articles are available on intervention, but most of the methods and techniques of intervention are not based on research, and little empirical evidence supports any forms of child and adolescent intervention. The lack of empirical research on child interventions calls attention to another key role of the supervisor in monitoring practitioner intervention with children and adolescents; that is, the supervisor must ensure that the techniques being used are producing results. If no progress is being made, the supervisor has a responsibility to review with the supervisee different approaches.

New clinicians and seasoned practitioners who have just started treatment of children will need much supervisory assistance, and no professional should attempt to supervise child and adolescent therapists without substantial experience in working with this population. The limitations of the practitioner entering child intervention for the first time were made clear to the author when an experienced colleague requested a consultation session with me. She started the session by saying that her practice was declining because of the decreased referrals from managed cost organizations. She had decided to "take up the slack by starting to see children." She had received several referrals but was finding the work difficult. She was surprised that children were different from adults, and she thought that buying some toys to use with the children might help. She wanted the consultation with me to get ideas about what toys to buy. This encounter highlighted the need for specialty training requirements for mental health professionals before beginning work with children. Doing child intervention is more complicated than knowing what toys to have in the office.

The main task of the supervisor with the clinician new to child treatment is to assist the worker in how to understand the child's view of the world and how to then relate to the child's world. Most adults are used to talking to adults and treat children as little adults. Therapists are trained mostly in direct means of intervention, which is talking with clients. With children the therapist must rely more on indirect means of intervention; that is, the therapist must use play and games to access the child's world. The use of indirect interventions makes it much more difficult to interpret the meaning of the client's responses. The supervisor must spend time analyzing the accuracy of the supervisee's interpretation of the meaning that has been applied to symbolic material. The clinician must rely more on collateral contacts (parents, caregivers, teachers, probation officers, siblings, playmates, etc.) to confirm interpretations.

Assessment of children is different from that of adults. Any diagnosis or assessment of a child should include an evaluation of the child's developmental level of functioning. Most children entering treatment today have suffered trauma or maltreatment. If these events occur over time and at an early age (prior to age ten), they most likely will produce developmental delays in physical development, language skills, academic skills (reading, writing, and mathematics), interpersonal skills, communication, and intelligence. Most developmental delays caused by trauma and maltreatment can be overcome if the child receives early intervention. For example, language skills are significantly influenced by abuse and trauma. In one of the few studies done of language skills of victimized children, it was found that 65 percent had receptive or expressive language delays (Munson, 2000a). This is significantly higher than the average rate of 20 percent found in public school settings. A significant number of children who receive a six- to eight-week remedial language program can overcome these language delays. This illustrates the importance of screening all children who enter therapy. One in five children who enter therapy and have not been victimized will have a language delay, and one in three children who have been victimized will have language delays. Therapists need to screen for language and other developmental delays and make referrals if delays are discovered. If the therapist does not have the ability to assess the child's development, then the child should be referred for a developmental assessment as part of the treatment plan. To treat children without knowledge of developmental level can, at best, result in no positive outcome and, at worst, cause further harm to the child through failing to provide developmentally focused intervention. The practitioner does not have to be a developmental psychologist to do basic developmental screening of children. Brief screening instruments and strategies can be learned and used by clinicians (Munson, 2001a). The supervisor should provide practitioners with the skills to do developmentally oriented assessment.

In the course of treating children and adolescents, the therapist will likely learn of abuse or neglect. Reporting of such information is mandatory (see Chapter 11 for information on reporting). Clinicians will often resist reporting abuse and neglect. Supervisors should review mandatory reporting requirements with supervisees for their jurisdiction and have a clear policy of the internal process for reporting. A clinician should not make a mandatory report without discussing it with the supervisor first, and a supervisor should not approve the reporting without first notifying the program director or agency director. Any action as significant as mandatory reporting should be reviewed at all levels of the organization before a report is made. This will ensure agency support for the action and prevent a higher-level administrator from receiving an telephone call from an abuse investigator, police officer, or reporter and having to admit that he or she has no knowledge of the situation. The clinician should be assisted in informing the child's nonoffending caregiver about the report and in how to review the report with the caregiver. The caregiver may want to change therapists after reviewing the report. This is rarely the case, but it should be an option offered to the person responsible for the child's care. If domestic violence has also been involved, the caregiver of the child may be at risk if the abuser has been violent with the caregiver in the past. In this situation, the therapist may have to offer protective assistance to the adult.

Supervisors have to be supportive of therapists in the process of intervention. Some therapists are task and goal oriented, and managed cost organizations pressure therapists to be completely goal and outcome oriented. Therapists in this position can become frustrated and feel that specific goals are not being reached with children. Play can be viewed as "unproductive." The supervisor should help the therapist appreciate that children do not subscribe to managed cost models and that the therapist needs to articulate why specific interventions are being made. For example, if puppet play is used as a technique, then the therapist should explain the specific content of the puppet interview. The therapist and supervisor should work out in advance what the theme of the puppet interview is to be and what questions will be asked of the child. Will the theme be, for example, sibling conflict, how to follow rules, being afraid of adults, or loss and grief? Once the theme is selected, the therapist will have to decide how follow-up of the activity will be conducted to measure the impact of the intervention. The supervisor and therapist can accomplish the intervention measurement in numerous ways (Munson, 2001a).

The Traumatized Child

Mental health practitioners are increasingly treating children who have suffered traumas, as society becomes more violent and less caring about the needs of children. The United States repeatedly ranks low among industrialized countries when it comes to the care and protection of children. The glaring lack of regard for children is readily documented, but generally ignored (Munson, 1994b).

Children who experience trauma rarely receive treatment. Most childhood trauma goes undetected or unreported. When it is reported, the victim is not likely to be treated because the courts and child care agencies do not recognize the psychological effects of trauma. Ironically, in many instances in which a perpetrator is involved, that person gets more treatment than the victim. In cases of direct trauma, such as sexual assault, the victim is often referred for mental health treatment, but in many instances the family fails to follow through or terminates treatment after a brief period. Children who witness events that produce trauma are not usually referred for treatment because police, judges, and social workers do not recognize or understand the long-term effects of trauma resulting from witnessing events.

Supervisors must ensure that traumatized children are not subjected to subtle victimization by therapists who are not trained to treat trauma victims. Three brief case vignettes illustrate some of the problems that can arise:

> Barry is a ten-year-old who directly suffered and witnessed trauma while in the care of his alcohol- and drug-abusing parents. At age two, he was placed in the care of his grandmother, who has struggled to provide a normal childhood for Barry. Barry's father was recently released from prison after serving three years for assault with a deadly weapon. The grandmother has been trying to care for Barry and support her son until he is able to find work. The grandmother became ill, and her doctor told her that she must have bed rest at least twelve to sixteen hours per day. The grandmother is very upset because she cannot care for her grandson. Her therapist told her that the solution was to have Barry "take on more responsibility" and "do the cooking, cleaning of the house, and the laundry."

> Heather was repeatedly sexually abused by her father for six years, beginning when she was age six. She was practically held prisoner, and many days the father would keep her home from school to have sex with her. She was removed from the home and placed in residential care. She had a problem with masturbating through her clothes in public places, especially school. She was referred for therapy, and the therapist gave Heather a book on masturbation and instructed the child care worker in the facility to take Heather to her room and "teach her how to masturbate in private." The residential facility director was shocked and sought the advice of a consultant who specializes in child sexual abuse. The consultant advised against implementing this plan.

> Mary was repeatedly sexually abused from age three to six by her mother and the mother's boyfriends. The Department of Social Ser-

vices (DSS) permanently severed the mother's rights and placed Mary in foster care. Mary was in three different foster homes over four years. She adjusted nicely in a fourth foster home and was there for two years. The foster parents told Mary they were going to adopt her, but after an older child in the home committed suicide, the family changed their plans to adopt. Mary was taken to a mental health center for treatment. Mary was a pleasant and cooperative child. After two sessions the child was terminated from therapy because she was "adjusting to the loss and the changed adoption plans." Mary became oppositional at home and was later taken to a therapist who specialized in the treatment of traumatized children. The therapist did an extensive evaluation that included testing. It was discovered that Mary was depressed and had some symptoms of anxiety. She had expressive language delays that prevented her from adequately expressing to others how she felt about what had happened to her. She was immediately started in intensive psychotherapy.

These brief examples from complex cases illustrate the revictimization of children by professionals and highlight a number of problems that effective supervision could have prevented. In the case of Barry, the therapist failed to see how she was victimizing Barry by "parentifying" him, a strategy that when used by parents is viewed as dysfunctional by most therapists. Heather was being further "sexualized" by the therapist; she would be symbolically imprisoned by the child care worker, just as her father did, if the privacy plan were carried out; and her compulsive behavior would be reinforced by the therapist's strategy. In the case of Mary, the therapist assessed the child on the basis of her presenting demeanor and did not consider the underlying dynamics nor conduct a thorough evaluation to establish a treatment plan. Instead she had two sessions with the child and sent her away as "adjusted." These errors in child intervention can be attributed to lack of training in and understanding of childhood trauma.

In the United States, no educational programs focus exclusively on the needs of traumatized children, even though symptoms of trauma are present in the overwhelming majority of children receiving mental health treatment. The training of therapists in this area is inadequate, and many child therapists do not know how to recognize or diagnose childhood trauma. This inability to recognize trauma symptoms can subject the child to professional revictimization, as the practitioner treats the child for other symptoms or focuses on the child's problems in other areas, when instead these problems stem directly from the trauma. As long as the trauma remains untreated, such behaviors or symptoms persist.

There are no specialty licenses or credentials for doing child therapy with traumatized children, but numerous play therapy institutes are emerging. Although some of these institutes are quite good and offer quality programs, many are faddish and lack depth of training. Play therapy institutes usually focus on general play therapy techniques and offer little training in trauma work. In most disciplines, practitioners have little or no training in child development, developmental psychopathology, childhood disorders, or child treatment theory or practice. It is possible for graduates of MSW programs to enter child therapy work without taking a single course related to child intervention. There are no specializations in child treatment, and no courses in supervision of child treatment are offered in social work schools. This is difficult to understand, considering the highly technical and sensitive nature of child diagnosis and intervention and the fact that social workers come in contact with traumatized children more than professionals in any other discipline. The lack of training opportunities draws attention to the importance of the supervisor in child trauma work. Supervisors must be knowledgeable about child trauma because they may be the only source of learning and skill development available for the clinicians working with this population.

These failures are in part a reflection of the societal lip service with regard to children. The United States has a young-adult orientation that leads to little concern for the very old or the very young. This is reflected in all aspects of child intervention. Most diagnostic categories for children are based on adult models. This is especially true of trauma. In the APA's diagnostic and statistical manual, the only category relating to trauma in children is the post-traumatic stress disorder (PTSD) diagnosis. This diagnosis is based on research done with Vietnam veterans. Although this diagnosis is commonly given to children, its manifestations frequently do not pertain to the reactions that children present when entering treatment. Supervisors need to be sensitive to the importance of differential diagnosis in child trauma work. For example, only 13 percent of child trauma victims meet the criteria for PTSD, while major depressive disorder and dysthymic disorder are underdiagnosed in this population.

The medications used for childhood psychiatric disorders are usually hand-me-downs of medications developed for use with adults. This is illustrated by the widespread use of antidepressant medications with children. The same is true of theories of behavior and theories of intervention. Few theories focus exclusively on child development or child intervention. Currently, there is much criticism of psychoanalytic theory, but at least the psychoanalytic schools of thought have devoted more attention to child development. This grounding in child development could be a contributing factor to the decreased use of psychoanalytic theory in an era when brief therapy pervades mental health theory and service.

Supervisors need to help supervisees focus on the developmental aspects of assessment and intervention with this population. Clinicians should be encouraged to draw on diverse intervention theories based on the needs of the child. For example, even though psychoanalytic theory has been criticized, it has been found to be effective in work with conduct disordered children. This is most likely due to the theory's emphasis on the role of attachment, and conduct disordered children are prone to having attachment failures.

The decreased emphasis on psychoanalytic theory is also related to the increasing influence of managed cost organizations. Managed cost companies in many ways are replacing supervision. The managed care staff determine who will do the treatment, what interventions are acceptable, the length of treatment, what modalities are acceptable, and the cost of care, along with a host of other subtle control mechanisms that influence process and outcome. Such rigid control by external treatment managers leaves little time or desire for supervision. Some managed cost plans will not pay for child treatment or severely limit the amount and type of treatment. This is another mirroring of the general societal disregard of children. Severely traumatized children cannot be treated in the twelve to twenty sessions that most managed cost companies support. The staff of managed cost companies have little or no understanding of, experience working with, or education in children and trauma.

No research centers focus on traumatized children. Although the federal government does have a small program that supports research on childhood trauma. Most of the research on trauma in children deals with child physical and/or sexual abuse. The physical and sexual abuse research has focused almost exclusively on diagnosis, identification, demographics, and incidence of abuse, while little research has been done on effective intervention strategies. Child sexual abuse is one form of trauma in children, but it is not the only form. Trauma also results from witnessing violence, loss, separation, neglect, accidents, and natural disasters, though little research has been done in these areas. Research that has been conducted shows that many children suffer from multiple forms of trauma, and these severe cases produce different responses from those of children who experience single-incident traumas. Supervisors should monitor supervisee evaluations and establish that the clinician has done a thorough trauma history as part of the intake process, including a chronology and sequencing of the traumatic events, calculation of the intensity of each event, review of the severity of each event, determination of the duration of each event, and assessment of the event or events that are causing the most disturbance for the child currently. Increased knowledge about childhood trauma has shown that different traumas produce different reactions in children, and that a singular diagnostic classification such as PTSD does not adequately address the treatment planning needs of traumatized children.

It is difficult to understand or explain why, as practice becomes more complex and stressful, there is decreased emphasis on supervision of practice. Supervisors who are faced with supervising child therapists have limited literature to guide treatment and supervisory planning. Although there is an abundance of workshops on generic child therapy, no seminars focus on trauma treatment or supervision in this area. Child therapy with traumatized children can be one of the most demanding and stressful forms of psychotherapeutic work. The parallel process and countertransference issues that can occur in work with traumatized children are significant. The development of symptoms in the therapist that parallel the child's reaction is common, and identification with the vulnerable child is ever present. A sustained workload in this area can result in significant changes in the therapist's view of the world. Most therapists who work with traumatized children will have strong reactions to the suffering that children endure. Without competent supervision, the therapists can suffer significant psychological impairment. It is imperative that more adequate training for therapists and supervisors who work in this area be developed. Supervisors and supervisees who work with the traumatized child population need recurring support to prevent stress reactions.

SUGGESTED READINGS

Dutton, D. G. (1998). *The Abusive Personality: Violence and Control in Intimate Relationships.* New York: Guilford.
    Study of the personality features of men who commit violence in intimate relationships.

Gitterman, A. (1991). *Handbook of Social Work Practice with Vulnerable Populations.* New York: Columbia University Press.
    Coverage of social work practice with vulnerable and oppressed people.

Jacobson, N. and Gottman, J. (1998). *When Men Batter Women: New Insights into Ending Abusive Relationships.* New York: Simon and Schuster.
    Survey of major issues related to domestic violence based on empirical research.

National Association of Social Workers (1995). *Encyclopedia of Social Work,* Nineteenth Edition. Washington, DC: NASW Press.
    Contains articles on a vast array of practice settings in which social workers are employed.

Powell, D. J. and Brodsky, A. (1993). *Clinical Supervision in Alcohol and Drug Abuse Counseling: Principles, Models, Methods.* New York: Lexington.
    Supervision model focused on substance and alcohol abuse supervision

Trickett, P. K. and Schellenbach, C. J. (eds.) (1998). *Violence Against Children in the Family and the Community.* Washington, DC: American Psychological Association.
    Series of readings about various forms of violence against children.

> Clinical work is often more widely varying
> than our theories reflect.
>
> Fred Pine
> *Drive, Ego, Object, and Self*

Chapter 14

Supervision in Unique Situations

Supervisors encounter unique situations in supervision that require cultural awareness of race and ethnicity, or subcultural and individually sensitive situations such as supervising pregnant practitioners, physically disabled practitioners, and practitioners who are in therapy. Other situations that are discussed are family therapy supervision, use of family of origin material in supervision, and supervising cotherapist activity. These areas were selected for discussion because they are increasingly encountered by supervisors of clinical practitioners.

INTRODUCTION

Supervisors must be sensitive to unique and important variables that affect the treatment relationship in powerful ways. For example, a pregnant therapist or a pregnant client can arouse powerful emotions in the treatment. A handicapped therapist or client can also give rise to previously unrecognized feelings. When the practitioner and client are from different races or ethnic groups, different issues often arise. When the practitioner is much older or much younger than the client, a special set of difficulties can emerge.

In dealing with these unique situations, supervisors should give practitioners time to discuss their responses to what is taking place in the treatment. All of these special situations give rise to feelings that need to be explored because they can block practitioner's feelings, thoughts, and responses, which can affect the treatment and can cause it to break down. Supervisors have a responsibility to assist practitioners in such difficult situations.

CULTURALLY SENSITIVE PRACTICE

The U.S. population has become increasingly diverse, and during the next fifty years, projections are that racial and ethnic minorities will become the majority of U.S. citizens. The U.S. population is expected to grow by 50 percent from the 1995 population of 263 million by 2050, when the population will consist of 206 million Caucasians, 88 million Hispanics, 56 million African Americans, 38 million Asians, and 3.7 million Native Americans (Ozawa, 1997). At the same time, no trends exist to indicate that members of minority groups are increasingly entering the social work profession. Although no long-term projections of professional school enrollments are available, the enrollment trends of the past twenty years show no significant increase in minority enrollment, having remained essentially unchanged for the twenty-year period, with BSW graduates averaging 24.6 percent, MSW graduates averaging 17.1 percent, and DSW/PhD graduates averaging 18.6 percent. If demographic trends and professional school graduate composition continue at the current levels, dominant-culture professionals will be serving clients with varying cultural backgrounds in the short run. It is not clear in the long run whether increased presence of minorities in the population will result in more diversity in the social work profession. The demographic trends and factors that influence professional education choice will have significant implications for social work practice and supervision in the short and long term. Chetkow-Yanoov (1999) argues that new concepts and paradigms are needed by professionals to work with clients from different cultures and to work with different cultural groups that are in conflict. Modern individual, group, and community intervention by social workers and their supervisors require a different focus than in the past.

Supervisors increasingly will have to monitor practitioners' sensitivity to the beliefs, attitudes, behaviors, and needs of clients who are different from the practitioners. Schools of social work have increased content related to vulnerable populations (Gitterman, 1991), but practitioners entering supervision have limited practical preparation for working with culturally different and vulnerable populations (Jivanjee, 1999). More literature focuses on defining culturally sensitive intervention than on addressing the supervisory relationship from a culturally sensitive perspective (Batten, 1990; Bernard, 1994; Brown and Landrum-Brown, 1995; Cashwell, Looby, and Housley, 1997; Cook and Helms, 1988; Douglas and Rave, 1990; Fong and Lease, 1997; Gopaul-McNicol and Brice-Baker, 1998; Hipp and Munson, 1995; Lago and Thompson, 1997; Preist, 1994; Pope-Davis and Coleman, 1997; Ryan and Hendricks, 1989; Williams and Halgin, 1995). Key factors that supervisors need to monitor in culturally sensitive supervision are the following:

1. Differing perceptions of the meaning of functions, expectations, explanations, and behavior of the client, practitioner, and supervisor whenever difference is part of the client/practitioner/supervisor complex
2. Ensuring that respect and acceptance are shown for religious, spiritual, political, age, gender, and lifestyle differences
3. Differences in the assessment of communication during intervention. (For example, practitioner access to client perceptions may be impeded by differing views of language, styles of communication, valuing of socioeconomic and other statuses, acceptance of direct questioning, use of storytelling, role of privacy, work and leisure roles, family structure, authority, and importance of age.)

These are general guidelines. The key is for the supervisor to ensure that the practitioner recognizes each situation as unique and appreciates that any generalizations made about clients have the potential to produce bias in the practitioner and resistance in the client. Whenever a client is from a different background or group, the practitioner and supervisor must work to understand and assist the client within his or her own culture, and the client must be viewed in contrast to the dominant culture in which he or she functions. This orientation is a balancing act and creates conflicts, but it is essential if the professional is to aid the client. Only through such an orientation can persons from different cultures be comprehensively understood. Supervisors should be alert to uniqueness, diversity, and difference in clients, practitioners, and themselves as supervisors. Supervisors must be alert to bias and limitations in all aspects and in all levels of their organization. Supervisors have a responsibility to monitor ancillary staff, administrators, and policymakers regarding cultural issues (Jackson and Lopez, 1999). The range of uniqueness can include, but is not limited to, race, ethnicity, culture, subculture, age, sexual orientation, gender, physical and psychological limitations, and geographic location. Combinations of these categories can give rise to complex interactions among individuals and families that limit or enhance the intervention process, depending on how the differences are understood, accepted, and utilized. Each case explored in supervision should be screened and reviewed for differences and special circumstances that could be a source of communication and acceptance failure in the professional relationship. Uniqueness should not be assessed only in the context of identifying the difference, but once identified it should be interpreted in the context of its contribution to current functioning. If there is a functional problem, it must be determined whether it can be worked with through the dominant background culture. For example, acculturation and assimilation can produce stress in families that leads to specific functional problems. This is especially the case for mothers engaged in child rearing. In situations involving combinations of difference factors, supervisors must be alert to the practitioner's focusing on one factor at the expense of another factor. For example, an immigrant person with a severe physical disability may have a practitioner who focuses on the assimilation issues and neglects the disability difficulties, whereas another practitioner may emphasize assistance with the disability and fail to recognize the assimilation difficulties.

Assessment and diagnosis of clients from different cultural and ethnic backgrounds should be done by the practitioner and supervisor with sensitivity and vigilance for bias and lack of knowledge. This process requires openness and nondefensiveness about cultural difference, the practitioner's cultural identity, possible bias, awareness of dynamics of difference, recognition of the need for knowledge of research on cultural difference, and availability of specialized resources (Lum, 1999). Assessment and diagnosis must take into account that the concept of the individual has different meanings in different cultural contexts (Sue et al., 1996). Culturally focused assessments must consider factors beyond the traditional background variables associated with assessment. Lum (2000) identifies salient factors as newcomer syndrome, psychosomatic syndromes, identity issues, elderly concerns, family migration history, relocation history, loss issues, trauma history, cultural shock, adjustment problems, family acculturation rate, work stress, financial stress, place of residence analysis, community influences, family problems, family strengths, help-seeking history and attitude, expectations of treatment, and concept of mental illness. This last point goes to the heart of the issue: diagnosis of mental illness should always be done in the context of an overall assessment. Diagnosis from a cultural context can be done within the DSM-IV-TR diagnostic system through use of the culture-bound syndromes in Appendix I. Supervisors should be thoroughly familiar with this section of the DSM-IV-TR and use it with supervisees when doing culture-bound diagnosis.

The term *culture-bound syndrome* was coined by a Western-trained Chinese psychiatrist, Pow Meng Yap, in 1969 (Mezzich et al., 1996). Some have argued that use of this term in the DSM-IV-TR has limitations (Munson, 2000b), but inclusion of this section in the DSM-IV-TR is an attempt to focus the role of culture in functioning and to make clinicians more aware of cultural factors affecting behavior. Cultural influences on mental health diagnosis are included in the DSM-IV-TR for a few reasons: (1) the manual is used in many countries, (2) the increasing cultural diversity of the United States requires consideration of the role of culture in the production of symptoms, and (3) there is a need for differentiation of cultural behaviors and mental disorders.

The culture-bound syndrome appendix has two sections. The first section is an outline intended to supplement the multiaxial diagnosis through guidelines evaluating and recording an individual's cultural context. The second section is a listing of culture-bound syndromes with brief descriptions of their features.

The outline for cultural formulation supplements the multiaxial diagnostic assessment and addresses difficulties encountered in applying DSM-IV-TR criteria in multicultural environments. It is an outline for systematic evaluation of cultural factors that may influence the person's functioning and may impact the relationship between the client and the mental health professional. This section can be especially helpful when the person being evaluated and the mental health professional are from different cultures, and it should be used whenever the practitioner is encountering difficulty understanding a person's cultural context. The clinician can record the data gathered about a person's culture by doing a narrative summary for the following categories.

1. *Cultural identity of the client.* The clinician should note
   a. ethnic or cultural group,
   b. degree of involvement with the culture of origin and host culture, and
   c. language skills and preferences.
2. *Cultural explanations of illness.* The clinician should note
   a. predominant forms of distress that convey symptoms or the need for social support,
   b. meaning and severity of symptoms in relation to cultural group and local illness type used by the individual's family and community to identify and explain the syndrome (derived from the sec-

ond section of Appendix I, which contains the definitions of culture-bound syndromes), and

   c. current preferences and past experiences with professional and common sources of intervention.

3. *Cultural factors in the psychosocial environment and levels of functioning.* The clinician should note

   a. interpretations of social stressors,

   b. social supports, and

   c. levels of functioning and disability, including local social environment stresses, religious factors, and kinship networks used to provide support.

4. *Cultural elements of the relationship between the client and clinician.* The clinician should describe

   a. differences in culture and social status of the client and clinician and

   b. problems cultural differences can cause in diagnosis and treatment.

5. *Overall cultural assessment related to diagnosis and care.* The clinician should conclude with a discussion of how cultural factors specifically influence comprehensive diagnosis and intervention.

Case Illustration:
Outline for Cultural Formulation of Mary Sanchez

1. *Cultural identity of the client*

An evaluation was done today of Mary Sanchez in our mental health center. Mary is twenty-three years old. She immigrated to Houston five years ago from her home in Reynosa, Mexico. Mary came to the United States with her husband and three children. Mary's husband has not permitted Mary to leave the home alone for any extended period of time since living in Houston. Mary has learned very little English, most likely due to her forced isolation by the husband. Mary's children have not been isolated, and they attend public school. Mary was accompanied to the evaluation by her oldest son, who is age sixteen. Her son Carlos speaks good English and was able to describe most of Mary's symptoms to me.

2. *Cultural explanations of illness*

Mary's primary reference group remains her family members who are living in Mexico. She has been back to visit them several times since living in the United States. Mary recently returned from a visit to Mexico. While in Mexico, she experienced a sudden onset of symptoms. She complained of stomachaches, headaches, sleep difficulty, and unexplained crying spells. She has had a significant appetite loss and is unable to concentrate on her household chores. Mary said that she has a bad case of "nerves" (nervios). Mary believes her "case of the nerves" is inherited and "runs in my family." She believes her symptoms are getting worse, and she does "not know what to do." She is fearful that her husband will find out she came to the center.

Mary will be further assessed for differential diagnosis of possible adjustment disorder, anxiety disorder, mood disorder, somatoform disorder, and acculturation problem. There is no evidence of dissociative disorder or psychotic disorder, but these disorders will continue to be reviewed as part of the rule-out process. The consideration of the culture-bound syndromes of nervios and possibly locura will be a key part of the comprehensive assessment.

3. *Cultural factors in the psychosocial environment and levels of functioning*

Mary reported that she has become more active in the church in the past year, and when her husband found this out, he became very angry with her and ordered her to stay away from the church. Mary had been planning to enroll in English classes that the church was sponsoring. Mary has no social supports or social contacts outside her family. During her return trip to Mexico, her family "pressured" her to do something about her situation with her husband. While in Mexico, Mary visited a curandero and received some herbal treatments.

4. *Cultural elements of the relationship between the client and clinician*

I was able to communicate with Mary minimally, but my Spanish is not good enough to do ongoing intervention with Mary. If her son had not been present, it would have been difficult for me to do the evaluation.

5. *Overall cultural assessment for diagnosis and care*

It is difficult to give Mary a DSM-IV-TR diagnosis at the present time. The stress-related factors in her life have been present for some time and could be indicative of a stress-related disorder. She denies that her symptoms are due to the stresses produced by the relationship with her husband, or by the pressure she is feeling from her family. I am concerned about the possibility of an eating disorder. I am reluctant to involve Mary in further appointments because of her fear of Mr. Sanchez's finding out about her evaluation visit to the center. I do not know to what degree Mary's situation may be made worse by acculturation issues. The role of religion needs to be considered in assisting Mary to get help, as well as its potential to cause more difficulties if her husband objects to her involvement in religion and treatment. I am reluctant to encourage Mary to involve Mr. Sanchez in the treatment. I will contact Mary's priest about the religious issues, and I will familiarize myself with the Catholic religion in order to better understand Mary in relation to her religious beliefs and the supports provided by the Church. I will contact a Spanish-speaking MSW therapist who works in an outreach facility that is part of our center and is located in Mary's neighborhood. I will have the therapist arrange further appointments for Mary. I will refer Mary to a primary care physician in her neighborhood to follow up on the physical symptoms and to evaluate the herbal treatments that were provided by the curandero. I believe more assessment of Mary's family situation and relationships needs to be done before family intervention is implemented. Diagnosis will be deferred until the precipitating factors are clarified. The differential diagnosis process described in item 2 above will be completed as part of the ongoing evaluation. I will consult with the Spanish-speaking MSW social worker who will be doing the intervention. Mary was provided a consent for treatment form, and she signed release of information forms. These forms were given to Mary in Spanish and were read to her by her son in my presence. Mary understands the treatment and evaluation plans described in this formulation and did agree to them.

The second section of Appendix I in the DSM-IV-TR, Glossary of Culture-Bound Syndromes, explains the twenty-five different syndromes. Culture-bound syndrome means recurrent, locality-specific patterns of aberrant behavior and troubling experience that can be linked to a particular DSM-IV-TR diagnostic category. These patterns can be considered indigenously to be "illnesses," or at least afflictions, and most have local names (APA, 2000a). Presentations conforming to the major DSM-IV-TR categories can be found throughout the world, but it must be recognized that the particular symptoms, course, and social response are very often influenced by local culture. Culture-bound syndromes are usually limited to specific societies or cultures and are localized, folk, diagnostic groupings that contain meanings for troubling symptoms and behaviors.

Rarely is equivalence established between culture-bound syndromes and DSM-IV-TR diagnostic classifications. Unusual behavior that might be observed by a clinician using the DSM-IV-TR and sorted into several categories may be included in a single folk category, and presentations that might be considered by a diagnostician using the DSM-IV-TR as belonging to a single category may be sorted into several categories by a clinician from the client's culture. Some conditions and disorders are culture-bound syndromes specific to industrialized societies (e.g., anorexia nervosa, dissociative identity disorder), given their rarity or absence in other less-developed cultures. Industrialized societies include distinctive and varied subcultures, including diverse immigrant groups that may have culture-bound syndromes.

PEOPLE WITH DISABILITIES

Oklin (1999) defines disability as a condition that limits functioning and may or may not be related to a physical or mental illness. People with disabilities are viewed by Oklin as members of a community with some common features. Members of this community should not be defined by a diagnosis or medical condition. Supervisors of clinicians who work with this community should ensure that the clinician is thoroughly familiar with the members' "history, language, perspectives, priorities, humor, norms, and sense of pride in its [the community's] identity." (Oklin, 1999:13). Historically there have been three models of disability: moral, medical, and minority. The moral model views disability as a result of immorality or "sins." The medical model is based on the conception that disability is the result of a medical condition that resides within the person. The newest model is the minority or social model, which holds that disability is a social construction in that society does not accommodate persons with disabilities and has negative attitudes toward them. This model holds that people with disabilities share many of the problems that people with cultural differences experience (Oklin, 1999). For this reason, many of the supervisory issues discussed in the previous section on culturally sensitive practice apply to disabilities. The practitioner who works with people with disabilities must have thorough training in the specifics of this practice specialty and cannot work with such persons as occasional cases in a general mental health practice. Oklin (1999), Hosie et al. (1989), and Livneh and Thomas (1997) have codified the key factors in training and supervision of practice related to persons with disabilities:

- Understanding of political, social, and physical environment impacts on persons with disabilities
- Recognition of the nature of stigma, prejudice, discrimination, status, and roles in relation to disability
- Knowledge of the disability rights movement, laws, legislation, and disability culture
- Knowledge of medical, developmental, psychological, family, ethnic, cultural, political, and spiritual contexts of people with disabilities as well as multiple minority statuses
- Recognition of the need for interdisciplinary collaboration for comprehensive disability intervention
- Expertise in assessment, diagnosis, case formulation, psychosocial intervention, and evaluation
- Knowledge of the independent living movement, supported employment, and transition from school to work status
- Knowledge of supportive technological advances and their application
- Knowledge of ethical mandates for work with disabled persons, including limitations of professional competence and scope of practice

PRACTITIONERS WHO ARE IN THERAPY

No reliable statistics are available, but indications are that a substantial number of practitioners have been in therapy. In one sample of graduate students surveyed, 52 percent of the students indicated that they had received treatment in the past, and 12 percent of this group were currently receiving treatment. A majority of those who had received treatment said that they decided to enter social work school because they identified with their therapists and had decided to use then as role models (Munson, Study A).

The important factor to be taken into account by the supervisor is how these practitioners' experiences with their therapists affect their own work. When therapists' role models are limited, as often is the case, the only role models available are their own therapists, which can result in distortions (Blumenfield, 1982:146). Most practitioners work alone and in isolation from others. The distortions that commonly occur are that the practitioner is being effective when in fact he or she is not, or that he or she is ineffective when performance is adequate. Practitioners who do not receive ample or adequate supervision are more likely to draw on their therapists as role models. They see their therapists in action more than they see their supervisors, and practitioners will develop whatever coping mechanisms they can to deal with the complexities of practice.

Practitioners do not discriminate how they use styles and techniques learned from their own therapists. Such carryover works and serves practitioners adequately as long as their clients have problems similar to those the practitioners present in their own therapy. It is natural for practitioners to think that if it works in their own situations, it will work satisfactorily for those they treat. However, practitioners must remember that such techniques and strategies are quite often appropriate only to the unique problems under treatment, and that adopting these strategies in a comprehensive fashion is eventually bound to fail. When practitioners have clients with backgrounds different from their own, the supervisor needs to be especially sensitive to these types of misapplication.

When a practitioner's own therapy is based on a theoretical orientation similar to the one the practitioner uses in his or her own practice, the natural tendency is to imitate the therapist who treated the practitioner. This can produce positive or negative results, depending on the situation. In some cases the practitioner uses a theory different from his or her own therapist's, and this most often results in clumsy performance in practice and frustration, especially at difficult points. There should be some exploration in supervision of the practitioner's therapist's styles and theoretical orientation, if the practitioner is open to such discussion involving his or her own therapy. The supervisor should do direct observation of the practitioner's work to detect any changes in style that could be detracting from performance. At the same time, a practitioner's own therapy can enhance practice in a number of ways, and this needs to be reinforced by the supervisor.

Such exploration does not have to involve the content of the practitioner's personal therapy, but it should focus on stylistic elements that carry over from therapy to practice. Dealing with this type of material requires much sensitivity and skill on the part of the supervisor. There must be clear boundaries about what is open to discussion and what is not. The supervisor should avoid judging or evaluating the practitioner's therapist. If the practitioner has lost confidence in the therapist and wants to talk about it, the supervisor can discuss this briefly and assist the practitioner in making a decision about how to deal with it, but that decision should be made solely by the practitioner.

FAMILY THERAPY SUPERVISION

Many supervisors assume that family therapy supervision is not different from individual therapy supervision. This belief usually grows out of supervisors' lack of skill in actually doing family therapy and social work's reliance on generic skills. Agencies should not place in supervisory positions staff who do not have substantial skill in doing family therapy if they are required to supervise family therapists. Theoretical grounding alone is not sufficient for effectively supervising family therapists. Although generic skills are necessary to any practice situation, they are not sufficient. For example, because more people are involved, family therapy automatically decreases the control the practitioner is able to exercise, as compared to the individual treatment situation. Visual 14.1 illustrates the increase in interactional combinations that can occur as the number of participants in the treatment group is increased. To make the treatment manageable, the supervisor and practitioner must make important decisions about how many family members and how many therapists to involve in the treatment. No amount of generic skills will help the therapist cope with a treatment group of unmanageable size. Bowen theoretically conceptualized the complexity of adding participants to the treatment situation. There is an actual exponential numerical increase as participants are added to the treatment (see Visual 14.1). Bowen believed that when the therapist who thinks in terms of individual therapy is presented clinically with families, he or she cannot "hear family concepts" (Haley, 1971:163-171).

Within the context of family therapy, each individual in treatment is part of an expanded, interactional system that is not compatible with individual treatment models. Bowen saw one difference as that of identifying family relationship patterns that do not emerge in individual treatment. The supervisor must be able to help the supervisee make this transition. For example, one pattern of family interactional relationship is for the family to put one member in the sick role or the patient role. In such dysfunctional systems, the person identified as sick will often eagerly fulfill this role outside and within the treatment. The unsuspecting practitioner with an individual orientation will adapt to this system and focus on treating the sick member, rather than focusing on the whole family in an attempt to break up this dys-

Portions of Family Therapy Supervision are reprinted from Carlton E. Munson, "Supervising the Family Therapist," *Social Casework* 61(March 1980), pp. 131-137. Reprinted by permission of the Family Service Association of America.

VISUAL 14.1. Combinations of Interactions for Treatment Situations

	One Worker		Two Workers	
Number of Clients	Two-Way Interaction	Three-Way Interaction	Two-Way Interaction	Three-Way Interaction
1	2	—	6	6
2	6	6	12	24
3	12	24	20	60
4	20	60	30	120
5	30	120	42	210
6	42	210	56	336
7	56	336	72	504

Source: Munson 1980c:132.

functional pattern. The supervisor must be alert to such manipulation of the practitioner by the family and help the therapist avoid conforming to the existing family interactional pattern.

At the other extreme, families may exclude a particular member from the interactional pattern. Family members will often subtly exclude members by trying to "rescue" them or by expressing painful feelings for them (Luthman and Kirschenbaum, 1974:77). It is easy for the unskilled practitioner to fail to recognize this pattern of exclusion. The supervisor must help the practitioner identify such patterns and assist the practitioner in aiding the excluded member to get back into the interactional system.

Interactional Issues

Families often avoid interactional issues, and the practitioner may not want to acknowledge this avoidance. The supervisor must be alert to such observational and interventive gaps and be prepared to discuss them with the supervisee. The best way for the supervisor to introduce the beginning family therapist to this method is to have the worker serve as cotherapist with the supervisor in treating families. The supervisor can help the worker gain direct experience by sharing strategies of intervention, techniques used, and skills employed.

If the supervisor is unable or unwilling to share his or her own practice, an alternative is to show the worker videotapes or play audiotapes of family therapy sessions. These can be tapes of sessions conducted in the agency or commercially produced tapes. The use of tapes to train family therapists must involve more than just allowing the worker to view or listen to the tapes. The supervisor must put the tapes in perspective before and after they are used. Differing styles and theoretical approaches must be explained, as must the reasons for specific interactions between the practitioners and family members. Family intervention is a process, and to observe segments of this process through tapes can be misleading. This is why actual involvement in the family therapy process is best. When tapes are used, the supervisor must fill in the gaps of the intervention process. Techniques learned out of context of the therapy process can lead the beginning therapist to develop a flippant attitude or a grab bag of techniques that can be confusing and, in some cases, detrimental to the families treated.

Audiovisual Devices

When one-way viewing mirrors and earphone devices are used, the supervisor needs to be aware of his or her own behavior and its impact on the practitioner. For example, the supervisor who is too active in using the earphone device to talk can confuse, frustrate, and limit the ability of the practitioner to carry out the therapy. This can be avoided if the supervisor seeks feedback from the practitioner about the amount of his or her involvement in the treatment as a "once-removed therapist." This form of live supervision must involve evaluation of the supervision as well as evaluation of the family treatment.

The use of audiovisual aids in supervising family therapists is a much more involved process than most supervisors realize. More planning needs to go into the use of such aids. Careful selection of aids is important. Orientation of the clients, practitioners, and supervisors to use of such aids is essential. Putting the use of aids in perspective before, during, and after their use is basic. Evaluation of the aids is as important as the evaluation of the treatment. Instructional aids cannot be used with all cases or for all supervision. The supervisor must carefully plan the use of segmental audiovisual aids so that the maximum benefit can be gained. The supervisor must be clear in advance about the objectives of the supervision, what the focus will be in the case material to be scrutinized, and procedures to be used in teaching the objectives of the supervision. The self-assessment instrument contained in Appendix VI can be a good aid in focusing the material that will be evaluated during supervision. (See Chapter 12 for the use of audiovisual techniques.)

Theory and Technique

Family therapists disagree about the use of theory versus technique in family treatment. This debate is not confined to family therapists and has been a factor in the evolution of other forms of therapy. Bowen viewed theory as important to family intervention (Haley, 1971:163); Whitaker believed the use of theory isolates the therapist, dichotomizes the treatment, makes the therapist an observer, and stifles practitioner creativity (Guerin, 1976:154-164). There has been little systematic study of how theory is actually used in family intervention and how it affects what is said and what gets done. There appears to be little conscious use of theory in the actual practice of family therapy. Beginning practitioners struggle with the intensity of the family therapy situation and have little energy to invest in the skilled use of theory; the experienced practitioner focuses on the interaction and issues to be explored without conscious consideration of the theoretical implications of his or her own activity. This does not mean that theory is not important in family intervention. What practitioners have been taught about family therapy does show up in their work, but this is seldom consciously recognized. For the purposes of supervision, this becomes an important point.

In order to give practitioners the technical skill to know how to deal with therapy content, the supervisor must have some way to organize the analysis of therapy content. Even though the practitioner may not always be aware of the use of theory in the practice situation, effective supervision for practice must be theoretically based. Whitaker argued that nontheoretical workers can be effective when given good supervision (Guerin, 1976:163). The more nontheoretical the therapy, the more important theory becomes in supervision. Opposition to the use of theory in supervision is often related to the fact that family dynamics change so much in the treatment process that it is very difficult to apply theory consistently. Because of the complexity of family interaction, it is important that theory be used to guide the supervision rather than be abandoned. Although it is hard work, consistent and clear use of theory can help to keep the treatment from becoming unfocused and nonspecific. Theory used in supervision must be related to the interaction process. Most family intervention theory has emerged from analysis of family interaction and fits the supervisory process quite well.

The supervisor must be careful of using theory in the abstract to avoid difficult or unfamiliar case material. The theoretical material must be related to clinical material. A good rule for the supervisor to follow is that no theoretical concept should be presented without the illustration of one or more clinical examples. It is easier for practitioners to handle criticism of their work when it is presented in relation to practice theory. It is easier for them to understand the implications of an action in theoretical terms, rather than simply in terms of therapist or supervisor behavior or feelings.

Theory and Diagnosis

In doing diagnosis in family therapy, theory is important. Some understanding of the theory in use must precede the diagnostic process. It is recommended that supervisors avoid teaching diagnosis before identifying the theoretical orientation of the supervisor or the agency. Diagnosis must be accomplished in relation to treatment. Minuchin (1974) pointed out that diagnosis and therapy are inseparable. When diagnosis and treatment goals are accomplished in theoretical harmony, the total treatment is more understandable and more easily adapted to by the clients, the practitioner, and the supervisor. When theory is not used in supervision, or when theory is applied inconsistently in diagnosis and treatment phases, there is more practitioner dissatisfaction with supervision, and it is more likely that the family will drop out of treatment.

When diagnosis and initial intervention are discussed and reviewed in a supervision session that does not have a theoretical focus, the practitioner may end up spending too much time in treatment merely giving the family information and gathering information about family history, systems, functioning, and symptoms. This lost time in treatment is usually a carryover from individual intervention, in which information is gathered and a label applied to it. Minuchin described the difference in approach in family therapy as follows: "a diagnosis is the working hypothesis that the therapist evolves from his experiences and observations upon joining the family" (Minuchin, 1974:129). A family diagnosis and treatment strategy emerge from the therapist's direct participation in the system. In family intervention, the diagnosis-treatment process is internally formulated and applied rather than externally imposed and preexisting, as in individual treatment. This difference makes the supervisor's task more difficult, but more effective and rewarding when logically and consistently applied.

Family therapy supervision is more complex and demanding than other forms of clinical supervision. There is necessarily more emphasis on live supervision and the use of audiovisual aids in supervision, which requires additional knowledge and skills on the part of the supervisor. Family therapy supervision should not be attempted by the nonpracticing supervisor.

The SEES System

Discovering the process of treatment and its relationship to technique is as important in learning family therapy as diagnosis and theory. The supervisor must find a way to integrate these concepts for the supervisee. The author has developed a conceptual scheme that is simple to learn and at the same time can convey how master family therapists integrate theory and practice (Munson, 1994a). The research that served as the basis for the conceptual model content analysis was applied to master family therapists' recorded videotape sessions, with a focus on identifying the purpose and function of intervention strategies used (Munson, Study II). This resulted in a classification system of four activities that appeared to be core techniques in each session the therapist conducted. The activities generally occurred in a flexible sequence that constituted a repeated process the therapist used to make interventions.

In this sequence, the practitioner analyzes the family's *style* of relating in the first part of the session. The therapist then moves to adjusting or adapting his or her own natural style of intervention to the family style, and this allows the practitioner to enter the family, join the family, or form an alliance with the family. This sets the stage for the therapist to *enable* individual family members to express themselves or to be protected from other family members or to assist the entire family to mobilize its resources to accomplish a task. Once this is done, the therapist then *encounters* the family by clarifying family patterns of relating and behaving. This is a form of confrontation without anger and is done in a caring way. After the encounter occurs, the practitioner guides the family to relate in a different way. This procedure is referred to as *shifting the dysfunction.* In shifting the dysfunction, the therapist goes through the steps of initiating the shift, implementing the shift, and implanting the shift. This involves setting up the situation as it would normally occur, then altering the pattern of interacting and working to make the alterations so powerful the family cannot return to the old pattern of relating. There are numerous ways of achieving a shift, for example, through the whole family participating or through one family member being encouraged not to respond in the usual manner. This process of style, enable, encounter, and shift dysfunction occurs repeatedly in master therapists' work, and it is evident in some of the earliest tapes of sessions done by pioneering family therapists in the 1960s, as well as in the latest models of family therapy (see, for example, Brendler et al., 1991).

The supervisor can use this system to assist beginning family therapists in their efforts to master this complex form of treatment. Visual 14.2 summarizes the SEES system for learning about family therapy by watching films of master therapists at work.

FAMILY OF ORIGIN MATERIAL IN SUPERVISION

The literature on family intervention can be confusing for beginning therapists, leaving them with the impression that "everything seems to work" (Kramer, 1980:281). This same confusion occurs in family therapy training programs. Supervisors need to help supervisees evaluate what works and what is ineffective. Younger practitioners are likely to have been exposed to family therapy theory and concepts as part of their professional training, but such exposure is often less than adequate and entered into before the practitioner is skilled at performing individual or group therapy (Kramer, 1980:275-276). Supervisors should remember that the beginning family therapist has only his or her own family of origin as a source of experience in family functioning, and this experience limits and blocks therapist appreciation of the diversity of family types and styles that exist.

VISUAL 14.2. SEES System for Analyzing Family Therapy Interactional Sequences

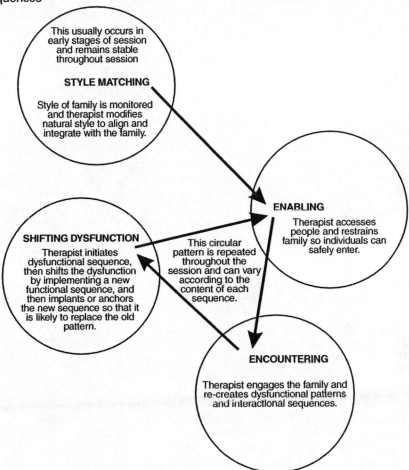

It is generally agreed that personal therapy associated with exploration of one's own family dynamics leads to one's being a better family therapist. Practitioners are encouraged to enter therapy to enhance their professional performance, and family therapy supervisors are encouraged "openly to discuss with students their experiences in current relationships with their own families" as a model for their supervisees' own practice (Goldenberg and Goldenberg, 1980:234-235). Kramer has argued that "the family therapist who has not himself experienced therapy is at a disadvantage," and that the family therapist "who has not worked on his own family relationships" is "handicapped" (1980:298).

Given these theoretical views, the confusion about what constitutes good treatment, and beginning practitioners' lack of adequate practice experience in doing family intervention, most inexperienced practitioners naturally have a tendency to commit to any strategy or technique that will aid them in coping with demanding and complex practice material. The use of family of origin material is one of these learning strategies. Exploration of personal experience is used as a means to learn about practice. This expectation is developed early in a therapist's career, during the training stage. One report in the literature on the use of family of origin material in a social work classroom setting illustrates this (Magee, 1982). The report reflects a trend to personalize for the student various forms of course content. This is based on the notion that having the student draw on personal experience to understand conceptual material fosters integration of content, development of self-awareness, and learning. No empirical evidence supports the view that this is the most effective and efficient way to promote learning, nor has any consideration been given to whether the use of such techniques impedes learning or, even more serious, violates students' right to privacy. Such exploration using students' personal lives to promote learning under any circumstances is unjustified. Haley has succinctly commented on such practices by observing that supervisees' personal lives are too important to be tampered with by supervisors (1976:187).

The only report on the use of family of origin groups in the field component of social work education is by Thistle (1981). She holds that students believe that "unashamed inquiry in [family] relationships is not only helpful but essential to the development of the family therapist," and she asserts that "the modification of the trainee's role in {the trainee's] family is one of the most dramatic and effective ways of teaching family therapy" (1981:248). Given these two statements, a basic contradiction emerges from the article that Thistle does not address. This contradiction is that the clients of the agency are severely mentally ill people who need inpatient psychiatric treatment, and their backgrounds are substantially different from the backgrounds of the therapist trainees. In spite of these major differences, the trainees are purported to learn about their clients by presenting "family albums and records and genograms" that make "the families come alive for group members" (Thistle, 1981:249). This type of exploration is justified on the grounds that individuals "attracted to the helping professions [are] often more comfortable looking at someone else's problems than [their] own" (Thistle, 1981:249). This view becomes the basis for the assertion that the main "task" of the group is for trainees to become "researchers in their own families" (Thistle, 1981:249). It is not clear how this relates to what the trainee does with his or her own clients.

History

Unlike that of many intervention techniques, the history of the use of family of origin material can be traced. It originated with Murray Bowen. The evolution of Bowen's ideas in this area is explained in his book *Family Therapy in Clinical Practice* (1978). A rather elaborate interweaving of points in the last fifty pages of the book describes this evolution. Bowen reports that he first learned to apply therapeutic dynamics to his family from a sickness perspective during his early psychoanalytic training. Later he began using his own theoretical formulations to study his own family. He worked through this by writing lengthy letters to his parents and siblings and calculated mailing them to coincide with trips to visit his family. This caused members of his family much anguish, and he reports that one brother was so angered that he threatened a libel suit (Bowen, 1978:513).

In 1967 Bowen began using his own family of origin experiences to teach psychiatric residents about treatment. These residents used these examples with their own families, and Bowen observed that these residents appeared to be "doing better clinical work as family therapists than any previous residents" (Bowen, 1978:531). Bowen began treating residents using this approach. He reported that in one "control" group he focused on extended family material but admitted that the results were disappointing. Bowen continued to use these techniques with residents and their wives as part of his training program. Hundreds of practitioners have participated in these training seminars. Many psychotherapists from various disciplines now use family of origin groups to train other therapists. These psychotherapists use the same techniques with their own supervisees that Bowen demonstrated and used with them, including exploration of family of origin material and letter-writing exercises.

There have been no empirical tests of what Bowen has produced as a participant observer in his own training seminars (Gurman, 1981b:355). No specific guidelines have been developed for the use of family of origin material with therapists in training. There are no reports in the literature of positive or negative outcomes or misapplications of this approach. Although reports identifying problems do occur in the literature, the tendency has been to overlook them and to emphasize the positive assumptions of the approach (see Gurman, 1981:352-364).

One case example that illustrates the lack of differential applications of family of origin material involved a student therapist:

> Mary was a second-year graduate student in an outpatient mental health clinic, where her supervisor was a strong advocate of family of origin groups for practitioners. The supervisor had participated in several seminars conducted by Bowenian trainers. The supervisor urged her supervisees to participate in a family of origin group she con-

ducted. Mary joined one of these groups and after several sessions was encouraged to present her family.

Mary presented her father as an aloof, stern businessman who did not communicate much. When her father tried to talk with her, Mary's mother would always interfere and accuse them of "plotting against her." Mary's mother had a lifelong history of mental illness, including a series of psychiatric hospitalizations. In order to avoid his wife's wrath, Mary's father gave up trying to communicate with Mary, which Mary found depressing. At the same time, she felt anger at her father for not confronting his wife with her "unfounded" accusations. Mary had left home over ten years ago and had visited her parents infrequently since leaving home. Mary's one younger sister had not attended college and had "never found her place in life." She described her parents, who lived over 500 miles away, as having settled into complacency about their life situation and acceptance of their daughter's loss of contact with them. Her parents remained reservedly proud of Mary's accomplishments. Mary desired to relate to her parents in a different way but did not know how to achieve this.

The family of origin group convinced Mary that she was engaged in a classic triangle with her parents and encouraged her to write a letter to her parents explaining this triangle and indicating that she wanted to break up this pattern of relating. After a holiday visit home, Mary, with much ambivalence, prepared a letter that she read to the group and subsequently mailed to her parents. The parents wrote back indicating that they did not understand Mary's comments, but that they still loved her and would like to fly in for her graduation because they were proud of her accomplishments. Mary took her parents' letter back to the family of origin group and was advised by the group to write to her parents indicating that she would refuse to see them if they came for her graduation, and that her achieving a graduate degree had been accomplished alone without help from them. It was the group's view that this would be a good way to break up the old pattern of "triangling." Mary followed through on this with another letter. The parents responded again with a long letter professing their love for her. They did not understand her position but would honor her feelings and not attend the graduation.

The question remains whether this was the best and most appropriate way to deal with Mary's situation, but the more important question concerns what this had to do with Mary's own development as a family therapist. None of it was ever related by the group to her own family practice. This entire process of family of origin work could be viewed as an unwarranted and unjustified intrusion into Mary's personal life.

Dynamics and Process

In groups in which family of origin material is explored extensively, it can become intertwined with group process and group dynamics that can give rise to therapeutic difficulties. Beck (1982) has reported an example of this in which a group member became reluctant to explore family of origin material, and this in turn gave rise to resentment on the part of other group members. This reaction of the group led the patient to withdraw from the group (it is not clear if these patients were therapists themselves in a supervision group). The question that emerges from this case example is, What is to become of participants who exercise their right to self-determination and do not agree to such a course of treatment or supervision?

The following case report illustrates how resistance can become problematic for the therapist in supervision:

> I was only married six months when my supervisor required me to participate in a family of origin group she was conducting. I didn't know much about it, but I thought I would give it a try. My husband is very involved with his family. This didn't particularly bother me, but the group pressed me about it. I've talked to my husband about it, but without much enthusiasm. He isn't into psychology, and he discounts this stuff. I did it because the group pushed me about it. I regret having done it. I want this marriage to work. It's the second marriage for both of us. My husband doesn't understand what I'm going through. I wish I would never have brought it up. I don't think it's that important. I don't see what it has to do with learning to do good therapy. I feel comfortable with our relationship as it is. I'm being more cautious about what I reveal in the group, but I can sense some of the other members don't like the way I'm reacting.

Supervisees become frustrated and disoriented when they fail to see the connection between actions of the family of origin group and their own families. Such experiences cause the therapist in training to become resentful and to view such efforts as being involuntarily forced into personal therapy. Also, in situations such as this, the therapist's learning is blocked because so much energy goes into resisting the group. When this occurs, the main objective of family of origin groups is thwarted—the supervisee ceases to learn about family therapy and how to become more skilled at doing it. Without adequate safeguards, personalizing family of origin material for the supervisee is a return to the former problematic practice of "psychologizing" the worker.

Relationship to Practice

The effect of family of origin emphasis in supervision has not been assessed from the perspective of its influence on practice activity. It has been shown that rarely is family of origin material applied in the supervision of the practitioner as it relates to the practitioner's clinical activity. When this gap exists, the potential is created for practitioners to misapply this material with their cases. There must be follow-up of such learning and its application as well as clinical demonstration of its relevance to clinical situations.

Overemphasis on family of origin material in supervision can lead the practitioner to a disproportionate focus on such material in cases. Dwelling on such material can fascinate but can lead to a narrow focus that detracts from a problem focus in the treatment. It can result in focusing on historical and inactive relationships at the expense of current relationship issues. Tangible problems and dysfunctional interactional and communication patterns in the family can be overlooked and avoided. This is especially the case in the diagnostic phase of intervention. If assessment of family functioning is inadequate or limited, the treatment will necessarily be distorted and misguided.

These issues remain unexplored in the use of family of origin material. Beck (1982) has alluded to the shortcomings of family of origin material in some situations. Supervisors who insist upon its use must be aware of these problems and develop strategies to combat them. Supervisors need to explore alternative means of promoting effective family treatment. For example, are there alternative methods of exploring family of origin material that put practitioners at less risk personally and are at the same time more practice relevant? Are other practice methods as effective, or more effective, in encouraging quality practice? Can the same ends be achieved through the use of cotherapists in family treatment? Clinical supervisors need to devote attention to appropriate differential application of family of origin material to supervisory and clinical practice situations.

Focus of Supervision

The amount of material that is revealed about one's family of origin should remain under the control of the supervisee and not the supervisor. To pressure supervisees to confront their own family of origin material distorts the learning process in supervision. Supervisors who press supervisees beyond the point of their comfort must ask why they are persisting in such a course of interaction. To guard against such a distortion of the supervisory learning experience, a good policy of the supervisor should be to explore family of origin material only after case material has been presented and problem areas in the case situation have been identified. The general rule being proposed here is that exploration of client dynamics should always precede exploration of therapist dynamics in the supervision. Such a policy ensures that the supervision will remain learning focused, and at any point at which therapists are reluctant to go further with personal material, they can fall back on the case material. When therapists' family of origin material is the exclusive focus in supervision, a feeling of being trapped can develop if a point is reached beyond which the therapists do not want to go. Dormant triangles should not be reestablished as a part of the supervisory experience; such actions should remain in the realm of therapy. The triangles in the families being treated by the practitioners should be the focus of the supervision.

COTHERAPIST ACTIVITY

Cotherapy work can be a totally rewarding experience, a completely devastating experience, or an alternately rewarding and devastating experience. These are generally the three categories of responses received when inquiring about practitioners' cotherapy experiences.

Cotherapists need some form of regular or periodic supervision. Cotherapy does not eliminate the need for supervision. It is not a good idea to expect cotherapy to serve as a form of mutual supervision. Cotherapy often results in difficulty if one of the participants seeks such activity as a source of supervision or consultation without making this explicit. The second therapist may be incapable or unwilling to fulfill this function.

Little solid empirical outcome research exists to confirm or refute the dichotomous claims of the effectiveness and inadequacy of cotherapy. The debate about its appropriateness in family therapy epitomizes the polarities that have been reached. Bowen described cotherapy as a method and technique that he viewed as "[o]ne of the major innovations and developments in family therapy" (1978:299). Haley holds that outcome studies show that cotherapy is not more effective, and he believes that "the use of a cotherapist is usually for the security of the clinician and not for the value of the client" (1976:16). Rabin (1967), in a survey of therapists, found that they preferred cotherapy but emphasized the importance of a "good" relationship between the therapists, although no clear definition of a "good" relationship was formulated. Research has indicated that therapist style (Rice et al., 1972) and theoretical orientation affect preference for cotherapy activity. Some research suggests that effectiveness is associated with comfort in the cotherapy situation, but as cotherapy activity increases, satisfaction with the method decreases (Gurman and Razin, 1977:212-213). A common theme in cotherapy research highlights the need for documenting sources and forms of conflict in this treatment practice.

Practitioners perceive that agencies are split evenly on whether to encourage cotherapy activity (Munson, Study F). In some agencies, acceptance of cotherapy is vague—practitioners are not encouraged to do cotherapy, but at the same time, it is not openly discouraged. Rarely do agencies have well-developed guidelines for the use of cotherapy. Generally, its use is left to practitioner interest, is undertaken at therapist initiative, and is not mandated by the agency. A strong agency expectation of cotherapy activity is usually related to a therapist training program in which a seasoned practitioner works with a student or an inexperienced practitioner.

Attitudes toward cotherapy conflict are related to differences in style or theoretical orientation. Personality differences and conflicts are occasionally a factor, but these are generally held to be of little significance and are easily resolved. Competition is expected more when both practitioners are very inexperienced or very experienced.

Conflict

Conflict is resolved more easily outside the treatment in meetings conducted immediately before or after the therapy sessions. Practitioners expect that they and their colleagues will make efforts to understand one another's style and orientation prior to entering cotherapy activity. Ironically, most practitioners do not mention supervision or consultation as an arena for dealing with cotherapy conflicts. This could be due to the emphasis on autonomy in practice and to the vague role and purpose of supervision and consultation in agencies. Cotherapy conflict is a legitimate concern in supervision.

When supervisees are doing cotherapy, the supervisor must be alert to potential for cotherapist conflict. Cotherapy activity and compatibility should be explored periodically to allow the practitioners to express and identify problem areas. It is rare that cotherapists are able to work together smoothly and effectively from the beginning. More often the cotherapists go through a period of struggling with compatibility of styles and strategies. Some cotherapists are able to work through these problems; others struggle to no avail and eventually go their separate ways. Supervision can often speed up the achievement of compatibility or help overcome what seem to be insurmountable differences. Supervision of cotherapy efforts aids in promoting effectiveness of therapy because clients frequently pick up on cotherapist conflict and use it to subvert the therapy.

Cotherapists who have substantial covert conflict act this out through interventions with clients, and they use clients to vie with each other and prove their respective views. Even though such problems can develop, cotherapy can benefit practitioners and clients in spite of the difficulties that can emerge.

Dominant Therapist

When cotherapy is attempted, usually one of the therapists emerges as dominant, based on experience, style, and amount or type of training. It has been observed that cotherapists are rarely equals (Grotjahn, 1977:248). This does not have to be a permanent state of affairs. When experience or amount or type of training interferes with equality, this can be brought into the open in supervision but minimized in the actual treatment situation. The less experienced or less trained practitioner can be encouraged to become more active, as this type of therapist tends to defer to the other therapist. The more experienced or more trained practitioner can be aided in monitoring interactions or interventions that promote the inequality. Dominant therapists can inadvertently reinforce the inequality in order to stay in control or to enhance their status in the treatment. The therapists can be assisted in ways of interacting directly in the treatment that conveys to the clients that they are genuinely working together. For those who believe that clients do not take cotherapists' styles of being active and passive into account, a story told by Carl Whitaker, the famous family therapist, is thought-provoking:

> The decision to use residents as co-therapists was also a deliberate one. I decided I could not tolerate playing games and trying to tease the residents into working with families. . . . They were free to participate or to watch. They automatically become part of the sessions, many times to their own amazement. I remember one resident who had said little or nothing for five interviews. When the . . . family came back for the sixth session, he wasn't there, having been up all night on call. They stayed for five minutes and then said, "Well, if Bill isn't going to be here, we might just as well come back next week," and walked out. This was a bit of a surprise to me, but it was a massive shock to the resident, who thought he was very unimportant. (Kopp, 1976:201)

Beginning practitioners show a tendency to need to be in control and to be overactive in the treatment. When two inexperienced practitioners do cotherapy, their combined need to be in control can lead to conflicts, especially when they disagree about how to direct and guide the therapy. In this situation, supervision by an experienced practitioner is important. The supervisor needs to assist such therapists directly with their specific interventions and to be involved in focusing the patterns that emerge in the treatment process and in designing the goals of the therapy.

When style promotes inequality, it can be handled through supervision/consultation intervention. Stylistic inequality is supported when one practitioner is more assertive than the other. Once this pattern is identified in supervision, techniques can be recommended that promote reversal of the styles. With practice of the techniques, equality can be accomplished.

Access to Clients

Conflict can develop from inequality that arises when one practitioner has more access to some of the clients than the other therapist. For example, in group therapy and family intervention, one of the therapists sometimes sees certain members individually in treatment, and when the group or family meets, that therapist will have more information to use in planning and making interventions. The second therapist often becomes aware of this information after the intervention is made and must seek clarification inside or outside the joint treatment. The second therapist can develop feelings of isolation if this knowledge difference becomes a pattern. The supervisor can help with such conflict by discovering the origin of the knowledge difference and encouraging pre- and posttherapy session meetings in which the more involved therapist shares knowledge of the individual cases with the less involved practitioner. Also, during the treatment, the more involved therapist can share the information directly, explain it briefly, and put the material directly into the group or family therapy, rather than intervening without explanation, but this strategy must be weighed against concerns about protecting the confidentiality of the individual treatment.

When students are placed in a cotherapy situation with an experienced therapist, they have no real control over their role. There is an inherent tendency to be passive and to follow the lead of the experienced practitioner, rather than alternating activity levels. Only the most sensitive, experienced therapist should be asked to do cotherapy with a student. When a student is placed with a practitioner from a different discipline, special care must be taken. Not only will this student tend to be more passive; he or she often will not have the knowledge base to understand many of the interventions made by the other therapist. The experienced practitioner may not have the patience to explain to the student the background information essential to developing understanding. The problems of inequity and lack of knowledge are compounded when a student is placed in an existing group that the experienced practitioner has been conducting.

Decision Guidelines

Holt and Greiner (Guerin, 1976) have summarized five important questions that should be addressed before attempting cotherapy:

1. For what goals should cotherapy be used?
2. In what treatment situations should cotherapy be used?
3. With what type of clients should cotherapy be used?
4. With what type of practitioners should cotherapy be used?
5. With what theoretical orientations should cotherapy be used?

Practitioners considering this form of therapy can use and expand upon these five questions to avoid problems in advance. Usually, little pretreatment planning goes into cotherapy, and the attitude seems to be that "we can deal with problems if they develop." This is unfortunate. Planning can prevent problems from developing and lessen the shock and impact of problems when they do occur.

There needs to be assessment of the interactional impact of having more than one therapist. The interactional combinations increase as participants are added to the treatment (Munson, 1980c:132). The previous five questions can be helpful in exploring the interactional impact of an additional therapist. A major question becomes, Do complexity and dynamics, based on a diagnostic assessment of the case or group, warrant inclusion of an additional therapist? A second question is, Do the concerns of a single practitioner justify adding a cotherapist, and how will this contribute to a different outcome? In some situations, it is better to initiate single-therapist treatment and regulate the therapy process by increasing supervision. This approach can prevent the development of a situation in which cotherapy is sought to overcome a single therapist's feelings of inadequacy.

Evaluation

To guard against conflict, there must be as much evaluation of the cotherapy activity as there is of the treatment. For this reason, supervision of the cotherapy becomes important. The supervisor must be alert to unrecognized conflict, floundering on the part of both therapists, and unstated feelings of secondary status on the part of one of the therapists. An effective tool in dealing with this is to require each practitioner to record independently his or her feelings and thoughts about the therapy and the cotherapy work. This is referred to as self-monitoring. An excerpt from an individual supervisory session with one cotherapist illustrates this point:

> I never gave much thought to what was going on between us until you had me write down my observations and thoughts. When we started the group, the stated agreement was that we would be coequal therapists. As I reflect on what has taken place, this has not happened. I have fallen into or have been put in the position of not being as knowledgeable or skilled as Marvin. Through writing the notes, I know now that I do much better when Marvin misses a session and I have the group to myself. I think the group members know this. When he returns, I revert to my more passive role. I don't like this pattern, but I don't know what to do about it.

With the help of the supervisor, the practitioner was able to do something about the situation. The supervisor brought the practitioners together and raised this material. The dominant therapist was also aware that this was happening but did not know how to deal with it. The offended therapist was able to share examples of how the dominant therapist fostered the inequality interactionally. The dominant therapist was not aware of the impact of his behaviors and agreed to alter them, and the second therapist agreed to make efforts to be more active and assertive. Follow-up on this revealed that the cotherapists' relationship improved. This carried over to the therapy and resulted in more effectiveness, increased feelings of mutual support, and more compatible therapeutic efforts.

Supervision of cotherapists should be developed with the awareness that there is no supervision when authority is absent and that, therefore, self-monitoring should be emphasized whenever possible. When coequal practitioners work together, authority is absent, and a third person—a supervisor—is needed to mediate the relationship.

Self-monitoring by each practitioner should be encouraged to help focus the potential problems in the cotherapy relationship. Each therapist should be expected to undergo a process of self-monitoring before entering a formal supervisory session. Langs (1979) refers to "self-supervision" as "silent activities" during a therapy session. It can occur before, during, or after a treatment session, but before the supervisory session. Self-monitoring can occur during a multiperson supervisory session and should be encouraged by the supervisor. Self-monitoring prior to supervision can make supervision more effective and focused. Self-monitoring is rehearsal for the time when designated supervision is withdrawn or decreased. As therapist skill and experience increase, self-monitoring should also increase.

Theory and Cotherapy

There is disagreement about the importance of theory in learning and doing treatment. Little systematic study has considered how theory is actually used in therapy and how it affects what is said and done (Munson, 1980c: 136). Speculative positions have been taken that theory is essential to good practice (Guerin, 1976:42); others hold that theory is of no value to practice and, in many instances, can be inhibiting (Guerin, 1976:162). Theory does play an important role in cotherapy activity, but not in the sense that we normally use it. When attempting cotherapy, it is important that the therapists develop a basic compatibility of style and that each therapist be able to understand and anticipate a sequence of interaction in which the other engages. To promote this, the practitioners must share with each other their theoretical orientations and how these orientations guide the interventions they make. Therapists do not need to adhere to the same theory, but they must discuss with each other what theories they use and how these theories guide what they do. This is especially important during the early stages of the cotherapy, when the therapists are least familiar with each other's interactional style. When theory is used to promote understanding of the therapists' interactional style, compatibility develops more rapidly, and when incompatibility exists, it becomes apparent much earlier in the treatment. As cotherapists become comfortable working together, theoretical exploration becomes less important and planning specific interventions becomes the focus.

The emphasis on theory in use is beneficial to the overall effectiveness of the treatment. It places a form of control on the interaction that helps keep the treatment focused on problems and therapeutic efforts. Practitioners who have used this approach to cotherapy have reported that they have transferred this orientation to their individual treatment cases, which has resulted in more effective interventions throughout their practice, and not just in the cotherapy situation.

Joint Style

As part of the supervision of cotherapy, it is helpful to focus periodically on the joint style that emerges. Practitioner style is a neglected element in assessing treatment interventions and outcomes. Although each therapist who engages in the cotherapy has his or her own style, a unified style of working together can be identified. It is helpful to have the practitioners describe the combined style. Many times the descriptions of the unified style are very different from the styles of the individual practitioners, and the therapists may differ on what they perceive the unified style to be. Identification and discussion of the unified style can reinforce and advance the compatibility of the practitioners through the increased understanding and sense of accomplishment that results from such awareness. Striving for unity and cohesiveness of style and their articulation in supervision can be beneficial to the therapy outcome, since there are indications that therapist cohesion is correlated with a positive therapist-client relationship (Munson, Study F).

Client Perception

Clients accept cotherapy fairly readily and tend to view such efforts as being positive because more than one person is interested in their difficulties and because the agency is willing to commit adequate resources to ensure quality treatment. The view that the presence of an additional therapist gives rise to feelings within clients that their problems must be very bad is generally unfounded. If the clients sense conflict and animosity between the therapists, they will not commit themselves to the therapy and may withdraw from treatment completely. This does not mean that clients should be protected from any therapist disagreement. There is a difference between specific disagreement over an interactional sequence and persistent underlying conflict. It can be therapeutic for clients to hear therapists disagree or to hear therapists express divergent views about the meaning of behavior or interaction. Such disagreement can help to bring out inconsistencies in the clients' actions. Where persistent unstated conflict exists, the clients are usually the first to recognize and verbalize it in the therapy. This is especially the case when cotherapy is used in group treatment. When clients broach this topic, the therapists should encourage them to express their observations so that they can gain insight into how their performance is perceived by the clients. This type of interaction can also help the practitioners validate their assessment of the clients' general ability to perceive events, interactions, and meanings of behavior accurately.

CONSULTATION

Increasingly, social workers are called upon to provide consultation services within the agencies that employ them as well as for other agencies where they serve as outside consultants. Social workers provide consultation mainly to schools, social service agencies, law enforcement, and long-term care settings. These consultation services are provided primarily to other social workers, but also to nurses, teachers, psychologists, doctors, clergy, lawyers, police, and judges (Kadushin, 1977). When supervisors do consultation work for diverse agencies and different professions, they are required to assume new roles and orientations quite different from their supervisory roles. The emphasis in this section will be on the practical aspects of consultation rather than on theoretical models (for theoretical orientations, see O'Neill and Trickett, 1982; Gallessich, 1982).

A study by Wallace (1982) identified the demographic factors that are reportedly associated with successful consultation. Some of these factors are geographic location, working in full-time private practice, sex of the consultant, and development of community contacts. The emphasis in this section will focus on the actions taken and procedures used by the consultant in order to be successful at this activity. For example, developing good community contacts is more likely to occur through developing a quality reputation by providing sound consultation, rather than by having lunch frequently with various agency representatives.

Consultation is easy for an organization to arrange, but getting good consultation is much more difficult to achieve. The supervisor who is entering consultation work must recognize that consultation is different from supervision. Supervision is mandated, and the supervisor has power by virtue of agency sanction of the position. The supervisor can give directives and expect that they will be implemented. The consultant role necessitates dealing with an agency or organization that seeks guidance and direction voluntarily. The organization employing the consultant is in a position to utilize, reject, or simply ignore the advice of the consultant.

The consultant is in a position only to give advice and make recommendations. When this advice is followed, it is rewarding, but if recommendations are ignored, the consultant can become frustrated and angry and may lose commitment to aiding the organization and its clients. This loss of commitment to promoting changes and improvements can result in demoralization by staff who participate in the consultation process because the consultant is often perceived as an external ally who can advocate change without fear of sanction.

The consultant must accept the advisory role and offer recommendations firmly, consistently, and continually, regardless of whether they are implemented. In reality, some recommendations get implemented and, for various reasons, others do not. The consultant has a responsibility to follow up on all recommendations to determine barriers to unimplemented recommendations and to seek alternative ways to deal with problems. If the majority of recommendations are not implemented, the consultant does need to question the value of continuing the consultation within the existing framework.

The consultant should be direct and use an interventive approach, while remaining sensitive to the organizational complexities and the right of the organization to use the consultant's input voluntarily. As long as this basic premise regarding the difference between supervision and consultation is kept in mind, most of the principles covered in this book can be applied to clinical case consultation or programmatic-oriented consultation.

Type and Focus of Consultation

The consultant must be clear about the type of consultation that is to be provided. This is important because many organizations know that they need a consultant but are not sure why they need a consultant or what they need a consultant to do. If the consultant can draw distinctions for the client between the different types of consultation that are available, this can be helpful to the organization in specifying the purpose of the consultation. Generally, the types of consultation include organizational consultation, program consultation, case consultation, and a combination of organizational, program, and case consultation. Within these types of consultation, the consultant will need to give added specificity to the consultation through helping the client identify the focus.

Consultation can focus on programmatic implementation relationships or take a personal or clinical focus. Combinations of these activities can be used, but multiple foci can be confusing for the consultee. It is best to separate the different forms as much as possible, but under some conditions the consultant will be required to integrate these activities. The integration mode occurs when the consultant is aiding in planning new programming, planning organizational structure change, working to resolve conflict or confusion between departments or units, attempting to resolve disagreements between administrators and clinicians, or addressing client dissatisfaction.

Integration of activities is more likely to be necessary if the agency or organization has significant, systemwide dysfunction.

In the *programmatic implementation* form, the consultant focuses on what organizational participants should do and how they should do it. This model is often used when an organization is attempting to establish or to reorganize a program or a department. This model is also useful when those assigned to carry out a program have little experience or skill with the services the program is designed to deliver. When an agency is undergoing major restructuring, a good model to use to organize the focus of the consultation is Bridges' (1991) model for the process of organizational change. Bridges believes that organizations try to implement change without consideration of what is being dismantled. He points out that it is not change that causes problems, but the process of transition from the old to new system. He separates the concepts of change by noting that change is situational and transition is psychological. People do not accept or adjust to change easily. Change cannot begin by eliminating the old procedures and focusing on the new methods to be implemented. Rather than simply beginning the new, the process of change should start with conscious planning to end the old structures and policies. (See Chapter 11 for details of Bridges' model of managing organizational change.)

A *relationship* focus deals with improving communication within an organization or program staff. This model is most useful where there is much staff conflict or a mixture of old and new staff. In some agencies, reorganization requires staff who have been functioning independently to work more closely with others in a team effort, and these workers often need help in making this transition. When focusing on relationships, the consultant will need to be more concerned with how work gets done and with the nature of staff interaction.

The *personal* focus occurs when the agency manager or department head is provided with personalized consultation. The consultant serves as a highly individualized resource for the manager and is, in a sense, a sympathetic ear for the consultee. This form of consultation can result in an intense, highly personalized relationship in which recommendations of the consultant, if implemented, can have widespread effects.

Consultation with a *clinical* focus occurs when the consultant gives advice about service delivery in specific cases. This can take the form of case presentations or actual intervention provided by the consultant through working directly with clients.

Consultation Structure

Regardless of the type or form of consultation used with an organization, five structural elements should be part of the process.

The Contract

The consultant should have a contract with the organization and should insist on a written contract. In organizations where serious problems exist or where staff conflict is severe, the consultant can become the "scapegoat" or become caught up in the confusion and conflict. A written contract can help the consultant avoid straying or being subverted from the original purpose of the consultant role. Staff changes over time can result in confusion about the role of the consultant even in healthy organizations. A written contract can save time when new managers enter a situation where long-term consultation arrangements exist.

The written contract should include information about consultant compensation, frequency and duration of visits, time period of the contract, the individual with whom the consultant will have direct contact, requirements for written reports by the consultant, functions of the consultant, and tasks of the consultant. These are general items that should be included, and either party to the contract should be free to ask for inclusion of any items they feel important to providing clarity.

The Plan

The consultation plan should be developed early in the consultation process and after an initial assessment has been done by the consultant. Based on the contractual functions and tasks, the consultant should assess the needs of the organization. The plan should be performance oriented and stated in terms of goals and objectives, both short-term and long-term. The consultation plan should expand on the contractual agreement. Some consultants prefer to negotiate the written contract after this assessment and plan development stage is completed.

In developing the plan, the consultant should be sensitive to the nature and culture of the organization. The nature of the organization relates to the services, programs, policies, and procedures of the organization. The consultant must develop a plan that is consistent with the nature of the organization and that can be reasonably implemented. The culture of the organization includes its informal structures—the unwritten rules and interactional patterns of the staff. Although these elements would not necessarily be part of the written plan, they are essential to the type of plan the consultant develops. If these informal elements are not observed by the consultant in the plan development stage, they can later interfere with implementation of the formal plan.

Contact

The contract and plan should specify frequency and duration of consultant visits. The structure of consultant visits will depend on the nature of the agency and the purpose of the consultation. In some cases, it is better to plan infrequent visits for large blocks of time, whereas in others frequent visits for small blocks of time are preferable. As a general rule, the more serious the problems, the more frequent the visits should be. Also, educationally oriented (clinical) consultation is more easily adapted to infrequent visits in large time blocks, while administrative (program) consultation is better suited to frequent visits for small time periods.

The timing of the visits should be established in connection with the time required to implement recommendations of the consultant. The organization must be given time to implement recommendations before being required to attempt additional changes. Change takes place slowly, and the consultant needs to provide latitude in order to avoid frustration and poor adjustment to change on the part of the staff (see Bridges, 1991; also see Chapter 11).

The consultant needs to be clear about whom to contact during visits. It can be cumbersome to have too many staff involved and ineffective to have too few staff involved. All staff who will be required to implement recommendations should be involved. The critical point is to plan and think through in advance what changes are to be made and where they are to be made, and then include all staff who will be essential to implementing the changes.

Reporting

The consultant should provide a written report for each visit. This can aid the organization in documenting and justifying the consultation activity. The consultant can use reports to evaluate and plan the evolution of the consultation process as well as to keep track of the sequencing of the recommendations and their implementation. Written reports can provide continuity from visit to visit and help the staff understand that the consultant will follow up on actions that were discussed during visits. Written reports allow staff to refer to the consultant's suggestions between visits, rather than waiting for the consultant's next visit to seek clarification. The written report should include, but does not have to be limited to, information regarding date of visit, length of visit, names of people with whom the consultant had contact, clients discussed, problems addressed, accomplishments, list of recommendations, and date and time of next visit. Visual 14.3 contains a recommended consultation report form that is simple but covers the relevant areas of most consultation visits in clinical settings.

Evaluation

The consultation process should also be evaluated. Consultation work that is provided for one visit only should be evaluated at the conclusion of

VISUAL 14.3. Consultant Form

CONSULTATION REPORT FORM

CONSULTANT: _____

ORGANIZATION: _____

   Address: _____

                _____

   Telephone: _____

DATE: _____

TIME: IN: _____

      OUT: _____

TOTAL TIME: _____

PERSONS CONTACTED:

TOPICS DISCUSSED:

CLIENTS DISCUSSED:

RECOMMENDATIONS:

PLANS FOR NEXT CONSULTATION:

SIGNATURE OF CONSULTANT: _____

the visit. Open-ended consultation should be evaluated periodically. Evaluation should occur at least once annually. The evaluation should be written as well as verbal. It should be focused on goal attainment and based on the contract, the plan, and the visitation reports. It is reasonable to expect that not all goals will be achieved. A primary purpose of the evaluation is to determine what has been accomplished and what remains to be done. Unmet goals might have been unrealistic, or perhaps problems were misperceived initially and need to be reconceptualized.

Resistance

Organizations seek consultation for various reasons, ranging from a genuine desire to improve functioning to saving money and avoiding criticism by regulatory bodies. Consultation is frequently perceived as a refreshing, creative, innovative opportunity for change, but it can also be viewed with resistance and suspicion and as unnecessary. For consultation to have a positive outcome, it must be accepted in principle by all levels of authority in the organization, especially by the higher levels of power and authority.

Individuals within the organization will vary in their reactions to the consultant. Rarely will all elements of the organization have an equal and consistent reaction to the consultation process. Some people will resent the consultant and attempt to subvert the consultant's recommendations; others will accept the consultant but show no strong commitment to the recommendations; others will support the consultant and use advice effectively. Some individuals may view the consultant as a savior who will solve all the organization's ills. People with this perspective will make individual appeals to the consultant to solve various problems or to help overcome powerful or troublesome individuals in the organization. The consultant must use information obtained from such appeals in a cautious and sensitive manner. Such information should be considered only in the context of the specific role of the consultant and the specific tasks or problems that the consultant has been employed to address.

Consultants can inadvertently threaten directors, administrators, supervisors, and ineffective practitioners. Even effective practitioners can be threatened by consultants if the consultation process is not implemented openly and with a clear understanding of why consultation has been sought. The consultant should request that staff be prepared in advance but should also begin the consultation process with an explanation of his or her own conceptions of the consultation. Administrators can imply that a consultant is being brought in "to straighten things out" and set up the consultant as a quasi-manager. This is not an appropriate role for the consultant.

Rather than telling the staff what consultation is, it is better to inquire how they perceive it and what they expect to get from it. This approach allows the consultant to learn how consultation has been presented to staff by the administration, as well as how the staff perceive it personally. After exploring these perceptions, the consultant can correct any misperceptions the staff may have.

Organization staff can consciously and unconsciously use certain strategies to resist the consultant. The types and forms of resistance are as varied as the number of participants in the consultation process. Some of the more common direct reactions are such comments as, "The consultant does not understand our situation," "The consultant is not here often enough to know what is going on," or "You need to know about the history of this agency to understand why we do things the way we do." All of these responses are aimed at negating the consultant's knowledge base for intervention.

Rather than confronting such reactions or becoming defensive, the consultant should ask the participants to explain the situation or to describe the history of the agency so that the consultant's knowledge gap can be overcome. The consultant should acknowledge that he or she is less knowledgeable than the staff and then focus on getting the information needed to do the consultation work.

More subtle resistances are structural and interactional. For example, some agencies will flood the consultant with nonessential issues or they will change the agenda items for each visit. It is true that in some agencies activity is crisis oriented and changes from day to day, but the basic issues and problems remain. When these strategies are used, the consultant needs to observe the patterns and formulate ideas about the major problems and then reconceptualize the nonessential issues and specific agenda items in the context of the persistent and real issues.

GENDER AND SUPERVISION

Issues in clinical social work supervision related to the gender of the worker have received little empirical study, and there has been little theoretical writing on the subject. This neglect is ironic in that supervision is the arena in which issues regarding gender discrimination are usually encountered (Munson, 1997b). For example, salary increases, performance evaluations, employment decisions, and promotions are all components of supervision that have been identified as the major sources of discrimination based on gender (Munson, 1997b).

Discrimination in these areas is related to hierarchical organizational arrangements in which supervisors are paid more than clinicians and administrators are paid more than supervisors. Truly, power is position. Scotch (1971) holds that unless women are free to move up into supervisory and administrative positions, the hidden inequities become exaggerated. Although sex typing of positions has diminished, the salary and promotional inequities still exist, often leading to covert resentment and, in some instances, to open conflict. Women have fared badly in this hierarchical process that is generally attributed to socialization practices with respect to gender roles (Williams, Ho, and Fielder, 1974).

Social work has not been as vigorous as other disciplines in investigating and documenting expectations and performance that are based on sex role stereotypes of men and women. Most researchers have found that workers who had a male or female supervisor found no significant differences in satisfaction with their job, salary, or supervision, or in promotional opportunity (Bartol and Wortman, 1976). Changes in clinical practice and the role of women and men require reexamination of supervision, practice, and male-female practitioner relationships.

Background

From the beginning of the social work profession in the 1800s to the mid-1960s, most of the major works on supervision were written by women, but subsequently the reverse has been true. This has led to a male stereotype of the supervisory relationships. Psychiatry, psychology, and social work (the three major professions delivering psychotherapy services) have been slow to address issues related to gender, and almost completely lacking in attention to gender and supervision issues.

Trends indicate that the pool of available professionally trained practitioners increasingly will be female (Munson, 1998b). This has implications for supervision. Limited literature exists on the nature of supervision practice based on gender. No reliable statistics exist regarding the percentage of female practitioners and supervisors. A study conducted in the mid-1970s of a random sample of social work practitioners revealed that 66 percent of the practitioners were female and 57 percent of supervisors were female (Munson, 1979c:105). NASW statistics show that, in 1995, 78.5 percent of its MSW-level membership was female and 89.7 percent of its BSW-level membership was female (Gibelman and Schervish, 1997). In the 1970s study, 57 percent of supervisors were female; by 1988 the female supervisory proportion was 69 percent, and in 1995 it was 72.5 percent (Gibelman and Schervish, 1997).

Historically, there has been little exploration of the roles of males and females in supervision. In a study of males in social work, Kadushin (1976a) found that only 21 percent viewed being supervised by a female as a problem, but 37 percent preferred to be supervised by a male. Kadushin considers the movement of males toward administration in part as an attempt to resolve the concerns associated with being supervised by a female. He concludes that his findings support previous speculation that males resist subordination to women. Wilensky and Lebeaux (1975) also hold this point of view, arguing that men do not remain in direct service positions, and women are seldom assigned top administrative posts because of the conflicts that are created when males are subordinate to females. They point out that strains are created for both sexes in such positions, and they attribute the stress to cultural socialization processes that are carried over to the work relationships.

In supervision it has been pointed out that helping supervisees gain knowledge involves different processes than those required to change attitudes (Pettes, 1979:5). Acquiring knowledge and changing attitudes are fundamental in dealing with gender issues in supervision. Changing attitudes in large measure is dependent on acquisition of knowledge. Through the use of facts, concepts, theories, and guidelines, the conditions for developing positive attitudes toward supervision based on gender can be explored.

Women and the Evolution of Supervision

In the past, in the day-to-day life of agency practice, the average female practitioner and supervisee lived in a traditional society where women showed deference to men and were rarely afforded the professional promotional opportunities men experienced. Women supervising women was a common occurrence, but women supervising men was a unique, brief encounter in the men's rise to higher levels of administration (Reynolds, 1965/1942; Munson, 1997b).

Historically, the female supervisor's lot was difficult and her effectiveness suppressed. Many skilled, knowledgeable female supervisors and teachers had to live in the shadow of male psychiatrists, even though much of what the psychiatrists had to offer was at best ineffective and at worst inappropriate in meeting practice demands (Reynolds, 1965/1942; Munson, 1997b). Many of the inroads made and creative practice methods devised by females relied on the influence of psychiatrists, as illustrated by the wife of psychiatrist Adolf Meyer, who became the first psychiatric social worker in New York in 1907 (Munson, 1983a:43). Although this model prevailed for over a century, the modern women's movement has produced many changes and demands a new perspective of supervision.

Feminist Practice

Current supervisory practice and gender issues can be portrayed as centering around the emerging literature on a feminist approach to practice. Feminist therapy has emerged from the modern women's movement that began in the early 1960s (Sturdivant, 1980). The initial rejection of psychotherapy by the general feminist movement was subsequently refocused by therapists into a specific model of feminist therapy. Sturdivant (1980) has conceptualized feminist therapy around the idea of "philosophy of treatment." The core of feminist therapy is a set of values and attitudes that are translated into practice skill. Feminist practitioners reject traditional gender roles and view societal and cultural values as necessarily making traditional therapy sexist.

Since approximately 20 percent (about 34 million) of Americans subscribe to traditional values, the nascent practitioner following the feminist therapeutic approach can be subjected to many conflicting pressures, just as the population as a whole is caught up in conflicting expectations (Yankelovich, 1981; Munson, 1997b). This conflict increases the importance of the role of the supervisor. The supervisor must give the practitioner the opportunity to explore the philosophy of practice and how it is manifested in what the practitioner does with the client. Without the opportunity to explore these attitudes, values, thoughts, and actions, the treatment can be misguided and confusing for the client. Symptoms, problems, roles, and responsibilities take on different meanings when a feminist perspective is introduced into the professional relationship.

The literature on feminist practice does not mention supervision as a way to help one build a feminist perspective but implies that this can be done through reading, introspection, and drawing on life experiences (Gibbs, 1984:22; Munson, 1997b; Hipp and Munson, 1995). The literature suggests that the "going it alone" approach is necessary to emulating the male-dominated professions (Robbins and Siegel, 1983:1), and others have pointed out the loneliness, doubt, and fear that can accompany this solitary approach (Milwid, 1983:68). A paradox exists here. Since feminist theory and therapy are so new, "going it alone" will only isolate the practitioner and prevent the spread of the approach. Historically, supervision has been the source of theory development and the spread of theory (application) in practice. Supervision is the place where the inexperienced practitioner grapples with theory and case material to produce a rewarding, skilled, confident practice style.

The evolution of theory is essential. For example, modern research on psychoanalytic theory is confirming some of its tenets, modifying others, and discarding some. Some feminist therapists have attempted to build the theory by countering against psychoanalytic theory. This has not helped feminist theory, nor has it greatly altered psychoanalytic practices. Both approaches have much to offer, and the focus in supervision, research, and practice should be the advancement of each theory and differential application. There have been efforts to reconcile feminist perspectives with traditional psychoanalytic approaches (McGoldrick et al., 1991). In the process of forging a place for feminist theory in conjunction with earlier theories, disagreement has arisen over whether feminist approaches to therapy constitute a method, a modality, a theory, or a philosophy. Some have argued that feminist therapy is a philosophy that can be used to enhance other approaches (Porter, 1985:334). Much more research and application are needed before this process can be considered complete.

The practitioner cannot merge philosophy and practice of feminist treatment alone. To try to do so would be inconsistent with feminist theoretical conceptions. Commitment to the theory is not sufficient, and the supervisor plays a crucial role in the successful outcome of a course of treatment. Intervention based solely on academic abstractions can result in loss of confidence, disillusionment, and withdrawal from a feminist or any approach. Such shifts on the part of the practitioner can result in the client becoming discouraged, lapsing back into former ineffective coping strategies, or withdrawing from treatment. It has been pointed out that the feminist practitioner must be comfortable and secure in her own role (Sturdivant, 1980:152). The practitioner who adopts this perspective out of insecurity, rather than security, can do harm within treatment and expose the client to potential harm outside the treatment. The supervisor's role in monitoring such limitations is critical. Evidence suggests that supervision is essential to identifying feminist therapists' blind spots and the anger they "did not hear" in treating female clients (Kaplan et al., 1983:29).

The field of psychology views the trend of theory development as evolutionary and expansive, psychiatry is returning to biological explanations of behavior, and social work is moving to a diverse number of specializations with decreased emphasis on theoretical grounding. These trends are somewhat removed from the situational stresses clients face in a society undergoing exponential change and provide little support for translating theory into practical, useful information (see Steininger, Newell, and Garcia, 1984:146). Feminist therapy holds much reality-based assistance for many clients and deserves attention in educational programs and supervision.

Feminist Practice and Supervision

The emergence of feminist practice raises issues for supervision and practice. Debate centers on whether males should treat female clients, whether the supervisor of a feminist practitioner should necessarily be a woman, and whether men are capable of a feminist perspective. Another issue that needs exploration is the advisability of feminist therapists treating men. With so many new underlying issues, feminist therapists should undergo adequate supervision or consultation rather than being left to resolve these issues without support (Munson, 1997b).

Female practitioners are less likely to have experienced supervision by a female during training (Seiden, 1982:287), and given the high percentage of men who have moved into administrative and supervisory positions, the chances of a female practitioner having a female supervisor are limited. Male supervisors of women are inadequately prepared and unsuspecting of many relevant feminist practice issues because of lack of exposure to female supervisors or feminist issues. Some supervisees, both male and female, will not understand the value of a feminist approach with certain clients, and these supervisees offer a special challenge for the feminist supervisor.

Situations involving a male supervising a feminist practitioner have a high risk of surprise, confusion, frustration, and defensiveness (Keefe and Maypole, 1983:104) on the part of the supervisor, who lacks the feminist's insight into traditional male behavior. The female supervisee can experience the same reactions when having to deal with an insensitive male supervisor. In such a situation, it is incumbent upon the supervisor to be open and aware, to develop understanding of the supervisee's position, and to examine his own biases about women. The same advice holds for the female supervisor who does not subscribe to the feminist philosophy. It is unrealistic to expect that because the supervisor is a woman, she will necessarily accept, understand, and advocate a feminist view (Munson and Hipp, 1998). Although the effects of the women's movement on education and practice are growing, it has been pointed out that the theory of female sexuality and feminine development continues to be based on a conventional variation of the male model, which could result in history repeating itself (Gould, 1984).

Feminist therapists hold that more equality of power and authority between supervisor and supervisee is a basic notion, just as it is in the relationship between practitioner and client (Porter, 1985). Some have pointed out that the power relationship can be effectively reversed in some situations, such as when a male supervisor can be given insight about female clients by a female supervisee (Brodsky, 1980:513). The question that remains to be addressed is, How much equality is necessary for effective feminist supervision? If there is to be total equality, it is no longer supervision.

Agency Function

Supervision of a feminist-oriented practitioner must take into account the needs of the client and the function of the agency. Although there are feminist practitioners, there are few feminist-oriented agencies. If a client comes to a specific agency with a specific problem or set of problems, a feminist approach to service must be compatible with client needs and agency function. Service should be based on client problems and needs, not on practitioner interest. This does not mean agency function and intervention cannot be integrated with a feminist approach. It is critical that the feminist perspective, the agency function, and the client needs be parallel. This is identified by Niles in a case example in which a client had talked about her ex-husband being behind in support payments, a son's appearance in juvenile court, and a sister's illness; then the worker suggested that they discuss the woman's obesity and how the woman could be attractive if she lost weight (Keefe and Maypole, 1983:104). In this example, the worker is depicted as reflecting gender bias. Exploring the client's obesity is considered valid only if it is introduced as a problem by the client. This would be true of genuine specific feminist issues, which could be easily related to the three issues presented by the client. Another example of this would be the battered wife whose therapist recommends marital or family intervention when the client requires shelter and protection, which is consistent with a feminist perspective. The supervisor should conceptualize treatment issues in the context of client-identified problems and agency function. This should be the background consideration of any treatment issues in feminist-oriented supervision.

Supervision should focus on the interventions to be made by the practitioner. In analyzing these interventions, feminist supervision can be oriented toward (1) the practitioner, (2) the client, or (3) the context of the treatment. In discussing feminist material in supervision, the emphasis is on the practitioner or the client. The question remains whether this is the most efficient way to learn about or supervise treatment. Some theorists have placed more emphasis on the treatment context because it is a more comprehensive approach. In this approach the focus is on exposure, interventions, and techniques (Lecker, 1976:185). Any treatment supervision that fails to integrate all components of the treatment will be necessarily limited in utility (Gurman, 1981a:420-422). Haley (1967) goes so far as to say that self-expression of the client (and in the supervisory framework the self-expression of the supervisor) cannot be separated from the context of the treatment. For feminist material to be effective in treatment and supervision, this basic point is paramount. The main consideration is that any exploration of feminist material in supervision should be case-related to avoid the supervision going astray. This approach can help promote a feminist orientation, rather than detract from it. For example, Gould holds that the use of Freudian theory in practice prohibited the development of feminist psychology. This inhibiting factor was reinforced through extension of Freudian theory use in the supervisory relationship to promote self-awareness (Gould, 1984:101).

Feminist material in supervision is relevant in the context of other practice questions: What are the problems that face the client? What techniques are most appropriate in relating to client problems? What are the goals of the treatment? How will outcomes be measured? How will practitioner "blind spots" be identified and overcome? Within the framework of these questions and other similar questions, feminist material can ultimately benefit, help, and be useful to the practitioner and client.

Gender Bias

Gender bias in the practitioner-client relationship can be a difficult problem to deal with in supervision, whether it be a male practitioner with a female client or a female practitioner with a male client. Gender bias has been found to be inversely correlated with self-concept and positively correlated with homophobia. One study found that homophobia was lowest among psychologists, moderate among psychiatrists, and highest among social workers (Anderson and Henderson, 1985:522). In supervision, dealing with such issues can be clarified by supervising the *position,* not the *person.* To avoid conflict and combativeness, the supervisor can focus on the case, tasks to be carried out, goals to be accomplished, and problems to be solved, rather than on the personality, attitudes, and values of the practitioner. Awareness techniques and exercises have been developed to explore stereotypes and biases in relation to clients of the opposite sex (Brodsky, 1980: 518-520). In efforts to enhance feminist practice, it has been argued that feminists who supervise can use the supervisory relationship to foster a sensitivity to feminist issues in treatment in order to promote understanding among neophyte practitioners that a problem exists (Marecek and Kravetz, 1982:302). This approach can be helpful, but if the supervisor and supervisee are not clear about the objectives of such an approach, this can lead to conflict in supervision. To avoid supervisory conflict, any awareness development-oriented supervision must be client related and connected to specific case material. In some cases, avoidance of feminist issues in supervision is preferable. This is especially the case where authority is highly structured.

In highly structured organizations that emphasize authority, the potential for supervisory conflict is increased. For example, in hospitals, where authority is structurally defined and divided along the lines of professional disciplines (medicine, nursing, social work, psychology, etc.), supervisees are more acutely aware of authority division, and this awareness carries over to the supervisory relationships. In the normal course of events, these relationship issues get worked out. In the case of mild problems, passage of time and the skill of the supervisor are the crucial factors. The following case example illustrates this:

> Tim, an advanced graduate student placed in a large government hospital, was required to do three rotations of four weeks each. He began his first rotation with a sense of superiority and spent much supervisory time ridiculing the bureaucracy and being sarcastic about his perceived insensitivity of the staff. He manifested a need to convince the supervisor that he knew more than the regular staff, had insights into clients and the organization that others did not, and held an "existential view" of the plight of the clients, the staff, and himself in the situation. The supervisor, a seasoned feminist practitioner, allowed Tim to express these views and did not challenge his views or attempt to defend or explain the system. The supervisor used Tim's observations to help him learn about organizations, clients, and staff at a conceptual level. The supervisor managed each supervision session in a way that guided Tim to focus on the question, "Under these circumstances, what could be done to help the patient?" She led Tim to express his views in the context of specific cases and what could be done to aid the

patient and/or the family. By the middle of the second rotation, Tim talked less about organizational and staff issues and focused on patient dynamics and difficulties to be addressed. He began to identify skilled and committed staff who were important to learn from and observe working. By the end of the third rotation, all the "old bravado" was gone and was replaced with professional exploration of strengths, weaknesses, limitations, and problems to be managed.

The supervisor's patience and skill led to overcoming the student's defensiveness and anxiety produced by an underlying sense of inadequacy. The positive outcome in this case is best described in the words of the supervisor:

> I know Tim was feeling overwhelmed and needed to defend against it. I gave him the flexibility to express his views. I knew he would come around when he realized that superiority stuff would not get him very far around here.

The supervisor avoided conflict by not allowing this situation to become a sex-based power struggle and focused instead on the practice issues facing the supervisee.

Not all gender-linked supervisory authority relationships result in such positive outcomes. In cases in which supervisees have more authority-related issues and the supervisor is less skilled and not open to exploring feminist issues, the conflicts can escalate to a point at which resolution is impossible, and the struggles become upsetting to the entire staff. This is illustrated by the case of Pat, a graduate student receiving a fellowship in a large hospital:

> Pat was assigned several cases involving different services in the hospital. The situation was complicated by the student's husband being a radiologist in the cancer unit. Other staff complained to the supervisor about Pat "taking advantage" of her husband's status in the unit and using her position as a basis for going around the rules. The supervisor attempted to discuss this with Pat by telling her to "cool it" on the ward. Pat viewed this as the supervisor "picking" on her and being "jealous" of her status. This low-grade conflict continued for several weeks and reached crisis stage when the hospital implemented a regulation that each discipline wear a designated color lab coat in the hospital. Pat refused to wear the coat and said it "clashed with many of my clothes." Pat's husband, embarrassed by the situation, refused to get involved. The director of the social work department entered the conflict, and when Pat became verbally combative with him, he terminated her from the fellowship. The hospital administrator withdrew the fellowship and assigned it to another department.

The supervisor in this case was a traditional male who had little understanding of the worker, so he withdrew from her. He expressed little interest in the emotional content and felt "the rules are the rules." He saw the student as a "feminist" because she had raised some feminist issues in supervision. This was not the issue, but it became an excuse for the supervisor and further isolated the student. With more openness and looking beyond slogans, the supervisor could have avoided the extreme actions that resulted.

Feminist Family Therapy

One of the most significant modern developments in the helping professions has been the increase of family therapy, and it raises a number of questions to be addressed and interpreted for the feminist-oriented practitioner and supervisor: How does the feminist therapist foster equality of the sexes in family practice? What is the effect of a feminist perspective in family treatment regarding the treatment process and outcome? How does a supervisor who is not schooled in a feminist perspective supervise a practitioner with a feminist perspective? Another related question is, Because more practitioners are entering private practice and often seek supervision from practitioners from other male-dominated disciplines, how can a practitioner engage in a sustained career development process based on a feminist perspective? Because most psychiatrists are male, does the psychiatrist supervisor and psychotherapist supervisee constellation foster reinforcement of the traditional, potentially sexist model of supervision and practice? These questions need attention in the family therapy field, as well as in supervision in general.

In family therapy supervision, it has been pointed out that "the supervisory process will be most successful . . . if it constantly focuses on the skills that the practitioner in training needs and must gradually begin to demonstrate" (Clarkin and Glick, 1982:89). This is a good rule to follow in all forms of supervision to avoid conflict.

Administration

The feminist practitioner, as with any emerging approach, has to struggle to define and build a practice orientation, but this struggle is mild compared to that of the feminist practitioner who desires to move to administration. Given the rise in the number of female practitioners and the dramatic decline of males entering the social work profession, there is increased speculation about the nature of the opportunities for and role of women in administrative positions.

Social work has lagged behind other disciplines in providing opportunities for women to move into administrative positions, and there has been a concomitant lag in documenting and investigating women's aptitudes in this area (Munson, 1982a; Munson, 1997b; Munson and Hipp, 1998). As opportunities in administration expand for women, new issues and choices are produced. New role models must be developed and supervisory opportunities and experiences provided that encourage and support women to pursue administrative positions. Supervision can be an arena in which to identify women who desire administrative careers. The role of the supervisor as a model for aspiring female administrators needs more attention. The importance of this area is highlighted by one study (Munson, 1982a) that found that female social workers in nonadministrative positions who desire to be administrators experience more conflict and negative perceptions than other groups of women who have no desire to be administrators. This could be due to lack of encouragement, support, and adequate role models.

It is not safe to assume that because someone is a helping professional he or she will be free of gender biases. Because women in administrative positions is a relatively new development, women encounter biases on the part of "old-time" colleagues that can be distressing. Distortion can result, leading to lack of understanding of the basis of older colleagues' views and of actions by younger women seeking role models. In the general organizational world, the woman is readily and easily made aware of the odds, resistances, and lack of role models she faces in a "man's world" (Kanter and Stein, 1979). The female professional in the clinical organization faces a more bewildering situation in that she is part of a profession that is moving toward a female majority but still offers few female role models because males have gravitated to the majority of high-rank positions. Under these circumstances, the support group concept for women becomes just as important in clinical settings as in the business world (Faver, Fox, and Shannon, 1983:83). On the other hand, given the gender typing of occupations in society (Pogrebin, 1980:535), the new majority status of women could enhance women's efforts to overcome the traditional sex typing of occupations in their preparation for and movement into middle management and upper-level positions of leadership. In this effort, much could be learned from the patterns of women's work groups and support groups in the corporate world (Kanter, 1977:299-303).

Supervision for Career Advancement

In clinical practice it is appropriate for the supervisor of female practitioners not only to supervise job performance but also to assist the female supervisees in preparation for career advancement. Women need to be encouraged to pursue and trained to perform supervisory and management roles, and their own supervisory experience can be an excellent arena for such preparation.

The findings of one study (Munson, 1982a:56) reveal that women who are practitioners with ambition to be administrators believe sexist practices exist at a high level, feel they need to be aggressive to get ahead, undergo more professional conflict, and desire more organizational supports for their career goals compared to female practitioners who have no desire for administrative positions. That such perceptions exist at a significantly higher level for women with administrative ambitions raises questions for how supervision is conceptualized and delivered, since these women will be the clinical administrative leaders in the coming decades. The profession needs to establish training programs to aid women in achieving their career aspirations. Supervisors of women with clinical management career aspirations should take these aspirations into account in their supervisory practices. For example, assertiveness by women in clinical managerial positions has been described as difficult for many women to engage in, and for many other participants to accept (Drury, 1984:133-135). This is an example of one area in which supervisors can be helpful to supervisees with managerial ambitions. In order to do this, the supervisor must have experience and skill at being assertive.

Gender and Stress

The supervisor has to deal with a number of matters, but practitioner stress reactions are a significant factor. With increased practice demands brought about by more varied client problems, the practitioner today is vulnerable to work-related stress. Along with this, practitioners are expected to master more theories, develop more techniques, and possess an array of coping strategies, as illustrated by the discussion of operationalizing feminist practice. Although client problems have become more extensive and intensive, institutional resources are decreasing, causing many practitioners to internalize these inadequacies.

Given the practice demands and the conflicts associated with administrative opportunities that feminists experience, the supervisor must be concerned with the potential for stress among feminist-oriented practitioners. The empirical research on stress among clinical social workers is not extensive. The few data-based studies have produced interesting, but sometimes confusing, results. Reiter (1980), in a study of clinical social workers, found that 46 percent would not choose social work as a career if they had it to do over. This is interesting in light of the view that jobs and professions in society have always been sex typed, and social work has traditionally been considered a woman's profession (82 percent of the respondents in Reiter's study were women). Because socialization processes prepare people for these roles in conscious and unconscious ways (Pogrebin, 1980:535), the consciousness-raising of the feminist movement could increase sensitivity to this regretted career choice when the reality of the practice world turns out to be radically different from the theoretical expectations and supervisors provide little assistance in making genuine feminist practice a reality.

The question of importance to the supervisor, based on Reiter's findings, is, Do women practitioners suffer higher stress reactions? Three studies suggest the answer to this question is no. A study by Streepy (1981) notes that stress is associated with such variables as income level, educational level, attitude toward the profession, and amount of work experience, rather than gender of the worker. Studies of hospital social workers (Munson, 1983b) and graduate social work students (Munson, 1984) showed no significant differences between the levels of stress reactions suffered by females as compared to males. These findings are the opposite of those revealed in a study of the medical field in which females reported significantly higher stress than males (Huebner et al., 1981). Reasons for psychotherapy practitioners' and students' lower levels of stress remain in the realm of speculation. However, none of these studies controlled for feminist practice perspective. It is quite possible that feminists suffer more or less stress when compared to others. Currently not enough data are available to answer this question. In such unknown areas, the role of the supervisor in promoting prevention of stress is important.

The number of female students and practitioners is increasing dramatically, and the women's movement has presented new philosophical, theoretical, and practical demands, conflicts, and rewards in day-to-day practice activities. Increased expectations and opportunities for administrative and practice advancement are creating new career choices for women in practice organizations. The supervisor can and should be a source of support and role modeling for women. The role of the supervisor in promoting effective clinical feminist models is a fundamental one because research has demonstrated that educational programs are not fostering feminist orientations to practice, even though the majority of students at the graduate and undergraduate levels are female (Munson and Hipp, 1998).

Education and Feminist Theory

If supervision is going to contribute a feminist orientation to practice, then education programs will have to foster this orientation for the next generation of practitioners. The evidence suggests that this is not occurring. The lack of feminist influence in the educational arena is interesting in light of the fact that the social work profession has always been predominately female and is becoming increasingly more so. Social work education enrollment statistics show that the profession will be substantially female in the next decade if current trends continue. In 1972, MSW student enrollment was 64 percent female, and in 1995 it had reached 82 percent. In 1972, 45 percent of social work faculty were female, and in 1995, 59 percent of faculty were female. Of the male faculty in 1995, 75 percent were over forty-five years of age, and 70 percent of doctoral students were female. If the trend of the past twenty years continues, males will be a very small portion of the social work profession. This raises the fundamental question, What will be the guiding philosophical and theoretical principles for a profession and an academic community that will become almost exclusively female? If feminism is to reign, then steps must be taken to prepare practitioners for the feminist future (Munson, 1997b).

The Council on Social Work Education (CSWE)-mandated social work curriculum has not changed to reflect the shift in student population or to take into account the impact of the feminist movement and the increase in feminist literature on the role of the social worker. Efforts to introduce feminist materials into the CSWE-mandated curriculum and classroom are not extensively documented in the literature. Surveys of published social work articles and books found that less than 10 percent focused on women's issues. Studies have found that social work students have little knowledge of the foundation of feminist literature. The research shows that students do not possess the underlying knowledge of feminist theory needed to compare and contrast feminist theory with other traditional orientations when selecting a theory for professional practice use. Research findings suggest that social work students identify more strongly with the tenets of feminism than they are willing to declare. At the same time, students claim lack of knowledge of what feminism means while expressing much interest in feminism. Faculty's lack of promotion of feminist reading is the critical factor in students' low level of understanding. Given the role and function of social work historically, the issue is whether schools of social work should adopt models of feminist theory that provide an orientation beyond that of the general population (Munson and Hipp, 1998).

That the majority of social work faculty are female and the research shows that a significant number of graduate students have low levels of core feminist knowledge would suggest that women faculty are not focusing on feminist issues with a level of intensity that would assist in conceptualizing a social work curriculum based on a feminist perspective, even though the Council on Social Work Education (CSWE) curriculum policy requires that all schools include curriculum content on women.

The view among social work faculty appears to be that feminist perspectives have become so widespread and feminist tenets so consistent with social work values and ethics that there is no need to teach feminism as foundation learning in social work education. Research has demonstrated that the difference between the women's movement and feminist theory used as a practice orientation is not being conveyed to students (Munson and Hipp, 1998).

A review of the feminist social work practice literature reveals that many authors do not draw significantly on the classic feminist literature. It could be that feminist literature is not taught by faculty because it is difficult to read, understand, and master or risky to teach when faced with tenure decisions. If feminism is to be one of the primary theoretical perspectives in the social work curriculum, a body of core literature will have to be identified that contrasts feminist models of intervention and traditional models. A central question is, Can students of feminism master it and adopt it as a practice strategy without a foundation of classical core feminist understanding?

Schools of social work will have to find ways to teach a broad spectrum of feminist views that are inclusive and not exclusive and include a clearly articulated feminist theory of practice. The data indicate that such a centrist view is not emerging. The research suggests that foundation feminism practice theory does not have a central place in the perspectives of the next generation of social work practitioners who will eventually become supervisors.

Much academic work needs to be done before practitioners and supervisors can effectively integrate feminist theory and practice. The curriculum approach to feminism must be much more extensive, provide grounding in historical perspectives, contain clear foundation content, and be integrated with other curriculum components before feminism can genuinely be considered a successful theoretical orientation that will produce effective feminist practitioners and supervisors.

THE PARTNERSHIP MODEL OF FEMINIST SUPERVISION

Supervision Paradigm Shift

A feminist perspective of supervision has been slow to emerge because it requires a major paradigm shift that takes into account client need, agency function, and practitioner preferences. Feminist practice and supervision focuses on change in structures in order to alter unjust practices. Fostering a feminist perspective in supervision through the use of what is referred to as a partnership model (Hipp and Munson, 1995) can assist in overcoming some of the outmoded aspects of the traditional hierarchical model. A feminist-based partnership paradigm, although a departure from traditional models, is an attempt to modify and supplement existing models, rather than to replace them. At the same time, the partnership model is a way to enhance supervision.

Much supervision knowledge has been historically compatible with modern feminist theory, but it has not been framed in such a context that would permit comprehensive application in practice. What has been lacking are specific guidelines for practice and supervision application. The role of the supervisor using a partnership model is to foster comprehensive application. Eisler (1987) uses a reinterpretation of the past to develop a new paradigm through advocating a partnership model in which women, men, and nature are linked rather then ranked and it is more important to work together to create a better world than to dominate others. Eisler's partnership model views gender relations as basic to humanness. Shifting relations between males and females involves dealing with the most fundamental questions of values, ethics, and social structure. Eisler uses the dominator and partnership models to demonstrate that those working for a more human and ethical society need to give high priority to developing gender roles based on partnership rather than domination. (Eisler, 1992). This formulation is basic to conceptualizing feminist supervision and practice.

The partnership model from a feminist perspective focuses on the sexes working together for a different world. Feminists and psychotherapists have had a primary goal of establishing a better world through raising the quality of life to its highest level. The partnership model concentrates on the need for change in both women and men practitioners and supervisors as they work together. Although the partnership model is a major paradigm shift, it is not intended to create false dichotomies. Partnership is not the other side of the coin of the dominator model, and consequently one that would be equally limiting. It is a different view of the world. For example, competition and cooperation may be found in both models, but they are used and viewed differently. Visual 14.4 summarizes some of the differences between the dominator model and the partnership model in supervision and lists the operational terms used in the two models. These operational terms are explored further in the following sections.

Conceptualizing a feminist perspective of supervision using Eisler's (1987) model requires articulation of supervisory structural systems issues at four levels: societal, agency, supervisory, and client system. These will be explored in relationship to the partnership model.

Societal Structure

The concept of power is key to the dominator society and constitutes power over people rather than shared relationships. For example, a dominator model is enacted at the societal level in a social welfare system that asserts power over everyone involved, in a way that lauds individualist values and a patriarchal system while it devalues femininity. Society dictates roles and expectations that are expressed through interaction. These expectations are brought to supervision and overtly and covertly characterize the interaction of the supervisor and supervisee. Analysis of supervision conversations can reveal the underlying patterns that are the basis of a person's subjectivity and dominator worldview. In partnership oriented-supervision, there must be acknowledgement of these patterns and how they can foster or impede supervision work and practice. Men have difficulty moving from the "self-centered" mode, and women have difficulty moving into this mode. With concerted effort the change can be made. Recognition of the patterns and

VISUAL 14.4. Dominator and Partnership Models of Supervision

	Orientation	
Structure	**Dominator**	**Partnership**
Societal	Power	Relationship
	Patriarchal	Feminist
	Hierarchical	Egalitarian
	Individualist	Communal
	Violent	Nurturing
	Self-centered	Other-centered
	Feminine devalued	Feminine respected
Agency	Power	Relationship
	Authoritarian	Democratic
	Survival dependent	Survival dependent
	Task and function	Affiliation
	Separation	Cooperation
	Competition	Process
	Product	
Supervision	Power	Relationship
	Learning and support	Learning and support
	Dependence	Independence
	Compliance	Shared decisions
	Obedience	Initiative
	Authoritarian	Democratic
	Indoctrination	Education
Client	Powerless	Relationship
	Passive	Active
	Directive	Nurturing
	Concern	Caring
	Object/recipient	Subject
	Practitioner doing for, not with, client	Working through and with

willingness to work to change them set the stage for a genuine partnership model of supervision/consultation to occur.

Supervisors need to understand the difference in communication patterns between women and men. In supervision there is a need to discuss these differences and how they influence client communication styles and patterns. It is empowering to share knowledge with clients to help them learn to understand their own behavior. Knowledge sharing is a large part of empowerment that fosters a genuine partnership model in supervision.

Supervisors can foster the understanding of larger societal issues by discussing them as essential material for case consultation. Societal and cultural influences are appropriate topics in supervision, as Mary Richmond observed: "Good supervision must include this consideration of wider aspects" (1917:351).

Professional and Agency Structure

The focus on authoritarian (dominator) models in agencies and group practices where separateness is the rule means that survival is dependent on task and function. The emphasis is on power over others rather than on fostering interdependent relationships. A partnership model in organizations is more centered on relationships and less on task and function. The supervisor must be alert to how an agency may engage in dominator acts that limit client options. The supervisor must work to overcome the bias in individual cases and to change organizational bias at the policy, personnel, and operational levels. A partnership perspective must be part of a larger learning experience for both the supervisor and the supervisee. Education for psychotherapy practice has not moved to such a model of supervision/consultation. Most courses on feminism deal with women's issues from a societal context and offer little in the way of intervention strategies in professional relationships or supervisory or consultative practice. A number of strategies compatible with psychotherapy methods and a partnership model need to be developed in agency settings. One strategy involves greater use of groups in agencies. The rich tradition of group intervention is particularly suited to a partnership model of practice and supervision.

The group intervention model is as useful for practitioners working together on goals and issues as it is for working with clients. It also allows for a discussion of process as well as product. It fosters an opportunity to develop better relationships between women and men at various staff levels. The use of codirectors and cochairs in various positions can also foster a sharing of power and a stronger sense of relationship. Group methods can lead to greater cooperation and less competition. Supervisors with a partnership perspective can encourage, support, and promote these different agency structures. It is important to note that it is advantageous to have female-male teams operating in cofacilitation positions. The dichotomy between females and males is a primary factor in the dominator model. This can be changed only when the sexes see that working together as partners is more effective. This form of partnership model reconceptualizes power. This does not imply that a democratic structuring of power means that all are alike or equally powerful at all times, but it does mean that structures can be created to give everyone equal access to resources and information.

The majority of psychotherapists in practice are women, and the majority of administrators and supervisors are men. For example, in clinical social work, men hold two-thirds of the managerial jobs in a profession that is two-thirds women. As long as the primary recipients of psychotherapy services are women, the majority of practitioners are women, and the administrators and supervisors are men, there will be a gap in the empowerment of women. That missing link is a partnership model. In order for fundamental change to occur, women and men will need to develop more effective models of communication. A shift is essential for social change because if the recent trend in graduate school enrollments continues, in the next decade, the psychotherapy professions will be predominantly female. As this occurs, women will need to teach men about women and relationships. Men need to seek out women for this knowledge and develop a capacity to listen. Supervision is the arena in which to begin the dialogue. Women have much to offer men about the treatment of women clients. For example, women practitioners with a feminist perspective can help men supervisors understand how difficult it is for battered women to leave abusive situations. Psychotherapists need feminist mentors regardless of whether those persons are supervisors or supervisees. The essence of the partnership model is that both the supervisor and the supervisee share input and influence.

Supervisory Structure

Psychotherapy supervision structure has historically followed a dominator model and continues to do so. Practitioners cannot rely on the supervisor to learn and apply a feminist perspective unless there is an explicit request for such an approach. Professional, licensure, and agency supervisory requirements usually follow the dominator model. This is normally referred to as the authority model used in supervision.

The theoretical orientations of the supervisor and the supervisee are a component of the supervisory structure. There has not been much empirical research on the congruence between the theoretical orientations of the supervisor and supervisee, but it has been speculated that congruence is important to positive supervision outcome. Steinhelber et al. (1984), in a study of 237 psychotherapy clients, found that clients reported significantly greater improvement when the supervisor and supervisee theoretical orientations were congruent. This raises questions regarding how compatibility between supervisor and supervisee can be accomplished when either party to the supervisory relationship wishes to use a feminist orientation. The feminist-oriented supervisor of a nonfeminist supervisee must find a way to reconcile the differing perspectives, and the supervisee who desires to develop a feminist practice approach must accommodate to the methods of a nonfeminist supervisor. The partnership model includes an explanation and negotiation of the orientation that will be the focus of the supervision. Even if one party does not have a feminist orientation, when the desired model is made explicit, it is easier to overcome differences and to develop a new perspective.

Supervision and practice power can be misused as they are in dominator societies, or they can be reframed as a shared resource in a partnership model. The feminist partnership model reconceptualizes "power as affiliation." Eisler (1987) sees this nondestructive view of power as a "win-win" rather than a "win-lose" situation. A partnership model fosters supervisory relationships based on joining and sharing to meet client and professional needs for a more humane world, rather than on competitive activity. This is done in supervision through a respect for the sharing of different viewpoints as normative, cooperative, and constructive interaction.

Client System Structure

A partnership perspective in supervision can be viewed as an extension of a feminist practice perspective. No specific definition of practice is used by feminists, and this is true of partnership-based supervision. Feminism is a way of thinking and being that is constantly changing. The control aspects of a dominator model filter down to the client level and the authoritarian effect is cumulative. The power structure model results in those at the bottom being powerless, passive recipients who do not engage in the change process.

A central component of a partnership perspective is valuing the process as well as the outcome. A dominator model places emphasis and value on only the goal or product. The prevailing philosophy of the dominator model is product oriented, and the focus is on how goals are achieved rather than what happens to people in the process. The increased use of managed cost models in mental health practice is resulting in more focus on the product aspect of the dominator model. A partnership model considers the people in the process and seeks to empower them by encouraging their input. In supervision, this allows for greater focus on what is actually happening during intervention.

This valuing of the other is related to a caring ethic. Caring has been associated with feminine culture and minimized by dominator culture. A partnership model combines caring and justice. It allows for the valuing of feminine qualities and views feelings as a valid subject. Supervisors can facilitate the process of valuing by discussing the feeling ethic as it relates to work with clients. The feminine ethic of care is basic to supervisory inquiry and can be effectively related to supervision and practice activity.

A partnership model is based on an active, caring relationship that views the client as a participant in working through problems. A partnership model allows for deeper exploration of work with others in their daily lives. Caring and life-enhancing activities are at the core of a partnership model.

Practitioners should be gender specialists who work to change roles and not just role performance.

The practitioner faces many issues in the client relationship that can be better understood and more likely to be brought to supervisory discussion if a partnership perspective is openly shared. The female practitioner with a male client and the male practitioner with a female client will encounter conscious dynamics based on socialization processes that impede client change. This should be discussed in supervision/consultation. Gender role and power relationships need further exploration in terms of the limitations of the dominator model and the positive effects of the partnership model. This is especially true in the case of mixed-gender practice and supervisee-supervisor gender combinations.

Overview

The partnership model, based on a feminist perspective, is more compatible with the values and goals of the psychotherapy professions than the dominator model. The supervisory/consultative role is an excellent place for practitioners to assess and model their professional strengths as efforts are made to enhance the quality of life. There is much work to be done to affect social change at the foundation of relationships. A partnership model provides the conceptual framework for doing this. Some critical questions need further exploration: Do supervisors view themselves as feminists? How do supervisors present a feminist perspective and a partnership model? Can education or training alter the male socialization process to the extent that males could supervise from a partnership model? How can a partnership model be fostered across the curriculum in psychotherapy education? Can a partnership model be implemented and sustained within institutions that remain hierarchical in orientation and structure? Further research is needed on supervision from a partnership model to address these questions.

ERGONOMICS

The term *ergonomics* has been used generically to mean the relationship humans have with machines, and was derived from the term *biotechnology*. At the macro level of technology, Toffler (1980) introduced the concept of "electronic cottages" that use machines to eliminate the need for human contact in certain areas. In the 1980s, Naisbitt (1982) took a different view in exploring "megatrends." He argued that high technology produces a human counterdemand for "high touch," and that high technology with "low touch" would be rejected by the public and consumers. Naisbitt called this the "high-tech–high-touch formula." It was his view that much modern theory of therapy is associated with this formula. He believed that when new technology is applied to humans in institutions, it should include a built-in corresponding high-touch component. From this perspective, it might be beneficial to view clinical social work as the high-touch component that must accompany high technology. This is a revolutionary way of thinking of social work practice in relation to technology and requires supervisors to develop a different orientation toward technology, clients, and practitioners. Social workers are increasingly involved with technology through applications in their work with clients as well as in their personal and professional lives, and this requires new models for approaching practice and supervision. For example, cases are now being supervised through FAX machine exchanges (Rustin, 1998) and psychotherapy is done over the Internet.

Naisbitt's view regarding rejection of technology and services that do not have high-touch components has not occurred. The trend of high-tech–low-touch has continued unabated and is illustrated by automated telephone answering systems, e-mail, automated banking machines, and e-commerce. Consumers have been unable to reject these systems because high-touch alternatives are not available. For example, almost all businesses have automated telephone answering systems that make it nearly impossible for the consumer to have direct access to sales and service staff. Corporate mergers have created large monopolies controlling many services and products. These monopolies have eliminated jobs, cut salaries and benefits, and replaced workers with machines as a way to increase profits at the expense of service to consumers (for a detailed discussion of these changes, see Danaher, 1996; Madrick, 1995). These changes have not been limited to the business community but have also spread to every form of human services provided by social workers. The increase in technology has been so sweeping and pervasive that Naisbitt has changed his high-touch hypothesis completely and argues that a "Technologically Intoxicated Zone" exists in which "Americans are intoxicated by technology" and this "intoxication is squeezing out our human spirit, intensifying our search for meaning" (1999:1). Naisbitt's altered view is that through "conscious awareness of your relationship with technology you can see and feel the Technologically Intoxicated Zone and help yourself, your family, your community and business" (4). The increased low-touch and the unavailability of high-touch alternatives are especially important for social workers and their clients because the populations served by social workers—elderly, women, children, minorities, urban and rural poor—frequently do not have computers and other technological devices available to them for communication and acquiring needed services (Krager and Levine, 1999).

Ergonomics has other implications for clinical supervision that need elaboration. First, many clients have relationships with machines. This is especially the case in medical settings, where, for example, renal dialysis has become commonplace and, with current technology, artificial heart transplant patients live permanently attached to a machine. With the miniaturization of technology, more patients are surviving with machines implanted or strapped to their bodies.

Supervisors and practitioners need to be increasingly aware of the significance of ergonomics for clients. Social workers have been slow to accept and resistant to admitting that people have relationships with machines. Machines have dehumanizing effects, and chief among these has been the computer. This has blinded professionals to the positive aspects of machines and retarded advocacy for their use to benefit clients. For example, telephone electronics, hearing and sight devices, and computer hookups can have many advantages for the elderly and people with disabilities. In this electronic age, social workers will be required to change significantly their attitudes about technology and machines if they are to provide maximum assistance to clients.

Second, machines are becoming more a part of the clinical practice and supervisory situations. The use of audio and video machines to record therapy sessions for subsequent use in therapy and supervision is becoming more common. In clinical interviews, videotape and audiotape machines are a third party to the treatment. In some settings, videotaping is considered a valuable therapeutic agent. The guidelines for the use of such machines are very limited. Used properly, they can enhance treatment, but improper applications can cause unanticipated intrusions. The supervisor has a responsibility to be skilled in the use of electronic audio and visual equipment (see Chapter 12).

Another form of technology that social workers increasingly use is communications devices, such as paging instruments. These devices have become common in hospital settings, in child welfare services, in mental health agencies, and among private practitioners. There has been no study of the effects of these devices on the functioning of workers. In some cases, they are used by workers voluntarily, and in others, involuntarily. Also, no studies have considered whether these instruments in fact increase response time or effectiveness of workers. Supervisors need to be more cognizant of the use of such devices and how they can be most effectively employed by practitioners.

SUGGESTED READINGS

Brendler, J. et al. (1991). *Madness, Chaos, and Violence: Therapy with Families at the Brink*. New York: Basic Books.
  System of work with families with seriously emotionally disturbed members. The system used by the authors is highly compatible with the SEES system described in this chapter.

Freud, S. (1988). *My Three Mothers and Other Passions.* New York: New York University Press.

Description of one person's exploration of family of origin experience that could serve as a guide for others.

Lum, D. (1999). *Culturally Competent Practice: A Framework of Growth and Action.* Belmont, CA: Wadsworth Publishing Co.

Coverage of knowledge and research on culturally based practice. This book can serve as a companion volume for Lum's *Social Work Practice and People of Color.*

Lum, D. (2000). *Social Work Practice and People of Color: A Process-Stage Approach.* Belmont, CA: Wadsworth Publishing Co.

Overview of model for work with diverse populations.

Lynch, E. W. and Hanson, M. J. (eds.) (1998). *Developing Cross-Cultural Competence: A Guide for Working with Children and Their Families*, Second Edition. Baltimore, MD: Paul H. Brookes.

Overview of working with families from various cultures.

Munson, C. E. (1994). "Cognitive Family Therapy," in D. K. Granvold (ed.), *Cognitive and Behavioral Treatment: Methods and Applications.* Pacific Grove, CA: Brooks/Cole, pp. 202-221.

Summary of family therapy, including the SEES system explained in this chapter.

Munson, C. E. (1997). "Gender and Psychotherapy Supervision: The Partnership Model," in C. E. Watkins (ed.), *Handbook of Psychotherapy Supervision.* New York: John Wiley, pp. 549-569.

Review of feminist concepts described in this chapter.

We should argue with terms, not fight
over them.

C. Wright Mills
The Sociological Imagination

Chapter 15

Art and Science in Social Work Practice

In this chapter a perspective on the use of the terms *art* and *science* to describe social work is presented to aid the supervisor. The supervisor needs to be able to approach the concepts of art and science as a way to expose and explore practice issues rather than as a means of disguising them. To accomplish this, a modified conceptualization of artistic elements and scientifically based practice is substituted for art and science. The conventions of traditional art are discussed in a context that allows application in social work supervision and practice.

INTRODUCTION

This book ends on the same note on which it began. In Chapter 2, which deals with the history of supervision, it was argued that the ideas of art and science played a key role in the evolution of practice theory and supervision's natural connection to this evolution. In this chapter an attempt is made to be more precise in the use of these two concepts in the context of modern practice theory and supervision.

The concept of art has been used loosely in many areas. Social work, along with other professions, uses the term without much precision. *Merriam-Webster's Collegiate Dictionary* (1994) even includes a generic definition of the term as "skill acquired by experience, study, or observation," and then gives the example of "the [art] of making friends." The more specific definition of art when applying it to conveying information about clinical social work practice is used in this chapter, that is, "the conscious use of skill and creative imagination esp. in the production of aesthetic objects."

The key words in this definition are *conscious, skill, creative imagination*, and *objects*. If clinical practice is compared to art, it must be shown how conscious use of skill was employed to produce an aesthetic object. With some reservations, the concept of "object" has been broadened in this chapter to include experiences, utterances, and actions that occur in treatment.

The most difficult task in comparing social work practice to art is the explication of conscious use of skill in given aspects of practice that are referred to as art. A major thesis of this chapter is that, in the past, the opposite approach to art was used. Rather than using the idea of art to make known consciously used skill that resulted in an elegant treatment sequence, the term *art* has been used to justify the unknown, unexplained, unconscious, and unverified aspects of clinical work.

There is a difference between the act or process of creation and the resulting art object, but it must be remembered that the two are connected, and process and object in art do not exist unilaterally. One way to explore the process and object of art separately, as well as interrelating them, is to identify the conventions that surround art. Becker (1974) has pointed out that the creation of a work of art requires elaborate cooperation among many people with specialized knowledge and skill. In order for these specialized people to cooperate, certain conventions have evolved that guide their interaction and cooperative efforts, and to a large extent these conventions place strong constraints on the artist and frequently dictate what the artist does. A naive view of the artist and art produces the stereotype of the artist as an unrestrained, creative, aloof, single agent who, in a recondite way, produces objects of art. This innocent view stems from the typical childhood conception of art, in which a five-year-old confronted with a classic painting is likely to say it was produced in a factory (Gardner, 1982:103-104).

In comparing social work practice to art, the formulations in this chapter hold that there is a relationship between the creative process, works of art (objects), and conventions that surround artists and art. This constellation led to the conception of the elements of art explained in this chapter.

No attempt is made to detract from what practitioners do in calling attention to the vague use of the terms *art* and *artist*. What is argued is that the use of the term *art* must be based on a definable, measurable perspective that enhances what clinicians do. All of the strategies suggested in this book—from audiovisual techniques to questioning techniques, for example—are designed to promote an artistic orientation rather than detract from it.

TRADITIONS

Much has been written about the art and science of social work practice. Rarely does a book on practice fail to mention the role of art and science. The notion of social work practice as an art was fostered early in the profession:

> [S]ocial case work, like most professional activities, is an art, an art in which the practitioner makes use of all the knowledge, wisdom, and philosophy in his possession, but an art nevertheless whose practice cannot be patternized. Each separate bit of professional practice is a creation in itself. (Lee and Kenworthy, 1929:188)

This is the description of random activity mentioned at the beginning of this book. Mary Richmond first called attention to the difference between random activity and practice by observing that as far as social work was concerned, the public had not drawn the distinction "between going through the motions of doing things and actually getting them done" (Richmond, 1965/1917:25).

Social work has a long tradition of using the terms *art* and *science* as generalizations that are difficult to apply. In explaining social casework, Richmond said, "In any art the description of its processes is necessarily far more clumsy than are the processes themselves" (1965/1917:103). In the Report of the Milford Conference, a very elegant statement about art and science is made:

> Nowhere does the fact that social case work is an art appear more clearly than in treatment. Here is the blending of scientific knowledge, training and experience as in the finished picture. Here, too, the vision of the artist is made an actuality through his ability to combine in ef-

fective use—not only with skill but with genius—the separate units of his knowledge. But the social case worker has no passive canvas on which to paint his picture. The client himself must be a participant in the art of social case work. (NASW, 1974:30)

Florence Hollis wrote that "casework is both an art and a science: an art in that it requires individual creativeness and skill; a science in that it is a body of systematized knowledge based upon observation, study and experimentation" (1966:265). This was the basis for her view that "casework is a scientific art" (Parad and Miller, 1963:13). Perlman contributed to the mystique of social casework as art by stating, "the art of doing cannot be taught in any complete sense" (1957:vii). Turner questioned, "Might it be that the complete therapist is not the theoretician but the artist whose theory is his intuition and skills his natural endowment?" He goes on to suggest that "perhaps the state of practice is such that the artistic component is stronger than the knowledge base and for the present we should leave the two separate" (1979:9). On the other hand, Pincus and Minahan "view art and science as allies, rather than adversaries. Unfortunately they are often not seen this way" (1973:34).

In the 1930s, "art" based on "the utilization of human skill as opposed to nature" was considered one of the "attributes" of a profession. In this sense, it was observed at the time that social work was not "much understood or widely appreciated by the public" as an art, in spite of enormous success of the profession in meeting human needs. Another attribute of a profession was service based on science and learning. In this realm, social work was considered as having hopeful signs, given the technical content in the educational curricula and the emphasis on supervised field training (Chapin and Queen, 1972/1937:99-100).

These are not descriptions of practice; they are not even descriptions of art. This view was held up to the supervisor as essential to learning. Each student was "at the mercy of her own creative capacity," and this creative capacity could not be "produced by professional training"; its essence had to be found in the practitioner's personality (Lee and Kenworthy, 1929:188).

ART TERMINOLOGY CONFUSION

This view caused a conflict for the supervisor and the practitioner that persists. If practice is art, and if creativity is innate and not learned, there is very little logic for applying prolonged, intense supervision to the practitioner's work for the purpose of "developing the capacity . . . to deal . . . with face-to-face situations" (Lee and Kenworthy, 1929:188). Only if social work practice existed solely for the entertainment of the worker and client would this view of social work as art suffice.

Since past commentators have repeatedly compared the term *art* in social work to the fine arts, the same literary approach is used in the following paragraphs by taking the comparison further to promote better understanding of this term and how it relates to social work practice. Clarity is needed about this comparison if it to be used to improve practice. In the fine arts there is much disagreement about what constitutes art and its conventions (Schoenwald, 1976:32). The premise of this chapter is that if social work practice is to be viewed as artistic, then the quality of practice can be enhanced by adhering more closely to the conventions of art.

The tendency has been to use the terms *art* and *science* in conjunction with each other. For example, Siporin (1975:52-55), who did a detailed analysis of these terms, exemplifies this tendency to combine the terms in his statement that "social work is . . . a . . . scientific art of practice" (Siporin, 1975:3). This is a good beginning, but more specificity is needed. Before these two terms can be interrelated, there is a need to be clearer about what each term means independently.

ARTISTIC ELEMENTS AND
SCIENTIFICALLY BASED PRACTICE

The concepts of the artistic elements of what gets done in practice and scientifically based practice come closer to how art and science are and can be applied in supervision and practice in a helpful manner. These concepts can be defined in relation to what the practitioner does in clinical work and what the supervisor does in the process of supervising that clinical work. The reasons for these distinctions are explained in the following paragraphs.

Supervision is one of the conventions that accompanies the practitioner's artistic efforts. Supportive supervision can enhance practitioners' artistic work; overly critical supervision can hamper it, just as poor lighting can ruin an otherwise good stage performance.

Art is a means and an end. Art exists for itself. Social work practice does not exist for itself. Its purpose is to help people change or obtain resources. These efforts are constrained by time, money, physical facilities, and many other factors. Art flourishes where there are few constraints. Even the process of treatment places constraints on the practitioner. During the diagnostic phase, the practitioner is constricted in his or her ability to do many creative acts; the diagnostic assessment must be completed. Art cannot be forced or delayed, but practice acts can.

The mention of art seems to promote profound, comprehensive statements without much detailed or practical application. This chapter adds detail to the term where others have relied on global vagueness and abstraction. The idea of the art of practice is important to supervision because supervisors, when they encounter difficult and complex practice impasses, tend to rely on the "art of practice" abstractions about which they have read in the literature.

The relationship between artistic elements and scientifically based practice can be illustrated by an example from the family therapy field. If one surveys the work of the major family therapy theorists, almost all of them believe that an essential part of helping a troubled family is for the practitioner "to join" the family interactionally and, in the process of doing this, disrupt the dysfunctional interactional patterns. This basic, knowledge-based, routine activity applies to almost all family intervention and serves for scientifically based interventions. The interventions made by the practitioner are based on repeatedly applied and generally accepted interventions that have been applied to specific situations. How the practitioner "joins" the family and goes about dismantling the dysfunctional patterns are matters of artistic elements. The ways of doing this are limited only by the practitioner's and supervisor's creative capabilities. The science is the basis for the intervention, and the art is the manner in which the intervention is applied.

The connection between the two conceptions is also illustrated by Hamilton's view that "the art of taking histories is dependent upon the ability to relate questions to the main themes in the client's story" (Hamilton, 1951:59). The practitioner's scientifically based knowledge of human behavior determines what questions are asked. How they are asked and how they elicit understanding and change are the artistic elements of practice.

Social workers have tended to look at art as a totally creative process, and since there are few conventions to guide practice, artistic elements of practice are incomplete. Perceiving art only as a creative process surrounded by mysticism is erroneous. Art, in fact, is surrounded by rigid conventions that often dictate creative acts (see Becker, 1974:767-776). The conventions that surround art involve collective action by support personnel. In comparing art and its conventions to social work practice, it is not taken into account that receptionists, typists, administrators, and other staff members are part of the artistic elements of practice. By considering the conventions and social organization of artistic activities and making appropriate comparisons to social work, more understanding about why some of interventions work and others do not can be fostered. For example, an untrained receptionist who offends and upsets a client in the waiting room can detract from the subsequent strategies of the practitioner in the interview.

ELEMENTS OF ART

Social work practice does not meet the test of an art in the traditional sense. Art traditionally is defined as dance, writing, painting, music, and sports competition. All of these art forms, as well as others, share certain basic elements:

1. Creation
2. Discipline
3. Rehearsal
4. Audience and critics

Each of these elements is discussed separately here, after a discussion of some general principles related to art and practice.

There is no attempt to compare social work practice directly to conventional art forms; instead the comparison is of practice to the conventions that surround traditional art forms, that is, the four elements just mentioned. In performing an art, the artist is surrounded by this set of conventions. It is held that if practice were a true art and the practitioner were an artist, social work practice would be surrounded by these same conventions.

Although many modern-day practitioners claim to be artists, Freud did not hold this view of treatment; he said, "I am not an artist; I could never have depicted the effects of light and color, only hard outlines." Picasso presented this same observation from the artist's point of view when he stated, "Anyone can take a sun and make a yellow ball out of it, but to take a yellow ball and make a sun out of it—that is art!"

Creation

Artists create. All artists produce something—a painting, a novel, a film, an on-stage performance. All genuine art forms involve an act or object of creation. Social work practice is a process that cannot be viewed as a performance. Even a recorded session of treatment does not qualify as a performance because it is one segment of a much larger and more complicated whole. No play is ever judged or considered a play on the basis of a single act.

Practitioners do engage in this convention. Practitioners create in a modified form that qualifies practice as having an artistic—a creative—element, but it is not art. There are creative ways in which practitioners engage clients, help them gain insight, and apply techniques and theory in practice. From this perspective, the practitioner uses the same processes of perceptiveness, imagination, original thinking, and recording of experience that the traditional artist uses. Once the supervisor adopts this view of artistic components of treatment, he or she is in a position to help the practitioner use theoretical orientations and philosophies to perceive and understand therapeutic action in a manner that allows him or her to be creative. The practitioner must have a theory or philosophy to guide practice, but at the same time, he or she must possess an openness to experience in order to relate imaginatively to the uniqueness of the client. The practitioner must have a perspective that permits integration of an array of facts and actions that fit into a logical whole to make therapeutic change possible. This highlights another difference between the practitioner and the artist. The artist produces or, more accurately, promotes change. It is not accurate to say the practitioner creates change. Only the client can do that. In fact, from this view, the client is more the artist in treatment and the practitioner is the director, producer, or teacher of the artist. The true artist reflects and documents change and, at times, produces change through his or her art. Artists mirror change and are directly involved in change that advances society.

Comments about the creative process by creative people in the arts or sciences assign very little value to the epistemology of creativity as a concept. They espouse a certain mysticism and indescribable quality to the what-and-how of their creative work. They do not think that trying to understand it is a fruitful endeavor. Instead, they frequently mention the notion of curiosity—the desire to know more—as the more important concept. Curiosity is viewed as the necessary and knowable ingredient of creativity.

Can supervision knowledge be advanced by focusing on the idea of curiosity? What is the role of curiosity in doing good diagnosis and treatment? How can curiosity be utilized to let clients know clinicians really care? How can curiosity enrich and advance practice? Curiosity can be the factor that helps in entering the realm of more and better information in a case that gives all appearances of being just like the dozens of other cases treated in the past. Curiosity on the part of the supervisor can inspire the practitioner, and curiosity on the part of the practitioner can be the tool to more in-depth intervention that motivates the client to change.

One of the best discussions of the object in art is John Dewey's *Art As Experience* (1958). The reader who has special interest in interaction in the form of practice as art should read Dewey's extensive treatment of the topic. Dewey discusses experience (interaction) and object in art separately, but he does so only to illustrate that they are basic components of a unified whole. He rejects the view that experience alone or an object alone constitutes art. This leads him to reject the idea that art is some experience "in us"; but even the discussion of the concept of "in us" is based on a set of emotions that emerge from an object of art. Even though he uses examples from psychiatry, he does not equate treatment with art. In the context presented by Dewey, treatment falls short of being art. Dewey summarizes his stand quite clearly and illustrates the point that is the substance of the view presented in this chapter:

> Art denotes a process of doing or making. This is as true of fine as of technological art. Art involves molding of clay, chipping of marble, casting of bronze, laying on of pigments, construction of buildings, singing of songs, playing of instruments, enacting roles on the stage,

going through rhythmic movements in dance. Every art does something with some physical material, the body or something outside the body, with or without the use of intervening tools, and with a view to production of something visible, audible or tangible. (1958:47)

Dewey also makes a distinction between art and science that can be helpful with the often-heard, vague phrase "the art and science of practice." This statement is rarely followed by an empirical explanation and remains to be applied in any abstract sense the practitioner or supervisor chooses. Dewey's view is based on "drawing a distinction between expression and statement" in which "science states meanings; art expresses them." When this explanation is used as a guide, art and science can be empirically defined in clinical discussion. Science can be applied when attempts are made to assign meaning to events that relate to treatment. To the extent that clinicians can talk about art in therapy—that is, artistic activity—it occurs in relation to how one expresses feelings, thoughts, and events in treatment. This distinction can be a powerful way of organizing discussion of clinical material in supervision. Imagination combined with observation is the key to creativity in practice.

Sartre has given a microanalysis of the importance of the object in the novel, theater, and film. The object, whatever it might be, is a sterile thing that becomes the focus of the expression of the artist. Depending on the art form, the artist's treatment of the object determines the observer's response to and interpretation of the object in the particular sense. The only perception of the object the observer brings to the artistic situation is general recognition of the object. The particular response to the generalized object is controlled by the artist, and the amount of the artist's control over the response varies with the art form (Sartre, 1976:6-20).

Discipline

Artistic creativity requires discipline. A great deal of discipline must precede a creative act. Raw talent does not ensure creative success. Art involves the unique blending of creativity and discipline. Herb Alpert has called attention to the fact that there is more to art than being technically trained by observing that, when you are a musician, "you don't get credit for just knowing the notes." If treatment has an artistic component, the practitioner must develop skill at balancing discipline and technical skill with creative reactions. Artists, in a pure sense, have a faith in what they do, a commitment to advancing their art and their skill, and a devotion to their craft. Florence Nightingale understood the importance of devotion to art, and her following comment illustrates the point being made:

Nursing is an art; and if it is to be made an art, it requires as exclusive a devotion, as hard a preparation, as any painter's or sculptor's work; for what is the having to do with dead canvas or cold marble, compared with having to do with the living body.

In comparing this loyalty to the social work profession, clinicians fall short. A study of clinical practitioners has revealed that almost half are disillusioned about their choice of social work as a profession (Reiter, 1980). The question that remains is how such reactions among such a large number of social workers influence their performance from an artistic perspective. Artists become disillusioned, but study of disillusioned artists demonstrates that they deal with such feelings by turning inward and using their art as an outlet for these feelings. Evidence suggests that many creative people are the most productive when working their way out of an episode of depression and despair (Pickering, 1974).

It is unclear how, and if, social workers use their work as a source of overcoming psychological reactions. Some who have studied stress among practitioners have suggested that using work to resolve personal and professional despair leads to more stress, making such efforts self-defeating. More insight into this process could add much to understanding the connection between creativity and stress, as well as provide evidence that there is an artistic element to practice.

Rehearsal

In all true art forms, the artist engages in rehearsal for the performance. This is not an element of practice. If practitioners are to recognize the artistic elements of social work, they need to identify the equivalent of rehearsal and practice. Supervision is the place where this can occur. The use of videotape and audiotape recordings, process recordings, and case discussion can be regarded as forms of practice or rehearsal for future sessions. Rehearsal can take the form of planning a treatment sequence or treatment session. Rehearsal can involve reviewing the empirical literature in a particular practice area before meeting a client with a problem in that area. The supervisor plays an important role in this process.

Audience and Critics

All art forms have an audience. People visit galleries to view paintings; people attend plays and musical performances. The clinical practice situation normally has no audience other than the client. Traditional art forms face critics of the art—the audience as well as professional critics.

The term *audience,* with respect to social work, is being used in the conceptual and not the descriptive sense. Audience does not necessarily mean a group of people who sit in a music hall and observe a performance or a play. Audience in this context means the observers, the spectators, and the evaluators of the object of art. Although it is a point open to debate, art, in the generic sense of the term, cannot exist without an audience.

Social work treatment has few critics. As has been pointed out in this book, the supervisor to some extent should and does serve as a critic. Rarely does criticism or judgment go beyond the supervisor. There is very little evaluation of outcome by individual practitioners or by agencies. Until more systematic evaluation is instituted, art or artistic qualities in practice cannot be claimed. It is in this realm that, ironically, managed cost organizations are correct about the limits of practice from an outcome perspective. Artistic elements of practice and scientifically based practice are what the professions and managed cost organizations have been at odds about without consciously recognizing it.

Art is recognized and judged through acclaim and awards. For example, painters paint to express themselves, but museums and galleries exist to reward that expression. There are numerous prizes and awards for excellence in art. The social work profession is devoid of awards and recognition of excellence in practice. Social work professional organizations have no organized programs specifically aimed at recognizing such excellence. If the social work profession is to take its artistic conceptualization of practice seriously, it will have to develop conventions for recognizing and fostering excellence in practice.

ART AS DEFENSE

The term *art* has been used to conceal clinical scientific shortcomings, and many practitioners retreat into the defense of "art" when expected to account for their performance. Haley (1980) has pointed out that it is easier to use this strategy with colleagues than with clients, but practitioners develop strategies to deal with both groups. When dealing with colleagues, practitioners insist on the importance of confidentiality, shy away from use of recordings or observation in supervision, emphasize the importance of long-term therapy, champion the idea of science in practice, and note the importance of credentials and licensing for practice (Haley, 1980:386). To guard against this, the supervisor should avoid allowing supervisees to use the art defense. Supervisees should be required to justify and explain their interventions. This is a primary function of supervisors, and they should avoid shrinking from this responsibility. Some people abandon supervision rather than face this issue (see Simon, 1982:32).

At a difficult moment in treatment, the tendency is to withdraw or become creative rather than to muster the discipline to exercise the technical skill that is required. Liv Ullmann has beautifully and succinctly described this phenomenon in relation to acting: "I love technical challenge. Stop on a chalk mark in the middle of a difficult emotional scene" (Ullmann, 1978:298). The clinician must be aware of the chalk marks in treatment during powerful and significant exchanges. This takes discipline, and skill is a more constant ingredient of creative activity than cognitive insight (Abell, 1966:329). Too often supervisors emphasize cognitive insight at the expense of technical skill, and the act of creation in this context becomes a means of rationalizing intervention errors.

Treating therapy as art assumes a highly developed approach that can be studied, mastered, applied, and judged. The way social workers have used the concept of art is the exact opposite. It is used to obscure and to elevate what is done to the level of the intangible, the unknowable. What is done in practice and supervision is partially described, then the clinician reaches a level of abstraction in treatment that he or she can only call art. There is a trend away from this view in psychotherapy. For example:

> . . . We believe that avoiding investigation and explicit discussion of how therapists deal with their patients has helped maintain an unfortunate aura of obscure complexity and magic, in which the resolution of patients' problems necessarily is seen as an art. Instead we feel that treatment is, or at least should be, much more a craft, albeit one to which the individual therapist can lend any artistry she possesses. With artistry alone, one can only stand in awe of the "gifted" therapist; with therapy viewed as a craft, one can learn to replicate effective problem-solving techniques. (Fisch et al., 1982:xiii)

In some ways the mental health field has gone to the other extreme of having accountability for practice activity so involved in the small details that the relationship and artistic elements that play a crucial role in positive outcomes have been rejected and forgotten. The challenge is to utilize a proper balance between practical artistic elements and precise scientific applications.

Only through discipline developed over time can the practitioner be prepared to perform the task of treatment. To the extent that *creativity in use* (efforts to provide further insight, organization, and understanding of the dynamics) occurs in treatment, it should take place more at low points in the process than at high points.

PATTERNS AND ART

Patterns, although not always apparent, are the essence of art. As Ariete has pointed out, "What seems to be due to chance is totally or to a large extent the result of special combinations of biological circumstances and antecedent life experiences" (1976:7). At the same time, "the characteristic of uniqueness or originality in a sequence of mental events or in certain forms of behavior is not enough to qualify them as creative products" (1976:7). Ariete also makes a point about patterns in treatment that highlights the misguided view that creativity lacks patterns and is a single act. In discussing the technique of free association in psychoanalysis, Ariete observes:

> The aim of the technique is to remove conscious control and to allow images, feelings, and ideas to come freely into consciousness. From this free flow emerge patterns that will disclose the conflicts and then the personality of the patient. . . . These circumstances represent millions of separate events; and since they are never duplicated in their number, sequence, strength, and other characteristics, their combination is enough to explain the uniqueness or originality of the individual. When spontaneous ideas occur repeatedly or in cycles or special sequences, the analyst helps the patient recognize patterns in them. The patterns existed before; but without the intervention of the analyst, the patient would not have discovered them or at least would have discovered them only with great difficulty. (1976:7)

Early social workers were not wrong in their description of practice; they just did not go far enough in their explanations. Such shortcomings illustrated that, at the early stages of the development of social work practice, its essence was not understood, and because of these limitations, the idea of art was used to fill the gaps in knowledge. Ariete's description of the discovery of patterns in practice further limits the idea of art in social work practice. Art must be free to take any course that presents itself, but the process of discovering preexisting patterns in treatment places restrictions on the form and direction of the treatment if it is to be of value to the client.

A question that remains to be answered through research is, Does theorizing in supervision hamper practitioner creativity? It appears that the answer depends on how the theorizing is handled by the supervisor.

Certain basic, routine actions must be done in practice; other actions are left to the discretion and creativity of the practitioner. This was illustrated in a poignant and down-to-earth comment by a social work student to a supervisor: "In my cases I think I do pretty good at the initial phase, and I can handle the termination phase okay. It is the stuff in the middle I have trouble with." The worker was expressing that the more basic, routine actions had been mastered, but the essence of the creative aspects of treatment was causing her difficulty. The supervisor must be alert to this distinction and to how the creative elements of practice can be the most troublesome. The supervisor must be ready to assist the worker in balancing learning about both the routine and the creative components of practice. Mary Richmond called attention to this point in *Social Diagnosis:* "The method that ignores or hampers the individuality of the worker stands condemned not only in social work but in teaching, in the ministry, in art and in every form of creative endeavor" (1965/1917:10).

SCIENCE

Richard Cabot was one of the earliest commentators on the role of art and science in social work. In discussing "the craftsmanship of social work," he observed, "In social work the art has preceded the science, as it did in medicine and music; but neither science nor art can live well without the other. The science must back and direct the art" (1973:56). He went on to add that "the art exists, but the science has not yet gotten very far" in social work (1973:70). In Cabot's view the art must be founded on the science. This parallels the view expressed earlier that the basic and routine aspects of practice must be connected with the creative elements of practice. Science is not always the routine, and art is not always the creative. Pincus and Minahan have stated succinctly the connection between artistic elements and scientifically based practice: "Although science and art will merge in the style of a particular social worker, he needs to know when he is operating from the basis of knowledge and when from creativity and intuition" (1973:36). Hollis used an analogy to describe this process in a somewhat different manner:

> No blueprint of treatment can ever be given, any more than a skier can know the twists and turns he will have to take on a steep, unknown course toward a distant objective. Like the skier, the worker knows his general direction, but he can see only a little way ahead and must quickly adapt his technique to the terrain. To do this he must be a master of technique, know what to do to accomplish what, and when a given procedure is necessary. (1966:275)

Supervision is where the science of practice should be orchestrated to foster effective artistic elements in intervention. All that is known from research should be brought to bear on what is observed in the practice situation and then used to make sense of what is presented by the client. Supervision should be the arena in which the known and familiar are separated from the unknown and the unfamiliar. Through such a dichotomous analysis, supervision becomes the place where new knowledge is forged. Instead of hiding the unfamiliar under the cloak of "our art," this defense must be abandoned, and limitation of knowledge brought into the open for exploration and advancement of knowledge. One of science's blessings and reassurances is that failures can be transformed into successes if practitioners and supervisors are willing to trust in science and use it, rather than attributing to art and the private knowing of the clinical artist so much that goes un-explained. Once this view is adopted, the science of what is done in supervision and practice can become the source of fun and joy that the traditional scientist derives from the search for knowledge.

Science As Struggle

Judson has pointed out that "the other side of the fun of science, as of art, is pain. A problem worth solving will surely require weeks and months of lack of progress, whipsawn between hope and the blackest sense of despair" (1980:5). The guise of art in clinical work has been used to avoid this pain, causing practitioners to endure frustration and gradual cynicism that is projected onto clients.

Lewis Thomas has provided an excellent summary of the role of science that can be applied in supervision:

> Science . . . is a model system for collective human behavior and has value because of this for all of us, for it is an activity that can be scrutinized and studied. . . . For this reason, among others, there is a need of critics in science, in the sense that classical art and architecture needed the Ruskins, music the Toveys, and contemporary literature the Leavises, Eliots, and Wilsons. Practitioners need people who can explain how science is done, down to the finest detail, and also why it is done, how the new maps of knowledge are being drawn, and how to distinguish among good science, bad science, and nonsense. (quoted in Judson, 1980:x)

In some respects "our science" of social work has been confused with "the sciences." Sullivan points out that "the sciences" are most convincing when dealing with inanimate matter but are much less convincing when dealing with life and living (1963:125). It is interesting that social work has been labeled inadequate as a science simply because it deals with what is admitted by scientists to be a more complex problem. The social work profession makes this same error by confusing the problem with the process of dealing with the problem. When early social workers talked about science, they did not mean that the profession could or should adopt the methods of the pure sciences intact. At present, too much time is spent attempting to reform social work into a pure science. The profession's predecessors recognized and accepted the differences between social sciences and basic sciences in a way that could be revived and used to provide relevance and understanding to current practice and supervision demands. Brackett stated this in 1903 when discussing supervision:

> Good administration of public aid is a part of good government. . . .
> Whether there be a science in all this or not, the problems are to be
> studied and solved in scientific ways—by openmindness, by use of
> the teachings of experience, by efforts to see causes and results.
> (1903:212)

SOCIAL WORK AND ARTISTIC QUALITIES

The idea of art should not be used to shroud what clinicians do in mysticism and esoteric abstractions. Social work practice is not art, but it does have artistic qualities that can be specified on the basis of the criteria discussed in this chapter. Through this less general approach to practice, technique, theory, and function can be more clearly defined. Conventions from art can be borrowed to advance what is done in practice, without obscuring practice by calling it art.

Terms used in the world of art can be used to refine and define what practitioners do, and it is in this sense that art should be used to advance knowledge and practice. Burke (1975) argues that five terms can be identified as valuable in generating principles in art and science: *act, scene, agent, agency,* and *purpose.* These terms should be the supervisor's guide in promoting artistic elements, artisitic qualities, and scientifically based practice.

Another way to use ideas about art to further practice is the common theme of seeing the particular in the universal. Schopenhauer wrote that this is a fundamental characteristic of genius, a characteristic that is associated with art and artists (Ariete, 1976:341). Sartre stated this relationship another way:

> the only way I can be connected with the tree is to see a character sit
> down in its shade. It is not the sight of the character, therefore, that
> makes the settings, but gestures; and gestures create the general rather
> than the particular. (1976:11)

By exploring the idea of the particular and the general or universal in relationships with clients, social workers can gain insight into what is done in practice.

Many terms used in the arts can be applied to improve the understanding of social work practice. This view has been expressed in relation to psychoanalysis:

> The chief hope of realizing these possibilities lies, not in psycho-
> analytical studies pursued in isolation, but in the combined operation
> of psychoanalytical insights with those derived from other and en-
> tirely different fields of knowledge. (Abell, 1966:25)

More precision is needed in the use of the term *art* because a thin line exists between creativity and chaos. It has been observed that "art is demonic, but it is also disciplined" (Schoenwald, 1976:32). Every act committed by a practitioner will have support as well as opposition. Until common agreement about the basis of interventions is reached, practice is neither art nor science. The development of practice standards and practice parameters is important to forming this common agreement.

The propensity to confuse artistry with treatment grew out of Freud's interest in art and artists and their role in society and culture. The parallel between artists and practitioners emerged later. Freud's work gives no indication that this parallel was ever a part of his view of practice. Although there are many parallels between the lives and work of Freud and DaVinci, he made no effort to draw such connections in his study of DaVinci. In reading Freud's work on DaVinci, one is struck by his avoidance of such comparisons and his emphasis on the limitations of psychoanalysis in understanding the artist.

The traditional ideas of art and science have limited utility for social work, and the use of these terms in treatment and supervision ultimately presents a dilemma, an enigma that places psychotherapy somewhere between art and science. Jung summarized all of this:

> Since self-knowledge is a matter of getting to know the individual facts, theories help very little in this respect. For the more a theory lays claim to universal validity, the less capable it is of doing justice to the individual facts. Any theory based on experience is necessarily *statistical;* that is to say, it formulates an *ideal* average which abolishes all exceptions at either end of the scale and replaces them by an abstract mean. . . . The distinctive thing about real facts, however, is their individuality. . . . At the same time man, as member of a species, can and must be described as a statistical unit; otherwise nothing general could be said about him. For this purpose he has to be regarded as a comparative unit. . . . If I want to understand an individual human being, I must lay aside all scientific knowledge of the average man and discard all theories in order to adopt a completely new and unprejudiced attitude. Now whether it is a question of understanding a fellow human being or of self-knowledge, I must in both cases leave theoretical assumptions behind me. Since scientific knowledge not only enjoys universal esteem but, in the eyes of modern man, counts as the only intellectual and spiritual authority, understanding the individual obliges me to commit *lese majeste,* so to speak, to turn a blind eye to scientific knowledge. This is a sacrifice not lightly made, for the scientific attitude cannot rid itself so easily of its sense of responsibility. . . . This conflict cannot be solved by an either-or but only by a kind of two-way thinking: doing one thing while not losing sight of the other. (1957:16-19)

BOOK CONCLUSION

As a conclusion to this chapter and to the book, Visual 15.1 has been prepared to capture all the elements of practice style that practitioners and supervisors must take into account when analyzing supervision practices. The artistic qualities and scientific components of practice are part of each of the elements of style. Practice is not all artistic elements or completely scientifically based. Some elements of practice style are more amenable to empirical measurement and scientific orientations, while others are more in the realm of artistic endeavor.

As a way to unify much of the content of this book, the elements of practice style presented in Visual 15.1 are summarized in the following pages. This conceptualization of practice style can be used to explore many aspects of supervision. Whether one is trying simply to enhance and improve practice or is working to solve a specific treatment difficulty, this conceptualization can be an effective guide for conducting such analyses. It can be a valuable tool in dealing with what Greben (1985) has identified as the task of supervision that requires examination in psychotherapy of what is amiss with therapists, rather than what is wrong with clients. All clinicians go amiss from time to time in such a complex endeavor as clinical treatment, and guidelines are needed to organize thoughts regarding where the difficulties reside. Analyzing the elements of practice style can help identify the sources of the difficulty. The elements of practice style are as follows.

1. *Philosophy of life.* All practitioners have some philosophy of life that they can articulate in general or specific form. The person's philosophy of life can reveal much about orientation to practice. It can be helpful to practitioners to state a philosophy of life as they struggle with defining practice style. This element is predominantly in the realm of artistic qualities of practice.

2. *Philosophy of practice.* Whereas practitioners have a philosophy of life they can articulate if asked, they have much difficulty articulating their philosophy of practice. It is important that the practitioner be assisted in identifying and articulating philosophy of practice as an essential aspect of practice style. The philosophy of practice and the philosophy of life do not have to be identical and completely compatible, but when philosophy of practice and philosophy of life are very different, the practitioner may encounter difficulty, frustration, and callousness in practice. Philosophy of practice is primarily an artistic quality.

3. *Theory in use.* Connected to philosophy of practice is "theory in use," which was identified by Argyris and Schon (1980). This is the theory that the practitioner uses in the actual conduct of practice. It is what the practitioner does while face to face with clients. Theory in use cannot be described;

it can only be observed by others or captured on videotape (or on audiotape in a limited form). When recorded, theory in use can be considered artistic and subjected to scientific analysis.

4. *Espoused theory.* "Espoused theory" was also first defined by Argyris and Schon (1980). It is connected to theory in use in that it is an attempt to describe or explain what the practitioner does in the actual practice situation. It can be a recognized theory from the literature or an accumulation of practice wisdom developed by the individual. There should be consistency between theory in use and espoused theory. If much disparity exists between the two, the practitioner can become confused, can confuse clients, and can be ineffective in practice. Espoused theory is a scientific aspect of practice that can be subjected to scientific scrutiny.

5. *Technique.* This element of practice style can emerge from any of the elements listed previously, but should have some connection to espoused theory that can be described and explained by the practitioner. Technique has been covered in detail in this book, and it can be considered from both artistic and scientific perspectives.

6. *Understanding of the treatment process.* This element is complex and can take much time and experience to develop. It is connected to all of the previous elements. It is much more than recognizing that treatment has beginning, middle, and end phases. It is the understanding of how clients and therapists react to treatment; how trust is developed and that there are several levels of trust; how resistance occurs in the client and the therapist and the stages of this process; appreciating what dictates brief and long-term treatment; how different reactions at different stages of the treatment are connected to events inside and outside the treatment; recognizing and using the patterns of behavior the client presents; and many other factors. This understanding can have artistic qualities and can be subjected to scientific inquiry.

7. *Random activity.* Random activity involves the absence of coherent treatment activity that produces a change for the client. The therapist in this mode can have a pleasant conversation with the client but there is no identifiable focus or outcome. Some therapists spend their entire careers engaging in random activity, while good practitioners lapse into random activity from time to time because they are tired, upset, frustrated, frightened, or caught off guard. Random activity has no artistic elements or scientific basis, but some practitioners describe such activity in artistic terms. Random activity can be externally scientifically observed and measured, and it is the supervisor's responsibility to perform such observation and to make interventions with the practitioner when random activity occurs.

VISUAL 15.1. Elements of Practice Style

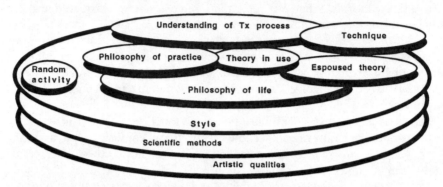

SUGGESTED READINGS

Abell, A. (1966). *The Collective Dream in Art: A Psycho Historical Theory of Culture Based on Relations Between the Arts, Psychology, and the Social Sciences.* New York: Schocken.
    Intellectual discussion of the connection between art and the behavioral sciences.

Ariete, S. (1976).*Creativity: The Magical Synthesis.* New York: Basic Books.
    A modern parallel to Dewey's *Art As Experience.* This book can serve as background for much of the discussion in this chapter on art and practice.

Booth, E. (1997). *The Everyday Work of Art. How Artistic Experience Can Transform Your Life.* Naperville, IL: Sourcebooks, Inc.
    Ideas and strategies for applying creativity to various tasks in life. Some of the strategies can be used in clinical social work practice. This book illustrates some of the points in this chapter related to the art and science of practice.

Burke, K. (1975). "The Five Key Terms of Dramatism," in D. Brissett and C. Edgley (eds.), *Life As Theater: A Dramaturgical Sourcebook.* Chicago: Aldine.
    A series of readings on the dramatic aspects of interaction with some discussion of their relationship to intervention. Many concepts can be used to expand on the points made in this chapter.

John Dewey, J. (1958). *Art As Experience.* New York: Capricorn.
    Classic book that discusses art with a focus on its relation to treatment as applied in this chapter.

Panter, B. M. et. al. (1995). *Creativity and Madness: Psychological Studies of Art and Artists.* Burbank, CA: AIMED Press.
    Collection of articles on creativity in the lives of sixteen artists, writers, and musicians. Introductory chapter on creativity.

Appendix I

Assessment Scale for Becoming a Clinical Supervisor (ASBCS)

ASSESSMENT SCALE FOR BECOMING A CLINICAL SUPERVISOR (ASBCS)

by Dr. Carlton E. Munson

Deciding to become a clinical supervisor can be a difficult decision. To offer some guides to consider, this instrument is provided. Check the response to the right of each factor.

FACTOR	RATING (Check one for each factor)	
The following is descriptive of me:	Column A	Column B
1. Enjoy teaching others	❑ Yes	❑ No
2. Patient when others do not understand	❑ Yes	❑ No
3. Skilled at indirect suggestion	❑ Yes	❑ No
4. Committed to helping others do better	❑ Yes	❑ No
5. Patient when listening to others' complaints	❑ Yes	❑ No
6. Enjoy planning ahead	❑ Yes	❑ No
7. Willing to decrease my own practice activity	❑ Yes	❑No
8. Enjoy answering questions	❑ Yes	❑No
9. Comfortable asking questions	❑ Yes	❑No
10. Can discuss organizational problems without anger	❑ Yes	❑No
11. Can tolerate others making mistakes	❑ Yes	❑No
12. Can accept criticism	❑ Yes	❑No
13. Can accept it when others do not take my advice	❑ Yes	❑No
14. Enjoy making decisions	❑ Yes	❑No
15. Like discussing theory	❑ Yes	❑No
16. Need support for decisions I make	❑ No	❑Yes
17. Dislike evaluating others' practice	❑ No	❑Yes
18. Prefer to work alone	❑ No	❑Yes
19. Find paperwork a source of frustration	❑ No	❑Yes
20. Prefer action to speculation	❑ No	❑Yes
TOTAL checks in each column	_____	_____

If the total of column A is larger than the total of column B, you will most likely find supervision rewarding. If column B exceeds column A, you should review the factors in column B and find ways to alter your views and behavior in these areas if you decide to enter supervision practice.

Appendix II

Educational Assessment Scale (EAS)

EDUCATIONAL ASSESSMENT SCALE (EAS)

by Dr. Carlton E. Munson

The following questions are to help your supervisor plan your supervisory learning needs. There are no correct or incorrect answers. Answer the questions factually. The objective is to be able to assess what you presently know and what areas need development. It is expected that there will be a number of areas in which you will have limited or no knowledge. Do not feel bad that you have limited knowledge in a given area. This instrument will be helpful only if you identify accurately what you know and do not know.

1. Previous Experience

Total years social work paid experience: _____
List job responsibilities:

Total years volunteer social work experience: _____
List job responsibilities:

Total years non-social work experience: _____
List job responsibilities:

2. Ethical Awareness

Have you read the social work code of ethics?   ❏No   ❏Yes

If yes, how many years has it been since you read
the code of ethics?_____

Have you taken the Munson Code of Ethics Scale?   ❏No   ❏Yes

If yes, give your score: _____
and the date taken: _____

Circle the number to the right in each area to indicate your level of knowledge or ability.

3. Theoretical Knowledge

	None	Little	Some		Moderate		Strong		Thorough	
Psychoanalytic	1	2	3	4	5	6	7	8	9	10
Adlerian	1	2	3	4	5	6	7	8	9	10
Jungian	1	2	3	4	5	6	7	8	9	10
Person-centered	1	2	3	4	5	6	7	8	9	10
Rational-emotive	1	2	3	4	5	6	7	8	9	10
Behavioral	1	2	3	4	5	6	7	8	9	10
Gestalt	1	2	3	4	5	6	7	8	9	10
Reality therapy	1	2	3	4	5	6	7	8	9	10
Existential	1	2	3	4	5	6	7	8	9	10
Transactional	1	2	3	4	5	6	7	8	9	10
Analysis	1	2	3	4	5	6	7	8	9	10
Psychodrama	1	2	3	4	5	6	7	8	9	10
Family therapy	1	2	3	4	5	6	7	8	9	10
Human potential	1	2	3	4	5	6	7	8	9	10
Communication	1	2	3	4	5	6	7	8	9	10

Indicate theories not listed above that you have utilized or know. Use the number scale to indicate your knowledge level for each theory listed:

4. Assessment and Diagnosis

	None	Some	Average	Extensive	Thorough
Social assessment	1	2	3	4	5
Use of DSM-IV-TR	1	2	3	4	5
Initial database	1	2	3	4	5
Initial treatment plans	1	2	3	4	5
Review treatment plans	1	2	3	4	5
Evaluating mental status	1	2	3	4	5
Interview evaluation	1	2	3	4	5
Social assessment	1	2	3	4	5
Psychological assessment	1	2	3	4	5

5. Intervention

	None	Some	Average	Extensive	Thorough
Forming alliances	1	2	3	4	5
Client engagement	1	2	3	4	5
Client confusion	1	2	3	4	5
Client hostility	1	2	3	4	5
Client resistance	1	2	3	4	5
Interpretations	1	2	3	4	5
Seeking clarification	1	2	3	4	5
Being supportive	1	2	3	4	5
Asking sensitive questions	1	2	3	4	5
Transference	1	2	3	4	5
Countertransference	1	2	3	4	5
Termination	1	2	3	4	5

6. Record Keeping

	None	Some	Average	Extensive	Thorough
Initial databases	1	2	3	4	5
Initial treatment plans	1	2	3	4	5
Review treatment plans	1	2	3	4	5
Progress notes	1	2	3	4	5
Invoicing	1	2	3	4	5
Outcome measures	1	2	3	4	5
Case management	1	2	3	4	5

7. Prior Supervisory Experience

List your past supervisory experiences. Include supervision of all types of past employment. Include in the listing your likes and dislikes in each supervisory experience.

8. Strengths and Limitations

Identify personal and professional strengths and limitations that could enhance or hinder your practice activity and performance in supervision.

9. View of Helping

What are your views and attitudes about clients and the helping relationship?

10. Goals

List your learning goals in supervision:

List your career goals and objectives:

What do you see as the relationship between your current learning goals and your career objectives?

Appendix III

Clinical Social Work Credentialing, Accrediting, and Professional Organizations

Clinical Social Work Credentialing, Accrediting, and Professional Organizations

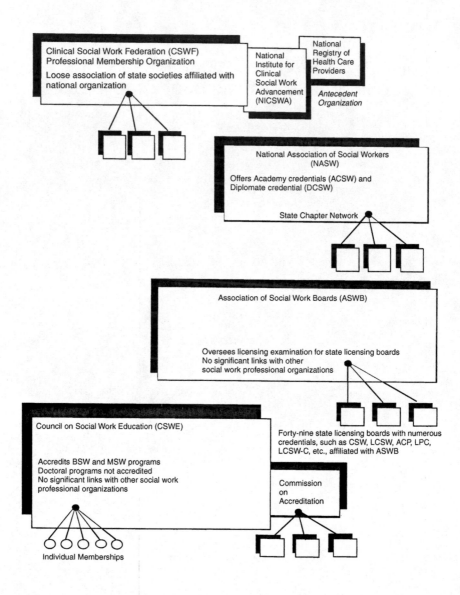

Appendix IV

Codes of Ethics of the National Association of Social Workers, the American Board of Examiners in Clinical Social Work, and the Clinical Social Work Federation

NATIONAL ASSOCIATION OF SOCIAL WORKERS CODE OF ETHICS

Overview

The *NASW Code of Ethics* is intended to serve as a guide to the everyday professional conduct of social workers. This *Code* includes four sections. The first section, "Preamble," summarizes the social work profession's mission and core values. The second section, "Purpose of the *NASW Code of Ethics*," provides an overview of the *Code's* main functions and a brief guide for dealing with ethical issues or dilemmas in social work practice. The third section, "Ethical Principles," presents broad ethical principles, based on social work's core values, that inform social work practice. The final section, "Ethical Standards," includes specific ethical standards to guide social workers' conduct and to provide a basis for adjudication.

Preamble

The primary mission of the social work profession is to enhance human well-being and help meet the basic human needs of all people, with particular attention to the needs and empowerment of people who are vulnerable, oppressed, and living in poverty. A historic and defining feature of social work is the profession's focus on individual well-being in a social context and the well-being of society. Fundamental to social work is attention to the environmental forces that create, contribute to, and address problems in living.

Social workers promote social justice and social change with and on behalf of clients. "Clients" is used inclusively to refer to individuals, families, groups, organizations, and communities. Social workers are sensitive to cultural and ethnic diversity and strive to end discrimination, oppression, poverty, and other forms of social injustice. These activities may be in the form of direct practice, community organizing, supervision, consultation, administration, advocacy, social and political action, policy development and implementation, education, and research and evaluation. Social workers seek to enhance the capacity of people to address their own needs. Social workers also seek to promote the responsiveness of organizations, communities, and other social institutions to individuals' needs and social problems.

The mission of the social work profession is rooted in a set of core values. These core values, embraced by social workers throughout the profession's history, are the foundation of social work's unique purpose and perspective:

- service
- social justice
- dignity and worth of the person
- importance of human relationships
- integrity
- competence

This constellation of core values reflects what is unique to the social work profession. Core values, and the principles that flow from them, must be balanced within the context and complexity of the human experience.

Purpose of the NASW Code of Ethics

Professional ethics are at the core of social work. The profession has an obligation to articulate its basic values, ethical principles, and ethical standards. The *NASW Code of Ethics* sets forth these values, principles, and standards to guide social workers' conduct. The *Code* is relevant to all social workers and social work students, regardless of their professional functions, the settings in which they work, or the populations they serve.

The *NASW Code of Ethics* serves six purposes:

1. The *Code* identifies core values on which social work's mission is based.
2. The *Code* summarizes broad ethical principles that reflect the profession's core values and establishes a set of specific ethical standards that should be used to guide social work practice.
3. The *Code* is designed to help social workers identify relevant considerations when professional obligations conflict or ethical uncertainties arise.
4. The *Code* provides ethical standards to which the general public can hold the social work profession accountable.
5. The *Code* socializes practitioners new to the field to social work's mission, values, ethical principles, and ethical standards.
6. The *Code* articulates standards that the social work profession itself can use to assess whether social workers have engaged in unethical conduct. NASW has formal procedures to adjudicate ethics complaints filed against its members.* In subscribing to this *Code*, social workers are required to cooperate in its implementation, participate in NASW adjudication proceedings, and abide by any NASW disciplinary rulings or sanctions based on it.

The *Code* offers a set of values, principles, and standards to guide decision making and conduct when ethical issues arise. It does not provide a set of rules that prescribe how social workers should act in all situations. Specific applications of the *Code* must take into account the context in which it is being considered and the possibility of conflicts among the *Code's* values, principles, and standards. Ethical responsibilities flow from all human relationships, from the personal and familial to the social and professional.

Further, the *NASW Code of Ethics* does not specify which values, principles, and standards are most important and ought to outweigh others in instances when they conflict. Reasonable differences of opinion can and do exist among social workers with respect to the ways in which values, ethical principles, and ethical standards should be rank ordered when they conflict. Ethical decision making in a given situation must apply the informed judgment of the individual social worker and should also consider how the issues would be judged in a peer review process where the ethical standards of the profession would be applied.

---

*For information on NASW adjudication procedures, see *NASW Procedures for the Adjudication of Grievances*.

Ethical decision making is a process. There are many instances in social work where simple answers are not available to resolve complex ethical issues. Social workers should take into consideration all the values, principles, and standards in this *Code* that are relevant to any situation in which ethical judgment is warranted. Social workers' decisions and actions should be consistent with the spirit as well as the letter of this *Code*.

In addition to this *Code*, there are many other sources of information about ethical thinking that may be useful. Social workers should consider ethical theory and principles generally, social work theory and research, laws, regulations, agency policies, and other relevant codes of ethics, recognizing that among codes of ethics social workers should consider the *NASW Code of Ethics* as their primary source. Social workers also should be aware of the impact on ethical decision making of their clients' and their own personal values and cultural and religious beliefs and practices. They should be aware of any conflicts between personal and professional values and deal with them responsibly. For additional guidance social workers should consult the relevant literature on professional ethics and ethical decision making and seek appropriate consultation when faced with ethical dilemmas. This may involve consultation with an agency-based or social work organization's ethics committee, a regulatory body, knowledgeable colleagues, supervisors, or legal counsel.

Instances may arise when social workers' ethical obligations conflict with agency policies or relevant laws or regulations. When such conflicts occur, social workers must make a responsible effort to resolve the conflict in a manner that is consistent with the values, principles, and standards expressed in this *Code*. If a reasonable resolution of the conflict does not appear possible, social workers should seek proper consultation before making a decision.

The *NASW Code of Ethics* is to be used by NASW and by individuals, agencies, organizations, and bodies (such as licensing and regulatory boards, professional liability insurance providers, courts of law, agency boards of directors, government agencies, and other professional groups) that choose to adopt it or use it as a frame of reference. Violation of standards in this *Code* does not automatically imply legal liability or violation of the law. Such determination can only be made in the context of legal and judicial proceedings. Alleged violations of the *Code* would be subject to a peer review process. Such processes are generally separate from legal or administrative procedures and insulated from legal review or proceedings to allow the profession to counsel and discipline its own members.

A code of ethics cannot guarantee ethical behavior. Moreover, a code of ethics cannot resolve all ethical issues or disputes or capture the richness and complexity involved in striving to make responsible choices within a moral community. Rather, a code of ethics sets forth values, ethical principles, and ethical standards to which professionals aspire and by which their actions can be judged. Social workers' ethical behavior should result from their personal commitment to engage in ethical practice. The *NASW Code of Ethics* reflects the commitment of all social workers to uphold the profession's values and to act ethically. Principles and standards must be applied by individuals of good character who discern moral questions and, in good faith, seek to make reliable ethical judgments.

Ethical Principles

The following broad ethical principles are based on social work's core values of service, social justice, dignity and worth of the person, importance of human relationships, integrity, and competence. These principles set forth ideals to which all social workers should aspire.

Value: *Service*

Ethical Principle: *Social workers' primary goal is to help people in need and to address social problems.*

Social workers elevate service to others above self-interest. Social workers draw on their knowledge, values, and skills to help people in need and to address social problems. Social workers are encouraged to volunteer some portion of their professional skills with no expectation of significant financial return (pro bono service).

Value: *Social Justice*

Ethical Principle: *Social workers challenge social injustice.*

Social workers pursue social change, particularly with and on behalf of vulnerable and oppressed individuals and groups of people. Social workers' social change efforts are focused primarily on issues of poverty, unemployment, discrimination, and other forms of social injustice. These activities seek to promote sensitivity to and knowledge about oppression and cultural and ethnic diversity. Social workers strive to ensure access to needed information, services, and resources; equality of opportunity; and meaningful participation in decision making for all people.

Value: *Dignity and Worth of the Person*

Ethical Principle: *Social workers respect the inherent dignity and worth of the person.*

Social workers treat each person in a caring and respectful fashion, mindful of individual differences and cultural and ethnic diversity. Social workers promote clients' socially responsible self-determination. Social workers seek to enhance clients' capacity and opportunity to change and to address their own needs. Social workers are cognizant of their dual responsibility to clients and to the broader society. They seek to resolve conflicts between clients' interests and the broader society's interests in a socially responsible manner consistent with the values, ethical principles, and ethical standards of the profession.

Value: *Importance of Human Relationships*

Ethical Principle: *Social workers recognize the central importance of human relationships.*

Social workers understand that relationships between and among people are an important vehicle for change. Social workers engage people as partners in the helping process. Social workers seek to strengthen relationships among people in a purposeful effort to promote, restore, maintain, and enhance the well-being of individuals, families, social groups, organizations, and communities.

Value: *Integrity*

Ethical Principle: *Social workers behave in a trustworthy manner.*

Social workers are continually aware of the profession's mission, values, ethical principles, and ethical standards and practice in a manner consistent with them. Social workers act honestly and responsibly and promote ethical practices on the part of the organizations with which they are affiliated.

Value: *Competence*

Ethical Principle: *Social workers practice within their areas of competence and develop and enhance their professional expertise.*

Social workers continually strive to increase their professional knowledge and skills and to apply them in practice. Social workers should aspire to contribute to the knowledge base of the profession.

Ethical Standards

The following ethical standards are relevant to the professional activities of all social workers. These standards concern (1) social workers' ethical responsibilities to clients, (2) social workers' ethical responsibilities to colleagues, (3) social workers' ethical responsibilities in practice settings, (4) social workers' ethical responsibilities as professionals, (5) social workers' ethical responsibilities to the social work profession, and (6) social workers' ethical responsibilities to the broader society.

Some of the standards that follow are enforceable guidelines for professional conduct, and some are aspirational. The extent to which each standard is enforceable is a matter of professional judgment to be exercised by those responsible for reviewing alleged violations of ethical standards.

1. SOCIAL WORKERS' ETHICAL RESPONSIBILITIES TO CLIENTS

1.01   Commitment to Clients

Social workers' primary responsibility is to promote the well-being of clients. In general, clients' interests are primary. However, social workers' responsibility to the larger society or specific legal obligations may on limited occasions supersede the loyalty owed clients, and clients should be so advised. (Examples include when a social worker is required by law to report that a client has abused a child or has threatened to harm self or others.)

1.02   Self-Determination

Social workers respect and promote the right of clients to self-determination and assist clients in their efforts to identify and clarify their goals. Social workers may limit clients' right to self-determination when, in the social workers' professional judgment, clients' actions or potential actions pose a serious, foreseeable, and imminent risk to themselves or others.

1.03   Informed Consent

(a) Social workers should provide services to clients only in the context of a professional relationship based, when appropriate, on valid informed consent. Social workers should use clear and understandable language to inform clients of the purpose of the services, risks related to the services, limits to services because of the requirements of a third-party payer, relevant costs, reasonable alternatives, clients' right to refuse or withdraw consent, and the time frame covered by the consent. Social workers should provide clients with an opportunity to ask questions.

(b) In instances when clients are not literate or have difficulty understanding the primary language used in the practice setting, social workers should take steps to ensure clients' comprehension. This may include providing clients with a detailed verbal explanation or arranging for a qualified interpreter or translator whenever possible.

(c) In instances when clients lack the capacity to provide informed consent, social workers should protect clients' interests by seeking permission from an appropriate third party, informing clients consistent with the clients' level of understanding. In such instances social workers should seek to ensure that the third party acts in a manner consistent with clients' wishes and interests. Social workers should take reasonable steps to enhance such clients' ability to give informed consent.

(d) In instances when clients are receiving services involuntarily, social workers should provide information about the nature and extent of services and about the extent of clients' right to refuse service.

(e) Social workers who provide services via electronic media (such as computer, telephone, radio, and television) should inform recipients of the limitations and risks associated with such services.

(f) Social workers should obtain clients' informed consent before audiotaping or videotaping clients or permitting observation of services to clients by a third party.

1.04   Competence

(a) Social workers should provide services and represent themselves as competent only within the boundaries of their education, training, license, certification, consultation received, supervised experience, or other relevant professional experience.

(b) Social workers should provide services in substantive areas or use intervention techniques or approaches that are new to them only after engaging in appropriate study, training, consultation, and supervision from people who are competent in those interventions or techniques.

(c) When generally recognized standards do not exist with respect to an emerging area of practice, social workers should exercise careful judgment and take responsible steps (including appropriate education, research, training, consultation, and supervision) to ensure the competence of their work and to protect clients from harm.

1.05   Cultural Competence and Social Diversity

(a) Social workers should understand culture and its function in human behavior and society, recognizing the strengths that exist in all cultures.

(b) Social workers should have a knowledge base of their clients' cultures and be able to demonstrate competence in the provision of services that are sensitive to clients' cultures and to differences among people and cultural groups.

(c) Social workers should obtain education about and seek to understand the nature of social diversity and oppression with respect to race, ethnicity, national origin, color, sex, sexual orientation, age, marital status, political belief, religion, and mental or physical disability.

1.06   Conflicts of Interest

(a) Social workers should be alert to and avoid conflicts of interest that interfere with the exercise of professional discretion and impartial judgment. Social workers should inform clients when a real or potential conflict of interest arises and take reasonable steps to resolve the issue in a manner that makes the clients' interests primary and protects clients' interests to the greatest extent possible. In some cases, protecting clients' interests may require termination of the professional relationship with proper referral of the client.

(b) Social workers should not take unfair advantage of any professional relationship or exploit others to further their personal, religious, political, or business interests.

(c) Social workers should not engage in dual or multiple relationships with clients or former clients in which there is a risk of exploitation or potential harm to the client. In instances when dual or multiple relationships are unavoidable, social workers should take steps to protect clients and are responsible for setting clear, appropriate, and culturally sensitive boundaries. (Dual or multiple relationships occur when social workers relate to clients in more than one relationship, whether professional, social, or business. Dual or multiple relationships can occur simultaneously or consecutively.)

(d) When social workers provide services to two or more people who have a relationship with each other (for example, couples, family members), social workers should clarify with all parties which individuals will be considered clients and the nature of social workers' professional obligations to the various individuals who are receiving services. Social workers who anticipate a conflict of interest among the individuals receiving services or who anticipate having to perform in potentially conflicting roles (for example, when a social worker is asked to testify in a child custody dispute or divorce proceedings involving clients) should clarify their role with the parties involved and take appropriate action to minimize any conflict of interest.

1.07 Privacy and Confidentiality

(a) Social workers should respect clients' right to privacy. Social workers should not solicit private information from clients unless it is essential to providing services or conducting social work evaluation or research. Once private information is shared, standards of confidentiality apply.

(b) Social workers may disclose confidential information when appropriate with valid consent from a client or a person legally authorized to consent on behalf of a client.

(c) Social workers should protect the confidentiality of all information obtained in the course of professional service, except for compelling professional reasons. The general expectation that social workers will keep information confidential does not apply when disclosure is necessary to prevent serious, foreseeable, and imminent harm to a client or other identifiable person or when laws or regulations require disclosure without a client's consent. In all instances, social workers should disclose the least amount of confidential information necessary to achieve the desired purpose; only information that is directly relevant to the purpose for which the disclosure is made should be revealed.

(d) Social workers should inform clients, to the extent possible, about the disclosure of confidential information and the potential consequences, when feasible before the disclosure is made. This applies whether social workers disclose confidential information on the basis of a legal requirement or client consent.

(e) Social workers should discuss with clients and other interested parties the nature of confidentiality and limitations of clients' right to confidentiality. Social workers should review with clients circumstances where confidential information may be requested and where disclosure of confidential information may be legally required. This discussion should occur as soon as possible in the social worker–client relationship and as needed throughout the course of the relationship.

(f) When social workers provide counseling services to families, couples, or groups, social workers should seek agreement among the parties involved concerning each individual's right to confidentiality and obligation to preserve the confidentiality of information shared by others. Social workers should inform participants in family, couples, or group counseling that social workers cannot guarantee that all participants will honor such agreements.

(g) Social workers should inform clients involved in family, couples, marital, or group counseling of the social worker's, employer's, and agency's policy concerning the social worker's disclosure of confidential information among the parties involved in the counseling.

(h) Social workers should not disclose confidential information to third-party payers unless clients have authorized such disclosure.

(i) Social workers should not discuss confidential information in any setting unless privacy can be ensured. Social workers should not discuss confidential information in public or semipublic areas such as hallways, waiting rooms, elevators, and restaurants.

(j) Social workers should protect the confidentiality of clients during legal proceedings to the extent permitted by law. When a court of law or other legally authorized body orders social workers to disclose confidential or privileged information without a client's consent and such disclosure could cause harm to the client, social workers should request that the court withdraw the order or limit the order as narrowly as possible or maintain the records under seal, unavailable for public inspection.

(k) Social workers should protect the confidentiality of clients when responding to requests from members of the media.

(l) Social workers should protect the confidentiality of clients' written and electronic records and other sensitive information. Social workers should take reasonable steps to ensure that clients' records are stored in a secure location and that clients' records are not available to others who are not authorized to have access.

(m) Social workers should take precautions to ensure and maintain the confidentiality of information transmitted to other parties through the use of computers, electronic mail, facsimile machines, telephones and telephone answering machines, and other electronic or computer technology. Disclosure of identifying information should be avoided whenever possible.

(n) Social workers should transfer or dispose of clients' records in a manner that protects clients' confidentiality and is consistent with state statutes governing records and social work licensure.

(o) Social workers should take reasonable precautions to protect client confidentiality in the event of the social worker's termination of practice, incapacitation, or death.

(p) Social workers should not disclose identifying information when discussing clients for teaching or training purposes unless the client has consented to disclosure of confidential information.

(q) Social workers should not disclose identifying information when discussing clients with consultants unless the client has consented to disclosure of confidential information or there is a compelling need for such disclosure.

(r) Social workers should protect the confidentiality of deceased clients consistent with the preceding standards.

1.08 Access to Records

(a) Social workers should provide clients with reasonable access to records concerning the clients. Social workers who are concerned that clients' access to their records could cause serious misunderstanding or harm to the client should provide assistance in interpreting the records and consultation with the client regarding the records. Social workers should limit clients' access to their records, or portions of their records, only in exceptional circumstances when there is compelling evidence that such access would cause serious harm to the client. Both clients' requests and the rationale for withholding some or all of the record should be documented in clients' files.

(b) When providing clients with access to their records, social workers should take steps to protect the confidentiality of other individuals identified or discussed in such records.

1.09 Sexual Relationships

(a) Social workers should under no circumstances engage in sexual activities or sexual contact with current clients, whether such contact is consensual or forced.

(b) Social workers should not engage in sexual activities or sexual contact with clients' relatives or other individuals with whom clients maintain a close personal relationship when there is a risk of exploitation or potential harm to the client. Sexual activity or sexual contact with clients' relatives or other individuals with whom clients maintain a personal relationship has the potential to be harmful to the client and may make it difficult for the social worker and client to maintain appropriate professional boundaries. Social workers— not their clients, their clients' relatives, or other individuals with whom the client maintains a personal relationship—assume the full burden for setting clear, appropriate, and culturally sensitive boundaries.

(c) Social workers should not engage in sexual activities or sexual contact with former clients because of the potential for harm to the client. If social workers engage in conduct contrary to this prohibition or claim that an exception to this prohibition is warranted because of extraordinary circumstances, it is social workers—not their clients—who assume the full burden of demonstrating that the former client has not been exploited, coerced, or manipulated, intentionally or unintentionally.

(d) Social workers should not provide clinical services to individuals with whom they have had a prior sexual relationship. Providing clinical services to a former sexual partner has the potential to be harmful to the individual and is likely to make it difficult for the social worker and individual to maintain appropriate professional boundaries.

1.10 Physical Contact

Social workers should not engage in physical contact with clients when there is a possibility of psychological harm to the client as a result of the contact (such as cradling or caressing clients). Social workers who engage in appropriate physical contact with clients are responsible for setting clear, appropriate, and culturally sensitive boundaries that govern such physical contact.

1.11   Sexual Harassment

Social workers should not sexually harass clients. Sexual harassment includes sexual advances, sexual solicitation, requests for sexual favors, and other verbal or physical conduct of a sexual nature.

1.12   Derogatory Language

Social workers should not use derogatory language in their written or verbal communications to or about clients. Social workers should use accurate and respectful language in all communications to and about clients.

1.13   Payment for Services

(a) When setting fees, social workers should ensure that the fees are fair, reasonable, and commensurate with the services performed. Consideration should be given to clients' ability to pay.

(b) Social workers should avoid accepting goods or services from clients as payment for professional services. Bartering arrangements, particularly involving services, create the potential for conflicts of interest, exploitation, and inappropriate boundaries in social workers' relationships with clients. Social workers should explore and may participate in bartering only in very limited circumstances when it can be demonstrated that such arrangements are an accepted practice among professionals in the local community, considered to be essential for the provision of services, negotiated without coercion, and entered into at the client's initiative and with the client's informed consent. Social workers who accept goods or services from clients as payment for professional services assume the full burden of demonstrating that this arrangement will not be detrimental to the client or the professional relationship.

(c) Social workers should not solicit a private fee or other remuneration for providing services to clients who are entitled to such available services through the social workers' employer or agency.

1.14   Clients Who Lack Decision-Making Capacity

When social workers act on behalf of clients who lack the capacity to make informed decisions, social workers should take reasonable steps to safeguard the interests and rights of those clients.

1.15   Interruption of Services

Social workers should make reasonable efforts to ensure continuity of services in the event that services are interrupted by factors such as unavailability, relocation, illness, disability, or death.

1.16 Termination of Services

(a) Social workers should terminate services to clients and professional relationships with them when such services and relationships are no longer required or no longer serve the clients' needs or interests.

(b) Social workers should take reasonable steps to avoid abandoning clients who are still in need of services. Social workers should withdraw services precipitously only under unusual circumstances, giving careful consideration to all factors in the situation and taking care to minimize possible adverse effects. Social workers should assist in making appropriate arrangements for continuation of services when necessary.

(c) Social workers in fee-for-service settings may terminate services to clients who are not paying an overdue balance if the financial contractual arrangements have been made clear to the client, if the client does not pose an imminent danger to self or others, and if the clinical and other consequences of the current nonpayment have been addressed and discussed with the client.

(d) Social workers should not terminate services to pursue a social, financial, or sexual relationship with a client.

(e) Social workers who anticipate the termination or interruption of services to clients should notify clients promptly and seek the transfer, referral, or continuation of services in relation to the clients' needs and preferences.

(f) Social workers who are leaving an employment setting should inform clients of appropriate options for the continuation of services and of the benefits and risks of the options.

2. SOCIAL WORKERS' ETHICAL RESPONSIBILITIES TO COLLEAGUES

2.01 Respect

(a) Social workers should treat colleagues with respect and should represent accurately and fairly the qualifications, views, and obligations of colleagues.

(b) Social workers should avoid unwarranted negative criticism of colleagues in communications with clients or with other professionals. Unwarranted negative criticism may include demeaning comments that refer to colleagues' level of competence or to individuals' attributes such as race, ethnicity, national origin, color, sex, sexual orientation, age, marital status, political belief, religion, and mental or physical disability.

(c) Social workers should cooperate with social work colleagues and with colleagues of other professions when such cooperation serves the well-being of clients.

2.02 Confidentiality

Social workers should respect confidential information shared by colleagues in the course of their professional relationships and transactions. Social workers should ensure that such colleagues understand social workers' obligation to respect confidentiality and any exceptions related to it.

2.03   Interdisciplinary Collaboration

(a) Social workers who are members of an interdisciplinary team should participate in and contribute to decisions that affect the well-being of clients by drawing on the perspectives, values, and experiences of the social work profession. Professional and ethical obligations of the interdisciplinary team as a whole and of its individual members should be clearly established.

(b) Social workers for whom a team decision raises ethical concerns should attempt to resolve the disagreement through appropriate channels. If the disagreement cannot be resolved, social workers should pursue other avenues to address their concerns consistent with client well-being.

2.04   Disputes Involving Colleagues

(a) Social workers should not take advantage of a dispute between a colleague and an employer to obtain a position or otherwise advance the social workers' own interests.

(b) Social workers should not exploit clients in disputes with colleagues or engage clients in any inappropriate discussion of conflicts between social workers and their colleagues.

2.05   Consultation

(a) Social workers should seek the advice and counsel of colleagues whenever such consultation is in the best interests of clients.

(b) Social workers should keep themselves informed about colleagues' areas of expertise and competencies. Social workers should seek consultation only from colleagues who have demonstrated knowledge, expertise, and competence related to the subject of the consultation.

(c) When consulting with colleagues about clients, social workers should disclose the least amount of information necessary to achieve the purposes of the consultation.

2.06   Referral for Services

(a) Social workers should refer clients to other professionals when the other professionals' specialized knowledge or expertise is needed to serve clients fully or when social workers believe that they are not being effective or making reasonable progress with clients and that additional service is required.

(b) Social workers who refer clients to other professionals should take appropriate steps to facilitate an orderly transfer of responsibility. Social workers who refer clients to other professionals should disclose, with clients' consent, all pertinent information to the new service providers.

(c) Social workers are prohibited from giving or receiving payment for a referral when no professional service is provided by the referring social worker.

2.07 Sexual Relationships

(a) Social workers who function as supervisors or educators should not engage in sexual activities or contact with supervisees, students, trainees, or other colleagues over whom they exercise professional authority.

(b) Social workers should avoid engaging in sexual relationships with colleagues when there is potential for a conflict of interest. Social workers who become involved in, or anticipate becoming involved in, a sexual relationship with a colleague have a duty to transfer professional responsibilities, when necessary, to avoid a conflict of interest.

2.08 Sexual Harassment

Social workers should not sexually harass supervisees, students, trainees, or colleagues. Sexual harassment includes sexual advances, sexual solicitation, requests for sexual favors, and other verbal or physical conduct of a sexual nature.

2.09 Impairment of Colleagues

(a) Social workers who have direct knowledge of a social work colleague's impairment that is due to personal problems, psychosocial distress, substance abuse, or mental health difficulties and that interferes with practice effectiveness should consult with that colleague when feasible and assist the colleague in taking remedial action.

(b) Social workers who believe that a social work colleague's impairment interferes with practice effectiveness and that the colleague has not taken adequate steps to address the impairment should take action through appropriate channels established by employers, agencies, NASW, licensing and regulatory bodies, and other professional organizations.

2.10 Incompetence of Colleagues

(a) Social workers who have direct knowledge of a social work colleague's incompetence should consult with that colleague when feasible and assist the colleague in taking remedial action

(b) Social workers who believe that a social work colleague is incompetent and has not taken adequate steps to address the incompetence should take action through appropriate channels established by employers, agencies, NASW, licensing and regulatory bodies, and other professional organizations.

2.11   Unethical Conduct of Colleagues

(a) Social workers should take adequate measures to discourage, prevent, expose, and correct the unethical conduct of colleagues.

(b) Social workers should be knowledgeable about established policies and procedures for handling concerns about colleagues' unethical behavior. Social workers should be familiar with national, state, and local procedures for handling ethics complaints. These include policies and procedures created by NASW, licensing and regulatory bodies, employers, agencies, and other professional organizations.

(c) Social workers who believe that a colleague has acted unethically should seek resolution by discussing their concerns with the colleague when feasible and when such discussion is likely to be productive.

(d) When necessary, social workers who believe that a colleague has acted unethically should take action through appropriate formal channels (such as contacting a state licensing board or regulatory body, an NASW committee on inquiry, or other professional ethics committees).

(e) Social workers should defend and assist colleagues who are unjustly charged with unethical conduct.

**3. SOCIAL WORKERS' ETHICAL RESPONSIBILITIES
   IN PRACTICE SETTINGS**

3.01   Supervision and Consultation

(a) Social workers who provide supervision or consultation should have the necessary knowledge and skill to supervise or consult appropriately and should do so only within their areas of knowledge and competence.

(b) Social workers who provide supervision or consultation are responsible for setting clear, appropriate, and culturally sensitive boundaries.

(c) Social workers should not engage in any dual or multiple relationships with supervisees in which there is a risk of exploitation of or potential harm to the supervisee.

(d) Social workers who provide supervision should evaluate supervisees' performance in a manner that is fair and respectful.

3.02   Education and Training

(a) Social workers who function as educators, field instructors for students, or trainers should provide instruction only within their areas of knowledge and competence and should provide instruction based on the most current information and knowledge available in the profession.

(b) Social workers who function as educators or field instructors for students should evaluate students' performance in a manner that is fair and respectful.

(c) Social workers who function as educators or field instructors for students should take reasonable steps to ensure that clients are routinely informed when services are being provided by students.

(d) Social workers who function as educators or field instructors for students should not engage in any dual or multiple relationships with students in which there is a risk of exploitation or potential harm to the student. Social work educators and field instructors are responsible for setting clear, appropriate, and culturally sensitive boundaries.

3.03 Performance Evaluation

Social workers who have responsibility for evaluating the performance of others should fulfill such responsibility in a fair and considerate manner and on the basis of clearly stated criteria.

3.04 Client Records

(a) Social workers should take reasonable steps to ensure that documentation in records is accurate and reflects the services provided.

(b) Social workers should include sufficient and timely documentation in records to facilitate the delivery of services and to ensure continuity of services provided to clients in the future.

(c) Social workers' documentation should protect clients' privacy to the extent that is possible and appropriate and should include only information that is directly relevant to the delivery of services.

(d) Social workers should store records following the termination of services to ensure reasonable future access. Records should be maintained for the number of years required by state statutes or relevant contracts.

3.05 Billing

Social workers should establish and maintain billing practices that accurately reflect the nature and extent of services provided and that identify who provided the service in the practice setting.

3.06 Client Transfer

(a) When an individual who is receiving services from another agency or colleague contacts a social worker for services, the social worker should carefully consider the client needs before agreeing to provide services. To minimize possible confusion and conflict, social workers should discuss with potential clients the nature of the clients' current relationship with other service providers and the implications, including possible benefits or risks, of entering into a relationship with a new service provider.

(b) If a new client has been served by another agency or colleague, social workers should discuss with the client whether consultation with the previous service provider is in the client's best interest.

3.07   Administration

(a) Social work administrators should advocate within and outside their agencies for adequate resources to meet clients' needs.

(b) Social workers should advocate for resource allocation procedures that are open and fair. When not all clients' needs can be met, an allocation procedure should be developed that is nondiscriminatory and based on appropriate and consistently applied principles.

(c) Social workers who are administrators should take reasonable steps to ensure that adequate agency or organizational resources are available to provide appropriate staff supervision.

(d) Social work administrators should take reasonable steps to ensure that the working environment for which they are responsible is consistent with and encourages compliance with the *NASW Code of Ethics*. Social work administrators should take reasonable steps to eliminate any conditions in their organizations that violate, interfere with, or discourage compliance with the *Code*.

3.08   Continuing Education and Staff Development

Social work administrators and supervisors should take reasonable steps to provide or arrange for continuing education and staff development for all staff for whom they are responsible. Continuing education and staff development should address current knowledge and emerging developments related to social work practice and ethics.

3.09   Commitments to Employers

(a) Social workers generally should adhere to commitments made to employers and employing organizations.

(b) Social workers should work to improve employing agencies' policies and procedures and the efficiency and effectiveness of their services.

(c) Social workers should take reasonable steps to ensure that employers are aware of social workers' ethical obligations as set forth in the *NASW Code of Ethics* and of the implications of those obligations for social work practice.

(d) Social workers should not allow an employing organization's policies, procedures, regulations, or administrative orders to interfere with their ethical practice of social work. Social workers should take reasonable steps to ensure that their employing organizations' practices are consistent with the *NASW Code of Ethics*.

(e) Social workers should act to prevent and eliminate discrimination in the employing organization's work assignments and in its employment policies and practices.

(f) Social workers should accept employment or arrange student field placements only in organizations that exercise fair personnel practices.

(g) Social workers should be diligent stewards of the resources of their employing organizations, wisely conserving funds where appropriate and never misappropriating funds or using them for unintended purposes.

3.10 Labor–Management Disputes

(a) Social workers may engage in organized action, including the formation of and participation in labor unions, to improve services to clients and working conditions.

(b) The actions of social workers who are involved in labor–management disputes, job actions, or labor strikes should be guided by the profession's values, ethical principles, and ethical standards. Reasonable differences of opinion exist among social workers concerning their primary obligation as professionals during an actual or threatened labor strike or job action. Social workers should carefully examine relevant issues and their possible impact on clients before deciding on a course of action.

4. SOCIAL WORKERS' ETHICAL RESPONSIBILITIES AS PROFESSIONALS

4.01 Competence

(a) Social workers should accept responsibility or employment only on the basis of existing competence or the intention to acquire the necessary competence.

(b) Social workers should strive to become and remain proficient in professional practice and the performance of professional functions. Social workers should critically examine and keep current with emerging knowledge relevant to social work. Social workers should routinely review the professional literature and participate in continuing education relevant to social work practice and social work ethics.

(c) Social workers should base practice on recognized knowledge, including empirically based knowledge, relevant to social work and social work ethics.

4.02 Discrimination

Social workers should not practice, condone, facilitate, or collaborate with any form of discrimination on the basis of race, ethnicity, national origin, color, sex, sexual orientation, age, marital status, political belief, religion, or mental or physical disability.

4.03   Private Conduct

Social workers should not permit their private conduct to interfere with their ability to fulfill their professional responsibilities.

4.04   Dishonesty, Fraud, and Deception

Social workers should not participate in, condone, or be associated with dishonesty, fraud, or deception.

4.05   Impairment

(a) Social workers should not allow their own personal problems, psychosocial distress, legal problems, substance abuse, or mental health difficulties to interfere with their professional judgment and performance or to jeopardize the best interests of people for whom they have a professional responsibility.

(b) Social workers whose personal problems, psychosocial distress, legal problems, substance abuse, or mental health difficulties interfere with their professional judgment and performance should immediately seek consultation and take appropriate remedial action by seeking professional help, making adjustments in workload, terminating practice, or taking any other steps necessary to protect clients and others.

4.06   Misrepresentation

(a) Social workers should make clear distinctions between statements made and actions engaged in as a private individual and as a representative of the social work profession, a professional social work organization, or the social worker's employing agency.

(b) Social workers who speak on behalf of professional social work organizations should accurately represent the official and authorized positions of the organizations.

(c) Social workers should ensure that their representations to clients, agencies, and the public of professional qualifications, credentials, education, competence, affiliations, services provided, or results to be achieved are accurate. Social workers should claim only those relevant professional credentials they actually possess and take steps to correct any inaccuracies or misrepresentations of their credentials by others.

4.07   Solicitations

(a) Social workers should not engage in uninvited solicitation of potential clients who, because of their circumstances, are vulnerable to undue influence, manipulation, or coercion.

(b) Social workers should not engage in solicitation of testimonial endorsements (including solicitation of consent to use a client's prior statement as a testimonial endorsement) from current clients or from other people who, because of their particular circumstances, are vulnerable to undue influence.

4.08 Acknowledging Credit

(a) Social workers should take responsibility and credit, including authorship credit, only for work they have actually performed and to which they have contributed.

(b) Social workers should honestly acknowledge the work of and the contributions made by others.

5. SOCIAL WORKERS' ETHICAL RESPONSIBILITIES TO THE SOCIAL WORK PROFESSION

5.01 Integrity of the Profession

(a) Social workers should work toward the maintenance and promotion of high standards of practice.

(b) Social workers should uphold and advance the values, ethics, knowledge, and mission of the profession. Social workers should protect, enhance, and improve the integrity of the profession through appropriate study and research, active discussion, and responsible criticism of the profession.

(c) Social workers should contribute time and professional expertise to activities that promote respect for the value, integrity, and competence of the social work profession. These activities may include teaching, research, consultation, service, legislative testimony, presentations in the community, and participation in their professional organizations.

(d) Social workers should contribute to the knowledge base of social work and share with colleagues their knowledge related to practice, research, and ethics. Social workers should seek to contribute to the profession's literature and to share their knowledge at professional meetings and conferences.

(e) Social workers should act to prevent the unauthorized and unqualified practice of social work.

5.02 Evaluation and Research

(a) Social workers should monitor and evaluate policies, the implementation of programs, and practice interventions.

(b) Social workers should promote and facilitate evaluation and research to contribute to the development of knowledge.

(c) Social workers should critically examine and keep current with emerging knowledge relevant to social work and fully use evaluation and research evidence in their professional practice.

(d) Social workers engaged in evaluation or research should carefully consider possible consequences and should follow guidelines developed for the protection of evaluation and research participants. Appropriate institutional review boards should be consulted.

(e) Social workers engaged in evaluation or research should obtain voluntary and written informed consent from participants, when appropriate, without any implied or actual deprivation or penalty for refusal to participate; without undue inducement to participate; and with due regard for participants' well-being, privacy, and dignity. Informed consent should include information about the nature, extent, and duration of the participation requested and disclosure of the risks and benefits of participation in the research.

(f) When evaluation or research participants are incapable of giving informed consent, social workers should provide an appropriate explanation to the participants, obtain the participants' assent to the extent they are able, and obtain written consent from an appropriate proxy.

(g) Social workers should never design or conduct evaluation or research that does not use consent procedures, such as certain forms of naturalistic observation and archival research, unless rigorous and responsible review of the research has found it to be justified because of its prospective scientific, educational, or applied value and unless equally effective alternative procedures that do not involve waiver of consent are not feasible.

(h) Social workers should inform participants of their right to withdraw from evaluation and research at any time without penalty.

(i) Social workers should take appropriate steps to ensure that participants in evaluation and research have access to appropriate supportive services.

(j) Social workers engaged in evaluation or research should protect participants from unwarranted physical or mental distress, harm, danger, or deprivation.

(k) Social workers engaged in the evaluation of services should discuss collected information only for professional purposes and only with people professionally concerned with this information.

(l) Social workers engaged in evaluation or research should ensure the anonymity or confidentiality of participants and of the data obtained from them. Social workers should inform participants of any limits of confidentiality, the measures that will be taken to ensure confidentiality, and when any records containing research data will be destroyed.

(m) Social workers who report evaluation and research results should protect participants' confidentiality by omitting identifying information unless proper consent has been obtained authorizing disclosure.

(n) Social workers should report evaluation and research findings accurately. They should not fabricate or falsify results and should take steps to correct any errors later found in published data using standard publication methods.

(o) Social workers engaged in evaluation or research should be alert to and avoid conflicts of interest and dual relationships with participants, should inform participants when a real or potential conflict of interest arises, and should take steps to resolve the issue in a manner that makes participants' interests primary.

(p) Social workers should educate themselves, their students, and their colleagues about responsible research practices.

6. SOCIAL WORKERS' ETHICAL RESPONSIBILITIES TO THE BROADER SOCIETY

6.01 Social Welfare

Social workers should promote the general welfare of society, from local to global levels, and the development of people, their communities, and their environments. Social workers should advocate for living conditions conducive to the fulfillment of basic human needs and should promote social, economic, political, and cultural values and institutions that are compatible with the realization of social justice.

6.02 Public Participation

Social workers should facilitate informed participation by the public in shaping social policies and institutions.

6.03 Public Emergencies

Social workers should provide appropriate professional services in public emergencies to the greatest extent possible.

6.04 Social and Political Action

(a) Social workers should engage in social and political action that seeks to ensure that all people have equal access to the resources, employment, services, and opportunities they require to meet their basic human needs and to develop fully. Social workers should be aware of the impact of the political arena on practice and should advocate for changes in policy and legislation to improve social conditions in order to meet basic human needs and promote social justice.

(b) Social workers should act to expand choice and opportunity for all people, with special regard for vulnerable, disadvantaged, oppressed, and exploited people and groups.

(c) Social workers should promote conditions that encourage respect for cultural and social diversity within the United States and globally. Social workers should promote policies and practices that demonstrate respect for difference, support the expansion of cultural knowledge and resources, advocate for programs and institutions that demonstrate cultural competence, and promote policies that safeguard the rights of and confirm equity and social justice for all people.

(d) Social workers should act to prevent and eliminate domination of, exploitation of, and discrimination against any person, group, or class on the basis of race, ethnicity, national origin, color, sex, sexual orientation, age, marital status, political belief, religion, or mental or physical disability.

AMERICAN BOARD OF EXAMINERS
IN CLINICAL SOCIAL WORK
Code of Ethics

As an organization fundamentally concerned with the health and well-being of persons served by social work professionals, the American Board of Examiners in Clinical Social Work (the Board) establishes and promulgates standards of conduct and practice for its certificants. This Code of Ethics, rooted in the fundamental humane values of the social work profession, sets forth ethical principles which are intended to guide clinical social workers in their professional roles, relationships, and responsibilities. Advanced clinical social workers who hold board certification agree thereby to abide by the principles enunciated in this Code of Ethics and the procedures and policies set forth therein.

The principal aim of social work is to serve people by (1) recognizing and enhancing the inherent worth, integrity, dignity, and well-being of each individual, (2) upholding the right to self-determination, and (3) affirming the right to freedom from discrimination on grounds of age, race, religion, nationality, sex or sexual preference, as an essential part of the doctrine of equal opportunity for all.

The following codified ethical principles are intended to govern clinical social workers in their various professional roles and relationships and at the various levels of responsibility in which they function in their work. These principles also serve as a basis for the Board to adjudicate allegations of their violation.

In subscribing to and abiding by this Code, the clinical social worker must take into consideration those principles that may have a bearing upon any situation in which ethical judgement is to be exercised or professional intervention or conduct may be planned. The course of action that the social worker chooses must adhere to the letter of this Code, as well as be consistent with the spirit of the responsibilities contained therein.

This Code sets forth general principles of conduct, and the judicious appraisal of conduct, in matters which have ethical implications. The Code does not cover every possible set of circumstances in which the social worker must take action or exercise judgement, and specific applications of ethical principles must be judged within context. However, in order to be permissible, the actions taken and determinations made in a given situation must satisfy not only the judgement of the individual social worker who is involved directly, but also the judgement of an unbiased jury of professional peers.

In subscribing to this Code, a clinical social worker certified by the Board is required to cooperate in its implementation and abide by any disciplinary rulings based on it. She or he shall also take adequate measures to discourage, prevent, and correct the unethical conduct of colleagues.

Reprinted by permission of the American Board of Examiners in Clinical Social Work.

I.   Responsibility to Clients

1. Service to clients is the primary responsibility of the clinical social worker.
2. At introduction to a client, the clinical social worker shall identify himself or herself as such, and shall accurately present professional qualifications, including education, training and experience.
3. The clinical social worker shall:
    1. inform the client of the nature and extent of his or her services;
    2. set fair and reasonable fees and fully inform the client of such fees;
    3. refrain from engaging in illegal or unethical fee splitting;
    4. explain in advance the obligations of both the social worker and the client in their interactions;
    5. judiciously terminate the client relationship when therapeutic services and relationships are no longer required or desired by the client.
4. In instances where the clinical social worker judges that there is a threat to the safety of the client or others, the clinical social worker must take all reasonable steps to prevent the client from causing harm to self or others.
5. Communication between the clinical social worker and the client shall be privileged to the maximum extent permitted by law, including observance of the following:
    1. Confidential information revealed to the social worker shall be released only when there is a clear necessity, such as when required by law; when specifically requested by the client for specified purposes; or when the information reveals a clear and imminent danger to the individual or others. The clinical social worker shall inform clients, during initial contact, of any limitations of confidentiality.
    2. Prior to release of confidential material, the client shall be apprised, and client consent shall be obtained, except under constraints of law or safety.
    3. When information is used for purposes of professional education or research, the clinical social worker shall maintain confidentiality, and shall conceal the identity of the client unless the client gives explicit written informed consent to reveal such identity.
6. Professional services shall be based on competent diagnostic and treatment skills for improving the mental health and social functioning of the client(s), whether individuals, couples, families, or groups.
7. As an employee, employer, or practitioner the clinical social worker shall not engage in or condone practices that are inhumane or that result in illegal or unjustifiable actions. Such practices include, but are not limited to, those based on considerations of race, handicap, age, gender, sexual preference, religion, or national origin in hiring, promotion, or training.
8. The clinical social worker recognizes that personal problems and conflicts may interfere with professional effectiveness. Accordingly, he or she must refrain from undertaking any activity in which the clinician's personal problems are likely to lead to inadequate performance or harm to a client, colleague, student, or research participant. If, during the course of the discharge of professional duties, the clinical social worker becomes aware of his/her personal matters impeding the discharge of those duties, competent professional assistance shall be sought to determine whether the clini-

cal social worker should suspend, terminate, or limit the scope of the professional and/or scientific activities.

9. The clinical social worker shall be responsible for monitoring the quality of the services offered, and for the continued evaluation of the effectiveness of those services for each individual client.

10. The clinical social worker shall constantly strive to increase knowledge and skills and seek consultation and continuing education and training as appropriate to remain competent, accurate, and aware of current knowledge in the profession.

11. The clinical social worker shall not misuse relationships with clients for personal advantage, profit, or interest.

12. Treatment of members of one's own family, relatives, or close friends, shall be avoided.

13. The clinical social worker shall refrain from engaging in social relationships with clients which interfere with clinical service provision.

14. The clinical social worker shall not exploit in any way his or her professional relationships with clients, supervisees, students, employees, or research participants. Clinical social workers shall not condone or engage in sexual harassment. Sexual harassment is defined as deliberate or repeated comments, gestures, or physical contacts of a sexual nature that are unwanted by the recipient. Under no circumstances shall any clinical social worker engage in a sexual relationship with a client, supervisee, student, employee, or research participant.

15. The clinical social worker shall not knowingly participate in, condone, or be associated with dishonesty, fraud, deceit, or misrepresentation in carrying out professional responsibilities.

16. The clinical social worker shall maintain the highest standards of ethical business practice and conduct.

II. Responsibility to Profession

1. The clinical social worker shall function within the legal restraints of his or her state license or registration, where such licensure or registration is required.

2. The clinical social worker must adhere to the standards prescribed by other legitimate professional organizations in which they maintain membership, and to the licensing and certification requirements of public regulatory bodies where they practice.

3. The clinical social worker shall act in a manner that will promote and preserve the values and standards of the profession.

4. In all interactions with colleagues, and when serving in an educational or consultative role, or in any public appearance, the clinical social worker shall clearly stipulate whether he or she is speaking as an individual or as a representative of the organization.

5. The clinical social worker shall not offer professional services in such a manner that the service is harmful to client's legitimate therapeutic involvement with other professionals. If approached by an individual already receiving similar services from another professional, consideration for the clients' welfare requires that the clinical social worker carefully consider both the exist-

ing professional relationship and the therapeutic issues involved, and that these be coordinated as necessary.

III. Responsibility to Society

1. As part of the clinical social worker's commitment to the promotion of the general welfare, he or she shall be alert to the purposes and consequences of policies of an employing institution. Where institutional practices conflict with the standards of the profession, change shall be sought in an appropriate manner.
2. The clinical social worker shall assume responsibility for identifying, developing, and fully utilizing knowledge for professional practice.
3. The clinical social worker shall maintain the values and standards applicable to clinical practice when engaging in any research endeavors intended to further professional knowledge. He or she will give careful consideration not only to the possible consequences of the research findings for the general welfare, but also to the effects such research might have on the subjects involved. The clinical social worker is aware of the need to obtain the informed consent of such individuals; to protect their right to privacy, confidentiality, and personal dignity; and to protect their persons from possible unwarranted mental or bodily harm. All of these considerations shall be attended to in the preparation of material of such research for oral or written presentation to peer groups, or for wider dissemination.
4. The clinical social worker shall not discriminate in the practice of social work on grounds of age, race, religion, nationality, gender, or sexual preference.

IV. Disciplinary Proceedings

Subject to its adjudication procedures, the Board of Directors, on the affirmative vote of a majority of its members then serving, may reprimand or censure any certificant of this organization, or may suspend or revoke a certificate if the certificant:

1. fraudulently or deceptively obtains or attempts to obtain a certificate or misrepresents his or her credentials;
2. is addicted to any narcotic or is habitually intoxicated;
3. misrepresents an unauthorized person as one who is certified;
4. is convicted of a felony or a crime involving moral turpitude, or any misdemeanor related to his or her qualifications or functions in the profession;
5. is professionally incompetent;
6. is mentally incompetent;
7. submits a false statement to collect a fee;
8. is disciplined by a licensing or disciplinary authority of any other organization, state, or country, resulting in expulsion from the said organization or revocation of licensure or certification; or
9. violates any provision of this Code of Ethics.

CLINICAL SOCIAL WORK FEDERATION
CODE OF ETHICS, REVISED 1997

PREAMBLE

The principal objective of the profession of clinical social work is the enhancement of the mental health and the well-being of the individuals and families who seek services from its practitioners. The professional practice of clinical social workers is shaped by ethical principles which are rooted in the basic values of the social work profession. These core values include commitment to the dignity, well-being, and self-determination of the individual; a commitment to professional practice characterized by competence and integrity, and a commitment to a society which offers opportunities to all its members in a just and nondiscriminatory manner. Clinical social workers examine practice situations in terms of the ethical dilemmas that they present, with a critical analysis of how the formulation of a solution fulfills the core requirements of ethical practice; non-malfeasance (doing no harm to clients); beneficence (helping clients); and autonomy (enhancing the self-determination of clients).

The following represents a specific codification of those ethical principles. It is intended to serve as a standard for clinical social workers in all of their professional functions, and to inspire their will to act in a manner consistent with those tenets. The clinical social worker is expected to take into consideration all principles in this code that have a bearing upon any situation in which ethical judgment is to be exercised, and to select a course of action consistent with the spirit, as well as the letter of the code.

Individual members of the Clinical Social Work Federation and of the various State Societies for Clinical Social Work agree to adhere to the precepts expressed in this Code, and to practice in a manner which is consistent with them. When the practice of a member is alleged to deviate from the Code of Ethics, the Code is to be used as a standard for the evaluation of the nature and seriousness of the deviation.

I. GENERAL RESPONSIBILITIES OF CLINICAL SOCIAL WORKERS

Clinical social workers maintain high standards in all of their professional roles, and value professional competence, objectivity, and integrity. They accept responsibility for the consequences of their work, and ensure that their services are used in an appropriate manner.

a) Clinical social workers bear a heavy professional responsibility because their actions and recommendations may significantly affect the lives of others. They practice only within their sphere of competence, and maintain and enhance that competence through participation in continuing professional development throughout their careers. They refrain from undertaking or continuing any professional activity in which their personal difficulties, or any other limitations, might lead to the inadequate provision of service.

---

b) Clinical social workers do not exploit professional relationships sexually, financially, or for any other professional and/or personal advantage. They maintain this standard of conduct toward all those who may be professionally associated with them.

c) Clinical social workers often function as employees in clinics, hospitals, and agencies, or as providers on managed care panels. In these positions, they are responsible for identifying and actively working to modify policies or procedures which may come into conflict with the standards of their profession. If such a conflict arises, the primary responsibility of the clinical social worker is to uphold the ethical standards of the profession. These standards require that commitment to the welfare of the client(s) is the primary obligation.

d) Clinical social workers have an additional responsibility, both to the profession which provides the basis of their practice, and to those who are entering that profession. As teachers, supervisors, and mentors, they are responsible for maintaining high standards of objectivity and scholarship. In all of their professional activities they consistently examine, and attempt to expand, the knowledge base on which practice in the profession is centered.

II.   RESPONSIBILITY TO CLIENTS

The primary responsibility of the clinical social worker is to the individual client, the family or the group with whom he or she has a professional relationship. Clinical social workers respect the dignity, protect the welfare, and maximize the self-determination of the clients with whom they work.

1. INFORMED CONSENT TO TREATMENT

a) Clinical social work treatment takes place within a context of informed consent. This requires that the client(s) be informed of the extent and nature of the services being offered as well as the mutual limits, rights, opportunities, and obligations associated with the provision of and payment for those services. In order for the consent be valid, the client(s) must be informed in a manner which is clear to them, must choose freely and without undue influence, and must have the capacity to make an informed choice. In instances where clients are not of legal age or competent to give a meaningful consent they will be informed in a manner which is consistent with their level of understanding. In such situations, authorization for treatment will be obtained from an appropriate third party, such as a parent or other legal guardian.

b) Clinical social workers have a duty to understand the potential impact on all aspects of treatment resulting from participation in various third party payment mechanisms, and to disclose fully their knowledge of these features to the client. Such features might include, but are not limited to; limitations of confidentiality; payment limitations related to provider choice; a summary of the treatment review process required by the plan; the comparative treatment orientations of the plan and of the clinical social worker; the possibility that benefits may be limited under the plan; the clinical social worker's relationship to the plan and any incentives to limit or deny care; and, the availability of alternative treatment options.

2. PRACTICE MANAGEMENT AND TERMINATION

a) Clinical social workers enter into and/or continue professional relationships based on their ability to meet the needs of clients appropriately. The clinical social worker terminates services and relationships with clients when such services and relationships are no longer in the client's best interest. Clinical social workers do not abandon clients by withdrawing services precipitously, except under extraordinary circumstances.

Clinical social workers give careful consideration to all factors involved in termination and take care to minimize the possible adverse effects it might have on the client(s). When interruption or termination of service is anticipated, the clinical social worker gives reasonable notification and provides for transfer, referral, or continuation of service in a manner as consistent as possible with the client's needs and preferences.

b) Clinical social workers providing services which are reimbursed by third party payers continue to have primary responsibility for the welfare of the client(s). The failure of the third party to authorize continued benefits does not remove the obligation of the clinical social worker to assure necessary treatment, if this is in the client's best interests. When benefits are ended, the clinical social worker has a number of options including; acceptance of private payment for continued services, at either regular or reduced rates; provision of services on an unpaid basis; and, referral to appropriate alternative treatment sources.

c) A clinical social worker who disagrees with the denial of continued benefits by a third party payer is responsible for discussing this action with the client(s), and for devising a clinically appropriate plan, which may or may not include appeal of the decision. Further pursuit of the appeals process will be based on such factors as; the degree to which the clinical social worker believes that further treatment is necessary for the client's well-being; the degree to which the client(s) wishes to pursue the appeals process, and; the degree to which there are alternative means available for the client(s) to continue treatment.

d) Clinical social workers keep records for each individual and family they treat which reflect relevant administrative rules, contractual obligations, and local and federal statutes. They are required to be knowledgeable about statutes relating to client access to records, and to fulfill their responsibility as required by law. When access to records is permitted, the clinical social worker will take appropriate, legally permitted steps to protect the privacy of all third parties who may be named in the records.

e) All requirements regarding the establishment, maintenance, and disposal of records relate equally to written and to electronic records.

Clinical social workers establish a policy on record retention and disposal, or are aware of agency policies regarding these issues, and communicate it to the client. In the event of the death or incapacity of a client, they safeguard the record, within existing statues, and the information contained therein. Clinical social workers have a plan or procedure for the proper handling of client records in the event of their own death or disability which both protects privacy, and ensures that legitimate access functions can be properly carried out.

3. RELATIONSHIPS WITH CLIENTS

a) Clinical social workers are responsible for setting clear and appropriate professional boundaries, especially in those instances in which dual or multiple relationships are unavoidable. They do not engage in dual or multiple relationships in which there is any risk of their professional judgment being compromised, or of the client being harmed or exploited. When clinical social workers provide services to two or more persons who have a relationship with each other, they clarify with all parties the nature of the professional responsibilities to each of them, and the ways in which appropriate boundaries will be maintained.

b) Clinical social workers do not, under any circumstances, engage in romantic or sexual contact with either current or former clients. Clinical social workers are also mindful of how their relationship with the family and/or friends of their clients might affect their work with the client. Consequently, they also avoid romantic or sexual involvements with members of the client's family, or with others with whom the client has a close, personal relationship.

c) Clinical social workers are aware of the authority which is inherent in their professional role. They do not engage in any activity that will abuse their professional relationships or exploit others for personal, political, or business interests. As practitioners, supervisors, teachers, administrators, and researchers their primary professional responsibility is always the welfare of the client(s) with whom they work.

d) When the clinical social worker must act on behalf of a client, that action should always safeguard the interests and concerns of that client. When another person has been authorized to act on behalf of a client, the clinical social worker should deal with that person in a manner which will safeguard the interests and concerns of the client.

e) Clinical social workers recognize and support the right to self-determination of clients who may choose not to relinquish their privacy by pursuing third party reimbursement for treatment, even when they are eligible for such reimbursement. In such instances, the clinical social worker makes every effort to assist the client in making alternative financial arrangements so that treatment can proceed.

f) When a clinical social worker determines that a conflict potentially detrimental to the treatment process has arisen, he or she should inform the individual(s) to whom he or she has a professional responsibility of the nature of the conflict and the way in which it might affect the provision of service.

4. COMPETENCE

a) Clinical social workers are aware of the scope in which they are entitled to practice. This scope is defined by their areas of personal competence; by their license or other legal recognition; and by their training and/or experience. They are responsible for confining their practice to those areas in which they are legally authorized and in which they are qualified to practice. When necessary, they utilize the knowledge and experience of members of other professions. In using such consultants or supervisors, the clinical social worker is responsible for ensuring that they are recognized members of their own profession, and are qualified and competent to carry out the service required.

b) Clinical social workers recognize that the privacy and intimacy of the therapeutic relationship may unrealistically intensify the client's feelings for them. The maintenance of professional boundaries and objectivity is crucial to effective and responsible treatment. Clinical social workers maintain self awareness and take care to prevent the possible harmful intrusion of their own unresolved personal issues into the therapeutic relationship. They take appropriate steps to resolve the situation when there is a danger of this occurring. Such steps could include, but are not limited to; seeking additional supervision or consultation; seeking additional personal treatment; and, if necessary, making alternative arrangements for the treatment of the client(s).

c) Clinical social workers recognize the responsibility to remain abreast of knowledge and developments in the field which may benefit their client(s). Ongoing involvement in supervision, consultation, and continuing education are some of the ways in which this responsibility can be fulfilled. It is particularly important for the clinical social worker to secure appropriate training, supervision, or consultation when attempting to use a treatment technique with which he or she is unfamiliar.

III. CONFIDENTIALITY

Clinical social workers have a primary obligation to maintain the privacy of both current and former clients, whether living or deceased, and to maintain the confidentiality of material that has been transmitted to them in any of their professional roles. Exceptions to this responsibility will occur only when there are overriding legal or professional reasons and, whenever possible, with the written informed consent of the client(s).

a) Clinical social workers discuss fully with clients both the nature of confidentiality, and potential limits to confidentiality which may arise during the course of their work. Confidential information should only be released, whenever possible, with the written permission of the client(s). As part of the process of obtaining such a release, the clinical social worker should inform the client(s) about the nature of the information being sought, the purpose(s) for which it is being sought, to whom the information will be released, how the client(s) may withdraw permission for its release, and, the length of time that the release will be in effect.

b) Clinical social workers know and observe both legal and professional standards for maintaining the privacy of records, and mandatory reporting obligations. Mandatory reporting obligations may include, but are not limited to; the reporting of the abuse or neglect of children or of vulnerable adults; the duty to take steps to protect or warn a third party who may be endangered by the client(s); and, any duty to report the misconduct or impairment of another professional.

Additional limits to confidentiality may occur because of parental access to the records of a minor, the access of legal guardians to the records of some adults, access by the courts to mandated reports, and access by third party payers to information for the purpose of treatment authorization or audit. When confidential information is released to a third party, the clinical social worker will ensure that the information divulged is limited to the minimum amount required to accomplish the purpose for which the release is being made.

c) Clinical social workers treating couples, families, and groups seek agreement among the parties involved regarding each individual's right to confidentiality, and the mutual obligation to protect the confidentiality of information shared by other parties to the treatment. Clients involved in this type of treatment should, however, be informed that the clinical social worker cannot guarantee that all participants will honor their agreement to maintain confidentiality.

d) When confidential information is used for purposes of professional education, research, or publication, the primary responsibility of the clinical social worker is the protection of the client(s) from possible harm, embarrassment, or exploitation. When extensive material is used for any of these purposes the clinical social worker makes every effort to obtain the informed consent of the client(s) for such use, and will not proceed if the client(s) denies this consent. Whether or not a consent is obtained, every effort will be made to protect the true identity of the client. Any such presentation will be limited to the amount necessary for the professional purpose, and will be shared only with other responsible individuals.

e) The development of new technologies for the storage and transmission of data poses a great danger to the privacy of individuals. Clinical social workers take special precautions to protect the confidentiality of material stored or transmitted through computers, electronic mail, facsimile machines, telephones, telephone answering machines, and all other electronic or computer technology. When using these technologies, disclosure of identifying information regarding the client(s) should be avoided whenever possible.

IV. RELATIONSHIPS WITH COLLEAGUES

Clinical social workers act with integrity in their relationships with colleagues and members of other professions. They know and take into account the traditions, practices, and areas of competence of other professionals and cooperate with them fully for the welfare of clients.

a) Clinical social workers represent accurately the views, qualifications and findings of colleagues. When expressing judgment on these matters they do so in a manner that is sensitive to the best interests of both colleagues and clients.

b) If a clinical social worker's services are sought by an individual who is already receiving similar services from another professional, consideration for the client's welfare is the primary concern. This concern requires that the clinical social worker proceed with great caution, carefully considering the existing professional relationship, the therapeutic issues involved, and whether it is therapeutically and ethically appropriate to be involved in the situation.

c) As supervisors, consultants, or employers, clinical social workers are responsible for providing competent professional guidance and a role model to colleagues, employees, and students. They foster working conditions that assure consistency, respect, privacy, and protection from physical or mental harm. Clinical social workers do not abuse the authority of their position by harassing or pressuring colleagues, employees, or students for sexual reasons, financial gain, or any other purpose. They refrain from actions that are unwanted by the recipient, and can reasonably be interpreted as pressuring or intimidating the recipient.

d) Clinical social workers carry out their responsibility to both clients and the profession by maintaining high standards of practice within the professional community. They take appropriate measures to discourage, prevent, expose, and correct unethical or incompetent behavior by colleagues, and also assist and defend colleagues believed to be unjustly charged with such conduct. They discourage the practice of clinical social work by those who fail to meet accepted standards of training and experience, or who are practicing outside of their area of competence.

e) Clinical social workers who have knowledge of a colleague's impairment, misconduct, or incompetence attempt to bring about remediation through whatever means is appropriate. Such actions may include, but are not limited to; direct discussion with the colleague, with permission from the client(s) if this is needed; a report, if mandatory, to a regulatory body, professional organization, or employer; a report to a supervisor, or other agency administrator.

V.   FEE ARRANGEMENTS

When setting fees, clinical social workers should give consideration to the client's ability to pay and make every effort to establish fees that are fair, reasonable, and commensurate with the value of the service performed.

a) In the initial contact with the client(s) fees for services and policies regarding fee collection should be clarified. This clarification should also take into account any financial constraint which may affect the treatment process.

b) It is unethical for a clinical social worker to offer, give, solicit, or receive any fee or other consideration to or from a third party for the referral of a client. They accept reimbursement from clients and from third party payers only for services directly rendered to the client(s). Clinical social workers may, however, participate in contractual arrangements in which they agree to discount their fees.

c) A clinical social worker who contracts with a third party payer agrees to abide by the conditions of the contract. If, however, the clinical social worker believes the contract contains elements which violate the ethics of the profession, the clinical social worker seeks to redress this situation through appropriate courses of action which may include; obtaining the other party's agreement to delete the clause; or, refusing to sign the contract.

d) Barter arrangements, in which goods or services are accepted from clients as payment for professional services, should be avoided as much as possible. Such plans, especially when they involve provision of services by the client(s), have the potential to constitute dual relationships which will damage the treatment. Barter arrangements may be entered into only in rare situations, and may only involve provision of goods, as opposed to services, in exchange for treatment. Such arrangements can only be entered into upon the specific request of the client, and when the following additional criteria are met; traditional payment methods are not possible; the client(s) is not coerced or exploited in any way, and; the arrangement is not detrimental to the client(s) or to the professional relationship.

e) Clinical social workers employed by an agency or clinic, and also engaged in private practice, conform to contractual agreements with the employing facility. They do not solicit or accept a private fee or consideration of any kind for providing a service to which the client is entitled through the employing facility.

VI. CLINICAL SOCIAL WORKERS' RESPONSIBILITIES TO THE COMMUNITY

Clinical social workers are aware of the social codes and ethical expectations in their communities, and recognize that violation of accepted societal, ethical, legal, and moral standards on their part may compromise the fulfillment of their professional responsibilities and/or reduce public trust in the profession.

a) Clinical social workers do not, in any of their capacities, practice, condone, facilitate, or collaborate with any form of discrimination on the basis of race, religion, color, national origin, gender, sexual orientation, age, socioeconomic status, or physical or emotional disability.

b) Clinical social workers practice their profession in compliance with legal standards, and do not participate in arrangements or activities which undermine or violate the law. When they believe, however, that laws or community standards are in conflict with the principles and ethics of the profession, they make known the conflict and work responsibly toward change that is in the public interest.

c) Clinical social workers recognize a responsibility to participate in activities leading toward improved social conditions. They should advocate and work for conditions and resources that give all persons equal access to the services and opportunities required to meet basic needs and to develop to the fullest potential.

VII. RESEARCH AND SCHOLARLY ACTIVITIES

In planning, conducting, and reporting a study, the investigator has the responsibility to make a careful evaluation of its ethical acceptability, taking into account the following additional principles for research with human subjects. To the extent that this appraisal, weighing scientific and humane values, suggests a compromise of any principle, the investigator incurs an increasingly serious obligation to observe stringent safeguards to protect the rights and well-being of research participants.

a) In conducting research in institutions or organizations, clinical social workers obtain appropriate authority to carry out their work. Host organizations are given proper credit for their contributions to the project.

b) Ethically acceptable research begins with the establishment of a clear and fair agreement between the investigator and the research participant that clarifies the responsibilities of each. The investigator has the obligation to honor all commitments included in that agreement.

c) Responsibility for the establishment and maintenance of acceptable ethical practice in research always remains with the investigator. The investigator is also responsible for the ethical treatment of research participants by collaborators, assistants, students, and employees, all of whom incur parallel obligations.

d) Ethical practice requires the investigator to inform the participant of all features of the research that might reasonably be expected to influence willingness to participate, and to explain all other aspects of the research about which the participant inquires. After the data are collected, the investigator provides the participant with information about the nature of the study in order to remove any misconceptions that may have arisen.

e) The ethical investigator protects participants from physical and mental discomfort, harm, and danger. If a risk of such consequences exists, the investigator is required to inform the participant of that fact, secure consent before proceeding, and take all possible measures to minimize distress. A research procedure must not be used if it is likely to cause serious or lasting harm to a participant.

f) The methodological requirements of the study may necessitate concealment, deception, or minimal risk to participants. In such cases, the investigator must be able to justify the use of these techniques and to ensure, as soon as possible, the participant's understanding of the reasons and sufficient justification for the procedure in question.

g) Ethical practice requires the investigator to respect the individual's freedom to decline to participate in, or withdraw from, research and to so inform prospective participants. The obligation to protect this freedom requires special vigilance when the investigator is, in any manner, in a position of authority over the participant. It is unethical to penalize a participant in any way for withdrawing from or refusing to participate in a research project.

h) Information obtained about the individual research participants during the course of an investigation is confidential unless otherwise agreed to in advance.

i) Investigation of human subjects in studies which use drugs, are conducted only in conjunction with licensed physicians.

j) Clinical social workers take credit only for work actually done in scholarly and research projects, and give appropriate credit to the contributions of others in a manner which is proportional to the degree to which those contributions are represented in the final product.

k) Research findings must be presented accurately and completely with full discussion of both their usefulness and their limitations. Clinical social workers are responsible for attempting to prevent any distortion or misuse of their findings.

VIII. PUBLIC STATEMENTS

Public statements, announcements of services, and promotional activities of clinical social workers serve the purpose of providing sufficient information to aid consumers in making informed judgments and choices. Clinical social workers state accurately, objectively, and without misrepresentation their professional qualifications, affiliations, and functions as well as those of the institutions or organizations with which they or their statements may be associated. In addition, they should correct the misrepresentations of others with respect to these matters.

a) In announcing availability for professional services, protection of the public is the primary concern. A clinical social worker may use any information so long as it describes his or her credentials and the services provided accurately and without misrepresentation. Information usually found helpful by the public includes the name of the professional; highest relevant academic degree from an accredited institution; specialized post-graduate training; type and level of state certification or license; any advanced certifications held; address and telephone number; office hours; type of service provided; languages spoken; and policy with regard to third party payments.

b) In announcements of available professional services, information regarding fees and fee policies may also be found helpful by prospective clients. Appropriate announcements of this type could include such general terms as "moderate fees." It is unethical to make statements regarding fees or fee policies which are deceptive, or misrepresent the actual fee arrangements.

c) The clinical social worker is responsible for assuring that all advertising is in conformity with the ethical standards of the profession. Publications announcing any type of clinic social work service describe those services accurately. They do not falsely or deceptively claim or imply superior personal or professional competence.

d) Clinical social workers are free to make public appearances and engage in public discussion regarding issues such as, for example, the relative value of alternative treatment approaches. Diagnostic and therapeutic services for clients, however, are rendered only in the context of a professional relationship. Such services are not given by means of public lectures, newspaper or magazine articles, radio or television programs, or anything of a similar nature. Professional use of the media or of other public forums is appropriate when the purpose is to educate the public about professional matters regarding which the clinical social worker has special knowledge or expertise.

e) Clinical social workers respect the rights and reputation of any professional organization with which they are affiliated, and do not falsely imply sponsorship or certification by any organization. When making public statements, the clinical social worker will make clear which are personal opinions, and which are authorized statements on behalf of the organization.

Appendix V

Ethics Knowledge Survey (EKS) for the NASW Code of Ethics

ETHICS KNOWLEDGE SURVEY (EKS)
FOR THE NASW CODE OF ETHICS

Complete the following scale of knowledge of the NASW Code of Ethics. The scoring key is printed at the conclusion of the questions.

The following true-false questions are to measure your familiarity with the NASW Code of Ethics. This is not a test. Answer all questions. If you do not know the answer to a question, select what you consider the most reasonable answer. Check the box to the left of the question to indicate your answer.

Name:_____

Have you read the NASW Code of Ethics?   ❑ Yes ❑ No

If yes, how long ago did you read it?_____

Were you required to read the NASW Code of Ethics as part of your social work education program?   ❑ Yes ❑ No

CHECK √ YOUR ANSWER IN THE BOX TO THE LEFT OF EACH QUESTION.

The NASW Code of Ethics . . .

TRUE ❑   FALSE ❑   01.   is based on six core values that guide the social work profession.

TRUE ❑   FALSE ❑   02.   defines a social worker's primary responsibility as service to clients.

TRUE ❑   FALSE ❑   03.   views informed consent of clients as an agency responsibility and does not provide directives regarding this area.

TRUE ❑   FALSE ❑   04.   requires social workers to foster self-determination of clients.

TRUE ❑   FALSE ❑   05.   requires involuntary clients be informed of their rights regarding services, and the extent of their right to refuse service.

TRUE ❑   FALSE ❑   06.   mandates informed consent if clients are video- or audiotaped.

TRUE ❑   FALSE ❑   07.   urges social workers to accept only jobs they have skills to perform.

TRUE ❑   FALSE ❑   08.   declares social workers should practice only in areas for which they are trained, except when the service is considered experimental.

TRUE ❑   FALSE ❑   09.   makes clear the confidentiality rule is absolute.

TRUE ❑   FALSE ❑   10.   mandates clients' access to records concerning them or any of their immediate family members on demand without condition.

TRUE ❑   FALSE ❑   11.   discourages, but allows, social workers to have sexual contact with relatives of clients.

TRUE ❑   FALSE ❑   12.   states sexual contact is permitted with clients six months after the client is terminated from service.

TRUE ❑   FALSE ❑   13.   permits a social worker to have a former friend as a client if the two have not had sexual contact in the past year.

TRUE ❑   FALSE ❑   14.   prohibits physical contact with clients under any circumstances.

TRUE ❑   FALSE ❑   15.   requires practitioner's fees be fair and based on client's income.

TRUE ❑   FALSE ❑   16.   does not address how social workers obtain income, since this is private.

TRUE ❑   FALSE ❑   17.   allows social workers to terminate clients for nonpayment of fees if certain conditions are met.

TRUE ❑   FALSE ❑   18.   cautions against making negative comments about colleagues to clients and other professionals, except when such comments are justified.

TRUE ❑   FALSE ❑   19.   requires respecting confidences shared by colleagues without exception.

TRUE ❑   FALSE ❑   20.   requires social workers to confront psychiatrists and psychologists on interdisciplinary teams who violate NASW Code of Ethics principles.

TRUE ❑   FALSE ❑   21.   encourages seeking client input to resolve disputes with colleagues.

TRUE ❑   FALSE ❑   22.   prohibits practitioners from receiving fees for making referrals.

TRUE ❑   FALSE ❑   23.   states supervisors should not have sexual contact with supervisees.

TRUE ❑   FALSE ❑   24.   requires reporting impaired colleagues to the state licensing board within five working days of observing the impaired functioning.

TRUE ❑   FALSE ❑   25.   requires reporting unethical colleagues to NASW staff within seven days of the alleged offense.

TRUE ❑   FALSE ❑   26.   requires supervisors to have training for their supervisory roles.

TRUE ❑   FALSE ❑   27.   does not permit dual or multiple relationships between supervisors and supervisees under any circumstances.

TRUE ❑   FALSE ❑   28.   indicates performance evaluations are based only on practice criteria.

TRUE ❑   FALSE ❑   29.   requires supervisors to inform clients when students are providing services to them.

TRUE ❑   FALSE ❑   30.   holds supervisors responsible for avoiding potentially harmful dual relationships with supervisees.

TRUE ❑   FALSE ❑   31.   requires keeping client records for a lengthy period after service ends.

TRUE ❑   FALSE ❑   32.   provides guidelines for how to handle clients who desire to transfer from one agency to another.

TRUE ❑   FALSE ❑   33.   requires administrators to take reasonable measures to ensure adequate supervision is available to practitioners.

TRUE ❑   FALSE ❑   34.   urges social workers to honor commitments made to employers.

TRUE ❑   FALSE ❑   35.   does not require practitioners' involvement in improving agency policy.

TRUE ❑   FALSE ❑   36.   states that social workers should not allow employing agency policies to interfere with the ethical practice of social work.

TRUE ❑   FALSE ❑   37.   discourages social workers' accepting jobs in agencies under NASW sanction for employment practices inconsistent with the NASW code.

TRUE ❑   FALSE ❑   38.   warns against refusing to treat someone because the person believes in a fundamental religion.

TRUE ❑   FALSE ❑   39.   considers private conduct outside the realm of professional concern and, therefore, has no commentary on private conduct.

TRUE ❑   FALSE ❑   40.   holds social workers responsible for monitoring their own potential for impaired functioning that could interfere with service to clients.

TRUE ❑   FALSE ❑   41.   requires social workers to distinguish statements as private and professional persons.

TRUE ❑   FALSE ❑   42.   prohibits soliciting the clients of colleagues.

TRUE ❑   FALSE ❑   43.   encourages social workers to participate in professional conferences.

TRUE ❑   FALSE ❑   44.   requires social workers to keep current on practice knowledge.

TRUE ❑   FALSE ❑   45.   makes exceptions of confidentiality rules when clients are participating in federally funded research projects.

TRUE ❑   FALSE ❑   46.   requires social workers to provide services during public emergencies.

TRUE ❑   FALSE ❑   47.   encourages political participation in shaping social policy through support of efforts to promote employment and access to resources.

TRUE ❑   FALSE ❑   48.   requires that judgment of ethical behavior be conducted by a jury of professional peers appointed by the state licensing board.

TRUE ❑   FALSE ❑   49.   urges against advertising/marketing of services by social workers.

TRUE ❑   FALSE ❑   50.   requires practitioners to seek the advice of supervisors whenever they are in doubt about a practice situation.

NASW CODE OF ETHICS KNOWLEDGE SURVEY
ANSWER KEY

Question Number	Correct Answer	Page Number	Section Number
1	True	1	Preamble
2	True	7	1.01
3	True	7	1.02
4	False	7	1.03
5	True	8	1.03 (d)
6	True	8	1.03 (f)
7	False	8/22	1.04 (a)/4.01
8	False	9	1.04 (f)
9	False	10	1.07 (c)
10	False	11/12	1.07 (f)/1.08 (b)
11	False	13	1.09 (b)
12	False	13	1.09 (c)
13	False	13	1.09 (d)
14	False	13	1.10
15	False	14	1.13 (a)
16	False	14	1.13 (b)
17	True	15	1.16 (c)
18	True	15	2.01 (b)
19	False	16	2.02
20	True	16	2.03 (b)
21	False	16	2.04 (b)
22	True	17	2.06 (c)
23	True	17	2.07 (a)
24	False	17	2.09 (a)
25	False	18	2.11 (b)
26	True	19	3.01 (a)
27	False	19	3.01 (c)
28	False	19	3.01 (d)
29	True	19	3.02 (c)

30	True	19	3.02 (d)
31	True	20	3.04 (d)
32	True	20	3.06 (b)
33	True	21	3.07 (d)
34	True	21	3.09 (a)
35	False	21	3.09 (b)
36	True	21	3.09 (d)
37	True	22	3.09 (f)
38	True	23	4.02
39	False	23	4.03
40	True	23	4.05 (a/b) 23
41	True	23	4.06 (a)
42	True	24	4.07 (a)
43	False	24	5.01 (d)
44	True	25	5.02 (c)
45	False	26	5.02 (l)
46	True	27	6.03
47	True	27	6.04 (b)
48	False	00	Not in code
49	False	00	Not in code
50	False	00	Not in code

After you calculate the total number correct, multiple the number of correct answers by 2, and that will be the percentage of correct answers. On average, supervisors score 59.9 percent and social work students score 70.1 percent correct on this scale.

Appendix VI

Practitioner Self-Assessment Form (PSAF)

PRACTITIONER SELF-ASSESSMENT FORM (PSAF)

This form is designed for use prior to supervison/consultation regarding a clinical case focusing on a particular session. Answer each question from the perspective of using this form as a working document to plan your next steps in this case based on your feelings, thoughts, and behaviors during the interview that is the focus of this questionnaire.

1. How long did the interview last? _____

2. Do you feel the interview was:

    a. too short?
    b. too long?
    c. just about right?

If you checked a or b, explain what factors contributed to the interview being too short or too long.

Who contributed most to this?

What could have been done to overcome this?

3. Did the interview have a focus?   ❏ Yes ❏ No

    If yes, what was the focus?

    If no, what prevented a focus from being developed?

    What could have been done to focus the interview more?

4. Do you feel the client/clients got what he or she came for?   ❏ Yes ❏ No

    If yes, what did he or she get?

    If no, what prevented it?

5. Did the interview have a flow of interaction or continuity?   ❑ Yes ❑ No

   If yes, generally describe this flow and how it was achieved.

   If no, what prevented flow and continuity?

6. Describe generally how you felt prior to the interview:

7. Describe generally how you felt during the interview:

8. Describe generally how you felt after the interview:

9. Describe your behaviors during the interview that you felt good about:

10. Describe client behaviors during the interview that you felt good about:

11. Describe your behaviors during the interview that you felt were not effective:

12. Describe client behaviors during the interview that you felt were distracting or disturbing:

13. Which of your gestures or behaviors do you believe enhanced the communication process?

14. Which client gestures or behaviors enhanced the communication process?

15. Which of your gestures or behaviors distracted from the communication process?

16. Which client gestures or behaviors distracted from the communication process?

17. Are there any problems associated with this interview with which you would like help?

18. What would you do differently if you could do the interview again?

19. Based on this interview, what client actions are needed to make significant changes?

20. Based on what you know now, what are the plans for the next interview?

Appendix VII

Short Form Stress Scale (SFSS)

SHORT FORM STRESS SCALE (SFSS)

This questionnaire measures stress associated with your work. The instrument has a self-scoring component. The scale is for assessment purposes only and is not intended to substitute for diagnosis or treatment of stress reactions. Persons who score high on the scale are encouraged to seek professional help. When stress reactions are recognized early and treated, positive outcomes are more likely.

Section 1: Background Information

Name: _____

Sex: ☐Female ☐Male   Age: _____

Religious preference: _____

Marital status: ☐Single ☐Married ☐Divorced ☐Widowed
    ☐Other: _____

Number of children: _____

How often do you attend religious services? _____

Education: ☐High school graduate ☐Bachelor's degree
    ☐Master's degree ☐Doctoral degree

Current job title: _____

Years employed in current agency: _____

Do you think your job is stressful?	☐ No ☐ Yes
Do you believe your job has caused you to develop physical symptoms?	☐ No ☐ Yes
Do you believe your job has caused you to have psychological symptoms?	☐No ☐ Yes
Have you ever considered quitting your job because of stress?	☐No ☐ Yes
Have you ever argued with a spouse/friend/family member about your job?	☐No ☐ Yes
Have you ever regretted your choice of the social work profession?	☐No ☐ Yes

Section 2: Stress Symptoms (SS)

In the following sections, circle the number to the right of the question that best describes your experience (1 = never; 2 =rarely; 3 = sometimes; 4 = often; 5 = always). How often do you have the following symptoms?

1. headaches	1	2	3	4	5
2. colds	1	2	3	4	5
3. stomachaches	1	2	3	4	5
4. dizzy spells	1	2	3	4	5
5. crying spells	1	2	3	4	5
6. muscle tension	1	2	3	4	5
7. cramps	1	2	3	4	5
8. sleep disturbance	1	2	3	4	5
9. memory problems	1	2	3	4	5
10. anxiety/worry	1	2	3	4	5

SYMPTOMS TOTAL =
(ITEMS 1 to 10)   ___ + ___ + ___ + ___ + ___   = ___

Section 3: Unhealthy Activities (UA)

How often do you engage in the following activities?

11. drink too much	1	2	3	4	5
12. smoke too much	1	2	3	4	5
13. use substances (drugs)	1	2	3	4	5
14. fail to engage in daily exercise	1	2	3	4	5
15. watch too much television	1	2	3	4	5
16. do not eat balanced meals	1	2	3	4	5
17. eat meals in a hurry	1	2	3	4	5
18. try to do too many things at once	1	2	3	4	5

19. spend too much time alone	1	2	3	4	5
20. watch TV, listen to radio, or read to go to sleep	1	2	3	4	5

UNHEALTY ACTIVITIES TOTAL =
(ITEMS 11 to 20)   __ + __ + __ + __ + __   = __

Section 4: Practice Performance (PP)

How often do you experience the following?

21. feel unappreciated and used by clients	1	2	3	4	5
22. feel clients create their own problems	1	2	3	4	5
23. feel apprehensive when meeting new clients	1	2	3	4	5
24. feel clients are making you nervous	1	2	3	4	5
25. get angry when clients do not comply	1	2	3	4	5
26. daydream while interviewing clients	1	2	3	4	5
27. avoid helping clients with special problems	1	2	3	4	5
28. do not feel you understand a client's anger	1	2	3	4	5
29. avoid returning client telephone calls	1	2	3	4	5
30. feel clients really do not want to change	1	2	3	4	5

PRACTICE PERFORMANCE TOTAL =
(ITEMS 21 to 30)   __ + __ + __ + __   __   = __

Section 5: Work Attitudes (WA)

How often do you experience the following?

31. feel my job is boring	1	2	3	4	5
32. feel trapped in my job	1	2	3	4	5

33.	become irritated by my work	1	2	3	4	5
34.	let experiences at work depress me	1	2	3	4	5
35.	feel overwhelmed by my job	1	2	3	4	5
36.	feel my training is not adequate to do my job	1	2	3	4	5
37.	believe my job tasks are not clearly defined	1	2	3	4	5
38.	work overtime or take work home	1	2	3	4	5
39.	believe it is best to just avoid co-workers	1	2	3	4	5
40.	feel my life would be better if I quit this job	1	2	3	4	5

WORK ATTITUDES TOTAL =   __ + __ + __ + __ + ____ = __
(ITEMS 31 to 40)

Section 6: Work Setting (WS)

How often would you describe your workplace as follows?

41.	not a good place to work	1	2	3	4	5
42.	the office has constant problems	1	2	3	4	5
43.	my supervision is not adequate	1	2	3	4	5
44.	the paperwork is excessive	1	2	3	4	5
45.	there is no positive office support group	1	2	3	4	5
46.	hate going to work	1	2	3	4	5
47.	do not have privacy in my office	1	2	3	4	5
48.	administrators do not care about workers	1	2	3	4	5
49.	have a feeling of dislike for co-workers	1	2	3	4	5
50.	working conditions are bad	1	2	3	4	5

WORK SETTING TOTALS=   __ + __ + __ + __ + ____ = __
(ITEMS 41 to 50)

TOTAL STRESS SCORE (TSS) = _____

Scoring Instructions

In each section total the numbers for the five columns and enter the numbers in the blanks at the bottom of the column. Then add the numbers across from left to right and enter the total in the blank after the equal sign at the far right of the page. That number is the score for that subscale of the stress scale. Do this procedure for each of the subscales. Add the subscale scores that are in each far right space and enter the total score in the space to the right of TOTAL STRESS SCORE. This is your total combined stress score. Each subscale score can be interpreted individually as well. Enter each score on the set "stress thermometers" on the following page.

STRESS SCALE SCORE SUMMARY SHEET

Enter your scores from each section of the Stress Scale on the appropriate "stress thermometer" below. Enter the "TOTAL STRESS SCORE" (TSS) in the TSS thermometer. You will have a numeric visual measurement of your stress level for each subscale, as well as an overall stress score. A score over 30 on any subscale should be considered elevated and worthy of attention. A Total Stress Score above 175 should be considered elevated and worthy of attention.

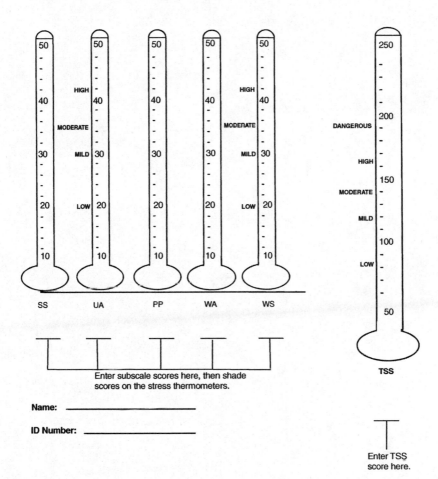

Enter subscale scores here, then shade scores on the stress thermometers.

Name: _____

ID Number: _____

Enter TSS score here.

Appendix VIII

Supervision Analysis Questionnaire (SAQ)

SUPERVISION ANALYSIS QUESTIONNAIRE (SAQ)

Please fill in or check the appropriate blank for each question.

1. Name of Practitioner: _____

    Name of Supervisor: _____
2. Sex of Practitioner: ❑Male ❑Female

    Sex of Supervisor: ❑Male ❑Female
3. Age of Practitioner: _____

    Age of Supervisor: _____

Answer the following questions by circling the response category below each question that best describes how you feel about the question (SD = strongly disagree; D = disagree; MD = mildly disagree; MA = mildly agree; A = agree; SA = strongly agree).

Answer all questions on the basis of your experience with your current supervisor named above. Scoring directions are at the end of the questionnaire.

Section A

1. Overall, I am satisfied with my supervisory experience.

    SD   D   MD   MA   A   SA
2. I usually come out of my supervisory conferences or groups feeling pretty good.

    SD   D   MD   MA   A   SA
3. I look forward to my supervisory sessions.

    SD   D   MD   MA   A   SA
4. My supervisor does not assume that I know a lot more than I really do and does not talk "over my head."

    SD   D   MD   MA   A   SA
5. My supervisor does not assume that I know a lot less than I believe I know.

    SD   D   MD   MA   A   SA
6. When one of my cases drops out of treatment, my supervisor is *not* more interested in how I contributed to this than in what motivated the client.

    SD   D   MD   MA   A   SA
7. My supervisor has helped to improve my efficiency as a practitioner.

    SD   D   MD   MA   A   SA
8. My supervisor has improved my effectiveness as a practitioner.

    SD   D   MD   MA   A   SA

9. When I go home at the end of the day, and I have had supervision, I can feel pretty good about my day's efforts.

SD   D   MD   MA   A   SA

10. My supervisor is sensitive to the size of my caseload.

SD   D   MD   MA   A   SA

11. My values about what constitutes good treatment are similar to those of my supervisor.

SD   D   MD   MA   A   SA

12. I do not have to seek the advice of my co-workers rather than take a problem up with my supervisor.

SD   D   MD   MA   A   SA

13. I rarely try to avoid conferences with my supervisor.

SD   D   MD   MA   A   SA

14. I can confront my supervisor with an issue.

SD   D   MD   MA   A   SA

15. My supervisor is sensitive to work-related stresses.

SD   D   MD   MA   A   SA

SCORE: _____

Section B

1. My supervisor does not let me do my work the way I think is best.

SD   D   MD   MA   A   SA

2. My supervisor does not respect me as a professional.

SD   D   MD   MA   A   SA

3. My supervisor rules with an iron hand.

SD   D   MD   MA   A   SA

4. My supervisor insists that everything be done his or her way.

SD   D   MD   MA   A   SA

5. My supervisor likes to give directions.

SD   D   MD   MA   A   SA

6. My supervisor has a "just pay attention and listen" attitude.

SD   D   MD   MA   A   SA

7. My supervisor seems more concerned that I deal with my cases according to the rules and regulations rather than being concerned that I do the best to aid my clients.

SD   D   MD   MA   A   SA

SCORE: _____

Section C

1. I feel my supervisor has contributed to my professional growth.
   SD   D   MD   MA   A   SA
2. My supervisor knows how to set priorities.
   SD   D   MD   MA   A   SA
3. My supervisor is good at organizing work.
   SD   D   MD   MA   A   SA
4. My supervisor knows how to teach techniques.
   SD   D   MD   MA   A   SA
5. My supervisor seems to know what he or she is talking about when it comes to dealing with case material.
   SD   D   MD   MA   A   SA
6. My supervisor has adequate knowledge to function as a good supervisor as far as his or her teaching role is concerned.
   SD   D   MD   MA   A   SA
7. My supervisor has helped me develop more self-awareness.
   SD   D   MD   MA   A   SA

SCORE: _____

Section D

1. I think my supervisor's assessment of my work is fair.
   SD   D   MD   MA   A   SA
2. My supervisor's assessment of my work is accurate.
   SD   D   MD   MA   A   SA
3. My supervisor expresses appreciation when I do a good job.
   SD   D   MD   MA   A   SA
4. My supervisor's written and oral evaluations of my performance are similar to my self-evaluations of my level of performance.
   SD   D   MD   MA   A   SA
5. What my supervisor says about my work and what goes into my written evaluation are consistent.
   SD   D   MD   MA   A   SA

SCORE: _____

Section E

1. My supervisor is very accepting of new ideas.
   SD   D   MD   MA   A   SA

2. My supervisor talks about theory and can apply the theory to the practice component of my cases.

   SD   D   MD   MA   A   SA

3. My supervisor does not try to analyze me rather than my cases.

   SD   D   MD   MA   A   SA

4. My supervisor is friendly.

   SD   D   MD   MA   A   SA

5. My supervisor is easy to approach about issues.

   SD   D   MD   MA   A   SA

6. My supervisor encourages me to talk openly and freely with him or her.

   SD   D   MD   MA   A   SA

7. My supervisor makes me feel at ease when talking with him or her.

   SD   D   MD   MA   A   SA

8. My supervisor communicates clearly in supervisory conversations.

   SD   D   MD   MA   A   SA

                                        SCORE: _____

Section F

1. My supervisor is usually looking for some issue to discuss in our conferences, and the best policy is to reveal as little as possible.

   SD   D   MD   MA   A   SA

2. My supervisor allows me to observe directly his or her own methods of working with cases through allowing me to sit in on some of his or her interviews.

   SD   D   MD   MA   A   SA

3. My supervisor sits in on some of my interviews as a means of gathering data to help me develop my professional skills.

   SD   D   MD   MA   A   SA

4. My supervisor uses audiotape recordings of interviews in our supervisory conferences or groups.

   SD   D   MD   MA   A   SA

5. My supervisor uses videotaped interviews as supervisory material in our conferences or groups.

   SD   D   MD   MA   A   SA

6. My supervisor requires me to process record case material for use in supervisory conferences or groups.

   SD   D   MD   MA   A   SA

7. My supervisor observes me through a one-way mirror.

SD   D   MD   MA   A   SA

SCORE: _____

Section G

1. I often become annoyed with my supervisor.

SD   D   MD   MA   A   SA

2. I often become angry with my supervisor.

SD   D   MD   MA   A   SA

3. I often have to confront my supervisor.

SD   D   MD   MA   A   SA

4. I often avoid my supervisor because I am angry with him or her.

SD   D   MD   MA   A   SA

5. I often leave the agency and take breaks because of anger at my supervisor.

SD   D   MD   MA   A   SA

SCORE: _____

Section H

1. My supervisory experience has been of limited value because of the agency confines.

SD   D   MD   MA   A   SA

2. My supervisor emphasizes the quantity of work while I am more interested in the quality of my work.

SD   D   MD   MA   A   SA

3. It is no use trying to do something creative or innovative in this agency because someone is always ready to put you down.

SD   D   MD   MA   A   SA

4. The administrators in this agency are only concerned with output and really show little concern for the welfare of the practitioners.

SD   D   MD   MA   A   SA

5. This agency seems to be constantly in a state of crisis; we simply just go from one crisis to another.

SD   D   MD   MA   A   SA

6. This agency has so many problems that I avoid them and devote my time to doing a good job with my clients.

SD   D   MD   MA   A   SA

7. All in all this agency is a pretty good place to work.

SD   D   MD   MA   A   SA

SCORE: _____

Section I

In percent, on the average, the proportioning of time in my supervisory sessions is:

1. _____ % discussing supervisor's personal problems
2. _____ % discussing supervisor's cases
3. _____ % discussing my personal problems
4. _____ % discussing administrative matters
5. _____ % discussing case material
6. _____ % discussing my growth and development of self-awareness
7. _____ % discussing everyday small talk that is unrelated to my work

_____ TOTAL = 100%

8. Conferences with my supervisor are held *(check one)*:

   ❑ Never   ❑Monthly or Less   ❑Biweekly   ❑ Weekly   ❑ Daily

9. Supervisory conferences are usually held:

   ❑ at my request   ❑ at the request of my supervisor

10. If I had my choice, I would prefer:

    ❑ individual one-to-one supervision

    ❑ group supervision

    ❑ combination individual and group supervision

    ❑ no supervision

Section J

1. On the average I conduct_____interviews each day.

2. On the average each interview lasts_____.

In percent, on the average, my work load is proportioned:

3. _____ % doing therapy
4. _____ % dictation

5. _____ % staff meetings
6. _____ % community work
7. _____ % other

_____ TOTAL = 100%

Section K

In the space provided, check the box for the model of supervision that most closely describes the model used in your supervision:

❏ A. Emphasis in supervision is placed on the three-part process of help, teaching, and administration. Clinicians are expected to develop self-awareness. Regularly scheduled individual conferences are used to manage the flow and content of work of supervisees.

❏ B. Supervision is viewed as strictly an administrative and teaching process. The supervisor avoids psychologizing the worker. The structure of supervision is regularly scheduled conferences with a specific agenda.

❏ C. Emphasis in supervision is placed on teaching, and administration latitude is provided for a variety of supervisory styles adapted to individual practitioner needs. Clinicians are allowed to choose among available experts for advice. Individual conferences are used sparingly. There is some use of group seminars.

❏ D. Role of individual supervisor is played down. The specific work group, which is set up on specialized skills and/or services, is the main supervisory unit and has virtually replaced the individual conference for supervisory decision making and problem solving.

❏ E. The individual supervisor supervises several practitioners in a group arrangement. The group works together to establish the direction and content of supervision. Learning experiences are provided mainly through members of the group sharing ideas, information, and observations with one another.

❏ F. Clinicians function completely independently and only answer to their own consciences. No direct control is exercised over the clinician, who is treated as a mature, experienced professional without need of supervision.

Section L

All supervisors are required to exercise authority and control in supervision from time to time. This question deals with how you view the source of authority and control used by your supervisor. Check the box for the description that *most closely parallels* the source of authority used by your supervisor.

❏ A. Administratively assigned and agency-sanctioned authority presides over practitioners.

❏ B. Authority rests in the ability to require or expect practitioners to reveal much about themselves in the supervisory relationship.

❏ C. In part, authority depends on the ability to have influence beyond the job situation through, for example, evaluations.
❏ D. Authority derives from the role as mediator of the relationship between clinician and the agency.
❏ E. Authority derives from the fact that the supervisor knows more about some things than the clinician does.
❏ F. Authority grows out of the personality of the supervisor and his or her ability to achieve cooperation from practitioners through diplomacy and skill in handling.

Section M

Along with their other duties, supervisors are required to perform teaching functions. This question deals with the teaching models used in your supervision. Check the box for the description of the teaching model that *most closely parallels* the one used by your supervisor.

❏ A. Basically the Socratic method is used. That is, supervisees are skillfully asked leading questions until they identify and recognize the material sought. The supervisor talks very little. The practitioner does most of the talking.
❏ B. The major thrust of teaching is to provide information that will help clinicians avoid making errors, and emphasis is placed on what not to do so as to avoid grave situations. This method is used to foster as much as possible the growth and self-expression of the clinician. The main function of teaching is viewed as provision for self-expression and development of self-awareness of the clinician.
❏ C. Teaching in supervision centers around whatever experiences emerge from the client treatment demands and the development of the essential skills necessary to provide treatment. Emphasis is placed on the relationship between knowing, feeling, and doing in practice.

Section N

1. Rank your supervisor from 1 to 10 (1 = low, 10 = high) according to how good a supervisor you think he or she is. *(Circle one)*

      1   2   3   4   5   6   7   8   9   10

2. Rank yourself from 1 to 10 (1 = low, 10 = high) in terms of how good a clinician you think you are. *(Circle one)*

      1   2   3   4   5   6   7   8   9   10

3. Do you think supervision has helped you improve your effectiveness and efficiency as a clinician?   ❏ Yes ❏ No

   Explain:

4. List what you like about your supervisor:

5. List what you dislike about your supervisor:

6. What do you see as the chief value of supervision?

7. Comments:

SAQ SCORING DIRECTIONS
AND INTERPRETATION OF RESULTS

Introduction

This questionnaire has fifteen sections that deal with various aspects of supervision structure and satisfaction. Following the background information section are fourteen sections that provide data for analysis of supervision:

Section A: General Supervisory Satisfaction (GSS)
Section B: Supervisory Exercise of Authority (SEA)
Section C: Supervisor Knowledge (SK)
Section D: Supervisory Evaluation of Practice (SEP)
Section E: Supervisory Style Satisfaction (SSS)
Section F: Supervisory Sharing of Practice (SSP)
Section G: Supervisory Anger Confrontation (SAC)
Section H: Supervision External Limitations (SEL)
Section I: Supervisory Interaction Analysis (SIA)
Section J: Daily Workload Activity (DWA)
Section K: Supervisory Structural Model (SSM)
Section L: Supervisor Source of Authority (SSA)
Section M: Supervisory Teaching Model (STM)
Section N: Supervisor Overall Ranking (SOR)

Scoring

Sections A through H are scored using the following scoring method. Each response item has a numeric value:

Response Code	Response Meaning	Code Value
SD	Strongly Disagree	1
D	Disagree	2
MD	Mildly Disagree	3
MA	MA Mildly Agree	4
A	Agree	5
SA	Strongly Agree	6

In each section the response items for each question should be totaled using the numeric code values. The totals for each section should be entered in the scoring blank at the end of the section.

The following sections provide information on interpretation of each section of the questionnaire.

Section A: General Supervisory Satisfaction (GSS)

This section measures the supervisee's general satisfaction with supervision. It is a global measure and covers a number of domains. Scores can range from 15 to 90. Categories of score interpretations are:

Score Range	Level of Supervision Satisfaction
15 to 30	Very low
31 to 45	Low
46 to 60	Moderate
61 to 75	High
76 to 90	Very high

Scores below 45 indicate the need for intervention to prevent the supervisory process from becoming totally ineffective and unproductive.

Section B: Supervisory Exercise of Authority (SEA)

This section provides a score that measures the degree of authority exercises over the supervisor. A high score indicates a supervisor who exercises much control over the practitioner and allows little autonomy or independence for the clinician. Scores can range from 7 to 42. Categories of score interpretations are:

Score Range	Level of Supervisor Exercise of Authority
7 to 14	Very high
15 to 21	High
22 to 28	Moderate with some autonomy
29 to 35	Moderate autonomy
36 to 42	High autonomy

High levels of control do not always indicate problematic supervision, and high levels of autonomy do not always indicate good supervision. Scores must be interpreted within the context of the actual supervision process. Good supervision contains a balance of authority and autonomy. Extreme high or low scores require analysis as to whether undue rigid control is being applied to the practitioner or whether complete autonomy is due to supervisor neglect or unavailability.

Section C: Supervisor Knowledge (SK)

This subscale measures the supervisee's perception of the supervisor's level of knowledge. Scores can range from 7 to 42. Categories of score interpretations are:

Score Range	Level of Supervisor Knowledge
7 to 14	Very low
15 to 21	Modest
22 to 28	Moderate
29 to 35	Adequate
36 to 42	High

Scores below 21 should be considered reason for concern and should lead to analysis of what the problem may be and how it could be improved.

Section D: Supervisory Evaluation of Practice (SEP)

This domain is a measure of the supervisee's view of the fairness, accuracy, and congruence of the supervisor's evaluation of the practitioner's performance. Scores can range from 5 to 30. Categories of score interpretations are:

Score Range	Level of Evaluation Satisfaction
5 to 10	Very low
11 to 15	Low
16 to 20	Moderate
21 to 25	High
26 to 30	Very high

Scores below 15 in this domain should be a focus of attention in supervision, and efforts should be made to clarify and resolve the difference of perception.

Section E: Supervisory Style Satisfaction (SSS)

Satisfaction with the supervisor's style of relating is measured by this subscale. Scores can range from 5 to 30. Categories of score interpretations are:

Score Range	Level of Style Satisfaction
5 to 10	Very low
11 to 15	Low
16 to 20	Moderate
21 to 25	High
26 to 30	Very high

Section F: Supervisory Sharing of Practice (SSP)

The sharing of practice subscale measures the extent to which the supervisee and supervisor directly share clinical material through various means such as video- and audiotaping. Scores can range from 7 to 42. Categories of score interpretations are:

Score Range	Level of Practice Sharing
7 to 14	Very low
15 to 21	Modest
22 to 28	Moderate
29 to 35	Adequate
36 to 42	High

Scores below 21 should alert the supervisor and practitioner to review the amount of case sharing done in supervision and assess whether increased sharing is needed. Low scores in this domain do not mean that increased sharing is necessary. Other forms of sharing and other factors in the amount of sharing may make the clinical sharing rate adequate to accomplish effective supervision.

Section G: Supervisory Anger Confrontation (SAC)

This domain measures the degree of anger the supervisee experiences in relation to the supervisor. Scores can range from 5 to 30. Categories of score interpretations are:

Score Range	Level of Anger
5 to 10	Very low
11 to 15	Low
16 to 20	Moderate
21 to 25	High
26 to 30	Very high

Scores above 15 should result in analysis of the source and nature of the anger. Scores above 21 have the potential to significantly disrupt the supervisory process.

Section H: Supervision External Limitations (SEL)

This section documents the supervisee's perception of constraints external to the supervision process that may lead to negative outcomes within the supervision process. Scores can range from 7 to 42. Categories of score interpretations are:

Score Range	Level of External Limitations
7 to 14	Very low
15 to 21	Modest
22 to 28	Moderate
29 to 35	High
36 to 42	Very high

Scores above 21 should be reviewed by the supervisor and supervisee. The limitations may be at a level that they are impacting or have the potential to impact the supervision process. Review of the limitations may lead to possible solutions to the limitations or result in strategies to work within the confines of the limitations. The identification and awareness of the limitations fostered by the completion of this scale may prevent the limitations from negatively influencing the supervision process.

Section I: Supervisory Interaction Analysis (SIA)

This section is not a subscale. It is a measure of how supervisory time is allocated, how often it occurs, and how supervision sessions are initiated. The data generated by this section can assist in analyzing the supervision interaction and content as part of a monitoring process. The responses in this section can be used in connection with the results on scaled sections A through H.

Section J: Daily Workload Activity (DWA)

In this section, daily workload activity is recorded and can be used in connection with the results on scaled sections A through H. The data in this section can also be used to monitor general workload activity periodically.

Section K: Supervisory Structural Model (SSM)

This section is not scaled. It can be used to identify the specific model used in supervision and to plan supervisory structure. The response of the supervisee can be used by the supervisor to assess congruence of the supervisor's and supervisee's perceptions of the supervision model in use.

Section L: Supervisor Source of Authority (SSA)

This section is not scaled. It can be used to identify the specific model of authority used in supervision and to plan supervisory structure. The response of the supervisee can be used by the supervisor to assess congruence of the supervisor's and supervisee's perceptions of the authority model used by the supervisor. The supervisee's perception can be used in connection with the results of the Section B: Supervisory Exercise of Authority (SEA) subscale.

Section M: Supervisory Teaching Model (STM)

This section is not scaled. It can be used to identify the specific teaching model used in supervision and to plan supervisory teaching activity. The response of the supervisee can be used by the supervisor to assess congruence of the supervisor's and supervisee's perceptions of the supervision teaching model in use.

Section N: Supervisor Overall Ranking (SOR)

This section includes a scale for ranking the supervisor's overall performance and a scale for the supervisee to rank self-perception of clinical skills. The narrative section is for indicating likes and dislikes related to supervision as well as identifying the value of supervision. Content of this section can be used in analysis of other sections of this instrument.

Appendix IX

Short Form Supervision Satisfaction Questionnaire (SFSSQ)

SHORT FORM SUPERVISION SATISFACTION QUESTIONNAIRE (SFSSQ)

1. Name of Practitioner: _____

    Name of Supervisor: _____

2. Sex of Practitioner: ❑ Male ❑ Female

    Sex of Supervisor: ❑ Male ❑ Female

3. Age of Practitioner: _____

    Age of Supervisor: _____

Answer the following questions by circling the response category below each question that best describes how you feel about the question (SD = strongly disagree; D = disagree; MD = mildly disagree; MA = mildy agree; A = agree; SA = strongly agree).

1. My supervisor respects me as a professional.

    SD   D   MD   MA   A   SA

2. My supervisor gives me appropriate autonomy to accomplish my work.

    SD   D   MD   MA   A   SA

3. I feel my supervisor has contributed to my professional growth.

    SD   D   MD   MA   A   SA

4. My supervisor is good at organizing work.

    SD   D   MD   MA   A   SA

5. My supervisor knows how to teach.

    SD   D   MD   MA   A   SA

6. My supervisor has helped me develop more self-awareness.

    SD   D   MD   MA   A   SA

7. I think my supervisor's assessment of my work is fair.

    SD   D   MD   MA   A   SA

8. My supervisor's assessment of my work is accurate.

    SD   D   MD   MA   A   SA

9. Overall, I am satisfied with my supervisory experience.

    SD   D   MD   MA   A   SA

10. I look forward to my supervisory sessions.

    SD   D   MD   MA   A   SA

11. My supervisor has helped to improve my efficiency as a practitioner.

SD   D   MD   MA   A   SA

12. My supervisor has improved my effectiveness as a practitioner.

SD   D   MD   MA   A   SA

13. My values about what constitutes good treatment are similar to those of my supervisor.

SD   D   MD   MA   A   SA

14. I can confront my supervisor with an issue.

SD   D   MD   MA   A   SA

15. My supervisor is accepting of new ideas.

SD   D   MD   MA   A   SA

16. My supervisor talks about theory and can apply the theory to the practice component of my cases.

SD   D   MD   MA   A   SA

17. My supervisor is friendly.

SD   D   MD   MA   A   SA

18. My supervisor makes me feel at ease when talking with him or her.

SD   D   MD   MA   A   SA

19. My supervisor communicates clearly in supervisory conversations.

SD   D   MD   MA   A   SA

20. My supervisor uses audiotapes and videotapes of interviews, one-way mirrors, or process recording as supervisory material in our supervisory conferences.

SD   D   MD   MA   A   SA

21. This agency is a good place to work.

SD   D   MD   MA   A   SA

22. I rarely become angry at my supervisor.

SD   D   MD   MA   A   SA

23. I rarely have to confront my supervisor.

    SD   D   MD   MA   A   SA

                                    SCORE: _____

24. Rank your supervisor from 1 to 10 (1 = low, 10 = high) according to how good a supervisor you think he or she is. *(Circle one)*

    1   2   3   4   5   6   7   8   9   10

25. Rank yourself from 1 to 10 (1 = low, 10 = high) in terms of how good a clinician you think you are. *(Circle one)*

    1   2   3   4   5   6   7   8   9   10

26. Do you think supervision has helped you improve your effectiveness and efficiency as a clinician?   ❑ Yes❑ No

Explain:

27. List what you like about your supervisor:

28. List what you dislike about your supervisor:

29. What do you see as the chief value of supervision?

30. Comments:

SFSSQ SCORING DIRECTIONS
AND INTERPRETATION OF RESULTS

Introduction

This questionnaire has thirty items that deal with various aspects of supervision structure and satisfaction. The first twenty-three questions are the short form supervision satisfaction scale that is derived from the parent instrument, the Supervision Analysis Questionnaire (SAQ).

Scoring

Items 1 through 23 are scored using the following scoring method. Each response item has a numeric value. The numeric values are:

Response Code	Response Meaning	Code Value
SD	Strongly Disagree	1
D	Disagree	2
MD	Mildly Disagree	3
MA	Mildly Agree	4
A	Agree	5
SA	Strongly Agree	6

The response numeric value for each question should be totaled using the numeric code values. The total should be entered in the scoring blank at the end of item 23.

The respondent's score is a global measure and covers a number of domains. Scores can range from 23 to 138. Categories of score interpretations are:

Score Range	Level of Supervision Satisfaction
23 to 46	Very low
47 to 69	Low
70 to 92	Moderate
93 to 115	High
116 to 138	Very high

Scores below 70 should be considered worthy of intervention to prevent significant disruption of the supervisory process.

Appendix X

Individual and Group Supervision Report Form

INDIVIDUAL AND GROUP SUPERVISON REPORT FORM

SUPERVISOR: _____

SUPERVISEE(S): _____

ORGANIZATION: _____

    Address: _____

                  _____

    Telephone:_____

DATE: _____

TIME IN: _____

OUT: _____

TOTAL TIME: _____

PERSONS PRESENT:

PURPOSE OF SESSION:

GOALS OR FOCUS OF SESSION:

TOPICS DISCUSSED:

CLIENTS DISCUSSED:

RECOMMENDATIONS:

PLANS FOR NEXT SESSION:

SIGNATURE OF SUPERVISOR: _____

This form is designed to comply with state social work licensing board requirements for documenting and reporting supervisor contact for licensure. Persons
documenting supervision for licensure should contact the state licensing board
for approval before using this form to document supervision.

References

Abell, W. (1966). *The Collective Dream in Art: A Psycho-Historical Theory of Culture Based on Relations Between the Arts, Psychology, and the Social Sciences.* New York: Schocken.

Ackley, D. C. (1997). *Breaking Free of Managed Care: A Step by Step Guide to Regaining Control of Your Practice.* New York: Guilford.

Adler, M. I. (1981). *Six Great Ideas: Truth, Goodness, Beauty, Liberty, Equality, Justice.* New York: Macmillan.

Ajemian, I. and Mount, B. M. (1980). *The Royal Victoria Hospital Manual on Palliative/Hospice Care.* New York: Arno.

Allman, W. F. (1994). *The Stone Age Present: How Evolution Has Shaped Modern Life from Sex, Violence, and Language to Emotions, Morals, and Communities.* New York: Simon and Schuster.

Alonso, A. (1985). *The Quiet Profession: Supervisors of Psychotherapy.* New York: Macmillan.

Alperin, R. M. and Phillips, D. G. (1997). *The Impact of Managed Care on the Practice of Psychotherapy: Innovation, Implementation, and Controversy.* New York: Brunner/Mazel.

Altheide, D. L. (1995). *An Ecology of Communication: Cultural Formats of Control.* New York: Aldine de Gruyter.

Amada, G. (1995). *A Guide to Psychotherapy.* New York: Ballentine.

American Association of State Social Work Boards (1998). *Social Work Laws and Board Regulations: A Comparison Guide.* Culpeper, VA: American Association of State Social Work Boards.

American Board of Examiners in Clinical Social Work (1989). *The Diplomate* 2 (June).

American Psychiatric Association (1994). *Diagnostic and Statistical Manual of Mental Disorders,* Fourth Edition. Washington, DC: American Psychiatric Association.

American Psychiatric Association (1996). *Practice Guidelines.* Washington, DC: American Psychiatric Association.

American Psychiatric Association (2000a). *Diagnostic and Statistical Manual of Mental Disorders,* Fourth Edition, Text Revision (DSM-IV-TR). Washington, DC: American Psychiatric Association.

American Psychiatric Association (2000b). *Practice Guidelines for the Treatment of Psychiatric Disorders: Compendium 2000.* Washington, DC: American Psychiatric Association.

Anderson, S. C. and Henderson, D. C. (1985) "Working with Lesbian Alcoholics." *Social Work* 30 (Summer), pp. 518-524.

Anonymous (1929). "Supervision." *The Family* 10 (April), pp. 35-45.

Anonymous (1973). "Position Statement of Family Service Agencies Regarding Graduate Schools of Social Work." *Smith College Studies in Social Work* 44 (February), pp. 108-110.

Argyris, C. and Schon, D. A. (1980). *Theory in Practice: Increasing Professional Effectiveness.* San Francisco: Jossey-Bass.

Ariete, S. (1976). *Creativity: The Magic Synthesis.* New York: Basic Books.

Aronson, J. (1996). *Inside Managed Care: Family Therapy in a Changing Environment.* New York: Brunner/Mazel.

Austad, C. S. (1996). *Is Long-Term Psychotherapy Unethical? Toward a Social Ethic in an Era of Managed Care.* San Francisco: Jossey-Bass.

Bagg, A. R. (1980). "AV Presentations: Step by Step, Inch by Inch." *AudioVisual Communications* 14 (January), pp. 35-39.

Bailey, J. (1980). *Ideas and Intervention: Social Theory for Practice.* London: Routledge and Kegan Paul.

Ball, J. C. et al. (1974). "The Heroin Addicts' View of Methadone Maintenance." *British Journal of Addiction* 69 (March), pp. 89-95.

Barber, B. (1963). "Some Problems in the Sociology of the Professions." *Daedalus* 92 (Fall), pp. 669-688.

Bartlett, H. (1970). *The Common Base of Social Work Practice.* Washington, DC: National Association of Social Workers.

Bartol, K. M. and Wortman, M. S. (1976). "Sex Effects in Leader Behavior Self-Description and Job Satisfaction." *Journal of Psychology* 94, pp. 177-183.

Barton, W. E. (1987). *The History and Influence of the American Psychiatric Association.* Washington, DC: American Psychiatric Press.

Batten, C. (1990). "Dilemmas of Cross-Cultural Psychotherapy Supervision." *British Journal of Psychotherapy,* 7, pp.129-140.

Beck, R. L. (1982). "Process and Content in the Family of Origin Group." *International Journal of Group Psychotherapy* 32 (April), pp. 233-244.

Becker, H. S. (1974). "Art As Collective Action." *American Sociological Review* 39 (December), pp. 767-776.

Berger, M. M. (ed.) (1978). *Videotape Techniques in Psychiatric Training and Treatment.* New York: Brunner/Mazel.

Bergin, A. E. and Garfield, S. L. (eds.) (1971). *Handbook of Psychotherapy and Behavior Change.* New York: Wiley.

Bergin, A. F. and Strupp, H. H. (1972). *Changing Frontiers in the Science of Psychotherapy.* Chicago: Aldine-Atherton.

Bernard, J. M. (1994). "Multicultural Supervision: A Reaction to Leong and Wagner, Cook, Priest, and Fukuyama." *Counselor Education and Supervision,* 34, pp. 159-171.

Berry, D. B. (1998). *The Domestic Violence Sourcebook: Everything You Need to Know*. Los Angeles: Lowell House.

Beukenkamp, C. (1956). "Clinical Observations on the Effect of Analytically Oriented Group Therapy and Group Supervision on the Therapist." *The Psychoanalytic Review* 43 (January), pp. 82-90.

Birenbaum, A. et al. (1979). "Training Medical Students to Appreciate the Special Problems of the Elderly." *The Gerontologist* 19 (December), pp. 575-579.

Bissell, L. et al. (1980). "The Alcoholic Social Worker: A Survey." *Social Work in Health Care* 5 (Summer), pp. 421-432.

Bloom, F. (1980). "Psychotherapy and Moral Culture: A Psychiatrist's Field Report." In T. J. Cottle and P. Whitten (eds.), *Psychotherapy: Current Perspectives*. New York: New Viewpoints.

Bloom, M. (1975).*The Paradox of Helping: Introduction to the Philosophy of Scientific Practice*. New York: Wiley.

Blumenfield, M. (1982). *Applied Supervision in Psychotherapy.* New York: Grune and Stratton.

Booth, E. (1997). *The Everyday Work of Art: How Artistic Experience Can Transform Your Life*. Naperville, IL: Sourcebooks, Inc.

Bowen, M. (1978). *Family Therapy in Clinical Practice*. New York: Jason Aronson.

Boyer, R. (1975). *An Approach to Human Services*. San Francisco: Canfield.

Boyers, R. (ed.) (1971). *R. D. Laing and Anti-Psychiatry*. New York: Harper and Row.

Brackett, J. R. (1903). *Supervision and Education in Charity*. New York: Macmillan.

Bradley, L. J. and Ladany, N. (eds.) (2001). *Counselor Supervison: Principles, Processes, and Practice*. Philadelphia: Brunner-Routledge.

Brager, G. A. (1968). "Advocacy and Political Behavior." *Social Work* 13 (April), pp. 5- 15.

Bramhall, M. and Ezell, S. (1981a). "How Agencies Can Prevent Burnout." *Public Welfare* 39 (Summer), pp. 33-47.

Bramhall, M. and Ezell, S. (1981b). "How Burned Out Are You?" *Public Welfare* 39 (Winter), pp. 23-55.

Bramhall, M. and Ezell, S. (1981c). "Working Your Way Out of Burnout." *Public Welfare* 39 (Spring), pp. 32-47.

Brandt, A. (1980). "Self-Confrontation." *Psychology Today* 14 (October), pp. 78-101.

Brendler, J. et al. (1991). *Madness, Chaos, and Violence: Therapy with Families at the Brink*. New York: Basic Books.

Brennan, E. C. (1976). "Expectations for Baccalaureate Social Workers." *Public Welfare* 34 (Summer), pp. 19-23.

Briar, S. (1970). "The Current Crisis in Social Casework." In Robert W. Klenk and Robert M. Ryan (eds.), *The Practice of Social Work*. Belmont, CA: Wadsworth, pp. 85-96.

Briar, S. and Miller, H. (1971). *Problems and Issues in Social Casework.* New York: Columbia University Press.

Bridges, W. (1991). *Managing Transitions: Making the Most of Change.* Reading, MA: Addison-Wesley.

Brodsky, A. M. (1980). "Sex Role Issues in the Supervision of Therapy." In A. K. Hess (ed.), *Psychotherapy Supervision: Theory, Research and Practice.* New York: John Wiley, pp. 509-522.

Brown, E. L. (1936). *Social Work As a Profession.* New York: Russell Sage Foundation.

Brown, M. T. and Landrum-Brown, J. (1995). "Counselor Supervision: Cross Cultural Perspectives." In J.G. Ponterotto and J. M. Casas (eds.), *Handbook of Multicultural Counseling.* Thousand Oaks, CA: Sage, pp.263-286.

Browning, C. H. and Browning, B. J. (1996). *How to Partner with Managed Care.* New York: Wiley.

Burgoyne, R. W. et al. (1976). "Who Gets Supervised? An Extension of Patient Selection Inequity." *American Journal of Psychiatry* 133 (November), pp. 1313-1315.

Burke, K. (1975). "The Five Key Terms of Dramatism." In D. Brissett and C. Edgely (eds.), *Life As Theater: A Dramaturgical Sourcebook.* Chicago: Aldine, pp. 370-375.

Butler, R. N. (1969). "Age-ism: Another Form of Bigotry." *The Gerontologist* 9 (Winter), pp. 243-246.

Cabot, R. C. (1915a). "Address," Proceedings of the National Conference of Charities and Corrections, Baltimore.

Cabot, R. C. (1915b). *Social Service and the Art of Healing.* New York: Moffat, Yard.

Cabot, R. C. (1973). *Social Service and the Art of Healing,* Reprinted Edition. Washington, DC: National Association of Social Workers.

Caligor, L., Bromberg, P. M., and Meltzer, J. D. (1984). *Clinical Perspectives on the Supervision of Psychoanalysis and Psychotherapy.* New York: Plenum.

Calsyn, R. J. et al. (1999). "Evaluating Team Leaders and Peers in Group Supervision." *The Clinical Supervisor* 18(2), pp. 203-210.

Caplow, T. (1976). *How to Run Any Organization: A Manual of Practical Sociology.* Hinsdale, IL: Dryden Press.

Cashwell, C. S., Looby, and Housley, (1997). "Appreciating Cultural Diversity Through Clinical Supervision." *The Clinical Supervisor* 15(1), pp.75-85.

Cervantes, S. M. (1950/1605). *The Ingenious Gentleman Don Quixote de la Mancha,* Reprint Edition. New York: Modern Library.

Chaiklin, H. (1978). "Role and Utilization of the Social Worker in Clinical Practice." In G. U. Balis (ed.), *Psychiatric Clinical Skills in Medical Practice,* Boston: Butterworth.

Chance, P. (1981). "That Drained-Out, Used-Up Feeling." *Psychology Today* 15 (January), pp. 88-95.

Chapin, F. S. and Queen, S. A. (1972/1937). *Research Memorandum on Social Work in the Depression.* New York: Social Science Research Council, Reprint Edition. New York: Arno.

Cherniss, C. and Egnatios, E. (1978). "Clinical Supervision in Community Mental Health." *Social Work* 23 (May), pp. 219-223.

Chescheir, M. W. (1979). "Social Role Discrepancies As Clues to Practice." *Social Work* 24 (March), pp. 89-94.

Chessick, R. (1977). *Great Ideas in Psychotherapy.* New York: Jason Aronson.

Chetkow-Yanoov, B. (1999). *Celebrating Diversity: Coexisting in a Multicultural Society.* Binghamton, NY: The Haworth Press.

Clark, R. W. (1980). *Freud: The Man and the Cause.* New York: Random House.

Clarkin, J. F. and Glick, I. D. (1982). "Supervision of Family Therapy." In M. Blumenfield (ed.), *Applied Supervision in Psychotherapy.* New York: Grune and Stratton, pp. 87-106.

Cohen, B. Z. and Laufer, H. (1999). "The Influence of Supervision on Social Workers' Perception of Their Profession." *The Clinical Supervisor* 18(2), pp. 39-50.

Commission on Accreditation (1994). *Handbook of Accreditation Standards and Procedures,* Fourth Edition. Alexandria, VA: Council on Social Work Education.

Comstock, G. A. and Tonascia, J. A. (1977). "Education and Mortality in Washington County, Maryland." *Journal of Health and Social Behavior* 18 (March), pp. 54-61.

Congress, E. P. (1999). *Social Work Values and Ethics: Identifying and Resolving Professional Dilemmas.* Chicago: Nelson-Hall.

Conyngton, M. (1971/1909). *How to Help: A Manual of Practical Charity,* Reprint Edition. New York: Arno.

Cook, D.A. and Helms, J. E. (1988). "Visible Racial/Ethnic Group Supervisees' Satisfaction with Cross-Cultural Supervision As Predicted by Relationship Characteristics." *Journal of Counseling Psychology* 35, pp. 268-274.

Coppedge, R. O. and Davis, C. G. (eds.) (1977). *Rural Poverty and the Policy Crisis.* Ames, IA: Iowa State University Press.

Corpt, E. A. and Reison, M. (1994). "Behaviorizing Your Clinical Language." *Managed Care News,* pp. 1-5.

Corsini, R. J. (ed.) (1986). *Current Psychotherapies.* Itasca, IL: Peacock.

Cottle, T. J. and Whitten, P. (1980). *Psychotherapy: Current Perspectives.* New York: New Viewpoints.

Dalali, I. et al. (1976). "Training of Paraprofessionals: Some Caveats." *Journal of Drug Education* 6, pp. 105-112.

Daley, M. R. (1979). "'Burnout': Smoldering Problem in Protective Services." *Social Work* 24 (September), pp. 375-379.

Danaher, K. (ed.) (1996). *Corporations Are Gonna Get Your Mama: Globalization and the Downsizing of the American Dream.* Monroe, ME: Common Courage Press.

Davies, J. F. (1974). "The Country Mouse Comes into Her Own." *Child Welfare* 53 (October), pp. 509-513.

Davis, S. (1991). "Violence by Psychiatric Inpatients: A Review." *Hospital and Community Psychiatry* 42 (June), pp. 585-589.

Day, P. J. (1997). *A New History of Social Welfare.* Boston: Allyn and Bacon.

Day, R. C. and Hamblin, R. L. (1967). "Some Effects of Close and Punitive Styles of Supervision." In G. D. Bell (ed.), *Organizations and Human Behavior: A Book of Readings.* Englewood Cliffs, NJ: Prentice-Hall, pp. 172-181.

DeSchweinitz, K. (1924). *The Art of Helping People Out of Trouble.* Boston: Houghton Mifflin.

Dewey, J. (1958). *Art As Experience.* New York: Capricorn.

Dinerman, M. and Geismar, L. L. (1984). *A Quarter-Century of Social Work Education.* Washington, DC: National Association of Social Workers.

Donahue, J. D. (1989). *The Privatization Decision: Public Ends, Private Means.* New York: Basic Books.

Douglas, M. A. D. and Rave, E. J. (1990). "Ethics of Feminist Supervision of Psychotherapy." In H. Lerman and N. Porter (eds), *Feminist Ethics in Psychotherapy.* New York: Springer, pp. 137-146.

Doverspike, W. F. (1999). *Ethical Risk Management: Guidelines for Practice.* Sarasota, FL: Professional Resource Exchange.

Dressler, D. M. et al. (1975). "Clinical Attitudes Toward the Suicide Attempted." *Journal of Nervous and Mental Disease* 160 (February), pp. 146-155.

Drury, S. S. (1984). *Assertive Supervision: Building Involved Teamwork.* Champaign, IL: Research Press.

Durkheim, E. (1933). *The Division of Labor in Society.* New York: Macmillan.

Dutton, D. G. (1998). *The Abusive Personality: Violence and Control in Intimate Relationships.* New York: Guilford.

Earle, R. H. and Barnes, D. J. (1999). *Independent Practice for the Mental Health Professional: Growing a Private Practice for the 21st Century.* Philadelphia: Brunner/Mazel.

Edelwich, J. and Brodsky, A. (1980). *Burnout: Stages of Disillusionment in the Helping Professions.* New York: Human Sciences.

Edelwich, J. and Brodsky, A. (1982). *Sexual Dilemmas for the Helping Professional.* New York: Brunner/Mazel.

Efran, J. S., Lukens, M. D., and Lukens, R. J. (1990). *Language Structure and Change: Frameworks of Meaning in Psychotherapy.* New York: Norton.

Ehrenreich, J. H. (1985). *The Altruistic Imagination: A History of Social Work and Social Policy in the United States.* Ithaca, NY: Cornell University Press.

Eisler, R. (1987). *The Chalice and the Blade.* New York: Harper and Row.

Eisler, R. (1992). Lecture. Chicago, IL: Association of Humanist Psychology.

Eldridge, W. D. (1982). "Coping with Accountability: Guidelines for Supervisors." *Social Casework* 63 (October), pp. 489-496.

Endress, A. H. (1981). "Being and Becoming a Professional." *Social Casework* 62 (May), pp. 305-308.

Epstein, L. (1973). "Is Autonomous Practice Possible?" *Social Work* 18 (March), pp. 5-12.

Ericsson, K. A. and Simon, H. A. (1993). *Protocol Analysis: Verbal Reports As Data*. Cambridge, MA: The MIT Press.

Etcheverry, R. et al. (1980). *The Uses and Abuses of Role Playing*. Paper presented at Second Group Work Symposium, Arlington, TX, November, pp. 1-19.

Ewalt, P. L. (ed.) (1980). *Toward a Definition of Clinical Social Work*. Papers from the NASW Invitational Forum on Clinical Social Work, June 7-9, 1979, Denver, CO. Washington, DC: National Association of Social Workers.

Famighetti, R. (ed.) (1999). *The World Almanac and Book of Facts 2000*. Mahwah, NJ: Primedia Reference, Inc.

Faver, C. A., Fox, M. F., and Shannon, C. (1983). "The Educational Process and Job Equity for the Sexes in Social Work." *Journal of Education for Social Work* 19 (3), pp. 78-87.

Feibleman, J. K. (1973). *Understanding Philosophy: A Popular History of Ideas*. New York: Horizon.

Feldman, J. L. and Fitzpatrick, R. J. (eds.) (1992). *Managed Mental Health Care: Administrative and Clinical Issues*. Washington, DC: American Psychiatric Press.

Finn, P. (1980). "Developing Critical Television Viewing Skills." *The Educational Forum* 44 (May), pp. 473-482.

Fisch, R. et al. (1982). *The Tactics of Change: Doing Therapy Briefly*. San Francisco: Jossey-Bass.

Fisher, J. (1975). "Training for Effective Therapeutic Practice." *Psychotherapy: Theory, Research and Practice* 12 (Spring), pp. 118-123.

Fisher, J. (1980). *The Response of Social Work to the Depression*. Cambridge, MA: Schenkman.

Flach, F. (1998). *A Comprehensive Guide to Malpractice Risk Management in Psychiatry*. New York: Hatherleigh.

Fong, M. L. and Lease, S. H. (1997). "Cross-Cultural Supervision: Issues for the White Supervisor." In D. B. Pope-Davis and H. L. K. Coleman (eds.), *Multicultural Counseling Competencies: Assessment, Education and Training, and Supervision*. Thousand Oaks, CA: Sage, pp. 387-405.

Fortune, A. E. (1985). *Task-Centered Practice with Families and Groups*. New York: Springer.

Fosdick, H. E. (1943). *On Being a Real Person*. New York: Harper and Row.

Freeman, L. (1980). *Freud Rediscovered*. New York: Arbor House.

Freud, S. (1967/1939). *Moses and Monotheism*, Reprint Edition. New York: Vintage.

Freud, S. (1988). *My Three Mothers and Other Passions*. New York: New York University Press.

Freudenberger, H. J. (1977). "Burnout: Occupational Hazard of the Child Care Worker." *Child Care Quarterly* 6 (Summer), pp. 90-99.

Freudenberger, H. J. and Richelsen, G. (1980). *Burn-Out: The High Cost of High Achievement.* New York: Anchor.

Fritz, G. K. and Poe, R. O. (1979). "The Role of a Cinema Seminar in Psychiatric Education." *American Journal of Psychiatry* 136 (February), pp. 207-210.

Gallant, J. P. and Thyer, B. A. (1989). "The 'Bug-in-the-Ear' in Clinical Supervision." *The Clinical Supervisor* 7 (Fall/Winter), pp. 43-58.

Gallessich, J. (1982). *The Professional Practice of Consultation.* San Francisco: Jossey-Bass.

Gardner, H. (1982). *Art, Mind and Brain: A Cognitive Approach to Creativity.* New York: Basic Books.

Garrett, A. (1954). *Learning Through Supervision.* Northampton, MA: Smith College Studies in Social Work.

Geiger, D. L. (1978). "Note: How Future Professionals View the Elderly: A Comparative Analysis of Social Work, Law, and Medical Students' Perceptions." *The Gerontologist* 18 (December), pp. 591-594.

Geismar, L. L. and Wood, K. M. (1982). "Evaluating Practice: Science As Faith." *Social Casework* 63 (May), pp. 266-272.

Gelfand, B. et al. (1975). "An Andragogical Application to the Training of Social Workers." *Journal of Education for Social Work* 11 (Fall), pp. 55-61.

Geller, J. L. (1996). "Mental Health Services of the Future: Managed Care, Unmanaged Care, Mismanaged Care." *Smith College Studies in Social Work* 66 (June), pp. 223-239.

Gibbs, M. S. (1984). "The Therapist As Imposter." In C. M. Brody (ed.), *Women Therapists Working with Women: New Theory and Process of Feminist Therapy.* New York: Springer Publishing Co., pp. 22-33.

Gibelman, M. (1995). *What Social Workers Do.* Washington, DC: NASW Press.

Gibelman, M. and Schervish, P. H. (1997). *Who We Are: A Second Look.* Washington, DC: NASW Press.

Ginsberg, L. (ed.) (1976). *Social Work in Rural Communities: A Book of Readings.* New York: Council on Social Work Education.

Gitterman, A. (ed.) (1991). *Handbook of Social Work Practice with Vulnerable Populations.* New York: Columbia University Press.

Goldenberg, I. and Goldenberg, H. (1980). *Family Therapy: An Overview.* Monterey, CA: Brooks/Cole.

Goldstein, E. G. (1980). "Knowledge Base of Clinical Social Work." *Social Work* 25 (May), pp. 173-178.

Goldstein, H. (1973). *Social Work Practice: A Unitary Approach.* Columbia, SC: University of South Carolina Press.

Goodman, M., Brown, J., and Deitz, P. (1992). *Managing Managed Care: A Mental Health Practitioner's Survival Guide.* Washington, DC: American Psychiatric Press.

Goodrich, T. J. et al. (1988). *Feminist Family Therapy: A Casebook.* New York: W.W. Norton and Company.

Gopaul-McNicol, S. A. and Brice-Baker, J. (1998). *Cross-Cultural Practice: Assessment, Treatment and Training.* New York: Wiley.

Gordon, W. E. (1981). "A Natural Classification System for Social Work Literature and Knowledge." *Social Work* 26 (March), pp. 134-138.

Gould, K. H. (1984). "Original Works of Freud on Women: Social Work References." *Social Casework,* 65, pp. 94-101.

Gould, S. J. (1980). *The Panda's Thumb: More Reflections in Natural History.* New York: Norton.

Greben, S. E. (1985). "Dear Brutus: Dealing with Unresponsiveness Through Supervision." *Canadian Journal of Psychiatry* 30 (February), pp. 48-53.

Greenberg, H. (1971). *Social Environment and Behavior.* New York: Schenkman.

Grinder, J. and Bandler, R. (1976). *The Structure of Magic II.* Palo Alto, CA: Science and Behavior Books.

Grinnell, R. M., Jr. (ed.) (1981). *Social Work Research and Evaluation.* Itasca, IL: Peacock.

Grosser, C. (1965). "Community Development Programs Serving the Urban Poor." *Social Work* 10 (July), pp. 15-21.

Grotjahn, M. (1977). *The Art and Technique of Analytic Group Therapy.* New York: Jason Aronson.

Groves, E. R. (1940). "A Decade of Marriage Counseling." *The Annals of the American Academy of Political and Social Science* 212 (November), pp. 72-80.

Guerin, P. J. (1976). *Family Therapy: Theory and Practice.* New York: Gardner.

Gurman, A. S. (1981a). "Integrative Marital Therapy: Toward the Development of an Interpersonal Approach." In S. H. Budman (ed.), *Forms of Brief Therapy.* New York: Guilford Press, pp. 415-457.

Gurman, A. S. (ed.) (1981b). *Questions and Answers in the Practice of Family Therapy.* New York: Brunner/Mazel.

Gurman, A. S. and Razin, A. M. (1977). *Effective Psychotherapy: A Handbook of Research.* New York: Pergamon.

Haley, J. (1967). "Marriage Therapy." In H. Greenwald (ed.), *Active Psychotherapy.* New York: Atherton, pp. 189-223.

Haley, J. (ed.) (1971). *Changing Families: A Family Therapy Reader.* New York: Grune and Stratton.

Haley, J. (1973). *Uncommon Therapy: The Psychiatric Techniques of Milton H. Erickson, MD.* New York: Norton.

Haley, J. (1976). *Problem-Solving Therapy: New Strategies for Effective Family Therapy.* New York: Harper Colophon.

Haley, J. (1980). "How to Be a Marriage Therapist Without Knowing Practically Anything." *Journal of Marital and Family Therapy* 6 (October), pp. 385-391.

Haley, J. (1996). *Learning and Teaching Therapy.* New York: Guilford.

Hall, C. S. and Lindzey, G. (1970). *Theories of Personality.* New York: Wiley.

Halmos, P. (1970). *The Faith of the Counsellors: A Study in the Theory and Practice of Social Case Work and Psychotherapy.* New York: Schocken.

Hamilton, G. (1951). *Theory and Practice of Social Case Work.* New York: Columbia University Press.

Hamlin, E. R. and Timberlake, E. M. (1982). "Peer Group Supervision for Supervisors." *Social Casework* 63 (February), pp. 82-87.

Handler, E. (1975). "Residential Treatment Programs for Juvenile Delinquents." *Social Work* 20 (May), pp. 217-222.

Handley, P. (1982). "Relationship Between Supervisors' and Trainees' Cognitive Styles and the Supervision Process." *Journal of Counseling Psychology* 29, pp. 508-515.

Handy, C. (1995). "Trust and the Virtual Organization." *Harvard Business Review* (May/June), pp. 40-50.

Handy, C. (1996). *Beyond Certainty: The Changing World of Organizations.* Boston, MA: Harvard Business School Press.

Hanna, E. A. (1992). "The Demise of the Field Advising Role in Social Work Education." *The Clinical Supervisor* 10(2), pp. 149-164.

Hansen, J. C. and Warner, R. W. (1971). "Review of Research on Practicum Supervision." *Counselor Education and Supervision* 10 (Spring), pp. 261-272.

Harrison, A. F. and Bramson, Robert M. (1982). *Styles of Thinking: Strategies for Asking Questions, Making Decisions, and Solving Problems.* Garden City, NY: Anchor Press/Doubleday.

Harrison, W. D. (1980). "Role Strain and Burnout in Child Protective Service Workers." *Social Service Review* 54 (March), pp. 31-44.

Hart, G. M. (1982). *The Process of Clinical Supervision.* Baltimore, MD: University Park Press.

Hart, H. and Hart, E. B. (1935). *Personality and the Family.* Boston: Heath.

Hawkins, D. (1944). "Mental Hygiene Problems of the Adolescent Period." *The Annals of the American Academy of Political and Social Service* 236 (November), pp. 128-135.

Hawthorne, L. (1975). "Games Supervisors Play." *Social Work* 20 (May), pp. 179-183.

Heidegger, M. (1968). *What Is Called Thinking?* New York: Harper and Row.

Hersen, M. and Barlow, D. H. (1976). *Single-Case Experimental Designs: Strategies for Studying Behavior Change.* New York: Pergamon.

Hess, A. K. (ed.) (1992). *Psychotherapy Supervision: Theory, Research, and Practice.* New York: Wiley.

Heston, A. H. (1929). "The Staff Conference As a Method of Supervision." *The Family* 10 (April), pp. 46-48.

Hewitt, J. P. (1976). *Self and Society: A Symbolic Interactionist Social Psychology.* Boston: Allyn and Bacon.

Hipp, J. L. and Munson, C. E. (1995). "The Partnership Model: A Feminist Supervision/Consultation Perspective." *The Clinical Supervisor* 13(1), pp. 23-38.

Hoffman, L. (1990). *Old Scapes, New Maps: A Training Program for Psychotherapy Supervisors.* Cambridge, MA: Milusik.

Hollis, E. V. and Taylor, A. L. (1951). *Social Work Education in the United States: The Report of a Study Made for the National Council on Social Work Education.* New York: Columbia University Press.

Hollis, F. (1966). *Casework: A Psychosocial Therapy.* New York: Random House.

Holloway, S. and Brager, G. (1989). *Supervising in the Human Services.* New York: The Free Press.

Holzner, B. and Marx, J. H. (1979). *Knowledge Application: The Knowledge System in Society.* Boston: Allyn and Bacon.

Homans, P. (1989). *The Ability to Mourn: Disillusionment and the Social Origins of Psychoanalysis.* Chicago: University of Chicago Press.

Horney, K. (1942). *Self-Analysis.* New York: Norton.

Hosie, T.W. et.al. (1989). "School and Rehabilitation Counselor Preparation: Meeting the Needs of Individuals with Disabilities." *Journal of Counseling Development* 68(1), pp. 68, 171.

Howe, D. (1989). *The Consumers' View of Family Therapy.* Hants, England: Gower.

Hudson, W. W. (1982). *The Clinical Measurement Package: A Field Manual.* Homewood, IL: Dorsey.

Huebner, L. et al. (1981). "Stress Management Training in Medical School." *Journal of Medical Education* 56, pp. 547-558.

Hughes, E. C. (1963). "Professions." *Daedalus* 92 (Fall), pp. 655-668.

Hutchinson, D. (1935). "Supervision in Social Case Work." *The Family* 16, pp. 44-47.

Jackson, V. H. and Lopez, L. (1999). *Cultural Competency in Managed Behavioral Healthcare.* Providence, RI: Behavioral Health Resource Press.

Jacobs, D., David, P. and Meyer, D. J. (1995). *The Supervisory Encounter: A Guide for Teachers of Psychodynamic Psychotherapy and Psychoanalysis.* New Haven, CT: Yale University Press.

Jacobson, N. and Gottman, J. (1998). *When Men Batter Women: New Insights into Ending Abusive Relationships.* New York: Simon and Schuster.

Jaffee, v. Special Administrator for Allen, Deceased v. Redmond et al., no. 95-266 (U.S. decided June 13, 1996).

Jayaratne, S. and Levy, R. L. (1979). *Empirical Clinical Practice.* New York: Columbia University Press.

Jivanjee, P. R. (1999). "Social Work Field Education to Serve Vulnerable Populations: A Case Study." *Journal of Teaching in Social Work* 18, pp. 185-207.

Jones, J. H. (1981). *Bad Blood: The Tuskegee Syphilis Experiment.* New York: The Free Press.

Jones, R. W. (1970). "Social Values and Social Work Education." In K. A. Kendall (ed.), *Social Work Values in an Age of Discontent.* New York: Council on Social Work Education, pp. 35-45.

Judson, H. F. (1980). *The Search for Solutions.* New York: Holt, Rinehart and Winston.

Jung, C. G. (1957). *The Undiscovered Self.* New York: Mentor.

Kadushin, A. (1968). "Games People Play in Supervision." *Social Work* 8 (March), pp. 23-32.

Kadushin, A. (1972). *The Social Work Interview.* New York: Columbia University Press.

Kadushin, A. (1974). "Supervisor-Supervisee." *Social Work* 19 (May), pp. 288-297.

Kadushin, A. (1976a). "Men in a Women's Profession." *Social Work* 21, pp. 440- 447.

Kadushin, A. (1976b). *Supervision in Social Work.* New York: Columbia University Press.

Kadushin, A. (1977). *Consultation in Social Work.* New York: Columbia University Press.

Kadushin, A. (1992). *Supervision in Social Work,* Third Edition. New York: Columbia University Press.

Kahn, A. (ed.) (1973). *Shaping the New Social Work.* New York: Columbia University Press.

Kahn, E. M. (1979). "The Parallel Process in Social Work Treatment and Supervision," *Social Casework* 60 (November), pp. 520-528.

Kanter, R. M. (1977). *Men and Women of the Corporation.* New York: Basic Books.

Kanter, R. M. and Stein, B. A. (1979). "The Gender Pioneers: Women in an Industrial Sales Force." In R. M. Kanter and B. A. Stein (eds.), *Life in Organizations: Work Places As People Experience Them.* New York: Basic Books, pp. 134-160.

Kaplan, A. (1964). *The Conduct of Inquiry: Methodology for Behavioral Science.* San Francisco: Chandler.

Kaplan, A. G. et al. (1983). "Women and Anger in Psychotherapy." In J. H. Robbins and R. L. Siegel (eds.), *Women Changing Therapy.* Binghamton, NY: The Haworth Press, pp. 29-40.

Kaplan, H. I. and Sadock, B. J. (1998). *Synopsis of Psychiatry: Behavioral Sciences/Clinical Psychiatry,* Eighth Edition. Baltimore, MD: Williams and Wilkins.

Karls, J. M. and Wandrei, K. E. (1994). *Person-in-Environment System: The PIE Classification System for Social Functioning Problems.* Washington, DC: NASW Press.

Kaslow, F. W. (ed.) (1972). *Issues in the Human Services.* San Francisco: Jossey-Bass.

Kaslow, F. W. (ed.) (1979). *Supervision, Consultation, and Staff Training in the Helping Professions.* San Francisco: Jossey-Bass.

Kazan, A. E. (ed.) (1992). *Methodological Issues and Strategies in Clinical Research.* Washington, DC: American Psychological Association.

Keefe, T. and Maypole, D. E. (1983). *Relationships in Social Service Practice.* Monterey, CA: Brooks/Cole.

Kendall, K. A. (1982). "A Sixty Year Perspective of Social Work." *Social Casework* 63 (September), pp. 424-428.

Kenemore, T. K. (1991). "Board Certified Diplomate: Who Cares?" *Clinical Social Work Journal* 19 (Spring), pp. 83-93.

Kennedy-Moore, E. and Watson, J. C. (1999). *Expressing Emotion: Myths, Realities, and Therapeutic Strategies*. New York: Guilford.

Kessler, R. C., McGonagle, K.O., and Zhao, S. (1994). "Lifetime and 12-Month Prevalence of DSM-III-R Psychiatric Disorders in the United States." *Archives of General Psychiatry* 51, 8-19.

Kets de Vries, M. F. R. (ed.) (1984). *The Irrational Executive: Psychoanalytic Studies in Management*. New York: International Universities Press.

Kets de Vries, M. F. R. and Miller, D. (1984). *The Neurotic Organization: Diagnosing and Revitalizing Unhealthy Companies*. New York: Harper Business.

Kirk, S. A. and Fischer, J. (1976). "Do Social Workers Understand Research?" *Journal of Education for Social Work* 12 (Winter), pp. 63-70.

Knapp, S. and Vandecreek, L. (1997). "Ethical and Legal Aspects of Clinical Supervision." In C. E. Watkins (ed.), *Handbook of Psychotherapy Supervision*. New York: John Wiley, pp. 589-599.

Knowles, M. (1970). *The Modern Practice of Adult Education: Andragogy versus Pedagogy*. New York: Association Press.

Koocher, G. P., Norcross, J. C., and Hill, S. S. (1998). *Psychologists' Desk Reference*. New York: Oxford University Press.

Kopp, S. (1976). *The Naked Therapist: A Collection of Embarrassments*. San Diego: EDITS.

Krager, H. J. and Levine, J. (1999). *The Internet and Technology for the Human Services*. New York: Longman.

Kramer, C. H. (1980). *Becoming a Family Therapist: Developing an Integrated Approach to Working with Families*. New York: Human Sciences Press.

Krause, E. A. (1977). *Power and Illness: The Political Sociology of Health and Medical Care*. New York: Elsevier.

Lachman, R. et al. (1979). *Cognitive Psychology and Information Processing: An Introduction*. Hillside, NJ: Lawrence Erlbaum.

Lago, C. and Thompson, J. (1997). "The Triangle with Curved Sides: Sensitivity to Issues of Race and Culture in Supervision." In G. Shipton (ed.), *Supervision of Psychotherapy and Counseling: Making A Place to Think*. Buckingham, England: The Open University, pp. 119-130.

Lane, R. C. (ed.) (1990). *Psychoanalytic Approaches to Supervision*. New York: Brunner/Mazel.

Langs, R. (1976). *The Therapeutic Interaction, Volume 11: A Critical Overview and Synthesis*. New York: Jason Aronson.

Langs, R. (1979). *The Supervisory Experience*. New York: Jason Aronson.

Langs, R. (1982). *The Psychotherapeutic Conspiracy*. New York: Jason Aronson.

Lasch, C. (1979). *The Culture of Narcissism: American Life in an Age of Diminishing Expectations*. New York: Norton.

Lastrucci, C. L. (1967). *The Scientific Approach: Basic Principles of the Scientific Method*. Cambridge, MA: Schenkman.

Lecker, S. (1976). "Family Therapies" In B. B. Wolman (ed.), *The Therapist's Handbook: Treatment Methods of Mental Disorders.* New York: Van Nostrand Reinhold, pp. 184-198.

Lee, P. R. and Kenworthy, M. E. (1929). *Mental Hygiene and Social Work.* New York: Commonwealth Fund.

Lerner, M. (1986). *Surplus Powerlessness: The Psychodynamics of Everyday Life and Psychology of Individual Transformation.* Atlantic Highlands, NJ: Humanities Press International.

Levi-Strauss, C. (1978). "Science: Forever Incomplete." *Johns Hopkins Magazine* 39 (July), p. 30.

Levy, C. (1973). "The Ethics of Supervision." *Social Work* 18 (March), pp. 14-21.

Lewin, K. K. (1970). *Brief Psychotherapy: Brief Encounters.* St. Louis, MO: Warren H. Green.

Lichter, S. R. et al. (1991). *Watching America: What Television Tells Us About Our Lives.* New York: Prentice-Hall.

Lief, A. (1948). *The Commonsense Psychiatry of Dr. Adolf Meyer.* New York: McGraw-Hill.

Linzer, N. (1999). *Resolving Ethical Dilemmas in Social Work Practice.* Boston: Allyn and Bacon.

Livneh, H. and Thomas, K. R. (1997). "Psychosocial Aspects of Disability." *Rehabilitation Education* 11(3), pp. 173-183.

Lowe, J. I. and Austin, M. J. (1997). "Using Direct Practice Skills in Administration." *The Clinical Supervisor* 15(2), pp. 129-145.

Lowenburg, F. et al. (2000). *Ethical Decisions for Social Work Practice,* Sixth Edition. Itasca, IL: Peacock.

Lowy, L. (1979). *Social Work with the Aging: The Challenge and Promise of the Later Years.* New York: Harper and Row.

Luborsky, L. and Crits-Christoph, P. (1990). *Understanding Transference: The CCRT Method.* New York: Basic Books.

Lum, D. (1999). *Culturally Competent Practice: A Framework of Growth and Action.* Belmont, CA: Wadsworth Publishing Co.

Lum, D. (2000). *Social Work Practice and People of Color: A Process-Stage Approach.* Belmont, CA: Wadsworth Publishing Co.

Lundblad, K. S. (1995). "Jane Addams and Social Reform: A Role Model for the 1990s." *Social Work* 40, pp. 661-669.

Luthman, S. G. and Kirschenbaum, M. (1974). *The Dynamic Family.* Palo Alto, CA: Science and Behavior Books.

Lynch, E. W. and Hanson, M. J. (ed.) (1998). *Developing Cross-Cultural Competence: A Guide for Working with Children and Their Families,* Second Edition. Baltimore, MD: Paul H. Brookes.

Macbeth, J. E. et al. (1995). *Legal and Risk Management Issues in the Practice of Psychiatry.* Washington, DC: Psychiatrists' Purchasing Group.

Madrick, J. (1995). *The End of Affluence: The Causes and Consequences of America's Economic Dilemma*. New York: Random House.

Magee, J. J. (1982). "Integrating Research Skills with Human Behavior and Social Environment: Assessing Historical and Cultural Influences on Students' Family Structure." *Journal of Education for Social Work* 18 (Winter), pp. 14-19.

Mandell, B. (1973). "The 'Equality' Revolution and Supervision." *Journal of Education for Social Work* 9 (Winter), pp. 43-54.

Marcus, P. M. and Marcus, D. (1972). "Control in Modern Organizations." In M. B. Brinkenhoff and P. R. Kung (eds.), *Complex Organizations and Their Environments*. Dubuque, IA: W. C. Brown, pp. 234-243.

Marecek, J. and Kravetz, D. (1982). "Women and Mental Health: A Review of Feminist Change Efforts." In H. Rubenstein and M. H. Bloch (eds.), *Things That Matter*. New York: Macmillan, pp. 296-303.

Margolin, G. (1998). "Effects of Domestic Violence on Children." In P. K. Trickett, and C. J. Shellenbach, *Violence Against Children in the Family and the Community*. Washington, DC: American Psychological Association, pp. 57-100.

Marsh, R. C. (ed.) (1971). *Bertrand Russell: Logic and Knowledge*. New York: Capricorn.

Marshall, R. J. and Marshall, S. V. (1988). *The Transference Countertransference Matrix: The Emotional-Cognitive Dialogue in Psychotherapy, Psychoanalysis, and Supervision*. New York: Columbia.

McGoldrick, M. et. al. (1991). *Women in Families: A Framework for Family Therapy*. New York: W.W. Norton and Company.

Mead, D. E. (1990). *Effective Supervision: A Task-Oriented Model for Mental Health Professions*. New York: Brunner/Mazel.

Melton, G. B. et. al. (1997). *Psychological Evaluation for the Courts: A Handbook for Mental Health Professionals and Lawyers*, Second Edition. New York: Guilford.

Merriam-Webster's Collegiate Dictionary (1994), Tenth Edition. Springfield, MA: Merriam-Webster, Inc.

Meyer, R. G. et. al. (1988). *Law for the Psychotherapist*. New York: W.W. Norton.

Mezzich, J. E. et. al. (eds.) (1996). *Culture and Psychiatric Diagnosis: A DSM-IV Perspective*. Washington, DC: American Psychiatric Press.

Miller, M. C. (1988). *Boxed In: The Culture of TV*. Evanston, IL: Northwestern University Press.

Mills, C. W. (1959). *The Sociological Imagination*. New York: Oxford University Press.

Milwid, B. (1983). "Breaking In: Experience in Male-Dominated Professions." In J. H. Robbins and R. J. Siegel (eds.), *Women Changing Therapy: New Assessments, Values and Strategies in Feminist Therapy*. Binghamton, NY: The Haworth Press, pp. 67-79.

Minahan, A. (1980). "What Is Clinical Social Work?" *Social Work* 25 (May), p. 171.

Minuchin, S. (1974). *Families and Family Therapy.* Cambridge, MA: Harvard University Press.

Mishne, J. (1980). *Psychotherapy and Training in Clinical Social Work.* New York: Gardner.

Moline, M. E. et. al. (1998). *Documenting Psychotherapy: Essentials for Mental Health Practitioners.* Thousand Oaks, CA: Sage.

Morgan, N. (1995). *How to Interview Sexual Abuse Victims.* Thousand Oaks, CA: Sage.

Morrison, M. R. and Stamps, R. F. (1998). *DSM-IV Internet Companion.* New York: Norton.

Motenko, A. K. et al. (1995). "Privatization and Cutbacks: Social Work and Client Impressions of Service Delivery in Massachusetts." *Social Work* 40, pp. 456-463.

Munson, C. E. (1974). "Definition of the Situation and Viewing Television Newscasts." *Sociological Research Symposium Proceedings* IV. Richmond, VA: Virginia Commonwealth University, pp. 452-459.

Munson, C. E. (1975). "The Uses of Structural, Authority and Teaching Models in Social Work Supervision." DSW dissertation, University of Maryland, 1975; Ann Arbor, MI: University Microfilms International.

Munson, C. E. (1976). "Professional Autonomy and Social Work Supervision." *Journal of Education for Social Work* 12 (Fall), pp. 95-102.

Munson, C. E. (1979a). "Applied Sociology and Social Work: Manpower and Theoretical Issues." *Journal of Sociology and Social Welfare* 6 (September), pp. 611-621.

Munson, C. E. (1979b). "Evaluation of Male and Female Supervisors." *Social Work* 24 (March), pp. 104-110.

Munson, C. E. (ed.) (1979c). *Social Work Supervision: Classic Statements and Critical Issues.* New York: The Free Press.

Munson, C. E. (1979d). "Supervision and Consultation in Rural Mental Health Practice." In *Proceedings, Fourth National Institute on Social Work in Rural Areas,* Laramie: University of Wyoming, pp. 87-93.

Munson, C. E. (1979e). "Symbolic Interaction and Social Work Supervision." *Journal of Sociology and Social Welfare* 6 (January), pp. 8-18.

Munson, C. E. (1980a). "Differential Impact of Structure and Authority in Supervision." *Arete* 6 (Spring), pp. 3-15.

Munson, C. E. (1980b). "Social Work in Aging." *Gerontology and Geriatrics Education* 1(1) (Fall), pp. 17-23.

Munson, C. E. (1980c). "Supervising the Family Therapist." *Social Casework* 61 (March), pp. 131-137.

Munson, C. E. (1980d). "Urban Rural Differences: Implications for Social Work Education and Training." *Journal of Education for Social Work* 16 (Winter), pp. 95-103.

Munson, C. E. (1981a)."Social Work Educational Consultation in Church-Related Nursing Homes." *Gerontology and Geriatrics Education* 1(3) (Spring), pp. 175-180.

Munson, C. E. (1981b). *Supervision for Clinical Practice.* Paper presented at Fifth Annual State Convention, National Association of Social Workers, El Paso, TX, October 21-23, pp. 1-16.

Munson, C. E. (1982a). "Perceptions of Female Social Workers Toward Administrative Positions." *Social Casework* 63, pp. 54-59.

Munson, C. E. (1982b). "A Study of Distress Reactions in Public Welfare Practitioners." Unpublished manuscript.

Munson, C. E. (1983a). *An Introduction to Clinical Social Work Supervision.* Binghamton, NY: The Haworth Press.

Munson, C. E. (1983b). "Stress Among Hospital Social Workers: An Empirical Study." Unpublished manuscript.

Munson, C. E. (1984). "Stress Among Graduate Social Work Students: An Empirical Study." *Journal of Education for Social Work* 20(3), pp. 20-29.

Munson, C. E. (1986). "Editorial: A Study of Ethics." *The Clinical Supervisor* 4 (Fall), pp. 1-5.

Munson, C. E. (1988). "Computers in Social Work Education." *Computers in Human Services* 3(1/2), pp. 143-157.

Munson, C. E. (1992). "Editorial: The Idea of Stress Revisited." *The Clinical Supervisor* 10(2), pp. 1-10.

Munson, C.E. (1993a). *Clinical Social Work Supervision,* Second Edition. Binghamton, NY: The Haworth Press.

Munson, C. E. (1993b). "The 'P' Word and Mental Health Services." *The Clinical Supervisor* 11(2), pp. 1-5.

Munson, C. E. (1994a). "Cognitive Family Therapy." In D. K. Granvold (ed.), *Cognitive and Behavioral Treatment: Methods and Applications.* Pacific Grove, CA: Brooks/Cole, pp. 202-221.

Munson, C. E. (1994b). "Editorial: Supervision and Revictimization of Children." *The Clinical Supervisor* 12(2), pp. 1-7.

Munson, C. E. (1995a). "Control and Authority in Mental Health Services." *Managed Care News* (March/May), pp. 2-4.

Munson, C. E. (1995b). *Foundation Concepts for Survival of Ethical Social Work Practice in the Health Care Environment.* Paper presented at National Institutes of Health, Bethesda, MD, September 15, pp. 1-15.

Munson, C. E.. (1996a). "Autonomy and Managed Care in Clinical Social Work Practice." *Smith College Studies in Social Work* 66 (June), pp. 241-260.

Munson, C. E. (1996b). "Autonomy and Managed Care in Clinical Social Work Practice." In G. Schamess (ed.), *The Corporate and Human Faces of Managed Health Care: The Interplay Between Mental Health Policy and Practice.* Northampton, MA: Smith College Studies in Social Work, pp. 241-260.

Munson, C. E. (1996c). *Clinical Supervision Curriculum Guide: Training Curriculum for Supervisors of Social Workers Seeking Licensure as Licensed Clinical Social Workers (LCSW's) by the Virginia Board of Social Work.* Culpeper, VA: Virginia Board of Social Work and American Association of Social Work Boards of Examiners.

Munson, C. E. (1996d). "Should Doctoral Programs Graduate Students Without Two Years Post-MSW Experience? NO!" *Journal of Social Work Education* 13(2), (Spring/Summer) pp. 158-172.

Munson, C. E. (1996e). "Technology, Change and the Clinical Social Work Practice Curriculum." In E. Torre (ed.), *Modes of Social Work Education II: The Electronic Social Work Curriculum in the Twenty-First Century.* New Orleans: Tulane Studies in Social Work, Tulane University Press, pp. 86-106.

Munson, C. E. (1997a). "The Future of Clinical Social Work and Managed Cost Organizations." *Psychiatric Services, A Journal of the American Psychiatric Association,* 48 (April), pp. 479-482.

Munson, C. E. (1997b). "Gender and Psychotherapy Supervision: The Partnership Model." In C. E. Watkins (ed.), *Handbook of Psychotherapy Supervision.* New York: John Wiley, pp. 549-569.

Munson, C. E. (1998a). "Evolution and Trends in the Relationship Between Clinical Social Work Practice and Managed Cost Organizations." In G. Schamess and A. Lightburn (eds.), *Humane Managed Care?* Washington, DC: NASW Press, pp. 308-324.

Munson, C. E. (1998b). "Social Work Students' Knowledge of Feminism." *Journal of Teaching in Social Work* 16(1/2) (Winter), pp. 57-73.

Munson, C. E. (1998c). "Societal Change, Managed Cost Organizations, and Clinical Social Work Practice." *The Clinical Supervisor* 17(2), pp. 1-41.

Munson, C. E. (2000a). "Language Delays and Child Trauma: The Clinical Supervisor's Role." *The Clinical Supervisor,* in press.

Munson, C. E. (2000b). *The Mental Health Diagnostic Desk Reference: Visual Guides and More for Learning to Use the Diagnostic and Statistical Manual (DSM-IV).* Binghamton, NY: The Haworth Press.

Munson, C. E. (2000c). "Supervision Standards of Practice in an Era of Societal Restructuring." In P. Allen-Meares and C. Garvin (eds.), *Handbook of Direct Practice in Social Work: Future Directions and Guidelines.* Beverly Hills, CA: Sage Publications, in press.

Munson, C. E. (2001a). *Assessment, Diagnosis and Treatment of the Traumatized Child.* Binghamton, NY: The Haworth Press.

Munson, C. E. (2001b). *The Mental Health Diagnostic Desk Reference: Visual Guides and More for Learning to Use the Diagnostic and Statistical Manual (DSM-IV-TR).* Binghamton, NY: The Haworth Press.

Munson, C. E. and Balgopal, P. (1978). "The Worker/Client Relationship: Relevant Role Theory." *Journal of Sociology and Social Welfare* 3 (May), pp. 404-417.

Munson, C. E. and Hipp, J. (1998). "Social Work Students' Knowledge of Feminism." *Journal of Teaching in Social Work* 16 (Winter), pp. 57-73.

Naisbitt, J. (1982). *Megatrends: Ten New Directions Transforming Our Lives*. New York: Warner Books.

Naisbitt, J. (1999). *High Tech-High Touch: Technology and Our Search for Meaning*. New York: Broadway Books.

National Association of Social Workers (1974). *Social Casework: Generic and Specific: A Report of the Milford Conference*. Washington, DC: NASW, Classic Series.

National Association of Social Workers (1982). "Ethics Violator Gets a Suspension," *NASW News* 27 (October), p. 12.

National Association of Social Workers (1987). *NASW Register of Clinical Social Workers, 1987*. Washington, DC: NASW.

National Association of Social Workers (1990). Code of Ethics. Washington, DC: NASW.

National Association of Social Workers (1991). *A Membership Sketch*. Washington, DC: NASW.

National Association of Social Workers (1995). *Encyclopedia of Social Work*, Nineteenth Edition. Washington, DC: NASW Press.

National Association of Social Workers (1996). Code of Ethics. Washington, DC: NASW.

National Association of Social Workers (1999). Code of Ethics. Washington, DC.

Nelson, G. L. (1978). "Psychotherapy Supervision from the Trainee's Point of View: A Survey of Preferences." *Professional Psychology* 10 (November), pp. 539-549.

Nicholson, J. et al. (1996). "Impact of Medicaid Managed Care on Child and Adolescent Emergency Mental Health Screening in Massachusetts." *Psychiatric Services* 47, pp. 1344-1350.

Oklin, R. (1999). *What Psychotherapists Should Know About Disability*. New York: Guilford.

Olin, J. T. and Keatinge, C. (1998). *Rapid Psychological Assessment*. New York: Wiley.

Olshevski, J. I., Katz, A. D., and Knight, B. G. (1999). *Stress Reduction for Caregivers*. Philadelphia: Brunner/Mazel.

O'Neil, J. V. (1999). "Profession Dominates in Mental Health." *NASW News* 44(6) (June), pp. 1-8.

O'Neill, P. and Trickett, E. J. (1982). *Community Consultation: Strategies for Facilitating Change in Schools, Hospitals, Prisons, Social Service Programs, and Other Community Settings*. San Francisco: Jossey-Bass.

Ozawa, M. N. (1997). "Demographic Changes and Their Implications." In M. Reisch and E. Gambrill (eds.), *Social Work in the 21st Century*. Thousand Oaks, CA: Pine Forge Press, pp. 8-27.

Panter, B. M. et. al. (1995). *Creativity and Madness: Psychological Studies of Art and Artists.* Burbank, CA: AIMED Press.

Parad, H. J. and Miller, R. R. (1963). *Ego-Oriented Casework: Problems and Perspectives.* New York: Family Service Association of America.

Parkinson, C. N. (1957). *Parkinson's Law and Other Studies in Administration.* Boston: Houghton Mifflin.

Parsons, T. (1937). *The Structure of Social Action.* New York: McGraw-Hill.

Parsons, T. (1951). *The Social System.* Glencoe, IL: The Free Press.

Patterson, J. and Kim, P. (1991). *The Day America Told the Truth.* New York: Prentice-Hall.

Pearlin, L. I. and Schooler, C. (1978). "The Structure of Coping." *Journal of Health and Social Behavior* 19 (March), pp. 2-21.

Perkins, J. F. (1944). "Common Sense and Bad Boys." *Atlantic Monthly* 173 (May), pp. 43-47.

Perlman, H. H. (1957). *Social Casework: A Problem-Solving Process.* Chicago: University of Chicago Press.

Perlman, H. H. (1969a). *Helping: Charlotte Towle on Social Work and Social Casework.* Chicago: University of Chicago Press.

Perlman, H. H. (1969b). *Social Casework: A Problem-Solving Process.* Chicago: University of Chicago Press.

Pettes, D. E. (1967). *Supervision in Social Work: A Method of Student Training and Staff Development.* London: Allen and Unwin.

Pettes, D.E. (1979). *Student and Staff Supervision: A Task-Centered Approach* London: Allen and Unwin.

Phillips, D. (1995). "Professional Standards and Managed Care." *National Federation of Societies for Clinical Social Work Progress Report* 13(1), pp. 11.

Pickering, G. (1974). *Creative Malady: Illness in the Lives and Minds of Charles Darwin, Florence Nightingale, Mary Baker Eddy, Sigmund Freud, Marcel Proust, Elizabeth Barrett Browning.* New York: Dell.

Pincus, A. and Minahan, A. (1973). *Social Work Practice: Model and Method.* Itasca, IL: Peacock.

Pine, F. (1990). *Drive, Ego, Object, and Self: A Synthesis for Clinical Work.* New York: Basic Books.

Plant, J. (1944). "Social Significance of War Impact on Adolescents." *The Annals of the American Academy of Political and Social Science* 236 (November), pp. 1-7.

Pogrebin, L. C. (1980). *Growing Up Free.* New York: Bantam.

Pollock, E. J. (1998). "With 'Case Rates' Cures Come Fast or the Doctor Incurs a Loss." *The Wall Street Journal* 231(2), p. A1.

Pope-Davis, D. B., and Coleman, H. L. K. (eds.) (1997*). Multicultural Counseling Competencies: Assessment, Education and Training, and Supervision.* Thousand Oaks, CA: Sage.

Porter, N. (1985). "New Perspectives on Therapy Supervision." In L. B. Rosewater and L. E. A. Walker (eds.), *Handbook of Feminist Therapy: Women's Issues in Psychotherapy*. New York: Springer, pp. 332-343.

Powell, D. J. and Brodsky, A. (1993). *Clinical Supervision in Alcohol and Drug Abuse Counseling: Principles, Models, Methods*. New York: Lexington.

Powicke, F. (1955). *Modern Historians and the Study of History*. London: Odhams, 1955.

Pratt, L. (1969). "Levels of Sociological Knowledge Among Health and Social Workers." *Journal of Health and Social Behavior* 10 (March), pp. 59-65.

Priest, R. (1994). Minority Supervisor and Majority Supervisee: Another Perspective of Clinical Reality. *Counselor Education and Supervision* 34, 152-158.

Pruger, R. (1973). "The Good Bureaucrat." *Social Work* 18 (July), pp. 26-32.

Psychotherapy Finances (1995a). "Managed Care Notes," 21(10), p. 5.

Psychotherapy Finances (1995b). "Special Report: What Is Your Professional Organization Doing for Your Practice?" 21(7), p. 6.

Psychotherapy Finances (1996). "Professional Notes: Mental Health Ranks Low on People's List of Health Care Priorities," 22(7), p. 10.

Public Health Service (1994). *Clinician's Handbook of Preventive Services*. Washington, DC: U.S. Department of Health and Human Services.

Rabin, H. M. (1967). "How Does Co-Therapy Compare with Regular Group Therapy?" *American Journal of Psychotherapy* 21 (April), pp. 244-255.

Ray, O. and Ksir, C. (1996). *Drugs, Society, and Human Behavior*. St Louis: Mosby.

Reamer. F. (1993). *The Philosophical Foundations of Social Work*. New York: Columbia University Press.

Reamer. F. (1995). *Social Work Values and Ethics*. New York: Columbia University Press.

Redl, F. and Wineman, D. (1951). *Children Who Hate*. New York: The Free Press.

Redl, F. and Wineman, D. (1952). *Controls from Within: Techniques for the Treatment of the Aggressive Child*. New York: The Free Press.

Reeser, J. C. and Epstein, I. (1990). *Professionalization and Activism in Social Work: The Sixties, the Eighties, and the Future*. New York: Columbia University Press.

Reeves, E. T. (1980). *So You Want to Be a Supervisor!* New York: AMACOM, American Management Associations.

Reid, W. J. (1978). *The Task-Centered System*. New York: Columbia University Press.

Reid, W. J. (1981). "Mapping the Knowledge Base of Social Work." *Social Work* 26 (March), pp. 124-132.

Reid, W. J. (1992). *Task Strategies: An Empirical Approach to Clinical Social Work*. New York: Columbia University Press.

Reid, W. J. and Epstein, L. (1972). *Task-Centered Casework*. New York: Columbia University Press.

Reisch, M. and Gambrill, E. (1997). *Social Work in the 21st Century.* Thousand Oaks, CA: Pine Forge Press.

Reiter, L. (1980). "Professional Morale and Social Work Training: A Study." *Clinical Social Work Journal* 8 (Fall), pp. 198-209.

Reynolds, B. C. (1965/1942). *Learning and Teaching in the Practice of Social Work,* Reprint Edition. New York: Russell and Russell.

Reynolds, B. C. (1973). *Between Client and Community: A Study in Responsibility in Social Casework,* Reprint Edition. New York: Oriole.

Rice, D. G. et al. (1972). "Therapist Experience and Style As Factors in Cotherapy." *Family Process* 11 (March), pp. 1-12.

Richmond, M. (1917). *Social Diagnosis.* New York: Russell Sage Foundation.

Richmond, M. (1965/1917). *Social Diagnosis.* New York: Russell Sage Foundation, Reprint Edition. New York: The Free Press.

Rippere, V. and Williams, R. (1985). *Wounded Healers: Mental Health Workers' Experiences of Depression.* New York: John Wiley and Sons.

Roazen, P. (1974). *Freud and His Followers.* New York: Knopf.

Robbins, J. H. and Siegel, R. J . (eds.) (1983). *Women Changing Therapy: New Assessments, Values and Strategies in Feminist Therapy.* Binghamton, NY: The Haworth Press.

Robinson, V. P. (1930). *A Changing Psychology in Social Case Work.* Chapel Hill, NC: University of North Carolina Press.

Robson, C. (1993). *Real World Research: A Resource for Social Scientists and Practitioner-Researchers.* Oxford, UK: Blackwell.

Rock, B. (1990). "Social Worker Autonomy in an Age of Accountability." *The Clinical Supervisor* 8 (Summer), pp. 19-31.

Rock, M. H. (ed.) (1997). *Psychodynamic Supervision: Perspectives of the Supervisor and the Supervisee.* Northvale, NJ: Jason Aronson.

Rosenbaum, M. and Ronen, T. (1998). "Clinical Supervision from the Standpoint of Cognitive-Behavior Therapy." *Psychotherapy* 35(2), pp. 220-230.

Rosenblatt, A. (1968). "The Practitioner's Use and Evaluation of Research." *Social Work* 13 (January), pp. 53-59.

Rossman, P. (1977). *Hospice.* New York: Fawcett.

Rubin, S. S. (1997). "Balancing Duty to Client and Therapist in Supervision: Clinical, Ethical and Training Issues." *The Clinical Supervisor* 16(1), pp. 1-23.

Ruckdeschel, R. A. and Farris, B. E. (1982). "Science: Critical Faith or Dogmatic Ritual." *Social Casework* 63 (May), pp. 272-275.

Rustin, M. (1998). "Observation, Understanding and Interpretation: The Story of a Supervision." *Journal of Child Psychotherapy* 24(3) (December), pp. 433-448.

Ryan, A.S. and Hendricks, C. O. (1989). "Culture and Communication: Supervising the Asian and Hispanic Social Worker." *The Clinical Supervisor* 7, pp. 27-40.

Sabin, J. E. (1997). "Managed Care: What Confidentiality Standards Should We Advocate for in Mental Health Care, and How Should We Do It?" *Psychiatric Services* 48(1), pp. 35-41.

Sales, E. and Navarre, E. (1970). *Individual and Group Supervision in Field Instruction: A Research Report.* Ann Arbor, MI: University of Michigan, School of Social Work.

Samantrai, K. (1991). "Clinical Social Work in Public Child Welfare Practice." *Social Work* 36 (July), pp. 359-361.

Sartre, J. P. (1976). *Sartre on Theater.* New York: Pantheon.

Schafer, R. (1976). *A New Language for Psychoanalysis.* New Haven, CT: Yale University Press.

Schamess, G. (1998). "Corporate Values and Managed Mental Health Care: Who Profits and Who Benefits?" In G. Schamess and A. Lightburn (eds.), *Humane Managed Care?* Washington, DC: NASW Press, pp. 23-35.

Schamess, G. and Lightburn, A. (1998). *Humane Managed Care.* Washington, DC: NASW Press.

Scheflen, A. E. (1972). *Body Language and the Social Order: Communication As Behavior Control.* Englewood Cliffs, NJ: Prentice-Hall.

Scheibe, K. E. (1970). *Beliefs and Values.* New York: Holt, Rinehart and Winston.

Schoenwald, R. L. (1976). "Belly Dancing or Baudelaire?" *The Chronicle of Higher Education* 13 (December 6), p. 32.

Schor, J. B. (1991). *The Overworked American: The Unexpected Decline of Leisure.* New York: Basic Books.

Schuler, E. A. et al. (eds.) (1971). *Readings in Sociology.* New York: Crowell.

Schumacher, E. F. (1977). *A Guide for the Perplexed.* New York: Perennial Library.

Schutz, B. M. (1982). *Legal Liability in Psychotherapy: A Practitioner's Guide to Risk Management.* San Francisco: Jossey-Bass.

Scotch, B. C. (1971). "Sex Status in Social Work: Grist for Women's Liberation." *Social Work* 16, pp. 5-11.

Seefeldt, C. et al. (1977). "Using Pictures to Explore Children's Attitudes Toward the Elderly." *The Gerontologist* 17 (December), pp. 506-512.

Seiden, A. M. (1982). "Overview: Research on the Psychology of Women." In H. Rubenstein and M. H. Bloch (eds.), *Things That Matter: Influences on Helping Relationships.* New York: Macmillan, pp. 285-295.

Selye, H. (1974). *Stress Without Distress.* New York: New American Library.

Sennett, R. (1980). *Authority.* New York: Knopf.

Sergiovanni, T. J. and Starratt, R. J. (1979). *Supervision: Human Perspectives.* New York: McGraw-Hill.

Sharp, A. M. et al. (2000). *Economics of Social Issues,* Fourteenth Edition. Boston: Irwin McGraw-Hill.

Shea, S. C. (1998). *Psychiatric Interviewing. The Art of Understanding: A Practical Guide for Psychiatrists, Psychologists, Counselors, Social Workers, Nurses, and Other Mental Health Professionals.* Philadelphia: W. B. Saunders.

Shorter, E. (1997). *A History of Psychiatry: From the Era of the Asylum to the Age of Prozac.* New York: Wiley.

Shulman, L. (1982). *Skills of Supervision and Staff Management*. Itasca, IL: Peacock.

Shulman, L. (1993). *Interactional Supervision*. Washington, DC: NASW Press.

Simon, B. K. (1977). "Diversity and Unity in the Social Work Profession." *Social Work* 22 (September), pp. 395-400.

Simon, R. (1982). "'Always with Guts': An Interview with Mara Selvini Palazzoli." *The Family Therapy Networker* 6 (May-June), pp. 29-32.

Siporin, M. (1956). "Dual Supervision of Psychiatric Social Workers." *Social Work* 1 (April), pp. 32-42.

Siporin, M. (1975). *Introduction to Social Work Practice*. New York: Macmillan.

Siporin, M. (1980). "Marriage and Family Therapy in Social Work." *Social Casework* 61 (January), pp. 11-21.

Sobel, D. (1980). "Psychotherapy from A to Z." *Houston Post* (November 16), p. 3.

Specht, H. and Courtney, M. (1994). *Unfaithful Angels: How Social Work Has Abandoned Its Mission*. New York: Free Press.

Spencer, H. (1902). *The Data of Ethics*. New York: P. F. Collier.

Stearns, P. N. and Lewis, J. (1998). *An Emotional History of the United States*. New York: New York University Press.

Stein, M. I. (ed.) (1961). *Contemporary Psychotherapies*. New York: The Free Press.

Stein, R. H. (1990). *Ethical Issues in Counseling*. New York: Prometheus.

Steinberg, R. J. and Davidson, J. E. (1982). "The Mind of the Puzzler." *Psychology Today* 16 (June), pp. 37-44.

Steinhelber, J. et al. (1984). "An Investigation of Some Relationship Between Psychotherapy Supervision and Patient Change." *Journal of Clinical Psychology* 40(6), pp. 1314-1353.

Steininger, M., Newell, J. D., and Garcia, L. T. (1984). *Ethical Issues in Psychology*. Homewood, IL: The Dorsey Press.

Stevenson, G. S. (1940). "Mental Hygiene of Children." *The Annals of the American Academy of Political and Social Science* 212 (November), pp. 130-137.

Stevenson, L. (1974). *Seven Theories of Human Nature*. New York: Oxford University Press.

Stoltenberg, C. D., McNeil, B., and Delworth, V. (1998). *IDM Supervision: An Integrated Developmental Model for Supervising Counselor Therapists*. San Francisco: Jossey-Bass.

Stone, M. H. (1997). *Healing the Mind: A History of Psychiatry from Antiquity to the Present*. New York: W.W. Norton.

Strean, H. S. (1978). *Clinical Social Work: Theory and Practice*. New York: The Free Press.

Strean, H. S. (1979). *Psychoanalytic Theory and Social Work Practice*. New York: The Free Press.

Streepy, J. (1981). "Direct-Service Providers and Burnout." *Social Casework* 62 (June), pp. 352-361.

Strupp, H. H. et al. (1977). *Psychotherapy for Better or Worse: The Problem of Negative Effects.* New York: Jason Aronson.

Sturdivant, S. (1980). *Therapy with Women: A Feminist Philosophy of Treatment.* New York: Springer.

Sue, D. W. et. al. (1996). *A Theory of Multicultural Counseling and Therapy.* Belmont, CA: Brooks/Cole.

Sullivan, H. S. (1954). *The Psychiatric Interview.* New York: Norton.

Sullivan, J. W. N. (1963). *The Limits of Science.* New York: New American Library.

Sullivan, W. M. (1995). *Work and Integrity: The Crisis and Promise of Professionalism in America.* New York: Harper Business.

Taft, J. (1940). "Foster Care for Children." *The Annals of the American Academy of Political and Social Science* 212 (November), pp. 179-185.

Tessler, R. C. and Polansky, N. A. (1975). "Perceived Similarity: A Paradox in Interviewing." *Social Work* 20 (September), pp. 359-363.

Thigpen, J. D. (1979). "Perceptional Differences in the Supervision of Paraprofessional Mental Health Workers." *Community Mental Health Journal* 15 (Summer), pp. 139-148.

Thistle, P. (1981). "The Therapist's Own Family: Focus of Training for Family Therapists." *Social Work* 26 (May), pp. 248-250.

Toffler, A. (1980). *The Third Wave.* New York: Bantam Books.

Tosone, C. (1998). "Countertransference and Clinical Social Work Supervision: Contributions and Considerations." *The Clinical Supervisor* 16(2), pp. 17-32.

Towle, C. (1965). *Common Human Needs.* Washington, DC: National Association of Social Workers.

Trader, H. (1974). "A Professional School's Role in Training Ex-Addict Counselors." *Journal of Education for Social Work* 10 (Fall), pp. 99-106.

Trattner, W. I. (1999). *From Poor Law to Welfare State: A History of Social Welfare in America,* Sixth Edition. New York: The Free Press.

Trickett, P. K. and Schellenbach, C. J. (eds.) (1998). *Violence Against Children in the Family and the Community.* Washington, DC: American Psychological Association.

Turner, F. J. (1978). *Psychosocial Therapy: A Social Work Perspective.* New York: The Free Press.

Turner, F. J. (ed.) (1979). *Social Work Treatment: Interlocking Theoretical Approaches.* New York: The Free Press.

Turner, F. J. (ed.) (1996). *Social Work Treatment: Interlocking Theoretical Approaches,* Fourth Edition. New York: The Free Press.

Ullmann, L. (1978). *Changing.* New York: Bantam.

U.S. Substance Abuse and Mental Health Services Administration (1998). *Mental Health in the United States, 1998.* Washington, DC: Government Printing Office.

Urdang, E. (1999). "The Video Lab: Mirroring Reflections of Self and the Other." *The Clinical Supervisor* 18(2), pp. 143-164.

Utz, P. (1980). *Video User's Handbook.* Englewood Cliffs, NJ: Prentice-Hall.

Veeder, N. (1990). "Autonomy, Accountability, and Professionalism: The Case Against Close Supervision in Social Work." *The Clinical Supervisor* 8 (Summer), pp. 33-65.

Veroff, J. et al. (1981). *Mental Health in America: Patterns of Help Seeking from 1957 to 1976.* New York: Basic Books.

Wallace, J. E. and Brinkerhoff, M. E. (1991). "The Measurement of Burnout Revisited." *Journal of Social Service Research* 14 (Spring/Summer), pp. 85-111.

Wallace, M. E. (1981). "A Framework for Self-Supervision in Social Work Practice." *Social Casework* 62 (May), pp. 293-304.

Wallace, M. E. (1982). "Private Practice: A Nationwide Study." *Social Work* 27 (May), pp. 262-267.

Warres, N. E. et al. (1996). "The Impact of Managed Care and Utilization Review: A Cross-Sectional Study in Maryland." *Psychiatric Services* 47(12), pp. 1319-1322.

Watkins, C. E. (ed.) (1997). *Handbook of Psychotherapy Supervision.* New York: John Wiley.

Watkins, C. E. (1999). "The Beginning Psychotherapy Supervisor: How Can We Help?" *The Clinical Supervisor* 18(2), (1999), pp. 63-72.

Webster, E. and Haler, P. (1989). "Effects of Two Types of Direct Supervisory Feedback on Student Clinicians' Use of Consequation." *The Clinical Supervisor* 7 (Spring 1989), pp. 7-26.

Weinberg, G. (1978). *Self-Creation.* New York: St. Martin's.

Weinberger, Paul E. (1974). *Perspectives on Social Welfare: An Introductory Anthology.* New York: Macmillan.

Weisinger, H. and Lobsenz, N. M. (1981). *Nobody's Perfect: How to Give Criticism and Get Results.* Los Angeles: Stratford.

Weisman, A. (1972). *On Dying and Denying.* New York: Behavioral Publications.

Wells, C. C. (1999). *Social Work Day to Day: The Experience of Generalist Social Work Practice.* New York: Longman.

Wells, S. J. (1995). "Child Abuse and Neglect Overview." In National Association of Social Workers (ed.), *Encyclopedia of Social Work,* Nineteenth Edition. Washington, DC: NASW Press.

Weppner, R. S. et al. (1976). "Effects of Criminal Justice and Medical Definitions of a Social Problem upon the Delivery of Treatment: The Case of Drug Abuse." *Journal of Health and Social Behavior* 17 (June), pp. 170-177.

Whiffen, R. and Byng-Hall, J. (1982). *Family Therapy Supervision: Recent Developments in Practice.* New York: Grune and Stratton.

Whyte, W. H. (1956). *The Organization Man.* New York: Simon and Schuster.

Widen, P. (1962). "Organizational Structure for Casework Supervision." *Social Work* 7 (October), pp. 78-85.

Wijnberg, M. H. and Schwartz, Mary C. (1977). "Models of Student Supervision: The Apprentice, Growth, and Role Systems Models." *Journal of Education for Social Work* 13 (Fall), pp. 110-112.

Wilensky, H. L. and Lebeaux, C. N. (1975). *Industrial Society and Social Welfare.* New York: The Free Press.

Williams, M., Ho, L., and Fielder, L. (1974). "Career Patterns: More Grist for Women's Liberation." *Social Work* 19, pp. 463-466.

Williams, R. H. (1982). "Is Plato Only Worth Five Points?" *The Educational Forum* 46 (Winter), pp. 167-179.

Williams, S. and Halgin, R. P. (1995). "Issues in Psychotherapy Supervision Between the White Supervisor and the Black Supervisee." *The Clinical Supervisor* 3, 39-61.

Wilson, S. J. (1978). *Confidentiality in Social Work: Issues and Principles.* New York: The Free Press.

Wilson, S. J. (1981). *Field Instruction: Techniques for Supervisors.* New York: The Free Press.

Winnicott, D. W. (1986). *Home is Where We Start From: Essays by a Psychoanalyst.* New York: W.W. Norton and Company.

Wiseman, C. (1979). Personal communication, August 9.

Wodarski, J. S. (1981). *The Role of Research in Clinical Practice: A Practical Approach for the Human Services.* Baltimore, MD: University Park Press.

Wolgein, C. S. and Coady, N. F. (1997). "Good Therapists' Beliefs About the Development of Their Helping Ability: The Wounded Healer Paradigm Revisited." *The Clinical Supervisor* 15(2), pp. 19-34.

Wolf, S. (1994). "Health Care Reform and the Future of Physician Ethics." *Hastings Center Report* 24(2), pp. 28-41.

Wolman, B. B. (1976). *The Therapist's Handbook: Treatment Methods of Mental Disorders.* New York: Van Nostrand Reinhold.

Woolf, V. (1960/1932). *The Second Common Reader,* Reprint Edition. New York: Harcourt Brace Jovanovich.

Wright, J.W. (ed.) (1999). *The New York Times 2000 Almanac.* New York: Penguin.

Yankelovich, D. (1981). *New Rules: Searching for Self-Fulfillment in a World Turned Upside Down.* New York: Random House.

Zischka, P. C. (1981)."The Effects of Burnout on Permanency Planning and the Middle Management Supervisor in Child Welfare Agencies." *Child Welfare* 60 (November), pp. 611-616.

Zuckerman, E. L. (1997). *The Paper Office: Forms, Guidelines and Resources,* Second Edition. New York: Guilford.

Index

HAWORTH Social Work Practice in Action
Carlton E. Munson, PhD, Senior Editor

DIAGNOSIS IN SOCIAL WORK: NEW IMPERATIVES by Francis J. Turner. (2002).

HUMAN BEHAVIOR IN THE SOCIAL ENVIRONMENT: INTERWEAVING THE INNER AND OUTER WORLD by Esther Urdang. (2002).

THE USE OF PERSONAL NARRATIVES IN THE HELPING PROFESSIONS: A TEACHING CASEBOOK by Jessica Heriot and Eileen J. Polinger. (2002).

CHILDREN'S RIGHTS: POLICY AND PRACTICE by John T. Pardeck. (2001) "Courageous and timely . . . a must-read for everyone concerned not only about the rights of America's children but also about their fate." *Howard Jacob Kerger, PhD, Professor and PhD Director, University of Houston Graduate School of Social Work, Texas*

BUILDING ON WOMEN'S STRENGTHS: A SOCIAL WORK AGENDA FOR THE TWENTY-FIRST CENTURY, SECOND EDITION by K. Jean Peterson and Alice A. Lieberman. (2001). "An indispensable resource for courses in women's issues, social work practice with women, and practice from a strengths perspective." *Theresa J. Early, PhD, MSW, Assistant Professor, College of Social Work, Ohio State University, Columbus*

ELEMENTS OF THE HELPING PROCESS: A GUIDE FOR CLINICIANS, SECOND EDITION by Raymond Fox. (2001). "Engages the reader with a professional yet easily accessible style. A remarkably fresh, eminently usable set of practical strategies." *Elayne B. Haynes, PhD, ACSW, Assistant Professor, Department of Social Work, Southern Connecticut State University, New Haven*

SOCIAL WORK THEORY AND PRACTICE WITH THE TERMINALLY ILL, SECOND EDITION by Joan K. Parry. (2000). "Timely . . . a sensitive and practical approach to working with people with terminal illness and their family members." *Jeanne A.Gill, PhD, LCSW, Adjunct Faculty, San Diego State University, California, and Vice President Southern California Chapter, AASWG*

WOMEN SURVIVORS, PSYCHOLOGICAL TRAUMA, AND THE POLITICS OF RESISTANCE by Norma Jean Profitt. (2000). "A compelling argument on the importance of political and collective action as a means of resisting oppression. Should be read by survivors, service providers, and activists in the violence-against-women movement." *Gloria Geller, PhD, Faculty of Social Work, University of Regina, Saskatchewan, Canada*

THE MENTAL HEALTH DIAGNOSTIC DESK REFERENCE: VISUAL GUIDES AND MORE FOR LEARNING TO USE THE DIAGNOSTIC AND STATISTICAL MANUAL (DSM-IV) by Carlton E. Munson. (2000). "A carefully organized and user-friendly book for the beginning student and less-experienced practitioner of social work, clinical psychology, of psychiatric nursing . . . It will be a valuable addition to the literature on clinical assessment of mental disorders." *Jerold R. Brandell, PhD, BCD, Professor, School of Social Work, Wayne State University, Detroit, Michigan and Founding Editor, Psychoanalytic Social Work*

HUMAN SERVICES AND THE AFROCENTRIC PARADIGM by Jerome H. Schiele. (2000). "Represents a milestone in applying the Afrocentric paradigm to human services generally, and social work specifically. . . . A highly valuable resource." *Bogart R. Leashore, PhD, Dean and Professor, Hunter College School of Social Work, New York, New York*

SOCIAL WORK: SEEKING RELEVANCY IN THE TWENTY-FIRST CENTURY by Roland Meinert, John T. Pardeck and Larry Kreuger. (2000). "Highly recommended. A thought-provoking work that asks the difficult questions and challenges the status quo. A great book for graduate students as well as experienced social workers and educators." *Francis K. O. Yuen, DSW, ACSE, Associate Professor, Division of Social Work, California State University, Sacramento*

SOCIAL WORK PRACTICE IN HOME HEALTH CARE by Ruth Ann Goode. (2000). "Dr. Goode presents both a lucid scenario and a formulated protocol to bring health care services into the home setting. . . . this is a must have volume that will be a reference to be consulted many times." *Marcia B. Steinhauer, PhD, Coordinator and Associate Professor, Human Services Administration Program, Rider University, Lawrenceville, New Jersey*

FORSENIC SOCIAL WORK: LEGAL ASPECTS OF PROFESSIONAL PRACTICE, SECOND EDITION by Robert L. Barker and Douglas M. Branson. (2000). "The authors combine their expertise to create this informative guide to address legal practice issues facing social workers." *Newsletter of the National Organization of Forensic Social Work*

SOCIAL WORK IN THE HEALTH FIELD: A CARE PERSPECTIVE by Lois A. Fort Cowles. (1999). "Makes an important contrition to the field by locating the practice of social work in health care within an organizational and social context." *Goldie Kadushin, PhD, Associate Professor, School of Social Welfare, University of Wisconsin, Milwaukee*

SMART BUT STUCK: WHAT EVERY THERAPY NEEDS TO KNOW ABOUT LEARNING DISABILITIES AND IMPRISONED INTELLIGENCE by Myrna Orenstein. (1999). "A trailblazing effort that creates an entirely novel way of talking and thinking about learning disabilities. There is simply nothing like it in the field." *Fred M. Levin, MD, Training Supervising Analyst, Chicago Institute for Psychoanalysis; Assistant Professor of Clinical Psychiatry, Northwestern University, School of Medicine, Chicago, IL*

CLINICAL WORK AND SOCIAL ACTION: AN INTEGRATIVE APPROACH by Jerome Sachs and Fred Newdom. (1999). "Just in time for the new millennium come Sachs and Newdom with a wholly fresh look at social work. . . . A much-needed uniting of social work values, theories, and practice for action." *Josephine Nieves, MSW, PhD, Executive Director, National Association of Social Workers*

SOCIAL WORK PRACTICE IN THE MILITARY by James G. Daley. (1999). "A significant and worthwhile book with provocative and stimulating ideas. It deserves to be read by a wide audience in social work education and practice as well as by decision makers in the military." *H. Wayne Johnson, MSW, Professor, University of Iowa, School of Social Work, Iowa City, Iowa*

GROUP WORK: SKILLS AND STRATEGIES FOR EFFECTIVE INTERVENTIONS, SECOND EDITION by Sondra Brandler and Camille P. Roman. (1999). "A clear, basic description of what group work requires, including what skills and techniques group workers need to be effective." *Hospital and Community Psychiatry (from the first edition)*

TEENAGE RUNAWAYS: BROKEN HEARTS AND "BAD ATTITUDES" by Laurie Schaffner. (1999). "Skillfully combines the authentic voice of the juvenile runaway with the principles of social science research." *Barbara Owen, PhD, Professor, Department of Criminology, California State University, Fresno*

CELEBRATING DIVERSITY: COEXISTING IN A MULTICULTURAL SOCIETY by Benyamin Chetkow-Yanoov. (1999). "Makes a valuable contribution to peace theory and practice." *Ian Harris, EdD, Executive Secretary, Peace Education Committee, International Peace Research Association*

SOCIAL WELFARE POLICY ANALYSIS AND CHOICES by Hobart A. Burch. (1999). "Will become the landmark text in its field for many decades to come." *Sheldon Rahan, DSW, Founding Dean and Emeritus Professor of Social Policy and Social Administration. Faculty of Social Work, Wilfrid Laurier University, Canada*

SOCIAL WORK PRACTICE: A SYSTEMS APPROACH, SECOND EDITION by Benyamin Chetkow-Yannov. (1999). "Highly recommended as a primary text for any and all introductory social work courses." *Ram A. Cnaan, PhD, Associate Professor, School of Social Work, University of Pennsylvania*

CRITICAL SOCIAL WELFARE ISSUES: TOOLS FOR SOCIAL WORK AND HEALTH CARE PROFESSIONALS edited by Arthur J. Katz, Abraham Lurie, and Carlos M. Vida. (1997). "Offers hopeful agendas for change, while navigating the societal challenges facing those in the human services today." *Book News Inc.*

SOCIAL WORK IN HEALTH SETTINGS: PRACTICE IN CONTEXT, SECOND EDITION edited by Tobra Schwaber Kerson. (1997). "A first-class document . . . It will be found among the steadier and lasting works on the social work aspects of American health care." *Hans S. Falck, PhD, Professor Emeritus and Former Chair, Health Specialization in Social Work, Virginia Commonwealth University*

PRINCIPLES OF SOCIAL WORK PRACTICE: A GENERIC PRACTICE AP-PROACH by Molly R. Hancock. (1997). "Hancock's discussions advocate reflection and self-awareness to create a climate for client change." *Journal of Social Work Education*

NOBODY'S CHILDREN: ORPHANS OF THE HIV EPIDEMIC by Steven F. Dansky. (1997). "Professional sound, moving, and useful for both professionals and interested readers alike." *Ellen G. Friedman, ACSW, Associate Director of Support Services, Beth Israel Medical Center, Methadone Maintenance Treatment Program*

SOCIAL WORK APPROACHES TO CONFLICT RESOLUTION: MAKING FIGHTING OBSOLETE by Benyamin Chetkow-yanoov. (1996). "Presents an examination of the nature and cause of conflict and suggests techniques for coping with conflict." *Journal of Criminal Justice*

FEMINIST THEORIES AND SOCIAL WORK: APPROACHES AND APPLI-CATIONS by Christine Flynn Salunier. (1996). "An essential reference to be read re-peatedly by all educators and practitioners who are eager to learn more about feminist theory and practice" *Nancy R. Hooyman, PhD, Dean and Professor, School of Social Work, University of Washington, Seattle*

THE RELATIONAL SYSTEMS MODEL FOR FAMILY THERAPY: LIVING IN THE FOUR REALITIES by Donald R. Bardill. (1996). "Engages the reader in quiet, thoughtful conversation on the timeless issue of helping families and individ-uals." *Christian Counseling Resource Review*

SOCIAL WORK INTERVENTION IN AN ECONOMIC CRISIS: THE RIVER COMMUNITIES PROJECT by Martha Baum and Pamela Twiss. (1996). "Sets a standard for universities in terms of the types of meaningful roles they can play in supporting and sustaining communities." *Kenneth J. Jaros, PhD, Director, Public Health Social Work Training Program, University of Pittsburgh*

FUNDAMENTALS OF COGNITIVE-BEHAVIOR THERAPY: FROM BOTH SIDES OF THE DESK by Bill Borcherdt. (1996). "Both beginning and experienced practitioners . . . will find a considerable number of valuable suggestions in Borcherdt's book." *Albert Ellis, PhD, President, Institute for Rational-Emotive Therapy, New York City*

BASIC SOCIAL POLICY AND PLANNING: STRATEGIES AND PRACTICE METHODS by Hobart A. Burch. (1996). "Burch's familiarity with his topic is evi-dent and his book is an easy introduction to the field." *Readings*

THE CROSS-CULTURAL PRACTICE OF CLINICAL CASE MANAGEMENT IN MENTAL HEALTH edited by Peter Manoleas. (1996). "Makes a contribution by bringing together the cross-cultural and clinical case management perspectives in working with those who have serious mental illness." *Disabilities Studies Quarterly*

FAMILY BEYOND FAMILY: THE SURROGATE PARENT IN SCHOOLS AND OTHER COMMUNITY AGENCIES by Sanford Weinstein. (1995). "Highly recomended to anyone concerned about the welfare of our children and the breakdown of the American family." *Jerold S. Greenberg, EdD, director of Community Service, College of Health & Human Performance, University of Maryland*

PEOPLE WITH HIV AND THOSE WHO HELP THEM: CHALLENGES, INTEGRATION, INTERVENTION by R. Dennis Shelby. (1995). "A useful and compassionate contribution to the HIV psychotherapy literature." *Public Health*

THE BLACK ELDERLY: SATISFACTION AND QUALITY OF LATER LIFE by Marguerite Coke and James A. Twaite. (1995). "Presents a model for predicting life satisfaction in this population." *Abstracts in Social Gerontology*

NOW DARE EVERYTHING: TALES OF HIV-RELATED PSYCHOTHERAPY by Steven F. Dansky. (1994). "A highly recommended book for anyone working with persons who are HIV positive. . . . Every library should have a copy of this book." *AIDS Book Review Journal*

INTERVENTION RESEARCH: DESIGN AND DEVELOPMENT FOR HUMAN SERVICE edited by Jack Rothman and Edwin J. Thomas. (1994). "Provides a useful framework for the further examination of methodology for each separate step of such research." *Academic Library Book Review*

CLINICAL SOCIAL WORK SUPERVISION, SECOND EDITION by Carlton E. Munson. (1993). "A useful, thorough, and articulate reference for supervisors and for 'supervisees' who are wanting to understand their supervisor or are looking for effective supervision...." *Transactional Analysis Journal*

IF A PARTNER HAS AIDS: GUIDE TO CLINICAL INTERVENTION FOR RELATIONSHIPS IN CRISIS by R. Dennis Shelby. (1993). "A women addition to existing publications about couples coping with AIDS, it offers intervention ideas and strategies to clinicians." *Contemporary Psychology*

GERONTOLOGICAL SOCIAL WORK SUPERVISION by Ann Burack-Weiss and Frances Coyle Brennan. (1991). "The creative ideas in this book will aid supervisiors working with students and experienced social workers." *Senior News*

THE CREATIVE PRACTITIONER: THEORY AND METHODS FOR THE HELPING SERVICES by Bernard Gelfand. (1988). "[Should] be widely adopted by those in the helping services. It could lead to significant positive advances by countless individuals." *Sidney J. Parnes, Trustee Chairperson for Strategic Program Development, Creative Education Foundation, Buffalo, NY*

MANAGEMENT AND INFORMATION SYSTEMS IN HUMAN SERVICES: IMPLICATIONS FOR THE DISTRIBUTION OF AUTHORITY AND DECISION MAKING by Richard K. Caputo. (1987). "A contribution to social work scholarship in that it provides conceptual frameworks that can be used in the design of management information systems." *Social Work*